Lecture Notes in Computer Science   10265

Commenced Publication in 1973
Founding and Former Series Editors:
Gerhard Goos, Juris Hartmanis, and Jan van Leeuwen

Editorial Board

More information about this series at http://www.springer.com/series/7412

Marc Niethammer · Martin Styner
Stephen Aylward · Hongtu Zhu
Ipek Oguz · Pew-Thian Yap
Dinggang Shen (Eds.)

Information Processing in Medical Imaging

25th International Conference, IPMI 2017
Boone, NC, USA, June 25–30, 2017
Proceedings

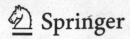 Springer

Editors

Marc Niethammer
University of North Carolina
Chapel Hill, NC
USA

Martin Styner
University of North Carolina
Chapel Hill, NC
USA

Stephen Aylward
Kitware Inc.
Carrboro, NC
USA

Hongtu Zhu
University of North Carolina
Chapel Hill, NC
USA

and

University of Texas
Houston, TX
USA

Ipek Oguz
University of Pennsylvania
Philadelphia, PA
USA

Pew-Thian Yap
University of North Carolina
Chapel Hill, NC
USA

Dinggang Shen
University of North Carolina
Chapel Hill, NC
USA

ISSN 0302-9743   ISSN 1611-3349   (electronic)
Lecture Notes in Computer Science
ISBN 978-3-319-59049-3   ISBN 978-3-319-59050-9   (eBook)
DOI 10.1007/978-3-319-59050-9

Library of Congress Control Number: 2017940845

LNCS Sublibrary: SL6 – Image Processing, Computer Vision, Pattern Recognition, and Graphics

Printed on acid-free paper

This Springer imprint is published by Springer Nature
The registered company is Springer International Publishing AG
The registered company address is: Gewerbestrasse 11, 6330 Cham, Switzerland

Preface

The 25th biennial international conference on Information Processing in Medical Imaging (IPMI 2017) was held at the Appalachian State University in Boone, North Carolina, USA, June 25–30, 2017. This conference was the latest in a series where novel developments in the acquisition, formation, analysis, and display of medical images were presented, discussed, dissected, and extended.

This year 147 manuscripts were submitted to IPMI. Of these, 53 were accepted, resulting in an acceptance rate of 36%. Out of the 53 accepted manuscripts, 24 were selected for oral presentation and 29 for poster presentation. All manuscripts were reviewed by exactly three reviewers. Based on these reviews, final acceptance and rejection decisions were made by the paper selection committee. The paper selection committee also discussed the overall program and decided whether a manuscript should be selected for an oral or for a poster presentation. Every effort was made to assure a fair selection process. In particular, the review process was double-blind. For the acceptance and rejection decisions, the paper selection committee was also blinded with respect to the authorship of manuscripts. Balancing with respect to research groups was not performed. Decisions were purely based on reviews and in-depth discussions of the paper selection committee. Owing to the large number of submissions, many good and promising manuscripts could unfortunately not be accepted to the final program of the conference.

Topics of interest of IPMI are diverse and have evolved over the past three decades in the medical imaging community that IPMI serves. This year's program covered topics that have become tradition at IPMI such as image registration, shape analysis, analysis on manifolds, and diffusion-weighted imaging. In addition, following the trend in computer vision and image analysis in general, a large number of submitted manuscripts explored machine-learning approaches, frequently in the form of deep learning, to address problems in the processing of medical imaging information.

As is tradition for IPMI, we put a strong emphasis on creating a vibrant atmosphere for in-depth research discussions. This included unlimited discussions for oral presentations as well as in-depth poster presentations. To foster a community spirit we, of course, also honored the traditional social components of IPMI, including spending as much time as possible together during the conference by staying on the campus of Appalachian State University, jointly exploring Boone, continuing discussion while hiking the beautiful Blue Ridge Mountains, and enjoying the IPMI choir.

IPMI 2017 also provided 16 scholarships to junior scientists from underrepresented populations. Of these scholarships, 15 went to junior female scientists and one to a junior scientist from an underrepresented racial or ethnic group. Furthermore, 18 out of the 24 oral presentations were eligible for the Erbsmann award, which is given in memory of Francois Erbsmann, one of the founders of IPMI. It is an award for the best oral presentation by a young scientist who is presenting for the first time at IPMI.

IPMI has always been a very special conference, combining a great scientific community, with discussions of the latest research, and a strong emphasis on nurturing the next generation of researchers. We feel grateful for having been able to continue this IPMI spirit.

June 2017

Marc Niethammer
Martin Styner
Stephen Aylward
Hongtu Zhu
Ipek Oguz
Pew-Thian Yap
Dinggang Shen

Organization

Chairs

General Chair
Martin Styner   University of North Carolina at Chapel Hill, USA

Program Chair
Marc Niethammer   University of North Carolina at Chapel Hill, USA

Program Co-chair
Dinggang Shen   University of North Carolina at Chapel Hill, USA

Venue/Event Chair
Stephen Aylward   Kitware Inc., USA

Venue/Event Co-chair
Ipek Oguz   University of Pennsylvania, USA

Discussion Chair
Hongtu Zhu   MD Anderson Cancer Center, USA

Website Chair
Greg Fleishman   University of Pennsylvania, USA

Proceedings Chair
Pew-Thian Yap   University of North Carolina at Chapel Hill, USA

Paper Selection Committee

Jorge Cardoso   University College London, UK
Jim Gee   University of Pennsylvania, USA
Polina Golland   Massachusetts Institute of Technology, USA
Xavier Pennec   Inria Sophia Antipolis, France
Baba Vemuri   University of Florida, USA

Scientific Committee

Daniel Alexander	University College London, UK
Stephanie Allassonniere	Ecole Polytechnique, France
Elsa D. Angelini	Columbia University, USA
John Ashburner	University College London, UK
Suyash P. Awate	Indian Institute of Technology Bombay, India
Meritxell Bach-Cuadra	Université de Lausanne, Switzerland
Christian Barillot	IRISA/CNRS, France
Pierre-Louis Bazin	Max Planck Institute for Human Cognitive and Brain Sciences, Germany
Sylvain Bouix	Brigham and Women's Hospital/Harvard Medical School, USA
M. Jorge Cardoso	University College London, UK
Gary Christensen	University of Iowa, USA
Albert Chung	Hong Kong University of Science and Technology, Hong Kong, SAR China
Ela Claridge	The University of Birmingham, UK
Olivier Commowick	Inria Rennes, France
Tim Cootes	Manchester University, UK
Benoit Dawant	Vanderbilt University, USA
Marleen de Bruijne	Copenhagen University, Denmark
Maxime Descoteaux	Université de Sherbrooke, Canada
Karen Drukker	University of Chicago, USA
Jim Duncan	Yale University, USA
Stanley Durrleman	Inria/ICM, France
Aaron Fenster	Robarts Research Institute, USA
Aasa Feragen	University of Copenhagen, Denmark
Thomas Fletcher	University of Utah, USA
Alejandro F. Frangi	University of Sheffield, UK
Mona K. Garvin	University of Iowa, USA
Guido Gerig	New York University, USA
Ben Glocker	Imperial College, UK
Polina Golland	Massachusetts Institute of Technology, USA
Miguel A. Gonzalez Ballester	Universitat Pompeu Fabra, Spain
Hayit Greenspan	Tel Aviv University, Israel
Matthias Guenther	Fraunhofer MEVIS, Germany
Boris Gutman	University of Southern California, USA
Justin Haldar	University of Southern California, USA
Dave Hawkes	University College London, UK
Tobias Heimann	Siemens AG, Germany
Mattias Heinrich	University of Lübeck, Germany
Yi Hong	University of Georgia, USA
Ivana Isgum	University Medical Center Utrecht, The Netherlands
Marie-Pierre Jolly	Siemens Corporate Research, USA

Anand Joshi   University of Southern California, USA
Boklye Kim   University of Michigan, USA
Andy King   Kings College London, UK
Stefan Klein   Erasmus University Medical Center, The Netherlands
Ender Konukoglu   ETH Zurich, Switzerland
Frithjof Kruggel   University of California Irvine, USA
Elizabeth Krupinski   Emory University, USA
Sebastian Kurtek   The Ohio State University, USA
Roland Kwitt   University of Salzburg, Austria
Jan Kybic   Czech Technical University, Czech Republic
Bennett Landman   Vanderbilt University, USA
Georg Langs   Medical University of Vienna, Austria
Tobias Lasser   Technical University of Munich, Germany
Boudewijn Lelieveldt   Leiden University Medical Center, The Netherlands
Christophe Lenglet   University of Minnesota, USA
Marius G. Linguraru   Children's National Medical Center, USA
Herve J. Lombaert   ETS Montreal, Canada
Cristian Lorenz   Philips Research, Germany
Marco Lorenzi   Inria Sophia Antipolis, France
Stephen Marsland   Massey University, New Zealand
Bjoern Menze   Technical University of Munich, Germany
Marc Modat   University College London, UK
Bernard Ng   Stanford University, USA
Alison Noble   University of Oxford, UK
Lauren O'Donnell   Harvard Medical School, USA
Ipek Oguz   University of Pennsylvania, USA
Sebastian Ourselin   University College London, UK
Xenophon Papademetris   Yale University, USA
Dzung Pham   Center for Neuroscience and Regenerative Medicine, USA
Stephen Pizer   The University of North Carolina at Chapel Hill, USA
Kilian Pohl   SRI/Stanford, USA
Marcel Prastawa   University of Utah, USA
Jerry Prince   Johns Hopkins University, USA
Yogesh Rathi   Brigham and Women's Hospital/Harvard Medical School,
                             USA
Joseph Reinhardt   University of Iowa, USA
Laurent Risser   University of Toulouse, France
Karl Rohr   University of Heidelberg, Germany
Daniel Rueckert   Imperial College London, UK
Olivier Salvado   Commonwealth Scientific and Industrial Research
                             Organisation, Australia
Benoit Scherrer   Boston Children's Hospital, USA
Christof Seiler   Stanford University, USA
Pengcheng Shi   Rochester Institute of Technology, USA
Kaleem Siddiqi   McGill University, Canada
Stefan Sommer   University of Copenhagen, Denmark

Lawrence Staib	Yale University, USA
Marius Staring	Leiden University Medical Center, The Netherlands
Colin Studholme	University of Washington, USA
Gabor Szekely	ETH Zurich, Switzerland
Chris Taylor	Manchester University, UK
Philippe Thevenaz	Ecole Polytechnique Federale de Lausanne, Switzerland
Carole Twining	The University of Manchester, UK
Gael Varoquaux	Inria, France
Tom Vercauteren	University College London, UK
Francois-Xavier Vialard	Paris Dauphine University, France
Tomaz Vrtovec	University of Ljubljana, Slovenia
Hongzhi Wang	IBM Almaden Research Center, USA
Simon Warfield	Harvard Medical School and Children's Hospital, USA
Demian Wassermann	Inria, France
Carl-Fredrik Westin	Harvard University, USA
Ross Whittaker	University of Utah, USA
Jianhua Yao	National Institutes of Health, USA
Pew-Thian Yap	The University of North Carolina at Chapel Hill, USA
Gary Zhang	University College London, UK
Miaomiao Zhang	Massachusetts Institute of Technology, USA
Kevin Zhou	Siemens Corporate Research, USA
Lilla Zollei	Harvard Medical School, USA
Reyer Zwiggelaar	University of Wales, UK

IPMI 2017 Board

Christian Barillot	IRISA Rennes, France
Randy Brill	Vanderbilt University, USA
Marleen de Bruijne	Erasmus MC Rotterdam, The Netherlands
Gary Christensen	University of Iowa, USA
James Duncan	Yale University, USA
Polina Golland	Massachusetts Institute of Technology, USA
Richard Leahy	University of Southern California, USA
Alison Noble	Oxford University, UK
Sebastien Ourselin	University College London, UK
Stephen Pizer	The University of North Carolina at Chapel Hill, USA
Josien Pluim	University of Utrecht, The Netherlands
Jerry Prince	Johns Hopkins University, USA
Gabor Szekely	ETH Zurich, Switzerland
Chris Taylor	University of Manchester, UK
Andrew Todd-Pokropek	University College London, UK
William Wells	Harvard Medical School, USA

Contents

Analysis on Manifolds

Shape Analysis

Disease Diagnosis/Progression

Brain Networks and Connectivity

Diffusion Imaging

Quantitative Imaging

Imaging Genomics

Image Registration

Segmentation

General Image Analysis

Analysis on Manifolds

Robust Fréchet Mean and PGA on Riemannian Manifolds with Applications to Neuroimaging

Monami Banerjee[1], Bing Jian[2], and Baba C. Vemuri[1(✉)]

[1] University of Florida, Gainesville, USA
monamie.b@gmail.com, baba.vemuri@gmail.com
[2] Google, Mountain View, CA, USA
jian.bing@gmail.com

Abstract. In this paper, we present novel algorithms to compute robust statistics from manifold-valued data. Specifically, we present algorithms for estimating the robust Fréchet Mean (FM) and performing a robust exact-principal geodesic analysis (ePGA) for data lying on *known* Riemannian manifolds. We formulate the minimization problems involved in both these problems using the minimum distance estimator called the L_2E. This leads to a nonlinear optimization which is solved efficiently using a Riemannian accelerated gradient descent technique. We present competitive performance results of our algorithms applied to synthetic data with outliers, the corpus callosum shapes extracted from OASIS MRI database, and diffusion MRI scans from movement disorder patients respectively.

1 Introduction

In this age of data deluge, manifold-valued features are widespread in Science and Engineering disciplines. As the amount of data to be processed grows by leaps and bounds, there is an obvious need to reduce the dimensionality of the data and provide some sort of statistics. To this end, Principal Component Analysis (PCA) has been employed as the main workhorse for data lying in vector spaces. However, when the input data reside on a smooth manifold, the nonlinear generalization called, Principal Geodesic Analysis (PGA) [7] is often employed. PGA in [7] makes use of the concept of linearization by first finding the intrinsic mean of the data lying on the smooth manifold and then makes use of the inverse Riemannian exponential (Exp) map, also called the Riemannian Log map, to map the data from the manifold to the tangent space anchored at the intrinsic mean of the data on the manifold. Then it performs PCA of this Log mapped data and projects the principal vectors back on to the manifold using the Exp map, obtaining the principal geodesic submanifolds. In order for this algorithm to work, it is assumed that the Rieamnnian Exp and Log maps exist in the desired neighborhood and can be computed efficiently. Although this linearized version of PGA is computationally efficient, it lacks in accuracy of the computed principal

This research was funded in part by, the NSF grant IIS-1525431 to BCV and the UFII fellowship to MB.

© Springer International Publishing AG 2017
M. Niethammer et al. (Eds.): IPMI 2017, LNCS 10265, pp. 3–15, 2017.
DOI: 10.1007/978-3-319-59050-9_1

components when the input manifold-valued data have a large variance. In order to cope with this issue, Sommer et al. [26] proposed to solve the problem without resorting to the aforementioned linearization. They called their algorithm, *exact-PGA*. In *exact-PGA* [26], the cost function being optimized involves minimization of the projection distance, also called the reconstruction error. This is a hard nonlinear optimization problem and a general efficient solution is lacking to date. Recently, Chakraborty et al. [3], proposed an efficient solution to the exact-PGA problem for constant curvature manifolds with several applications. There are several variants of the PGA algorithm in literature and we briefly discuss a few here. Authors in [23] presented a technique to compute the principal geodesics (without approximation) but only for the special Lie group, $SO(3)$. Geodesic PCA (GPCA) [15] solves a different optimization function namely, optimizing the projection error along the geodesics. GPCA does not use a linear approximation, but is restricted to manifolds where a closed form expression for the geodesics exists. More recently, a probabilistic version of PGA called PPGA was presented in [28], which is a nonlinear version of PPCA [27]. As an alternative to PGA, Hauberg [11] introduced a Riemannian version of the well known principal curves algorithm restricted to complete Riemannian manifolds. However, none of these methods are robust to outliers in the data.

In this paper, we present a statistically robust formulation for estimating the Fréchet mean (FM) [9] as well as for computing the *exact-PGA*. Our notion of robustness here implies relative "insensitivity (stickiness)" of the location of the estimated FM to outliers in the data. Further, our work here is restricted to smooth Riemannian manifolds and does not consider stratified spaces. For "sticky" and "non-sticky" FM of data in stratified spaces, we refer the reader to [13]. Our formulation makes use of the well known M-estimator in statistics called L_2E introduced by Scott [24]. In finding the FM from data, one minimizes the so called sum of squared geodesic distances between the unknown FM and the given data samples. Whereas, for estimating the principal components in the *exact-PGA* algorithm, one minimizes the sum of squared projection errors, defined by the geodesic distances between the data points and the geodesics emanating from the FM as a function of direction. In [8], authors proposed a geometric median formulation on Riemannian manifolds and have shown robustness of the median. *Though mean and median are distinct statistics, for the sake of completeness, we will compare our robust mean formulation with the intrinsic median.*

The robust formulation for estimating the FM and computing the PGA involves casting the aforementioned geodesic distance minimization costs in both problems into the L_2E based M-estimator framework. This is precisely what is achieved here in this paper. Note that there are no robust PGA methods in existing literature and the theory and algorithm presented here are the first to the best of our knowledge. Hence, we compare our work to one other method of achieving robust PGA, which is our own modification of the conventional non-robust PGA. This modification involves replacing the PCA in the tangent space at the FM performed in the conventional PGA [7] by an existing robust PCA algorithm [12].

The rest of this paper is organized as follows: Sect. 2 contains the theoretical formulation of the robust FM and PGA respectively. In Sect. 3, we present several examples on synthetic data, shapes extracted from OASIS MRI database, and diffusion MRI scans from movement disorder patients respectively. In Sect. 4, we draw conclusions.

2   Robust Statistics

In this section, first we present a novel formulation of, the robust FM followed by the robust PGA. In both these formulations, we will use the well known and statistically robust minimum distance estimator called the integral squared error (a.k.a. the L_2 error) denoted by L_2E [24].

2.1   Robust FM on a Riemannian Manifold: Using the L_2E

Computing the FM is a commonly encountered task in many application problems including but not limited to shape analysis [16], directional statistics [19], diffusion tensor analysis [17,20,22] and many others. In the following we will first define the FM and then present a formulation for computing it robustly from data corrupted with outliers.

Let $(\mathcal{M}^m, g)$ be a Riemannian manifold equipped with a Riemannian metric g [6], where $m = \dim(\mathcal{M})$. Given a point $p \in \mathcal{M}$ and the tangent vector $\mathbf{v} \in T_p\mathcal{M}$, there exists a unique geodesic α such that $\alpha(0) = p$ and $\alpha' = v$. In general, its existence however is only guaranteed locally. The Riemannian exponential map Exp at the point $p \in \mathcal{M}$ is a locally diffeomorphic map on to the neighborhood of p and is defined as $\mathsf{Exp}_p(\mathbf{v}) = \alpha(1)$, where, α is defined over $[0, 1]$. If $B(p)$ denotes the largest such neighborhood, then, the inverse of the Exp map, called the Riemannian Log map is well defined in this neighborhood. Let $d : \mathcal{M} \times \mathcal{M} \to \mathbf{R}$ be the distance induced by the metric g on $\mathcal{M}$. Then, for $p, q \in \mathcal{M}$, $d(p, q) = ||\mathsf{Log}_p(q)||_p$. Given the data $X = \{x_i\}_{i=1}^N \subset \mathcal{M}$, the FM μ is defined by the following minimization [9], $\mu = \mathrm{argmin}_{x \in \mathcal{M}} \sum_{i=1}^N d^2(x, x_i)$. The existence and uniqueness of the FM in general is only guaranteed within a geodesic ball of a certain radius [1,21]. As is usually the case in literature [3,7,26], we will also assume that the input data lie within this geodesic ball, so that FM exists and is unique. Our assumption about the data including the outliers lying inside a geodesic ball of an appropriate radius is in line with earlier work reported in [8].

We now propose a robust formulation to compute FM on a Riemannian manifold based on the well known robust L_2E estimator [24]. It is easy to show that minimizing the sum-of-squared function defined in the FM computation is equivalent to maximizing the likelihood of the distances (of sample points from the FM) being randomly drawn from a one-dimensional half-normal distribution. It is well known that maximum likelihood estimation (MLE) is well suited for estimation problems in which the model is a good descriptor for the data. However, it well known that the ML estimates are highly biased if the data contain outliers [2]. In [2], Basu et al. defined a single parameter family of divergences between distributions, termed the *density power divergence*. This family of divergences is controlled by a single parameter and includes the KL (Kullback-Leibler) divergence and the L_2 distance as limiting cases. Recognizing that the minimum density power divergence estimators can be interpreted as a particular case of M-estimators [14], Basu et al. [2] have shown that the L_2 estimator (L_2E) corresponding to L_2 distance is superior to MLE in terms of robustness. Scott [24] also exploited the applicability of L_2E to parametric modeling and demonstrated its robustness behavior and nice properties of practical importance.

In the parametric case, given the random variable $\epsilon \in \mathbf{R}$ with unknown density $g(\epsilon)$, and a model $f(\epsilon|\boldsymbol{\theta})$, with a parameter vector $\boldsymbol{\theta}$, we can write the L_2E criterion as, $L_2(f,g) = \int [f(\epsilon|\boldsymbol{\theta}) - g(\epsilon)]^2 \, d\epsilon$. Note that, in the expansion of this integral, the term $\int g(\epsilon)^2 \, d\epsilon$ does not depend on $\boldsymbol{\theta}$ and $\int f(\epsilon|\boldsymbol{\theta}) \, g(\epsilon) \, d\epsilon = E_g[f(\epsilon|\boldsymbol{\theta})]$ is the so called expected height of the density which can be approximated by the estimator $\frac{1}{N} \sum_{i=1}^{N} f(\epsilon_i|\boldsymbol{\theta})$. Hence, the proposed estimator minimizing the L_2 distance will be,

$$\hat{\boldsymbol{\theta}}_{\mathrm{L_2E}} = \arg \min_{\boldsymbol{\theta}} \left(\int f(\epsilon|\boldsymbol{\theta})^2 d\epsilon - \frac{2}{N} \sum_{i=1}^{N} f(\epsilon_i|\boldsymbol{\theta}) \right). \tag{1}$$

In the case of model being a Gaussian or mixture of Gaussians, we have a closed form expression for the integral in the bracketed quantity in (1) and hence can avoid numerical integration which severely limits the practical applications not only in computation time but also in accuracy.

Noting that the L_2E criterion does not require that the model $f(\epsilon|\mu)$ be a density, Scott [25] suggested a method for outlier detection and clustering by partial mixture modeling. A partial mixture model basically advocates the use of a small number of components in a "full" N-component Gaussian mixture model, thereby under fitting the outlier-corrupted data. One of the advantages of this model is that the weight w provides us the fraction of the data to which the component has been fitted. For example, using just a single component, this model will account for the largest fraction (cluster) of the data and thus accounting for the inliers (assuming that the outliers correspond to a smaller fraction). This is appropriate in our work because, our focus is on finding the FM (and later, PGA) of a single cluster of data possibly corrupted with outliers.

In our context, $\epsilon = d(\mu, x) \in [0, \infty)$. Note that, $\epsilon \in \mathbf{R}$ depends on the FM, $\mu \in \mathcal{M}$. Inspired by the ideas describe above, to model the density of the geodesic distances from the FM to the data, we chose a partial mixture of half-normal densities with mean $\sqrt{2}\sigma/\sqrt{\pi}$, and variance, $\sigma^2(1 - 2/\pi)$ (here σ is unknown parameter of the half-normal density), i.e., $f(\epsilon(\mu)) = w \phi(\epsilon(\mu)|\sigma^2)$. For simplicity of notation, we will drop the μ from $\epsilon(\mu)$ in the rest of the paper. Here, $\phi(\epsilon|\sigma^2)$ is the half-normal density and w denotes the weight of the partial mixture.

Lemma 1. *If the model density $f(\epsilon|\mu) = w \phi(\epsilon|\sigma^2)$, then the L_2E criterion is given by,*

$$L_2 E(\mu, w, \sigma^2) = \frac{w^2}{\sqrt{\pi\sigma^2}} - \frac{2\sqrt{2}w}{\sqrt{\pi}N\sigma} \sum_{i=1}^{N} \exp \left\{ -\frac{d^2(\mu, x_i)}{2\sigma^2} \right\}. \tag{2}$$

Proof.

$$\int f(\epsilon|\mu)^2 \, d\epsilon = \int w^2 \, \phi^2(\epsilon|\sigma^2) \, d\epsilon = w^2 \int \left[\exp\left(-\frac{\epsilon^2}{2\sigma^2}\right) \right]^2 d\epsilon$$

$$= w^2 \int \left[\exp\left(-\frac{\epsilon^2}{\sigma^2}\right) \right] d\epsilon = \frac{w^2}{\sqrt{\pi\sigma^2}}. \tag{3}$$

Substituting $\epsilon_i = d(\mu, x_i)$, we get $f(\epsilon_i|\mu) = \frac{\sqrt{2}w}{\sqrt{\pi}\sigma} \exp\left\{ -\frac{d^2(\mu, x_i)}{2\sigma^2} \right\}$. Now, using Eq. 1, we get the desired result in Eq. 2. ∎

Estimation of the parameters is then achieved by minimizing this L_2E criterion with respect to the parameters. We derived an analytic expression for gradient of the L_2E cost (not shown here due to lack of space) and employed it in a variant of the accelerated gradient descent (AGD) [10] adopted to Riemannian manifolds. This leads to the optimal set of parameters, $\hat{\mu}_{L_2E} \in \mathcal{M}, \hat{w} > 0, \hat{\sigma}^2 > 0$. In addition to the robust FM estimate, $\hat{\mu}_{L_2E}$, the partial weight $\hat{w}$ also indicates the fraction of the data being treated as outliers. In the following, we state and prove the robustness of the FM estimator formulated above.

Theorem 1. *The L_2E formulation to compute FM in Eq. 2 is robust to outliers.*

Proof. Let x_j be an outlier, for some j, i.e., $d(\mu, x_j)$ is very large. The *influence function* [14] of $L_2E(\mu, w, \sigma^2)$ is proportional to $\frac{\partial L_2E(\mu, w, \sigma^2)}{\partial d(\mu, x_j)}$. If we can show that as $d(\mu, x_j) \to \infty$, $\frac{\partial L_2E(\mu, w, \sigma^2)}{\partial d(\mu, x_j)} \to 0$, we can then claim that our formulation to compute FM, i.e., the L_2E criterion $L_2E(\mu, w, \sigma^2)$ is robust. Now, $\frac{\partial L_2E(\mu, w, \sigma^2)}{\partial d(\mu, x_j)} = \frac{-4\sqrt{2}w}{\sqrt{\pi}N\sigma} \exp\left\{ -\frac{d^2(\mu, x_j)}{2\sigma^2} \right\} \mathrm{Log}_{x_j}\mu$. So, in the limit as $d(\mu, x_j) \to \infty$, $\frac{\partial L_2E(\mu, w, \sigma^2)}{\partial d(\mu, x_j)} \to 0$, i.e., our formulation is robust. ∎

2.2 Principal Geodesic Analysis (PGA)

The goal of PGA is to find a set of $r < m$ orthogonal basis vectors of $T_\mu\mathcal{M}$, called principal vectors $\{\mathbf{v}_j\}_{j=1}^r$, such that the data variance along the geodesic submanifold spanned by these principal vectors is maximized [3,7]. An alternative definition of PGA [26] involves minimizing the reconstruction error, $\sum d^2(x_i, \hat{x}_i)$, where $\hat{x}_i$ is the ith reconstructed data point in the principal submanifold spanned by the basis vectors $\{\mathbf{v}_j\}_{j=1}^r$. These two formulations result in the same solution in $\mathbf{R}^n$ but not so on a general Riemannian manifold. In [3], the principal vectors $\{\mathbf{v}_j\}$ are defined recursively by,

$$\mathbf{v}_j = \underset{\|\mathbf{v}\|=1, \mathbf{v} \in V_{j-1}^\perp}{\mathrm{argmin}} \frac{1}{N} \sum_{i=1}^N d^2(x_i, \Pi_{S_j}(x_i)), \qquad S_j = \mathrm{Exp}_\mu(\mathrm{span}\{V_{j-1}, \mathbf{v}_j\}), \quad (4)$$

where, $V_{j-1} = \{\mathbf{v}_1, \cdots, \mathbf{v}_{j-1}\}$. S_j is the submanifold spanned by $V_j = \{V_{j-1}, \mathbf{v}_j\}$, and $\Pi_{S_j}(x)$ is the point in S_j closest to $x \in \mathcal{M}$. In this paper, we will use this alternative formulation to define a robust formulation of PGA on a Riemannian manifold.

2.3 Robust PGA on a Riemannian Manifold: Using L_2E

Equipped with a robust FM formulation and the basic PGA, we are now ready to propose a formulation for the robust PGA. Let the ith reconstructed data point be denoted by $\hat{x}_i$, then using an approach analogous to the one used to define robust FM, we model the density for the distance between x and $\hat{x}$ by a partial mixture of half-normal density with $\sqrt{2}\sigma'/\sqrt{\pi}$ mean and variance $\sigma'^2(1 - 2/\pi)$ (here σ' is unknown). Let $\epsilon' = d(x, \hat{x})$, using the same notation as in Eq. 4, $\hat{x} = \Pi_{S_j}(x)$ and $S_j = \mathsf{Exp}_\mu(\mathrm{span}\{V_{j-1}, \mathbf{v}_j\})$. Now to get the set of parameters $\{\hat{\mathbf{v}}_j\}, \hat{w}' > 0, \hat{\sigma}'^2 > 0$, we minimize the following L_2E criterion:

$$L_2E(\{\mathbf{v}_j\}, w', \sigma'^2) = \frac{w'^2}{\sqrt{\pi}\sigma'^2} - \frac{2\sqrt{2}w'}{\sqrt{\pi}N\sigma'} \sum_{i=1}^{N} \exp\left\{ -\frac{d^2(\hat{x}_i, x_i)}{2\sigma'^2} \right\}, \qquad (5)$$

with an added constraint to ensure that the principal vectors $\{\mathbf{v}_j\}$ are mutually orthogonal. In order to minimize the above function, we need an analytic expression for the projection, $\Pi_{S_j}(x)$. This analytic expression can either be exact or an approximation. We now present the derivations of the projection operator $\Pi_{S_j}(x)$.

Various Forms of the Projection Operator. In this section, we present a method to approximate $\Pi_{S_j}(x)$ on a Riemannian manifold $\mathcal{M}$. On manifolds with constant sectional curvature, we resort to the exact analytic form of $\Pi_{S_j}(x)$ derived in [3]. Let $\hat{x} = \Pi_{S_j}(x)$, then $\hat{x}$ can be expressed as $\mathsf{Exp}_\mu(\sum_j c(x, \mathbf{v}_j) \mathbf{v}_j)$ where the coefficient function $c : \mathcal{M} \times T_\mu\mathcal{M} \to \mathbf{R}$ can be defined as $c(x, \mathbf{v}_j) = \mathrm{sgn}(g_\mu(\mathbf{v}_j, \mathsf{Log}_\mu x)) \, d(\mu, \Pi_{\mathrm{span}\{\mathbf{v}_j\}}(x))$, where $\Pi_{\mathrm{span}\{\mathbf{v}_j\}}(x)$ returns the closest point of x on the geodesic of dim-1 submanifold spanned by $\mathbf{v}_j$. We use $\mathrm{sgn}(g_\mu(\mathbf{v}_j, \mathsf{Log}_\mu x))$ to define $c(x, \mathbf{v}_j)$, as the coefficient can be negative as well. Since, on a general Riemannian manifold, $\Pi_{\mathrm{span}\{\mathbf{v}_j\}}(x)$ is the solution of a hard optimization problem [26], here we approximate $c(x, \mathbf{v}_j)$ by $c(x, \mathbf{v}_j) = g_\mu(\mathsf{Log}_\mu x, \mathbf{v}_j)$.

Moving on to the case of non-zero constant curvature manifolds, it is possible to derive the exact analytic expression of the projection operator as was shown in [3]. These analytic expressions will considerably reduce the computational complexity involved in computing the projection operator. Equipped with these closed form expressions for $\Pi_{\mathrm{span}\{\mathbf{v}_j\}}(x)$ on constant curvature manifolds, we can compute $c(x, \mathbf{v}_j)$ analytically as $c(x_i, \mathbf{v}_j) = \mathrm{sgn}(g_\mu(\mathbf{v}_j, \mathsf{Log}_\mu x_i)) \, d(\mu, \Pi_{\mathrm{span}\{\mathbf{v}_j\}}(x_i))$ on constant curvature manifolds. Thus, we get $\hat{x}_i = \mathsf{Exp}_\mu\left(\sum_j c(x_i, \mathbf{v}_j) \mathbf{v}_j \right)$, for all i.

Theorem 2. *The L_2E formulation to compute the PGs in Eq. 5 is robust to outliers.*

Proof. We first observe that the minimization of $L_2E(\{\mathbf{v}_j\}, w', \sigma'^2)$ in Eq. 5 is equivalent to the maximization of

$$L_2\widetilde{E}(\{\mathbf{v}_j\}, w', \sigma'^2) = \frac{w'^2}{\sqrt{\pi}\sigma'^2} - \frac{2\sqrt{2}w'}{\sqrt{\pi}N\sigma'} \sum_{i=1}^{N} \exp\left\{ -\frac{d^2(\hat{x}_i, \mu)}{2\sigma'^2} \right\}$$

This follows from the fact that minimization of reconstruction error is equivalent to maximization of variance of the reconstructed point. This equivalence relation is exploited in literature [3,26]. Now, assume that x_j is an outlier for some j, i.e., $d(x_j, \mu)$ is very large. We can see that, for all $\mathbf{v}$, $c(x_j, \mathbf{v}) = g_\mu(\text{Log}_\mu x_j, \mathbf{v})$ is very large as norm of $\text{Log}_\mu x_j$ is very large. So, $d(\hat{x}_j, \mu) = \| \left(\sum_k c(x_j, \mathbf{v}_k) \mathbf{v}_k \right) \|$ is also very large, where $\|.\|$ is taken with inner product g_μ. Now, the influence function of $L_2\widetilde{E}(\{\mathbf{v}_j\}, w', \sigma'^2)$ is proportional to $\frac{\partial L_2\widetilde{E}(\{\mathbf{v}_j\}, w', \sigma'^2)}{\partial d(\hat{x}_j, \mu)}$. Using calculations analogous to those in the proof of Theorem 1, we can see that as $d(\hat{x}_j, \mu) \to \infty$, $\frac{\partial L_2\widetilde{E}(\{\mathbf{v}_j\}, w', \sigma'^2)}{\partial d(\hat{x}_j, \mu)} \to 0$, i.e., our formulation to compute the PGs is robust. ∎

Similar to the L_2E FM, we derived an analytic gradient for Eq. 5, and employed the manifold extension of a variant of AGD in [10]. However, due to lack of space, we do not include them here.

3 Experiments

In this section, we present results for data lying on two Riemannian manifolds namely: the hypersphere, $\mathbf{S}^m$ (with canonical metric), and the symmetric positive definite matrix manifold, SPD(m) (with GL(m) invariant metric). In all experiments, we randomly perturb some fraction of the data points in order to create outliers. We performed two sets of experiments for each data set which are described below:

- We compared our Robust L_2E-FM, μ^*, with the conventional FM, $\bar{\mu}$, and the Fréchet Median (FMe), $\tilde{\mu}$, [8,9] of the outlier added data set. Let the FM of the original data, i.e., without the outliers, be denoted by μ. Then, we compared $d(\mu, \mu^*)$ with $d(\mu, \tilde{\mu})$ and $d(\mu, \bar{\mu})$ respectively, where d is the geodesic distance on the manifold where the data reside. We also computed and compared the sample variances (s²) with μ^*, $\tilde{\mu}$ and $\bar{\mu}$ using the same geodesic distance.
- We compared the proposed L_2E-PGA, with a robust extension of the PGA algorithm in [7], where instead of PCA in the tangent space anchored at the FM, we use a robust PCA on the Log-mapped data in the tangent space anchored at the FMe, $\tilde{\mu}$, of the given data. The specific robust PCA algorithm used in this context is the one in [12], which uses trimmed-Grassmann averages to compute the principal components in the PCA algorithm. Robustness is achieved via the use of ℓ_1-norm. Hence, we call this the Grassmann-median PGA or simply GMPGA. We measured the reconstruction error, E_r, to assess performance of the methods. The original data without the outliers was used to compute the reconstruction error using just the leading principal vector. For the sake of completeness, a similar comparison with PGA [7] is also reported.

In both the above cases, we also report the computation time for each method. Now, we will separately discuss the results for the two commonly encountered manifolds namely, the $\mathbf{S}^m$ and the SPD(m).

3.1   Robust FM and PGA for Data on the Hypersphere $\mathbf{S}^m$

In this section, we first present the results for a synthetic data set on $\mathbf{S}^2$. In this data, we first generated 1000 samples on $\mathbf{S}^2$ by perturbing points along a chosen direction $(0, 1, 0)^t$, with the perturbation following a log-normal distribution in the tangent space at the north pole. This created a band of points along the aforementioned direction (see Fig. 1). Then we randomly select 5%, 10%, 15% and 20% of the data (percentage of outliers is denoted by ς), and overwrite them with points similarly generated but along a different direction vector anchored at the north pole, specifically the vector $(0, 1, 1)^t$. This produces the said amount of outliers as shown in Fig. 1. We then compared the performances of L_2E-PGA, GMPGA and PGA on this data set.

From the plots, it is evident that the L_2E-PGA outperforms the competition. The conventional PGA fails to detect outliers as expected. The detailed comparison results with GMPGA and PGA are shown in Table 1 (right). In Table 1 (on the left), we also present the comparative performances of L_2E-FM and $\tilde{\mu}$. We can see that for FM computation, L_2E-FM outperforms the non-robust FM, $\tilde{\mu}$. In the case of L_2E-PGA, it takes comparable time but gives the best performance compared to the two competitors.

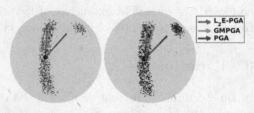

Fig. 1. Robust FM computation for the synthetic data on $\mathbf{S}^2$ with, *Left:* 10% and *Right:* 20% outliers.

Table 1. Synthetic data results on $\mathbf{S}^2$ for, *Left:* FM and *Right:* PGA.

ς (%)	μ^* $d(\mu, \mu^*)$	s^2	t(s)	$\bar{\mu}$ $d(\mu, \bar{\mu})$	s^2	t(s)	$\tilde{\mu}$ $d(\mu, \tilde{\mu})$	s^2	t(s)	L_2E-PGA E_r	t(s)	GMPGA E_r	t(s)	PGA E_r	t(s)
5	**0.04**	**0.24**	2.01	0.06	0.25	**0.01**	0.05	0.25	0.32	**0.01**	3.63	0.01	2.65	0.09	1.67
10	**0.07**	**0.24**	2.84	0.12	0.26	**0.01**	0.08	0.25	0.37	**0.01**	3.56	0.01	4.71	0.10	1.69
15	**0.12**	**0.25**	3.15	0.17	0.27	**0.01**	0.14	0.26	0.23	**0.01**	4.92	0.02	4.81	0.10	1.71
20	**0.16**	**0.26**	3.35	0.23	0.29	**0.01**	0.19	0.27	0.31	**0.01**	9.62	0.04	7.07	0.11	3.90

The poor performance of conventional PGA in the presence of outliers is not at all surprising because it can not cope with outliers. GMPGA however demonstrates comparable performance to our L_2E-PGA in the case of a small fraction of outliers but not for larger fractions.

OASIS Data [18]: We now compare the performance of the L_2E based FM and PGA with the competing methods on publicly available OASIS data. This dataset consists of T1-MR brain scans of subjects with ages in the range from 18 to 96 including individuals with early Alzheimer's Disease. We have identified an individual to be *Young* (with age between 10 to 40), *Middle Aged* (with age between 40 to 70) and *Old* (with age between 70 to 100).

Table 2. OASIS data results on $\mathbf{C}P^{250}$ for, *Left:* FM and *Right:* PGA

ς (%)	μ^*			$\bar{\mu}$			$\tilde{\mu}$			L$_2$E-PGA		GMPGA		PGA	
	$d(\mu,\mu^*)$	s^2	t(s)	$d(\mu,\bar{\mu})$	s^2	t(s)	$d(\mu,\tilde{\mu})$	s^2	t(s)	E_r	t(s)	E_r	t(s)	E_r	t(s)
5	**0.09**	1.13	4.69	0.19	1.16	**0.01**	0.16	1.14	0.07	**1.08**	1.04	1.11	0.85	1.11	**0.78**
10	**0.14**	1.14	6.83	0.26	1.17	**0.01**	0.23	1.15	0.07	**1.08**	3.91	1.13	0.93	1.13	**0.80**
15	**0.25**	1.15	21.76	0.47	1.26	**0.01**	0.37	1.19	0.08	**1.10**	4.60	1.24	0.97	1.13	**0.80**
20	**0.35**	1.19	22.11	0.48	1.27	**0.01**	0.43	1.25	0.08	**1.11**	4.60	1.25	2.63	1.13	**0.81**

We randomly picked 4 brain scans from within each decade, totalling 36 brain images. From each brain scan, we segmented the corpus callosum (CC) region. Then, we take a set of landmark points from the boundary of the CC shape and map it to *Kendall's shape space* [16], which is a complex projective space, $\mathbf{C}P^{250}$. The results are shown in the Table 2. Similar to before, this result indicates a superior performance of the L$_2$E-FM in comparable time. In the case of PGA, L$_2$E-PGA yields a smaller reconstruction error compared to GMPGA and the conventional (non-robust) PGA. This superior performance could be attributed to the fact that unlike in GMPGA, there is no linearization operation in the L$_2$E-PGA. Further, the L$_2$E formulation has no tuning parameters and is less prone to local minima due to the presence of a natural scale parameter σ' which is automatically adjusted starting at a large initial value permitting global search and gradually decreasing to small σ' that permits a precise approximation. For each of the three classes of individuals, i.e., Young, Middle aged and Old, we also present the reconstructed shape using first 34 principal geodesics in Fig. 2. In terms of shape reconstruction, PGA performs the worst,

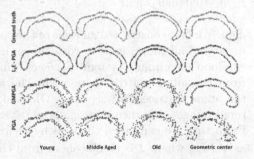

Fig. 2. Reconstruction results from the OASIS data

and L$_2$E-PGA performs the best. The last column of this figure depicts the mean shape computed using L$_2$E-FM, the conventional FM and FMe. As expected, FMe is better than FM but our L$_2$E-FM results in the "best" mean shape.

3.2 Robust FM and PGA on SPD(m)

Movement Disorder Data: In this experiment, the data consists of HARDI acquisitions from patients with Parkinsons disease (PD), essential tremor (ET). The goal here is to perform robust PGA and demonstrate the power of this representation via a depiction of the reconstruction error. All the HARDI data for full brain were acquired on a 3T Phillips MR scanner using a single-shot spin echo EPI sequence, with the following acquisition parameters: repetition time = 7748 ms, echo time = 86 ms, flip angle = 90, # of diffusion gradients: 64, field of view = 224 224 mm, in-plane resolution = 2 mm iso-tropic,

12   M. Banerjee et al.

slice-thickness $= 2\,\mathrm{mm}$, SENSE factor $= 2$. Data from 22 control and 26 PD patients were acquired using the above HARDI acquisition protocol. Distortions due to eddy currents and head motion was corrected by using the FSL software.

From previous studies, it is well known that, the basal ganglia region of the brain is significantly affected by Parkinson's disease, we chose our ROI for analysis to be this region in the brain. The image volume size we work with here is $(112 \times 112 \times 60)$ for each diffusion gradient direction.

Along with the diffusion images, for each data, we also have a mask defining the following region of interests (ROIs) in basal ganglia: left and right anterior substantia nigra, left and right posterior substantia nigra, left and right thalamus, and left and right puta-

Table 3. Movement disorder data results on the product manifold of SPD(3) for, *Top:* FM and *Bottom:* PGA

ς (%)	μ^*			$\bar{\mu}$			$\bar{\mu}$		
	$d(\mu,\mu^*)$	s^2	t(s)	$d(\mu,\bar{\mu})$	s^2	t(s)	$d(\mu,\bar{\mu})$	s^2	t(s)
5	1.40	0.01	3.11	31.63	998.32	1.99	16.26	264.14	4.07
10	1.47	0.01	10.64	42.94	1841.98	2.39	25.91	672.47	4.16
15	1.57	0.01	12.41	65.24	4294.63	2.70	53.97	2916.183	4.01
20	1.66	0.01	26.72	88.79	7889.97	2.88	73.74	4543.60	4.23

L_2E-PGA		GMPGA		PGA	
E_r	t(s)	E_r	t(s)	E_r	t(s)
0.19	151.96	1.93	43.47	8.26	10.50
0.22	153.74	7.96	51.82	6.63	22.49
0.22	156.50	13.74	59.39	13.06	43.00
0.22	157.21	14.96	62.68	16.79	58.99

men. We first constructed an atlas of the control population [5], and then affinely registered all the s_0 images, with the s_0 image of the atlas, to bring them to a common co-ordinate system. For each image, we used the rotation, computed from the affine matrix, to re-orient the 64 gradient directions. We also used the affine matrices to warp the ROI masks, so that they will match the registered images. We then non-rigidly registered each image to the atlas using [4]. From this, we computed the Cauchy Deformation Tensor (CDT) in each voxel as $\sqrt{JJ^T}$, where J is the Jacobian from the non-rigid registration.

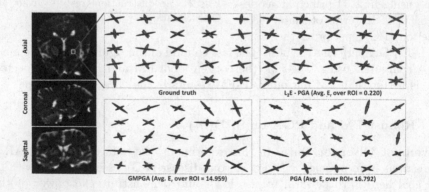

Fig. 3. CDT reconstruction results for the movement disorder data

Since CDT is a symmetric positive definite (SPD) matrix, the CDT field of each image lies on a product SPD manifold. We constructed a combined ROI mask, from the 22 initial ROI masks of the control population. In this combined

ROI mask, a voxel value is set to 1, if there is more than $\eta\%$ overlap of the initial ROIs, else it is set to 0. To emphasize the effect of the PD in the basal ganglia, among the $112 \times 112 \times 60$ voxels in each image, we considered the CDTs only in the voxels of the combined ROI mask. We chose $\eta = 50$ to get 864 voxels. It is not uncommon to misclassify between patients with essential tremor (ET) and PD patients, hence, we naturally have data samples from ET patients as an outlier. As before, we have reported results in Table 3 by varying the percentage of outliers present in the data, i.e., varying mis-labelled samples with ET. The results in Table 3 indicates superior E_r values from our formulation compared to the competitors. In Fig. 3, we have shown comparison results of reconstructed CDTs (with 20% outliers) of a 5×5 region inside the ROI (region colored red in the figure). Our visualization of the CDT (3×3 SPD matrices) presented here is as follows: eigen values are used as lengths of the axis of the ellipsoid and eigen vectors give the orientation of each ellipsoid. It is clear from the figure that our robust PGA formulation yields a better reconstruction.

4   Conclusions

In this paper, we presented novel algorithms to compute the robust FM, dubbed the L_2E-FM, and robust PGA, dubbed the L_2E-PGA, for data on Riemannian manifolds. In both these problems, we formulated the minimizations involved using an M-estimator called the L_2E. One of the key advantages of the proposed L_2E based formulation is that it is free of tuning parameters. Further, unlike the conventional PGA which uses a linear approximation of the manifold in the neighborhood of the FM, L_2E-PGA uses the exact-PGA cost function which yields more accurate results even in the case of data with large variance. Through an extensive set of synthetic and real experiments, we showed that our L_2E formulation achieves robustness in computing both the FM and PGA. Further, since there are no other robust PGA methods in literature to compare with, we developed the GMPGA method, which performs GMPCA (Grassmann averaging to compute PCA) [12] in the tangent space anchored at the FM. Finally, we presented experiments on MRI data from the publicly available OASIS database and diffusion MRI scans of movement disorder patients as well as synthetic data on the sphere with varying amounts of outliers to demonstrate superior performance of our robust algorithms in comparison to the competing methods.

Acknowledgements. Authors thank Drs. Vaillancourt, Okun and Ofori of the University of Florida, for providing us the movement disorder data used here.

References

1. Afsari, B.: Riemannian L_p center of mass: existence, uniqueness, and convexity. Proc. Am. Math. Soc. **139**(2), 655–673 (2011)
2. Basu, A., Harris, I.R., Hjort, N.L., Jones, M.: Robust and efficient estimation by minimising a density power divergence. Biometrika **85**(3), 549–559 (1998)

3. Chakraborty, R., Seo, D., Vemuri, B.C.: An efficient exact-PGA algorithm for constant curvature manifolds. In: IEEE CVPR (2016)
4. Cheng, G., Vemuri, B.C., Carney, P.R., Mareci, T.H.: Non-rigid registration of high angular resolution diffusion images represented by gaussian mixture fields. In: Yang, G.-Z., Hawkes, D., Rueckert, D., Noble, A., Taylor, C. (eds.) MICCAI 2009. LNCS, vol. 5761, pp. 190–197. Springer, Heidelberg (2009). doi:10.1007/978-3-642-04268-3_24
5. Cheng, G., Vemuri, B.C., Hwang, M.S., Howland, D., Forder, J.R.: Atlas construction from high angular resolution diffusion imaging data represented by gaussian mixture fields. In: ISBI, pp. 549–552 (2011)
6. DoCarmo, M.P.: Riemannian Geometry. Birkhauser, Basel (1992)
7. Fletcher, P.T., Lu, C., Pizer, S.M., Joshi, S.: Principal geodesic analysis for the study of nonlinear statistics of shape. IEEE TMI **23**(8), 995–1005 (2004)
8. Fletcher, P.T., Venkatasubramanian, S., Joshi, S.: The geometric median on Riemannian manifolds with application to robust atlas estimation. NeuroImage **45**(1), S143–S152 (2009)
9. Fréchet, M.: Les éléments aléatoires de nature quelconque dans un espace distancié. In: Annales de l'institut Henri Poincaré, vol. 10, pp. 215–310 (1948)
10. Ghadimi, S., Lan, G.: Accelerated gradient methods for nonconvex nonlinear and stochastic programming. Math. Program. Ser. A **156**(1), 59–99 (2016)
11. Hauberg, S.: Principal curves on Riemannian manifolds. IEEE TPAMI **38**(9), 1915–1921 (2015)
12. Hauberg, S., Feragen, A., Black, M.J.: Grassmann averages for scalable robust PCA. In: CVPR, pp. 3810–3817 (2014)
13. Hotz, T., Huckemann, S., Le, H., Marron, J.S., Mattingly, J.C., Miller, E., Nolen, J., Owen, M., Patrangenaru, V., Skwerer, S., et al.: Sticky central limit theorems on open books. Ann. Appl. Probab. **23**(6), 2238–2258 (2013)
14. Huber, P.J.: Robust statistics. In: Lovric, M. (ed.) International Encyclopedia of Statistical Science, pp. 1248–1251. Springer, Heidelberg (2011)
15. Huckemann, S., Hotz, T., Munk, A.: Intrinsic shape analysis: geodesic PCA for Riemannian manifolds modulo isometric lie group actions. Stat. Sin. **20**(1), 1–58 (2010)
16. Kendall, D.G.: Shape manifolds, procrustean metrics, and complex projective spaces. Bull. Lond. Math. Soc. **16**(2), 81–121 (1984)
17. Lenglet, C., Rousson, M., Deriche, R., Faugeras, O.: Statistics on the manifold of multivariate normal distributions: theory and application to diffusion tensor MRI processing. JMIV **25**(3), 423–444 (2006)
18. Marcus, D.S., Wang, T.H., Parker, J., Csernansky, J.G., Morris, J.C., Buckner, Y.L.: Open access series of imaging studies (OASIS): cross-sectional MRI data in young, middle aged, nondemented, and demented older adults. J. Cogn. Neurosci. **19**, 1498–1507 (2007)
19. Mardia, K., Dryden, I.: Shape distributions for landmark data. Adv. Appl. Probab. **21**, 742–755 (1989)
20. Moakher, M., Batchelor, P.G.: Symmetric positive-definite matrices: from geometry to applications and visualization. In: Weickert, J., Hagen, H. (eds.) Visualization and Processing of Tensor Fields, pp. 285–298. Springer, Heidelberg (2006)
21. Pennec, X.: Intrinsic statistics on Riemannian manifolds: basic tools for geometric measurements. JMIV **25**(1), 127–154 (2006)
22. Pennec, X., Fillard, P., Ayache, N.: A Riemannian framework for tensor computing. IJCV **66**(1), 41–66 (2006)

23. Said, S., Courty, N., Le Bihan, N., Sangwine, S.J.: Exact principal geodesic analysis for data on SO(3). In: EUSIPCO-2007, pp. 1700–1705 (2007)
24. Scott, D.W.: Parametric statistical modeling by minimum integrated square error. Technometrics **43**(3), 274–285 (2001)
25. Scott, D.W.: Outlier detection and clustering by partial mixture modeling. In: Antoch, J. (ed.) COMPSTAT 2004, pp. 453–464. Physica-Verlag HD, Heidelberg (2004). doi:10.1007/978-3-7908-2656-2_37
26. Sommer, S., Lauze, F., Hauberg, S., Nielsen, M.: Manifold valued statistics, exact principal geodesic analysis and the effect of linear approximations. In: Daniilidis, K., Maragos, P., Paragios, N. (eds.) ECCV 2010. LNCS, vol. 6316, pp. 43–56. Springer, Heidelberg (2010). doi:10.1007/978-3-642-15567-3_4
27. Tipping, M.E., Bishop, C.M.: Probabilistic principal component analysis. J. R. Stat. Soc. B **61**(3), 611–622 (1999)
28. Zhang, M., Fletcher, P.T.: Probabilistic principal geodesic analysis. In: Advances in Neural Information Processing Systems, pp. 1178–1186 (2013)

Inconsistency of Template Estimation
with the Fréchet Mean in Quotient Space

Loïc Devilliers[1]([⊠]), Xavier Pennec[1], and Stéphanie Allassonnière[2]

[1] Université Côte d'Azur, Inria, France
loic.devilliers@inria.fr
[2] Université Paris Descartes, INSERM UMRS 1138,
Centre de Recherche des Cordeliers, Paris, France

Abstract. We tackle the problem of template estimation when data
have been randomly transformed under an isometric group action in the
presence of noise. In order to estimate the template, one often minimizes the variance when the influence of the transformations have been
removed (computation of the Fréchet mean in quotient space). The consistency bias is defined as the distance (possibly zero) between the orbit of
the template and the orbit of one element which minimizes the variance.
In this article we establish an asymptotic behavior of the consistency
bias with respect to the noise level. This behavior is linear with respect
to the noise level. As a result the inconsistency is unavoidable as soon
as the noise is large enough. In practice, the template estimation with a
finite sample is often done with an algorithm called max-max. We show
the convergence of this algorithm to an empirical Karcher mean. Finally,
our numerical experiments show that the bias observed in practice cannot be attributed to the small sample size or to a convergence problem
but is indeed due to the previously studied inconsistency.

1 Introduction

The template estimation is a well known issue in different fields such as statistics on signals [12], shape theory, computational anatomy [6,8,10] etc. In these
fields, the template (which can be viewed as the prototype of our data) can be
(according to different vocabulary) shifted, transformed, wrapped or deformed
due to different groups acting on data. Moreover, due to a limited precision in the
measurement, the presence of noise is almost always unavoidable. These mixed
effects on data lead us to study the consistency of algorithms which claim to
compute the template. A popular algorithm consists in the minimization of the
variance, in other words, the computation of the Fréchet mean in quotient space.
This method has been already proved to be inconsistent [3,7,13]. One way to
avoid the inconsistency is to use another framework, for a instance a Bayesian
paradigm [4]. However, if one does not want to change the paradigm, then one
needs to have a better understanding of the geometrical and statistical origins
of the inconsistency.

© Springer International Publishing AG 2017
M. Niethammer et al. (Eds.): IPMI 2017, LNCS 10265, pp. 16–27, 2017.
DOI: 10.1007/978-3-319-59050-9_2

Notation: In this paper, we suppose that observations belong to a Hilbert space $(H, \langle \cdot, \cdot \rangle)$, we denote by $\| \cdot \|$ the norm associated to the dot product $\langle \cdot, \cdot \rangle$. We also consider a group of transformation G which acts isometrically on H the space of observations. This means that $x \mapsto g \cdot x$ is a linear automorphism of H, such that[1] $\|g \cdot x\| = \|x\|$, $g' \cdot (g \cdot x) = (g'g) \cdot x$ and $e \cdot x = x$ for all $x \in H$, $g, g' \in G$, where e is the identity element of G.

The generative model is the following: we transform an unknown template $t_0 \in H$ with ϕ a random and unknown element of the group G and we add some noise $\sigma \epsilon$ with a positive noise level σ, ϵ a standardized noise: $\mathbb{E}(\epsilon) = 0$, $\mathbb{E}(\|\epsilon\|^2) = 1$. Moreover we suppose that ϵ and ϕ are independent random variables. Finally, the only observable random variable is:

$$Y = \phi \cdot t_0 + \sigma \epsilon. \tag{1}$$

If we assume that the noise is independent and identically distributed on each pixel or voxel with a standard deviation s, then $\sigma = \sqrt{N}s$, where N is the number of pixels/voxels.

Quotient Space and Fréchet Mean: The random transformation of the template by the group leads us to project the observation Y into the quotient space defined as the set containing all the orbit $[x] = \{g \cdot x, g \in G\}$ for $x \in H$. Because the action is isometric, the quotient space H/G is equipped with a pseudometric[2] defined by:

$$d_Q([x],[y]) = \inf_{g \in G} \|x - g \cdot y\| = \inf_{g \in G} \|g \cdot x - y\|.$$

The quotient pseudometric is the distance between x and y' where y' is the registration of y with respect to x. We define the variance of the random orbit $[Y]$ as the expectation of the square pseudometric between the random orbit $[Y]$ and the orbit of a point x in H:

$$F(x) = \mathbb{E}(d_Q^2([x],[Y])) = \mathbb{E}(\inf_{g \in G} \|x - g \cdot Y\|^2) = \mathbb{E}(\inf_{g \in G} \|g \cdot x - Y\|^2). \tag{2}$$

Note that $F(x)$ is well defined for all $x \in H$ because $\mathbb{E}(\|Y\|^2)$ is finite. In order to estimate the template, one often minimizes this function. If $m_\star \in H$ minimizes F, then $[m_\star]$ is called a Fréchet mean of $[Y]$. The consistency bias, noted CB, is the pseudometric between the orbit of the template $[t_0]$ and $[m_\star]$: $CB = d_Q([t_0],[m_\star])$. If such a $m_\star$ does not exist, then the consistency bias is infinite.

Questions:

- What is the behavior of the consistency with respect to the noise?
- How to perform such a minimization of the variance? Indeed, in practice we have only a sample and not the whole distribution.

---

[1] Note that in this article, $g \cdot x$ is the result of the action of g on x, and $\cdot$ should not to be confused with the multiplication of real numbers noted $\times$.

[2] d_Q is called a pseudometric because $d_Q([x],[y])$ can be equal to zero even if $[x] \neq [y]$. If the orbits are closed sets then d_Q is a distance.

Contribution: In this article, we provide a Taylor expansion of the consistency bias when the noise level σ tends to infinity. As we do not have the whole distribution, we minimize the empirical variance given a sample. An element which minimizes the variance is called an empirical Fréchet mean. We already know that the empirical Fréchet mean converges to the Fréchet mean when the sample size tends to infinity [15]. Therefore our problem is reduced to find an empirical Fréchet mean with a finite but sufficiently large sample. One algorithm called the max-max algorithm [1] aims to compute such an empirical Fréchet mean. We establish some properties of the convergence of this algorithm. In particular, when the group is finite, the algorithm converges in a finite number of steps to an empirical Karcher mean (a local minimum of the empirical variance given a sample). This helps us to illustrate the inconsistency in this very simple framework.

Of course, generally people use a subgroup of diffeomorphisms which acts non isometrically on data such that images, landmarks etc. We believe that studying the inconsistency in this simplified framework will help us to better understand more complex situations. Moreover it is also possible to define and use isometric actions on curves [9,12] or on surfaces [11] where our work can be directly applied.

This article is organized as follows: in Sect. 2, we study the presence of the inconsistency and we establish the asymptotic behavior when the noise parameter σ tends to ∞. In Sect. 3 we detail the max-max algorithm and its properties. Finally, in Sect. 4 we illustrate the inconsistency with synthetic data.

2   Inconsistency of the Template Estimation

We start with the main theorem of this article which gives us an asymptotic behavior of the consistency bias when the noise level σ tends to infinity. One key notion in Theorem 1 is the concept of fixed point under the action G: a point $x \in H$ is a fixed point if for all $g \in G$, $g \cdot x = x$. We require that the support of the noise ϵ is not included in the set of fixed points. But this condition is almost always fulfilled. For instance in $\mathbb{R}^n$ the set of fixed points under a linear group action is a null set for the Lebesgue measure (unless the action is trivial $g \cdot x = x$ for all $g \in G$ but this situation is irrelevant).

Theorem 1. *Let us suppose that the support of the noise ϵ is not included in the set of fixed points under the group action. Let Y be the observable variable defined in Eq. (1). If the Fréchet mean of $[Y]$ exists, then we have the following lower and upper bounds of the consistency bias noted CB:*

$$\sigma K - 2\|t_0\| \leq CB \leq \sigma K + 2\|t_0\|, \tag{3}$$

where $K = \sup_{\|v\|=1} \mathbb{E} \left(\sup_{g \in G} \langle g \cdot v, \epsilon \rangle \right)$ is a constant which depends only on the standardised noise and on the group action. We have $K \in (0, 1]$. The consistency bias has the following asymptotic behavior when the noise level σ tends to infinity:

$$CB = \sigma K + o(\sigma) \text{ as } \sigma \to +\infty. \tag{4}$$

It follows from Eq. (3) that K is the consistency bias with a null template $t_0 = 0$ and a standardised noise $\sigma = 1$. We can ensure the presence of inconsistency as soon as the signal to noise ratio verifies $\frac{\|t_0\|}{\sigma} < \frac{K}{2}$. Moreover, if the signal to noise ratio verifies $\frac{\|t_0\|}{\sigma} < \frac{K}{3}$ then the consistency bias verifies $CB \geq \|t_0\|$. In other words, the Fréchet mean in quotient space is too far from the template: the template estimation with the Fréchet mean in quotient space is useless in this case. In [7] the authors also give lower and upper bounds as a function of σ but these bounds are less informative than our current bounds. Indeed, in [7] the lower bound goes to zero when the template becomes closed to fixed points. This may suggest that the consistency bias was small for this kind of template, which is not the case. The proof of Theorem 1 is postponed in Appendix A, the sketch of the proof is the following:

- $K > 0$ because the support of ϵ is not included in the set of fixed points under the action of G.
- $K \leq 1$ is the consequence of the Cauchy-Schwarz inequality.
- The proof of Inequalities (3) is based on the triangular inequalities:

$$\|m_\star\| - \|t_0\| \leq CB = \inf_{g \in G} \|t_0 - g \cdot m_\star\| \leq \|t_0\| + \|m_\star\|, \tag{5}$$

where $m_\star$ minimises (2): having a piece of information about the norm of $m_\star$ is enough to deduce a piece of information about the consistency bias.
- The asymptotic Taylor expansion of the consistency bias (4) is the direct consequence of inequalities (3).

Note that Theorem 1 is absolutely not a contradiction with [12] where the authors proved the consistency of the template estimation with the Fréchet mean in quotient space for all $\sigma > 0$. Indeed their noise was included in the set of constant functions which are the fixed points under their group action.

One disadvantage of Theorem 1 is that it ensures the presence of inconsistency for σ large enough but it says nothing when σ is small, in this case one can refer to [13] or [7].

3 Template Estimation with the Max-Max Algorithm

3.1 Max-Max Algorithm Converges to a Local Minima of the Empirical Variance

Section 2 can be roughly understood as follows: if we want to estimate the template by minimising the Fréchet mean with quotient space then there is a bias. This supposes that we are able to compute such a Fréchet mean. In practice, we cannot minimise the exact variance in quotient space, because we have only a finite sample and not the whole distribution. In this section we study the estimation of the empirical Fréchet mean with the max-max algorithm. We suppose that the group is finite. Indeed, in this case, the registration can always be found by an exhaustive search. In a compact group acting continuously, the registration also exists but is not necessarily computable without approximation. Hence, the numeric experiments which we conduct in Sect. 4 lead to an empirical Karcher mean in a finite number of steps.

If we have a sample: $Y_1, \ldots, Y_I$ of independent and identically distributed copies of Y, then we define the empirical variance in the quotient space:

$$F_I(x) = \frac{1}{I} \sum_{i=1}^{I} d_Q^2([x], [Y_i]) = \frac{1}{I} \sum_{i=1}^{I} \min_{g_i \in G} \|x - g_i \cdot Y_i\|^2 = \frac{1}{I} \sum_{i=1}^{I} \min_{g_i \in G} \|g_i \cdot x - Y_i\|^2.$$

(6)

The empirical variance is an approximation of the variance, indeed thanks to the law of large number we have $\lim_{I \to \infty} F_I(x) = F(x)$ for all $x \in H$. One element which minimizes globally (respectively locally) F_I is called an empirical Fréchet mean (respectively an empirical Karcher mean). For $x \in H$ and $\underline{g} \in G^I$: $\underline{g} = (g_1, \ldots, g_I)$ where $g_i \in G$ for all $i \in 1..I$ we define J an auxiliary function by:

$$J(x, \underline{g}) = \frac{1}{I} \sum_{i=1}^{I} \|x - g_i \cdot Y_i\|^2 = \frac{1}{I} \sum_{i=1}^{I} \|g_i^{-1} \cdot x - Y_i\|^2.$$

The max-max algorithms iteratively minimizes the function J in the variable $x \in H$ and in the variable $\underline{g} \in G^I$:

Algorithm 1. Max-Max algorithm

Require: A starting point $m_0 \in H$, a sample $Y_1, \ldots, Y_I$.
  $n = 0$.
  while Convergence is not reached **do**
    Minimizing $\underline{g} \in G^I \mapsto J(m_n, \underline{g})$: we get g_i^n by registering Y_i with respect to m_n.
    Minimizing $x \in H \mapsto J(x, \underline{g}^n)$: we get $m_{n+1} = \frac{1}{I} \sum_{i=1}^{I} g_i^n \cdot Y_i$.
    $n = n + 1$.
  end while
  $\hat{m} = m_n$

Note that the empirical variance does not increase at each step of the algorithm since: $F_I(m_n) = J(m_n, \underline{g}^n) \geq J(m_{n+1}, \underline{g}^n) \geq J(m_{n+1}, \underline{g}^{n+1}) = F_I(m_{n+1})$. This algorithm is sensitive to the the starting point. However we remark that $m_1 = \frac{1}{I} \sum_{i=1}^{I} g_i \cdot Y_i$ for some $g_i \in G$, then without loss of generality, we can start from $m_1 = \frac{1}{I} \sum_{i=1}^{I} g_i \cdot Y_i$ for some $g_i \in G$.

Proposition 1. *As the group is finite, the convergence is reached in a finite number of steps.*

Proof. The sequence $(F_I(m_n))_{n \in \mathbb{N}}$ is non-increasing. Moreover the sequence $(m_n)_{n \in \mathbb{N}}$ takes value in a finite set which is: $\{\frac{1}{I} \sum_{i=1}^{I} g_i \cdot Y_i, \ g_i \in G\}$. Therefore, the sequence $(F_I(m_n))_{n \in \mathbb{N}}$ is stationary. Let $n \in \mathbb{N}$ such that $F_I(m_n) =$

$F_I(m_{n+1})$. Hence the empirical variance did not decrease between step n and step $n + 1$ and we have:

$$F_I(m_n) = J(m_n, \underline{g}_n) = J(m_{n+1}, \underline{g}_n) = J(m_{n+1}, \underline{g}_{n+1}) = F_I(m_{n+1}),$$

as m_n is the unique element which minimizes $m \mapsto J(m, \underline{g}_n)$ we conclude that $m_{n+1} = m_n$. $\qquad\qquad\qquad\qquad\qquad\qquad\qquad\qquad\qquad\qquad\qquad\qquad\qquad$ $\square$

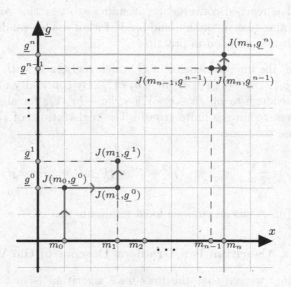

Fig. 1. Iterative minimization of the function J on the two axis, the horizontal axis represents the variable in the space H, the vertical axis represents the set of all the possible registrations G^I. Once the convergence is reached, the point (m_n, g_n) is the minimum of the function J on the two axis in green. Is this point the minimum of J on its whole domain? There are two pitfalls: firstly this point could be a saddle point, it can be avoided with Proposition 2, secondly this point could be a local (but not global), this is discussed in Subsect. 4.3. (Color figure online)

This proposition gives us a shutoff parameter in the max-max algorithm: we stop the algorithm as soon as $m_n = m_{n+1}$. Let call $\hat{m}$ the final result of the max-max algorithm. It may seem logical that $\hat{m}$ is at least a local minimum of the empirical variance. However this intuition may be wrong: let us give a simple counterexample (but not necessarily realistic), suppose that we observe $Y_1, \ldots, Y_I$, due to the transformation of the group it is possible that $\sum_{i=1}^{n} Y_i = 0$. We can start from $m_1 = 0$ in the max-max algorithm, as Y_i and 0 are already registered, the max-max algorithm does not transform Y_i. At step two, we still have $m_2 = 0$, by induction the max-max algorithm stays at 0 even if 0 is not a Fréchet or Karcher mean of $[Y]$. Because 0 is equally distant from all the points in the orbit of Y_i, 0 is called a focal point of $[Y_i]$. The notion of focal point is important for the consistency of the Fréchet mean in manifold [2]. Fortunately, the situation where $\hat{m}$ is not a Karcher mean is almost always avoided due to the following statement.

Proposition 2. *Let $\hat{m}$ be the result of the max-max algorithm. If the registration of Y_i with respect to $\hat{m}$ is unique, in other words, if $\hat{m}$ is not a focal point of Y_i for all $i \in 1..I$ then $\hat{m}$ is a local minimum of F_I: $[\hat{m}]$ is an empirical Karcher mean of $[Y]$.*

Note that, if we call z the registration of y with respect to m, then the registration is unique if and only if $\langle m, z - g \cdot z \rangle \neq 0$ for all $g \in G \setminus \{e\}$. Once the max-max algorithm has reached convergence, it suffices to test this condition for $\hat{m}$ obtained by the max-max algorithm and for Y_i for all i. This condition is in fact generic and is always obtained in practice.

Proof. We call g_i the unique element in G which register Y_i with respect to $\hat{m}$, for all $h \in G \setminus \{g_i\}$, $\|\hat{m} - g_i \cdot Y_i\| < \|\hat{m} - h_i \cdot Y_i\|$. By continuity of the norm we have for a close enough to m: $\|a - g_i \cdot Y_i\| < \|a - h_i \cdot Y_i\|$ for all $h_i \neq g_i$ (note that this argument requires a finite group). The registrations of Y_i with respect to m and to a are the same:

$$F_I(a) = \frac{1}{I} \sum_{i=1}^{I} \|a - g_i \cdot Y_i\|^2 = J(a, \underline{g}) \geq J(\hat{m}, \underline{g}) = F_I(\hat{m}),$$

because $m \mapsto J(m, \underline{g})$ has one unique local minimum $\hat{m}$. $\square$

3.2 Max-Max Algorithm Is a Gradient Descent of the Variance

In this Subsection, we see that the max-max algorithm is in fact a gradient descent. The gradient descent is a general method to find the minimum of a differentiable function. Here we are interested in the minimum of the variance F: let $m_0 \in H$ and we define by induction the gradient descent of the variance $m_{n+1} = m_n - \rho \nabla F(m_n)$, where $\rho > 0$ and F the variance in the quotient space. In [7] the gradient of the variance in quotient space for m a regular point was computed (m is regular as soon as $g \cdot m = m$ implies $g = e$), this leads to:

$$m_{n+1} = m_n - 2\rho \left[m_n - \mathbb{E}(g(Y, m_n) \cdot Y) \right],$$

where $g(Y, m_n)$ is the almost-surely unique element of the group which register Y with respect to m_n. Now if we have a set of data $Y_1, \ldots, Y_n$ we can approximated the expectation which leads to the following approximated gradient descent:

$$m_{n+1} = m_n(1 - 2\rho) + \rho \frac{2}{I} \sum_{i=1}^{I} g(Y_i, m_n) \cdot Y_i,$$

now by taking $\rho = \frac{1}{2}$ we get $m_{n+1} = \frac{1}{I} \sum_{i=1}^{I} g(Y_i, m_n) \cdot Y_i$. So the approximated gradient descent with $\rho = \frac{1}{2}$ is exactly the max-max algorithm. But the max-max algorithm is proven to be converging in a finite number of steps which is not the case for gradient descent in general.

4   Simulation on Synthetic Data

In this Section[3], we consider data in an Euclidean space $\mathbb{R}^N$ equipped with its canonical dot product $\langle \cdot, \cdot \rangle$, and $G = \mathbb{Z}/N\mathbb{Z}$ acts on $\mathbb{R}^N$ by circular permutation on coordinates:

$$(\bar{k} \in \mathbb{Z}/N\mathbb{Z}, (x_1, \ldots, x_N) \in \mathbb{R}^N) \mapsto (x_{1+k}, x_{2+k}, \ldots x_{N+k}),$$

where indexes are taken modulo N. This space models the discretization of functions with N points. This action is found in [1] and used for neuroelectric signals in [9]. The registration between two vectors can be made by an exhaustive research but it is faster with the fast Fourier transform [5].

4.1   Max-Max Algorithm with a Step Function as Template

We display an example of a template and the template estimation with the max-max algorithm on Fig. 2(a). Note that this experiment was already conducted in [1]. But no explanation of the appearance of the bias was provided. On the opposite, we know from the precedent Section that the max-max result is an empirical Karcher mean, and that this result can be obtained in a finite number of

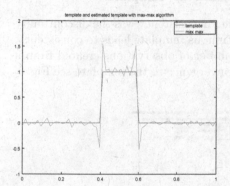 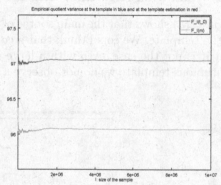

(a) Example of a template (a step function) and the template estimation with a sample size 10^5 in $\mathbb{R}^{64}$, ϵ is Gaussian noise and $\sigma = 10$. At the discontinuity points of the template, we observe a Gibbs-like phenomena.

(b) Variation of $F_I(t_0)$ (in blue) and of $F_I(\hat{m})$ (in red) as a function of I the size of the sample. Since convergence is already reached, $F(\hat{m})$, which is the limit of red curve, is below $F(t_0)$: $F(t_0)$ is the limit of the blue curve. Due to the inconsistency, $\hat{m}$ is an example of point such that $F(\hat{m}) < F(t_0)$.

Fig. 2. Template t_0 and template estimation $\hat{m}$ on Fig. 2(a). Empirical variance at the template and the template estimation with the max-max algorithm as a function of the size of the sample on Fig. 2(b). (Color figure online)

---

[3] The code used in this Section is available at http://loic.devilliers.free.fr/ipmi.html.

steps. Taking $\sigma = 10$ may seem extremely high, however the standard deviation of the noise at each point is not 10 but $\frac{\sigma}{\sqrt{N}} = 1.25$ which is not so high.

The sample size is 10^5, and the algorithm stopped after 94 steps, and $\hat{m}$ the estimated template (in red on the Fig. 2(a)) is not a focal points of the orbits $[Y_i]$, then Proposition 2 applies. We call empirical bias (noted EB) the quotient distance between the true template and the point $\hat{m}$ given by the max-max result. On this experiment we have $\frac{EB}{\sigma} \simeq 0.11$. Of course, one could think that we estimate the template with an empirical bias due to a too small sample size which induces fluctuation. To reply to this objection, we keep in memory $\hat{m}$ obtained with the max-max algorithm. If there was no inconsistency then we would have $F(t_0) \leq F(\hat{m})$. We do not know the value of the variance F at these points, but thanks to the law of large number, we know that:

$$F(t_0) = \lim_{I \to \infty} F_I(t_0) \text{ and } F(\hat{m}) = \lim_{I \to \infty} F_I(\hat{m}),$$

Given a sample, we compute $F_I(t_0)$ and $F_I(\hat{m})$ thanks to the definition of the empirical variance F_I (6). We display the result on Fig. 2(b), this tends to confirm that $F(t_0) > F(\hat{m})$. In other words, the variance at the template is bigger that the variance at the point given by the max-max algorithm.

4.2   Max-Max Algorithm with a Continuous Template

Figure 2(a) shows that the main source of the inconsistency was the discontinuity of the template. We could think that a continuous template leads to consistency. But it is not the case, even with a large number of observations created from a continuous template we do not observe a convergence to the template see Fig. 3,

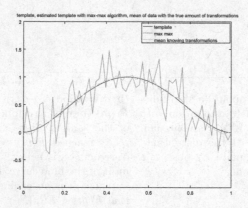

Fig. 3. Example of an other template (here a discretization of a continuous function) and the template estimation with a sample size 10^3 in $\mathbb{R}^{64}$ (in red), ϵ is Gaussian noise and $\sigma = 10$. Even with a continuous function the inconsistency appears. In green we compute the mean of data with the true amount of transformations. (Color figure online)

the empirical bias satisfies $\frac{EB}{\sigma} = 0.25$. If we knew the original transformations we could invert the transformations on data and take the mean, that is what we deed in green on Fig. 3. We see that with a sample size 10^3, the mean gives us almost the good result since we have in that case $\frac{EB}{\sigma} = 0.03$.

4.3 Does the Max-Max Algorithm Give Us a Global Minimum or only a Local Minimum of the Variance?

Proposition 2 tells us that the output of the max-max algorithm is a Karcher mean of the variance, but we do not know that if it is Fréchet mean of the variance. In other words, is the output a global minimum of the variance? In fact, F_I' has a lot of local minima which are not global. Indeed we can use the max-max algorithm with different starting points and we observe different outputs (which are all local minima thanks to Proposition 2) with different empirical variance (result non shown).

5 Discussion and Conclusion

We provided an asymptotic behavior of the consistency bias when the noise level σ tends to infinity, as a consequence, the inconsistency cannot be neglected when σ is large. However we have not answered this question: can the inconsistency be neglected? When the noise level is small enough, then the consistency bias is small [7,13], hence it can be neglected. Note that the quotient space is not a manifold, this prevents us to use *a priori* the Central Limit theorem for manifold proved in [2]. But if the Central Limit theorem could be applied to quotient space, the fluctuations induce an error which would be approximately equal to $\frac{\sigma}{\sqrt{I}}$ and if $K \ll \frac{1}{\sqrt{I}}$, then the inconsistency could be neglected because it is small compared to fluctuation.

If the Hilbert Space is a functional space, for instance $L^2([0, 1])$, in practice, we never observe the whole function, only a finite number values of this function. One can model these observable values on a grid. When the resolution of the grid goes to zero, one can show the consistency [14] by using the Fréchet mean with the Wasserstein distance on the space of measures rather than in the space of functions. But in (medical) images the number of pixels or voxels is finite.

Finally, in a future work one needs to study the template estimation with non isometric action. But we can already learn from this work: in the numerical experiments we led, we have seen that the template estimated is more detailed that the true template. The intuition is that the estimated template in computational anatomy with a group of diffeomorphisms is also more detailed. But the true template is almost always unknown. It is then possible that one think that the computation of the template succeeded to capture small details of the template while it is just an artifact due to the inconsistency. Moreover in order to tackle this question, one needs to have a good modelisation of the noise, for instance in [12], the observations are curves, what is a relevant noise in the space of curves?

A   Proof of Theorem 1

Proof. In the proof, we note by S the unit sphere in H. In order to prove that $K > 0$, we take x in the support of ϵ such that x is not a fixed point under the action of G. It exists $g_0 \in G$ such that $g_0 \cdot x \neq x$. We note $v_0 = \frac{g_0 \cdot x}{\|x\|} \in S$, we have $\langle v_0, g_0 \cdot x \rangle = \|x\| > \langle v_0, x \rangle$ and by continuity of the dot product it exists $r > 0$ such that: $\forall y \in B(x,r) \quad \langle v_0, g_0 \cdot y \rangle > \langle v_0, y \rangle$ as x is in the support of ϵ we have $\mathbb{P}(\epsilon \in B(x,r)) > 0$, it follows:

$$\mathbb{P}\left(\sup_{g \in G} \langle v_0, g \cdot \epsilon \rangle > \langle v_0, \epsilon \rangle \right) > 0. \tag{7}$$

Thanks to Inequality (7) and the fact that $\sup_{g \in G} \langle v_0, g \cdot \epsilon \rangle \geq \langle v_0, \epsilon \rangle$ we have:

$$K = \sup_{v \in S} \mathbb{E}\left(\sup_{g \in G} \langle v, g \cdot \epsilon \rangle \right) \geq \mathbb{E}\left(\sup_{g \in G} \langle v_0, g \cdot \epsilon \rangle \right) > \mathbb{E}(\langle v_0, \epsilon \rangle) = \langle v_0, \mathbb{E}(\epsilon) \rangle = 0.$$

Using the Cauchy-Schwarz inequality: $K \leq \sup_{v \in S} \mathbb{E}(\|v\| \times \|\epsilon\|) \leq \mathbb{E}(\|\epsilon\|^2)^{\frac{1}{2}} = 1$. We now prove Inequalities (3). The variance at λv for $v \in S$ and $\lambda \geq 0$ is:

$$F(\lambda v) = \mathbb{E}\left(\inf_{g \in G} \|\lambda v - g \cdot Y\|^2 \right) = \lambda^2 - 2\lambda \mathbb{E}\left(\sup_{g \in G} \langle v, g \cdot Y \rangle \right) + \mathbb{E}(\|Y\|^2). \tag{8}$$

Indeed $\|g \cdot Y\| = \|Y\|$ thanks to the isometric action. We note $x^+ = \max(x,0)$ the positive part of x and $h(v) = \mathbb{E}(\sup_{g \in G} \langle v, g \cdot Y \rangle)$. The $\lambda \geq 0$ which[4] minimizes (8) is $h(v)^+$ and the minimum value of the variance restricted to the half line $\mathbb{R}^+ v$ is $F(h(v)^+ v) = \mathbb{E}(\|Y\|^2) - (h(v)^+)^2$. To find $[m_\star]$ the Fréchet mean of $[Y]$, we need to maximize $(h(v)^+)^2$ with respect to $v \in S$: $m_\star = h(v_\star)v_\star$ with[5] $v_\star \in \operatorname{argmax}_{v \in S} h(v)$. As we said in the sketch of the proof we are interested in getting a piece of information about the norm of $\|m_\star\|$ we have: $\|m_\star\| = h(v_\star) = \sup_{v \in S} h$. Let $v \in S$, we have: $-\|t_0\| \leq \langle v, g\phi \cdot t_0 \rangle \leq \|t_0\|$ because the action is isometric. Now we decompose $Y = \phi \cdot t_0 + \sigma\epsilon$ and we get:

$$h(v) = \mathbb{E}\left(\sup_{g \in G} \langle v, g \cdot Y \rangle \right) = \mathbb{E}\left(\sup_{g \in G} \left(\langle v, g \cdot \sigma\epsilon \rangle + \langle v, g\phi \cdot t_0 \rangle \right) \right)$$

$$h(v) \leq \mathbb{E}\left(\sup_{g \in G} \left(\langle v, g \cdot \sigma\epsilon \rangle + \|t_0\| \right) \right) = \sigma\mathbb{E}\left(\sup_{g \in G} \langle v, g \cdot \epsilon \rangle \right) + \|t_0\|$$

$$h(v) \geq \mathbb{E}\left(\sup_{g \in G} \left(\langle v, g \cdot \sigma\epsilon \rangle \right) - \|t_0\| \right) = \sigma\mathbb{E}\left(\sup_{g \in G} \langle v, g \cdot \epsilon \rangle \right) - \|t_0\|.$$

---

[4] Indeed we know that $x \in \mathbb{R}^+ \mapsto x^2 - 2bx + c$ reaches its minimum at the point $x = b^+$ and $f(b^+) = c - (b^+)^2$.

[5] Note that we remove the positive part and the square because $\operatorname{argmax} h = \operatorname{argmax}(h^+)^2$ since h takes a non negative value (indeed $h(v) \geq \mathbb{E}(\langle v, \phi \cdot t_0 + \epsilon \rangle) = \langle v, \mathbb{E}(\phi \cdot t_0) \rangle$ and this last quantity is non negative for at least one $v \in S$).

By taking the biggest value in these inequalities with respect to $v \in S$, by definition of K we get:

$$- \|t_0\| + \sigma K \leq \|m_\star\| \leq \|t_0\| + \sigma K. \tag{9}$$

Thanks to (9) and to (5), Inequalities (3) are proved.   □

References

1. Allassonnière, S., Amit, Y., Trouvé, A.: Towards a coherent statistical framework for dense deformable template estimation. J. R. Stat. Soc.: Ser. B (Stat. Methodol.) **69**(1), 3–29 (2007)
2. Bhattacharya, R., Patrangenaru, V.: Large sample theory of intrinsic and extrinsic sample means on manifolds. Ann. Stat. **31**, 1–29 (2003)
3. Bigot, J., Charlier, B.: On the consistency of Fréchet means in deformable models for curve and image analysis. Electron. J. Stat. **5**, 1054–1089 (2011)
4. Cheng, W., Dryden, I.L., Huang, X.: Bayesian registration of functions and curves. Bayesian Anal. **11**(2), 447–475 (2016)
5. Cooley, J.W., Tukey, J.W.: An algorithm for the machine calculation of complex fourier series. Math. Comput. **19**(90), 297–301 (1965)
6. Cootes, T.F., Marsland, S., Twining, C.J., Smith, K., Taylor, C.J.: Groupwise diffeomorphic non-rigid registration for automatic model building. In: Pajdla, T., Matas, J. (eds.) ECCV 2004. LNCS, vol. 3024, pp. 316–327. Springer, Heidelberg (2004). doi:10.1007/978-3-540-24673-2_26
7. Devilliers, L., Allassonnière, S., Trouvé, A., Pennec, X.: Template estimation in computational anatomy: Fréchet means in top and quotient spaces are not consistent. ArXiv e-prints, August 2016
8. Guimond, A., Meunier, J., Thirion, J.P.: Average brain models: a convergence study. Comput. Vis. Image Underst. **77**(2), 192–210 (2000)
9. Hitziger, S., Clerc, M., Gramfort, A., Saillet, S., Bénar, C., Papadopoulo, T.: Jitter-adaptive dictionary learning-application to multi-trial neuroelectric signals. arXiv preprint arXiv:1301.3611 (2013)
10. Joshi, S., Davis, B., Jomier, M., Gerig, G.: Unbiased diffeomorphic atlas construction for computational anatomy. NeuroImage **23**, S151–S160 (2004)
11. Kurtek, S., Klassen, E., Ding, Z., Avison, M.J., Srivastava, A.: Parameterization-invariant shape statistics and probabilistic classification of anatomical surfaces. In: Székely, G., Hahn, H.K. (eds.) IPMI 2011. LNCS, vol. 6801, pp. 147–158. Springer, Heidelberg (2011). doi:10.1007/978-3-642-22092-0_13
12. Kurtek, S.A., Srivastava, A., Wu, W.: Signal estimation under random time-warpings and nonlinear signal alignment. In: Advances in Neural Information Processing Systems, pp. 675–683 (2011)
13. Miolane, N., Holmes, S., Pennec, X.: Template shape estimation: correcting an asymptotic bias. arXiv preprint arXiv:1610.01502 (2016)
14. Panaretos, V.M., Zemel, Y.: Amplitude and phase variation of point processes. Ann. Stat. **44**(2), 771–812 (2016)
15. Ziezold, H.: On expected figures and a strong law of large numbers for random elements in quasi-metric spaces. In: Kožešnik, J. (ed.) Transactions of the Seventh Prague Conference on Information Theory, Statistical Decision Functions, Random Processes and of the 1974 European Meeting of Statisticians, pp. 591–602. Springer, Dordrecht (1977)

Kernel Methods for Riemannian Analysis of Robust Descriptors of the Cerebral Cortex

Suyash P. Awate[1]([⊠]), Richard M. Leahy[2], and Anand A. Joshi[2]

[1] Computer Science and Engineering Department,
Indian Institute of Technology (IIT) Bombay, Mumbai, India
suyash@cse.iitb.ac.in
[2] Signal and Image Processing Institute (SIPI), University of Southern California,
Los Angeles, USA

Abstract. Typical cerebral cortical analyses rely on spatial normalization and are sensitive to misregistration arising from partial homologies between subject brains and local optima in nonlinear registration. In contrast, we use a descriptor of the 3D cortical sheet (jointly modeling folding and thickness) that is robust to misregistration. Our histogram-based descriptor lies on a *Riemannian manifold*. We propose new *regularized nonlinear methods* for (i) detecting group differences, using a *Mercer kernel* with an implicit lifting map to a reproducing kernel Hilbert space, and (ii) regression against clinical variables, using *kernel density estimation*. For both methods, we employ kernels that exploit the Riemannian structure. Results on simulated and clinical data shows the improved accuracy and stability of our approach in cortical-sheet analysis.

Keywords: Cortex · Folding · Thickness · Robustness · Riemannian space · Reproducing kernel hilbert space · Hypothesis tests · Kernel regression

1 Introduction

Cerebral cortical geometry holds key insights into development, aging, disease progression, and cognition. We propose a new framework to study *cortical sheet* geometry to detect inter-group differences and regress against clinical variables. Our model subsumes the complementary properties of folding and thickness.

Typical studies of the cortex focus either on folding [19,25,27] or thickness [9,14,23], but *not* both. They rely on spatial normalization and perform hypothesis tests at every cortical location in the normalized space. However, while the major sulcal patterns are similar across individuals, there is a large variation of the finer-scale cortical folding structure across individuals. This leads to a limited number of homologous features across subject brains [15,16,24], which compromises the precision of the spatial alignment. Moreover, the optimization underlying dense diffeomorphic nonlinear registration is challenged by multiple

Thanks to IIT-B Seed Grant 14IRCCSG010, NIH R01NS089212, NIH R01NS074980.

M. Niethammer et al. (Eds.): IPMI 2017, LNCS 10265, pp. 28–40, 2017.
DOI: 10.1007/978-3-319-59050-9_3

local optima. Thus, misregistration is inevitable and can inflate the variability of the cortical descriptors and, thereby, reduce the power of subsequent hypothesis tests. To alleviate problems of partial homology and local optima, we use local histogram-based descriptors that are robust to misregistration.

Our histogram-based descriptor lies on a Riemannian manifold. We propose novel *Riemannian statistical* methods for two typical studies: (i) detecting group differences, using *Mercer kernels* to fit compact models to non-Gaussian data distributions by implicitly employing a lifting map to a reproducing kernel Hilbert space (RKHS), and (ii) regression against clinical variables, using nonlinear regression via *kernel density estimation*. Our kernels exploit the Riemannian structure and enable us to effectively deal with (i) nonlinear variations in the data, i.e., within distributions of cortical descriptors, and (ii) dependencies of the cortical descriptors on clinical variables.

We present a new framework for two typical cortical analyses: (i) detecting group differences and (ii) regression against clinical variables. We use a neighborhood-based histogram feature of local cortical geometry, subsuming folding and thickness characteristics, which is robust to misregistration stemming from biology (partial homology) and numerical analysis (local optima). We propose *regularized nonlinear models* for both analyses, giving compact and reliable model fits, using *kernels* that exploit the Riemannian structure of the space of histograms. Results on simulated and clinical data shows the improved accuracy and stability of our approach cortical sheet analyses.

2   Related Work

Several cortical studies have focus on its thickness characteristics [9,14,23] or folding characteristics [19,25,27], relying on analyses of cortical features across subjects at every location on the cortical surface (typically, the inner/mid cortical surface). Unlike these studies, we model the 3D *cortical sheet* including the complementary characteristics of folding and thickness. There are many models for local cortical folding complexity. While [3] uses local curvature measures, [25] represents the cortical surface using spherical wavelets that lead to a set of wavelet coefficients capturing folding at every cortical location. Another method [26] uses spherical harmonic constructions and local fractal dimension to measure folding complexity. In contrast, we capture folding through curvedness and shape index that can lead to easier interpretation. Unlike other approaches, we perform pointwise studies using a local-histogram descriptor combining folding and thickness, which is robust to misregistration. Local histograms were used in [2] without Riemannian analyses and in [1] for linear Riemannian analyses.

Unlike other descriptors [2,3,25,26], our descriptor lies on a *Riemannian* manifold and we propose novel *kernel-based statistical* methods that exploit the Riemannian structure. Instead of learning a linear approximation to a manifold (e.g., using isomap) and then using Euclidean statistical analyses in the linearized space, we propose nonlinear statistical analysis directly in the (Riemannian) feature space. For group-difference analysis, we propose a *Mercer kernel* for modeling the (possibly non-Gaussian) distributions of the histograms within Riemannian space, along with regularized analysis in RKHS. For regression, we propose nonlinear *kernel regression* directly on the Riemannian manifold [21], and propose a data-driven consistent estimator of the bandwidth parameter.

3   Methods

We first describe our model for the 3D cortical sheet and the robust descriptor of local cortical geometry. We then describe the proposed Riemannian analyses, involving kernel methods, for hypothesis testing to (i) detect group differences in cortical geometry and (ii) regress cortical geometry against clinical variables.

3.1   A Geometrical Model for the Cerebral Cortical Sheet

We use a medial model for the 3D cortical sheet to represent its folding and thickness characteristics. We choose the mid-cortical surface $\mathcal{M}$ as the medial surface to model folding. In addition, we use pointwise thickness measurements on the medial surface to model the 3D sheet. At each point m on $\mathcal{M}$, the thickness measurement $t(m)$ gives the locations of the inner and outer (pial) cortical surfaces, at distances $t(m)/2$ along the inward and outward normals to $\mathcal{M}$ at m.

We compute cortical thickness based on an improved version of the diffusion-based method in [11], accounting for partial-volume effects by spatially modulating the diffusion strength proportionately. This also produces the mid-cortical surface $\mathcal{M}$ as a level set of the steady-state potential field. For each point m on $\mathcal{M}$, we model the local folding geometry through the principal curvatures determined by the first and second fundamental forms, by fitting a quadratic patch to the local surface around m. The principal curvatures $\kappa_{\min}(m)$ and $\kappa_{\max}(m)$ completely describe the local geometry (up to second order and up to a translation and rotation). We reparametrize the 2D space of $(\kappa_{\min}(m), \kappa_{\max}(m))$, via a polar transformation [13], into the orthogonal bases of curvedness $C(m) :=$ $(\kappa_{\min}(m)^2 + \kappa_{\max}(m)^2)^{0.5}$ and shape index $S(m) := \frac{1}{\pi} \arctan\left(\frac{\kappa_{\min}(m) + \kappa_{\max}(m)}{\kappa_{\min}(m) - \kappa_{\max}(m)}\right)$ that meaningfully separate notions of bending and shape for easier interpretation. The curvedness $C(m) \geq 0$ measures local patch bending at a particular patch scale/size, and is invariant to location and pose. The shape index $S(m) \in [-1, 1]$ is a pure measure of shape, modulo size, location, and pose.

A Robust Local Descriptor of Cortical Folding and Thickness. Nature limits the homology across human brains to about two dozen landmarks in each hemisphere [24]. In typical analyses relying on dense nonlinear diffeomorphic spatial normalization, this partial homology can lead to pointwise correspondences at non-homologous locations, e.g., a gyrus in one brain mapped to a sulcus in another. Such correspondences can inflate the variability of the cortical descriptors and reduce the power of the subsequent hypothesis tests.

One may consider, for a moment, a naive approach to reduce this variability by surface-based spatial smoothing of the descriptors at multiple scales. However, spatial averaging can reduce differences between the smoothed features across corresponding points in subject brains, because multiple spatial distributions of features can all yield the same average. This problem is serious for the brain cortex that is a complex convoluted structure with large variations in the local geometry over small displacements of surface location m. For instance, the value of the shape index drastically changes magnitude and sign as we traverse a surface path from a gyrus (-1) to a sulcus $(+1)$. Curvedness values, along the gyrus-to-sulcus path also changes drastically; from a large positive value to zero (at the inflection point) and back to a large positive value. Cortical thickness also exhibits a variation from gyrus to sulcus, where the crowns of gyri are typically 20% thicker than the fundi of sulci [7]. Indeed, Sect. 4 demonstrates the reduction in the quality of results from smoothing-based *multiscale* features.

Instead of averaging features across spatial neighborhoods, we propose to use the histograms of neighborhood features, which captures the higher-order statistics of the features. In this way, we extend the notion of histogram-based texture descriptors for images to histogram-based descriptors for the cortical sheet geometry; indeed the cortical sheet exhibits high-frequency spatial variations of features just like a textured image exhibits high-frequency spatial variation of intensity. We propose the local cortical descriptor at location m on the cortical surface to be the *joint histogram* of shape-index values $S(n)$, curvedness values $C(n)$, and thickness values $T(n)$ at locations n within a spatial neighborhood around location m. The neighborhood size depends on the typical size of *regions* (*not* individual points) in the cortex over which homologies can be reliably established (we take this as a region of diameter $1\,\mathrm{cm}$). This histogram is robust to the inevitable misregistration of sulci/gyri at fine scales. Moreover, unlike the neighborhood average that is a scalar, the histogram is a richer descriptor that restricts averaging to each histogram bin.

Riemannian Space of Histograms. We perform statistical analyses using the joint histograms $H_i(m)$ as the local feature descriptor for the cortex at location m for subject i. If the histogram has B bins, then $H_i(m) \in (\mathbb{R}_{\geq 0})^B$, $\|H_i(m)\|_1 = 1$, and $H_i(m)$ lies on a Riemannian manifold. To measure distance between two histograms $H_1(m)$ and $H_2(m)$, we use the Fisher-Rao distance metric $d_{\mathcal{H}}(H_1(m), H_2(m)) := d_{\mathcal{S}}(F_1(m), F_2(m))$, where $F_i(m)$ is the square-root histogram that is denoted $\sqrt{H_i(m)}$, with the value in the b-th bin $F_i(m, b) := \sqrt{H_i(m, b)}$, and $d_{\mathcal{S}}(F_1(m), F_2(m))$ is the geodesic distance between $F_1(m)$ and $F_2(m)$ on the unit hypersphere $\mathbb{S}^{B-1}$.

3.2 Group Analysis Using a Mercer Kernel in Riemannian Space

To detect differences between two groups of histograms, we need models for the distribution of histograms within each group. We propose a parametric and a nonparametric model, and associated test statistics for hypothesis testing.

Parametric Model. Modeling a parametric probability density function (PDF) on a hypersphere entails fundamental trade-offs between model generality and the viability of the underlying parameter estimation. For instance, although

Fisher-Bingham PDFs on $\mathbb{S}^d$ are able to model generic anisotropic distributions using $O(d^2)$ parameters, their parameter estimation may be intractable [17]. In contrast, parameter estimation for the $O(d)$-parameter von Mises-Fisher (vMF) PDF is tractable, but that PDF can only model isotropic distributions. We use a tractable approximation of a Normal law on a Riemannian manifold [22], modeling anisotropy through its covariance parameter in the tangent space at the mean. For a group with I subjects, at each cortical location m, we fit the approximate Normal law to the data $\{\sqrt{H_i(m)}\}_{i=1}^I$ as follows. We optimize for the Frechet mean $\mu \in \mathbb{S}^{B-1}$ via iterative gradient descent [4], where $\mu := \arg\min_\nu \sum_{i=1}^I d_{\mathcal{S}}^2(\nu, \sqrt{H_i(n)})$ under the constraint $\nu \in \mathbb{S}^{B-1}$. We use the logarithmic map $\mathrm{Log}_\mu(\cdot)$ to map the square-root histograms $\{\sqrt{H_i(m)}\}_{i=1}^I$ to the tangent space at the estimated Frechet mean μ and find the optimal covariance matrix C in closed form [8]. For any histogram H, we define the geodesic Mahalanobis distance between $\sqrt{H}$ and mean μ, given covariance C, as $d_{\mathcal{HM}}(\sqrt{H}; \mu, C) := (\mathrm{Log}_\mu(\sqrt{H})^\top C^{-1} \mathrm{Log}_\mu(\sqrt{H}))^{0.5}$.

Nonparametric Model. Our nonparametric modeling approach relies on the use of a Mercer kernel to map the square-root histograms on the hypersphere to a RKHS, followed by using (kernel) PCA to fit a multivariate Gaussian distribution to the mapped data in the RKHS. In this way, the Mercer kernel allows us to model nonlinear modes of variation in the data more effectively than the Normal-law approach. The kernel-based strategy has the potential to yield compact fits to the data, thereby being able to detect subtle differences, and detect cortical regions, more accurately. For this purpose, we choose a real-valued Mercer kernel that exploits the Riemannian structure of the space of histograms, which is the vMF Mercer kernel defined on the Riemannian space of histograms as follows: $K_{\mathrm{vMF}}(H_1, H_2; \gamma) := \exp(\gamma\langle\sqrt{H_1}, \sqrt{H_2}\rangle)$, where $\gamma > 0$ is a regularization parameter. We set γ to be the average of all intra-group pairwise inner products between the square-root histograms in the dataset.

Let the associated lifting map for the Mercer kernel be $\Phi(\cdot)$ that maps H to $\Phi(H) := k(\cdot, H)$ in a RKHS $\mathcal{F}$. Consider two vectors in RKHS: $f := \sum_{i=1}^I \alpha_i\Phi(H_i)$ and $f' := \sum_{j=1}^J \beta_j\Phi(H_j)$. The inner product $\langle f, f'\rangle_{\mathcal{F}} := \sum_{i=1}^I \sum_{j=1}^J \alpha_i\beta_j K_{\mathrm{vMF}}(H_i, H_j)$. The norm $\|f\|_{\mathcal{F}} := \sqrt{\langle f, f\rangle_{\mathcal{F}}}$. When $f, f' \in \mathcal{F}\backslash\{0\}$, let $f \otimes f'$ be the rank-one operator defined as $f \otimes f'(g) := \langle f', g\rangle_{\mathcal{F}} f$. The model fit via kernel PCA, to a sample of size N, gives a mean μ and a covariance operator C. The Mahalanobis distance relies on a regularized sample inverse-covariance operator [18] $C^{-1} := \sum_{q=1}^Q (1/\lambda_q) v_q \otimes v_q$, where λ_q is the q-th largest eigenvalue of the covariance operator C, v_q is the corresponding eigenfunction, and $Q < N$ is a regularization parameter. We choose Q to be the number of principal eigenfunctions that capture 90% of the energy in the eigenspectrum. Then, the square-root inverse-covariance operator is $C^{-1/2} := \sum_q (1/\sqrt{\lambda_q}) v_q \otimes v_q$ and the Mahalanobis distance of point $f \in \mathcal{F}$ from mean $\mu \in \mathcal{F}$ is $d_{\mathcal{FM}}(f; \mu, C) := \|C^{-1/2}(f - \mu)\|_{\mathcal{F}}$.

Test Statistics. For both parametric and nonparametric models, at each cortical location m, for two cohorts $\{H_i^X(m)\}_{i=1}^I$ and $\{H_j^Y(m)\}_{j=1}^J$, we obtain the means $\mu^X(m)$, $\mu^Y(m)$ and covariances $C^X(m)$, $C^Y(m)$. For the parametric model the means lie on the hypersphere and the covariances are defined on the tangent spaces at the means. For the nonparametric model, the means and the covariance operators lie in the RKHS associated with the Mercer kernel. To perform hypothesis testing for significant differences between the groups, we need test statistics for the parametric and nonparametric models. For both models, we propose a test statistic $t(m)$ to measure the dissimilarity between the two cohort distributions by adding the squared Mahalanobis geodesic distance between the group means with respect to each group covariance, i.e., $t(m) := d^2_{\mathcal{M}}(\mu^X(m); \mu^Y(m), C^Y(m)) + d^2_{\mathcal{M}}(\mu^Y(m); \mu^X(m), C^X(m))$. The Hotelling's 2-sample T^2 test statistic used in the usual Euclidean multivariate Gaussian case may be inapplicable in our parametric Riemannian case because the covariances $C^X(m)$ and $C^Y(m)$ are defined in two different (tangent) spaces.

3.3 Kernel Regression in Riemannian Space

To regress local cortical geometry against a clinical variable, we need a regressor in the Riemannian space of histograms. We propose a nonlinear regressor that relies on principles on kernel density estimation.

Regression Model. We propose an extension of the Nadaraya-Watson nonlinear kernel regressor [10] to the Riemannian space of histograms [21], with the kernel PDF as $P_K(H; \mu, c) := (1/\eta) \exp(c d_{\mathcal{H}}(H, \mu))$, where H and μ are histograms, μ is the mean parameter, c is the concentration parameter, and η is the normalization constant. Interestingly, this kernel PDF is equivalent to the vMF PDF on the hypersphere associated with square-root histograms. Given a cohort comprising the independent variables as the joint histograms $\{H_i(m)\}_{i=1}^I$ and the dependent variable as the clinical score $\{S_i\}_{i=1}^I$, the clinical score S for an arbitrary histogram H is given by $r(H; \{H_i, S_i\}_{i=1}^I, c) := \frac{\sum_{i=1}^I P_K(H; H_i, c) S_i}{\sum_{i=1}^I P_K(H; H_i, c)}$.

Data-driven selection of the bandwidth parameter $1/c$ is critical for reliable regression. We propose a leave-one-out (LOO) cross validation approach [10] to automatically optimize the bandwidth parameter based on the structure underlying the data. We optimize c by brute force; we first compute the mean squared error, in the LOO regression estimates across the dataset, for a sequence of discretized parameter values and then select the parameter value that minimizes this error. This estimate c_{CV} is guaranteed to be consistent [10].

Test Statistic. At each location m on the cortex, we want to test the hypothesis that the clinical variable is dependent on the local cortical descriptor. If the null hypothesis was true, i.e., the clinical variable was independent of the local cortical geometry, then the optimal regressor would be a constant function. We compare the sets of residual errors across the dataset $\{S_j - \widehat{r}(H_j(m); \{H_i(m), S_i\}_{i=1}^I)\}_{j=1}^I$, resulting under two regressors $\widehat{r}(\cdot)$, i.e., (i) the constant-function regressor $\widehat{r}(H) = \delta$ and (ii) the kernel regressor $\widehat{r}(H) = r(H; \{H_i(m), S_i\}_{i=1}^I, c_{\text{CV}})$. If the null hypothesis was true, then the two regressors will produce residuals that would appear to be drawn from the same distribution. If the null hypothesis was false, then the residuals from the kernel regressor would be significantly smaller than those from the constant-function regressor. Thus, we propose the test statistic as the well-known F statistic, i.e., the ratio of the sample variances of the two sets of residuals.

3.4 Permutation Testing and Stability Analysis Using Resampling

Voxel-wise parametric hypothesis testing in the framework of general linear models runs a test at each voxel and adjusts p-values to control for Type-I error arising from multiple comparisons, using Gaussian field theory. However, such parametric approaches make strong assumptions on the data distributions and the dependencies within neighborhoods. In contrast, permutation tests are non-parametric, rely on the generic assumption of exchangeability, lead to stronger control over Type-1 error, are more robust to deviations of the data and effects of processing from an assumed model, and yield multiple-comparison adjusted p values (controlling family-wise error rate through the permutation-distribution of the extremal test statistic). Under the null hypothesis, assuming exchangeability, in mappings between (i) cortical descriptors and (ii) group labels/clinical scores, we use permutation-based resampling to empirically compute the null distribution of the extremal (across all cortical locations) test-statistic values proposed in Sects. 3.2 and 3.3, to compute p values. To evaluate the *stability* of the p values under variation in cohorts, we compute a set of p values by bootstrap sampling the original cohort and analyzing the associated variation.

4   Results and Discussion

We evaluate our framework on MRI volumes from 2 large datasets: (i) OASIS, for the group-difference study, and (ii) Human Connectome Project (HCP), for the regression study. We use BrainSuite (http://brainsuite.org/) for computing the tissue segmentation, thickness (Fig. 1(a)), mid-cortical surface, shape index (Fig. 1(b)), curvedness (Fig. 1(c)), and spatial normalization [12].

Group-Difference Study: Validation with Simulated Differences. We randomly assigned 140 control subjects to 2 groups of 90 and 50 subjects. We treat the larger group as normal, mimicking practical scenarios. For the

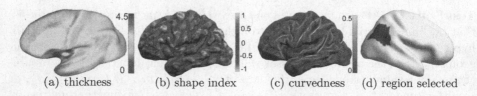

(a) thickness   (b) shape index   (c) curvedness   (d) region selected

Fig. 1. Cortical sheet model. Computed values of the cortical (a) thickness, (b) shape index, and (c) curvedness, at each point on the mid-cortical surface. Simulating cortical effects. (d) Selected region for simulating group effects.

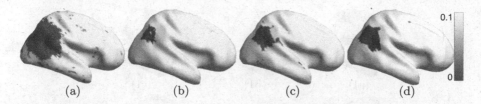

Fig. 2. Group-difference study: validation with simulated differences. permutation test p values with the following features: (a) joint multiscale descriptor, (b) joint histogram descriptor with Euclidean analysis, (c) joint histogram descriptor with Riemannian normal-law analysis, (d) joint histogram descriptor with Riemannian kernel-based analysis (*proposed*).

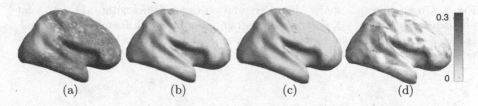

Fig. 3. Group-difference study: simulated differences, stability analysis. *Standard deviation* of p values, via *bootstrap sampling*, for: (a) joint multiscale descriptor, (b) joint histogram descriptor with Euclidean analysis, (c) joint histogram descriptor with Riemannian normal-law analysis, (d) joint histogram descriptor with Riemannian kernel-based analysis (*proposed*).

50 subjects, we simulated both cortical thinning (eroding the cortex segmentation) and flattening (smoothing the cortex segmentation) in a part of the right parietal lobe (Fig. 1(d)). This (i) reduced thickness and curvedness values and (ii) increased the concentration of shape index values around ±0.5 (corresponding to gyral ridges and sulcal valleys). We then tested for differences between cortices of these 2 cohorts. We compare our approach, i.e., using local joint-histogram descriptors and *nonparametric kernel-based* Riemannian statistical analysis (Sect. 3.2), against 3 other approaches: (i) *multiscale* joint descriptors of shape index, curvedness, and thickness (Sect. 3.1), with Euclidean analysis, (ii) histogram descriptors with Euclidean multivariate-Gaussian analysis, ignoring the Riemannian structure, and (iii) histogram descriptors with Riemannian *parametric Normal-law* modeling (Sect. 3.2).

The detection of group differences with multiscale descriptors (Fig. 2(a)) leads to many false positives. While the histogram-based Euclidean analysis (Fig. 2(b)) detects a region much smaller than the actual (false negatives), the histogram-based Riemannian Normal-law analysis detects a region larger than the actual (false positives). Detection accuracy is best with the proposed approach of Riemannian analysis with Mercer kernels (Fig. 2(d)) that leads to a compact region with very few false positives/negatives. The stability of all histogram-based analyses (Fig. 3) is significantly higher (lower variation in p

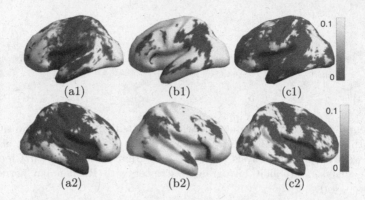

Fig. 4. Group-difference study: MCI. Permutation test p values with: (a1), (a2) joint multiscale descriptor, (b1), (b2) joint histogram descriptor with Riemannian Normal-law analysis, (c1), (c2) joint histogram descriptor with Riemannian kernel-based analysis (*proposed*).

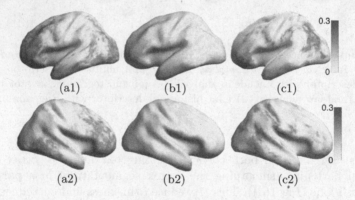

Fig. 5. Group-difference study: MCI, stability analysis. *Standard deviation* of permutation test p values, via *bootstrap sampling*, for: (a1), (a2) joint multiscale descriptor, (b1), (b2) joint histogram descriptor with Riemannian normal-law analysis, (c1), (c2) joint histogram with Riemannian kernel-based analysis (*proposed*).

values) than the multiscale-descriptor analysis. The stability of the proposed approach (Fig. 3(d)), in the affected region in the parietal lobe, is higher than the other histogram-based approaches (Fig. 2(b) and (c)).

Group-Difference Study: MCI Data. We tested for differences in 2 cohorts from the OASIS dataset: (i) 140 control subjects and (ii) 28 subjects with mild cognitive impairment (MCI) with a clinical dementia rating of 1. The histogram-based descriptors (Fig. 5(b) and (c)) give more stable results than the multiscale descriptors (Fig. 5(a)). The proposed kernel-based approach (Fig. 4(c)) is able to detect differences in more brain lobes, without significant reduction in stability, as compared to the histogram-based Riemannian Normal-law approach (Fig. 4(b)).

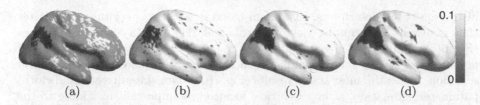

Fig. 6. Regression study: validation with simulated effects. Permutation test p values for: (a) joint multiscale descriptor with linear regression, (b) joint multiscale descriptor with kernel regression, (c) joint histogram descriptor with linear regression, (d) joint histogram descriptor with kernel regression in Riemannian space (*proposed*).

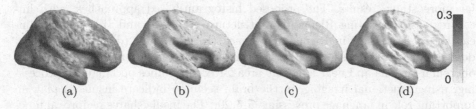

Fig. 7. Regression study: simulated effects, stability analysis. *Standard deviation* of p values, via *bootstrap sampling*, for: (a) joint multiscale descriptor with linear regression, (b) joint multiscale descriptor with kernel regression, (c) joint histogram descriptor with linear regression, (d) joint histogram descriptor with kernel regression in Riemannian space (*proposed*).

Regression Study: Validation with Simulated Effects. We took 200 MRI volumes from the HCP dataset along with clinical scores on a task. First, we randomly reassign the scores to subjects, to eliminate any existing dependencies between the score and cortical geometry. Then, for all the subjects, we simulated subtle relationships between the scores and the geometry of a part of the right parietal lobe (Fig. 1(d)), by cortical thinning (eroding the cortex segmentation) and flattening (smoothing the cortex segmentation) in amounts directly related to the score.

We compare our approach, i.e., using local joint-histogram descriptors and nonlinear kernel regression on Riemannian space (Sect. 3.3) with cross-validation based data-driven bandwidth estimation, against 3 other approaches: (i) multiscale joint descriptors (Sect. 3.1) with linear regression, (ii) multiscale joint descriptors with nonlinear regression with data-driven bandwidth estimation, and (iii) histogram descriptors with linear regression, ignoring Riemannian structure.

Linear regression with multiscale descriptors performs poorly, wrongly indicating relationships (Fig. 6(a)) with the entire cortex and with the worst stability under bootstrap sampling of the cohort (Fig. 7(a)). With multiscale descriptors, nonlinear regression improves over linear regression, but still leads to many false positive and false negatives (Fig. 6(b)) and has less stability (Fig. 7(b)) than histogram-based descriptors. Histogram-based descriptors perform much better that multiscale descriptors, yielding a coherent region with few false positives (Fig. 6(c) and (d)) and greater stability (Fig. 7(c) and (d)). Our histogram-based nonlinear-regression on Riemannian space, along with automatic bandwidth selection, yields the most stable results (Fig. 7(d)). Our data-driven bandwidth-parameter estimation, at every cortical location, is important in adding to the stability of the nonlinear regression approaches.

Regression: Task Score, Stability Analysis. We tested for dependencies between local cortical structure and the task score (average of language-based story and mathematics tasks) on 200 subjects in the HCP dataset. Analogous to the other results in the paper, the histogram-based descriptors (Fig. 9) give far more stable results. The proposed histogram-based approaches, with linear regression ignoring Riemannian structure (Fig. 8(a) and (b)) and nonlinear kernel regression in Riemannian space (Fig. 8(c) and (d)), seem to show dependencies of the task scores on the cortical structure around the insular and opercular regions and near language areas. Recent studies on language processing, using functional imaging, in the brain seem to indicate insula to play an important role in language processing [5,6,20]. The insula shares reciprocal functional and structural connections with linguistic, motor, limbic, and sensory brain areas.

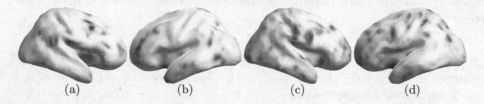

(a)   (b)   (c)   (d)

Fig. 8. Regression study: task score. Permutation test p values for the joint histogram descriptor with: (a) and (b) linear regression, and (c) and (d) kernel regression in Riemannian space, with data-driven bandwidth selection (*proposed*).

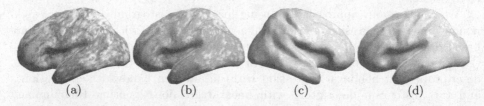

(a)   (b)   (c)   (d)

Fig. 9. Regression study: task score, stability analysis. *Standard deviation* of permutation test p values, via *bootstrap sampling*, for the: (a) joint multiscale descriptor with linear regression, (b) joint multiscale descriptor with kernel regression, (c) and (d) joint histogram descriptor with kernel regression in Riemannian space, with data-driven bandwidth selection (*proposed*).

Conclusion. We propose a framework for analysis of cortical geometry to (i) detect group differences and (ii) regress against clinical variables. We use a cortical descriptor that is *robust* to fine-scale misregistration, having a *Riemannian* structure. We propose novel *regularized nonlinear models* for analyses, giving compact and reliable model fits, using kernels that exploit the Riemannian structure. Our results show improved robustness and accuracy relative to (i) multiscale descriptors and (ii) linear analyses.

References

1. Awate, S.P., Leahy, R.M., Joshi, A.A.: Riemannian statistical analysis of cortical geometry with robustness to partial homology and misalignment. In: Ourselin, S., Joskowicz, L., Sabuncu, M.R., Unal, G., Wells, W. (eds.) MICCAI 2016. LNCS, vol. 9900, pp. 237–246. Springer, Cham (2016). doi:10.1007/978-3-319-46720-7_28
2. Awate, S.P., Yushkevich, P., Song, Z., Licht, D., Gee, J.: Cerebral cortical folding analysis with multivariate modeling and testing: studies on gender differences and neonatal development. Neuroimage **53**(2), 450–459 (2010)
3. Batchelor, P., Castellano-Smith, A., Hill, D., Hawkes, D., Cox, T., Dean, A.: Measures of folding applied to the development of the human fetal brain. IEEE Trans. Med. Imaging **21**(8), 953–965 (2002)
4. Buss, S., Fillmore, J.: Spherical averages and applications to spherical splines and interpolation. ACM Trans. Graph. **20**(2), 95–126 (2001)
5. Chee, M., Soon, C., Lee, H., Pallier, C.: Left insula activation: a marker for language attainment in bilinguals. Proc. Natl. Acad. Sci. **101**(42), 15265–15270 (2004)
6. Eickhoff, S., Heim, S., Zilles, K., Amunts, K.: A systems perspective on the effective connectivity of overt speech production. Phil. Trans. Royal Soc. **367**, 2399 (2009)
7. Fischl, B., Dale, A.: Measuring the thickness of the human cerebral cortex from magnetic resonance images. Proc. Natl. Acad. Sci. **97**(20), 11050–11055 (2000)
8. Fletcher, T., Lu, C., Pizer, S., Joshi, S.: Principal geodesic analysis for the study of nonlinear statistics of shape. IEEE Trans. Med. Imaging **23**(8), 995–1005 (2004)
9. Hardan, A., Muddasani, S., Vemulapalli, M., Keshavan, M., Minshew, N.: An MRI study of increased cortical thickness in autism. Am. J. Psychiatry **163**(7), 1290–1292 (2006)
10. Hardle, W.: Applied Nonparametric Regression. Cambridge University Press, Cambridge (1990)
11. Jones, S., Buchbinder, B., Aharon, I.: Three-dimensional mapping of cortical thickness using Laplace's equation. Hum. Brain Mapp. **11**(1), 12–32 (2000)
12. Joshi, A.A., Shattuck, D.W., Leahy, R.M.: A method for automated cortical surface registration and labeling. In: Dawant, B.M., Christensen, G.E., Fitzpatrick, J.M., Rueckert, D. (eds.) WBIR 2012. LNCS, vol. 7359, pp. 180–189. Springer, Heidelberg (2012). doi:10.1007/978-3-642-31340-0_19
13. Koenderink, J.J.: Solid Shape. MIT Press, Chichester (1991)
14. Luders, E., Narr, K., Thompson, P., Rex, D., Woods, R., Jancke, L., Toga, A.: Gender effects on cortical thickness and the influence of scaling. Hum. Brain Mapp. **27**, 314–324 (2006)
15. Lyttelton, O., Boucher, M., Robbins, S., Evans, A.: An unbiased iterative group registration template for cortical surface analysis. Neuroimage **34**, 1535–1544 (2007)

16. Mangin, J., Riviere, D., Cachia, A., Duchesnay, E., Cointepas, Y., Papadopoulos-Orfanos, D., Scifo, P., Ochiai, T., Brunelle, F., Regis, J.: A framework to study the cortical folding patterns. Neuroimage **23**(1), S129–S138 (2004)
17. Mardia, K., Jupp, P.: Directional Statistics. Wiley, Hoboken (2000)
18. Mas, A.: Weak convergence in the function autoregressive model. J. Multivar. Anal. **98**, 1231–1261 (2007)
19. Nordahl, C., Dierker, D., Mostafavi, I., Schumann, C., Rivera, S., Amaral, D., Van-Essen, D.: Cortical folding abnormalities in autism revealed by surface-based morphometry. J. Neurosci. **27**(43), 11725–11735 (2007)
20. Oh, A., Duerden, E., Pang, E.: The role of the insula in speech and language processing. Brain Lang. **135**, 96–103 (2014)
21. Pelletier, B.: Nonparametric regression estimation on closed Riemannian manifolds. J. Nonparametric Stat. **18**, 57–67 (2006)
22. Pennec, X.: Intrinsic statistics on Riemannian manifolds: basic tools for geometric measurements. J. Math. Imaging Vis. **25**(1), 127–154 (2006)
23. Redolfi, A., Manset, D., Barkhof, F., Wahlund, L., Glatard, T., Mangin, J.F., Frisoni, G.: Head-to-head comparison of two popular cortical thickness extraction algorithms: a cross-sectional and longitudinal study. Plos ONE **10**(3), e0117692 (2015)
24. Van-Essen, D., Dierker, D.: Surface-based and probabilistic atlases of primate cerebral cortex. Neuron **56**, 209–225 (2007)
25. Yeo, B.T.T., Yu, P., Grant, P.E., Fischl, B., Golland, P.: Shape analysis with overcomplete spherical wavelets. In: Metaxas, D., Axel, L., Fichtinger, G., Székely, G. (eds.) MICCAI 2008. LNCS, vol. 5241, pp. 468–476. Springer, Heidelberg (2008). doi:10.1007/978-3-540-85988-8_56
26. Yotter, R., Nenadic, I., Ziegler, G., Thompson, P., Gaser, C.: Local cortical surface complexity maps from spherical harmonic reconstructions. Neuroimage **56**, 961 (2011)
27. Yu, P., Grant, P., Qi, Y., Han, X., Segonne, F., Pienaar, R., Busa, E., Pacheco, J., Makris, N., Buckner, R., Golland, P., Fischl, B.: Cortical surface shape analysis based on spherical wavelets. IEEE Trans. Med. Imaging **26**(4), 582–597 (2007)

Conditional Local Distance Correlation
for Manifold-Valued Data

Wenliang Pan[1,2], Xueqin Wang[1,2], Canhong Wen[1,2], Martin Styner[3],
and Hongtu Zhu[4(✉)]

[1] Department of Statistical Science, Sun Yat-sen University, Guangzhou, China
[2] Southern China Research Center of Statistical Science, Sun Yat-sen University,
Guangzhou, China
[3] University of North Carolina at Chapel Hill, Chapel Hill, USA
[4] University of Texas MD Anderson Cancer Center, Houston, USA
htzhu@email.unc.edu, hzhu@mdanderson.org

Abstract. Manifold-valued data arises frequently in medical imaging,
surface modeling, computational biology, and computer vision, among
many others. The aim of this paper is to introduce a conditional local
distance correlation measure for characterizing a nonlinear association
between manifold-valued data, denoted by X, and a set of variables (e.g.,
diagnosis), denoted by Y, conditional on the other set of variables (e.g.,
gender and age), denoted by Z. Our nonlinear association measure is
solely based on the distance of the space that X, Y, and Z are resided,
avoiding both specifying any parametric distribution and link function
and projecting data to local tangent planes. It can be easily extended
to the case when both X and Y are manifold-valued data. We develop
a computationally fast estimation procedure to calculate such nonlinear
association measure. Moreover, we use a bootstrap method to determine
its asymptotic distribution and p-value in order to test a key hypothesis
of conditional independence. Simulation studies and a real data analysis
are used to evaluate the finite sample properties of our methods.

Keywords: Manifold-valued · Local distance correlation · Shape
statistics

1 Introduction

Manifold-valued data frequently arises in many domains, such as medical imaging,
computational biology, and computer vision, among many others [2,11,19,23,28].

Wang's research was partially supported by a grant from International Science &
Technology Cooperation Program (20163400042410001).

Styner's work was partially supported by grants R01-HD055741, R01-HD059854 and
U54-HD079124.

Zhu's work was partially supported by the US National Institutes of Health (grants
MH086633, EB021391-01A1), the National Science Foundation (grants SES-1357666
and DMS-1407655), and a senior investigator grant from the Cancer Prevention
Research Institute of Texas.

© Springer International Publishing AG 2017
M. Niethammer et al. (Eds.): IPMI 2017, LNCS 10265, pp. 41–52, 2017.
DOI: 10.1007/978-3-319-59050-9_4

Examples of manifold-valued data in medical imaging analysis include the Grassmann manifold, planar shapes, matrix Lie groups, deformation field, symmetric positive definite (SPD) matrices, and the shape representation of cortical and subcortical structures. Most manifold-valued objects are inherently nonlinear and high-dimensional (or even infinite-dimensional), so analysis of these complex objects presents many mathematical and computational challenges.

Motivated by shape analysis, the aim of this paper is to measure a linear/nonlinear association between manifold-valued data (e.g., shape representation) and a random vector/variable (e.g., diagnosis), while controlling for the other random vector (e.g., age). Specifically, consider n independent observations $\{(X_i, Y_i, Z_i)\}_{1 \leq i \leq n}$, where X_i, Y_i, and Z_i are elements in metric spaces $\mathscr{X}$, $\mathscr{Y}$, and $\mathscr{Z}$, respectively. In traditional statistics, these metric spaces are Euclidean spaces of arbitrary dimension. Correlation and regression analyses are the fundamental statistic techniques for quantifying the degree of association between X and Y, with/without the effect of a set of controlling random variables Z removed. For instance, Pearson correlation and its multivariate extension, so-called canonical correlation analysis (CCA), are powerful tools for measuring the degree of linear association between X and Y. Moreover, partial correlation measures the degree of linear association between two random variables, while controlling for a random vector. Alternatively, one may fit a regression with Y_i as response and both X_i and Z_i as covariates such that $Y_i = \beta_0 + X_i^T \beta_x + Z_i^T \beta_z + \epsilon_i$, where β_0, β_x, and β_z are regression coefficients and ϵ_i are measurement errors.

Generalizations of correlation and regression analyses to manifold-valued data are recently gaining popularity. Most existing methods for manifold-valued data are primarily on their mean and variation [5,6,10,12]. Some nonparametric methods were subsequently developed for the density estimation of manifold data [3,19,21]. Recently, in [14], a Riemannian CCA model was proposed to measure an intrinsically linear association between manifold-valued data and a random vector (or two manifold-valued objects). Furthermore, various intrinsic regression models have been developed for manifold-valued data [2–4,7,9,10,13,16,19,24,29]. Most of these regression methods often require specifying a link function, projecting manifold-valued data to local tangent planes for computing residuals, and transporting all residuals to a common space [7].

However, when X_i or/and Y_i are manifold-valued data, little has been done on the analysis of X and Y, while controlling for Z due to at least two major challenges. First, it is computationally challenging to optimize the objective function for the regression analysis of X and Y, when the dimension of X is relatively high. Such objective function is generally not convex and has a large number of parameters. Particularly, standard gradient-based optimization methods used in the literature strongly depend on the starting value of unknown parameters. Second, most intrinsic regression models for manifold-valued data require the specification of link functions (e.g., geodesic link), but it is conceptually challenging to choose a correct appropriate link function for any regression model that provides goodness of fit to a given data set. Due to these challenges, it is difficult to make further statistical inference (e.g., hypothesis test).

We propose a conditional local distance correlation to measure the nonlinear association between X and Y, while controlling for Z. Since such distance correlation measure solely requires the specification of the distances on the metric spaces $\mathscr{X}$, $\mathscr{Y}$, and $\mathscr{Z}$, it is applicable when both X and Y are manifold-valued data in different spaces. It also enjoys four major advantages. First, it avoids the optimization of a complex objective function, since empirical distance correlation measure is the function of pairwise distance between sample points. Second, it avoids the projection of manifold-valued data to local tangent planes. Third, it has a high statistical power of detecting complex and unknown nonlinear relationships between X and Y. Fourth, it is easy to make statistical inference on the nonlinear association between X and Y, while controlling for Z.

2   Methods

2.1   Conditional Local Distance Correlation

We review a novel distance correlation for characterizing statistical dependence between two random variables or two random vectors of arbitrary dimensions [25]. In [15], distance correlation was further extended to stochastic processes in metric spaces when such metric spaces are of strong negative type. Distance correlation as an extension of Pearson correlation has several important properties. The first and most important one is that it is zero if and only if two random vectors are independent. The second one is its computational simplicity, since empirical distance correlation is the function of pairwise distance between sample points.

We introduce a conditional local distance correlation to measure the nonlinear association between X and Y, while controlling for Z, when $\mathscr{X}$, $\mathscr{Y}$, and $\mathscr{Z}$ are metric spaces. Let $d_X(\cdot,\cdot)$, $d_Y(\cdot,\cdot)$, and $d_Z(\cdot,\cdot)$ be, respectively, the metrics of $\mathscr{X}$, $\mathscr{Y}$, and $\mathscr{Z}$. Let $M(\mathscr{X}|Z)$ (or $M(\mathscr{Y}|Z)$) denote the set of finite conditional probability measures on $\mathscr{X}$ (or $\mathscr{Y}$) given Z. We say that $\mu \in M(\mathscr{X}|Z)$ has a finite first moment if $\int_{\mathscr{X}} d_X(o,x)d|\mu|(x|z) < \infty$ for some $o \in \mathscr{X}$. Similarly, we can define $\nu \in M(\mathscr{Y}|Z)$. Define $a_\mu(x|z) := \int d_X(x,x')d\mu(x'|z)$ and $D_X(\mu|z) := \int d_X(x,x')d\mu(x'|z)d\mu(x|z)$ as finite functions when $\mu \in M(\mathscr{X}|Z)$ has a finite first moment. Also, we can define $a_\nu(y|z)$ and $D_Y(\nu|z)$ for $\nu \in M(\mathscr{Y}|Z)$ and Y.

Definition 1. *The local distance covariance $\mathcal{LDV}(X,Y|Z)$ between random processes X and Y with finite moments given Z is defined as the square root of*

$$\mathcal{LDV}^2(X,Y|Z) = E[\{d_X(X,X') - a_\mu(X|Z) - a_\mu(X'|Z) + D_X(\mu|Z)\} \\ \times \{d_Y(Y,Y') - a_\nu(Y|Z) - a_\nu(Y'|Z) + D_Y(\nu|Z)\}|Z],$$

where X' and Y' are the independent copies of X and Y, respectively.

By setting $X = Y$, we obtain the local distance variance as $\mathcal{LDV}(X|Z) = \mathcal{LDV}(X,X|Z)$.

Definition 2. *The local distance correlation between random processes X and Y with finite moments given Z is defined as the square root of*

$$\mathcal{LDC}^2(X,Y|Z) = \frac{\mathcal{LDV}^2(X,Y|Z)}{\sqrt{\mathcal{LDV}^2(X|Z)\mathcal{LDV}^2(Y|Z)}}$$

if $\mathcal{LDV}^2(X|Z)\mathcal{LDV}^2(Y|Z) > 0$, or 0 otherwise.

Under the condition that the metric spaces are of strong negative type, it can be shown that $\mathcal{LDC}^2(X,Y|Z=z) = 0$ if and only if X and Y given $Z = z$ are conditionally independent. This property distinguishes the local distance correlation from the existing methods in the literature [2–4,7,13,14,16,19,24,29]. As shown below, it is easy to estimate $\mathcal{LDC}^2(X,Y|Z)$ and use its estimate to make statistical inference.

2.2 Estimation Procedure

The next interesting question is to estimate the local distance covariance and correlation. The local distance dependence statistics are defined as follows. Let (X_i, Y_i, Z_i) for $i = 1, \ldots, n$ be a random sample of n independent and identically distributed random vectors from the joint distribution of random vectors (X, Y, Z). We compute two distance matrices $(a_{kl}) = d_X(X_k, X_l)$ and $(b_{kl}) = d_Y(Y_k, Y_l)$. For notational simplicity, it is assumed that $\mathscr{X} = R^r$ holds. We consider a kernel function $K(\cdot)$ on R^r satisfying two regularity conditions as follows:

(C1): $\int_{\mathbb{R}^r} z K(z) dz = \mathbf{0}$, $\int_{\mathbb{R}^r} K(z) dz = 1$, $\int_{\mathbb{R}^r} |K(z)| dz < \infty$, $\int_{\mathbb{R}^r} K^2(z) dz > 0$, and $\int_{\mathbb{R}^r} ||z||_2^2 K(z) dz < \infty$.
(C2): $h^r \to 0$ and $nh^r \to \infty$, as $n \to \infty$,

where the chosen bandwidth h is a smoothing parameter which has an influence on the resulting estimate.

Let $\omega_{h,k}(Z) = K_h(Z - Z_k)$, $\omega_{h,kl}(Z) = K_h(Z - Z_k)K_h(Z - Z_l)$, $\omega_{h,ijkl}(Z) = K_h(Z - Z_i)K_h(Z - Z_j)K_h(Z - Z_k)K_h(Z - Z_l)$, and $\omega_h(Z) = \sum_{k=1}^{n} \omega_{h,k}(Z)$, where $K_h(Z) = K((Z - Z_k)/h)/h^r$. We then introduce $A_{kl}(Z;h)$ as follows:

$$A_{kl}(Z;h) = a_{kl} - \bar{a}_{k\cdot}(Z;h) - \bar{a}_{\cdot l}(Z;h) + \bar{a}_{\cdot\cdot}(Z;h),$$

where $a_{kl} = d_X(X_k, X_l)$, $\bar{a}_{k\cdot}(Z;h) = \{\omega_h(Z)\}^{-1} \sum_{l=1}^{n} d_X(X_k, X_l)\omega_{h,l}(Z)$, $\bar{a}_{\cdot l}(Z;h) = \{\omega_h(Z)\}^{-1} \sum_{k=1}^{n} d_X(X_k, X_l)\omega_{h,k}(Z)$, and

$$\bar{a}_{\cdot\cdot}(Z;h) = \{\omega_h(Z)\}^{-2} \sum_{k,l=1}^{n} d_X(X_k, X_l)\omega_{h,kl}(Z).$$

Similarly, we can define $b_{kl} = d_Y(Y_k, Y_l)$ and $B_{kl}(Z;h)$. Then, the empirical local distance covariance can be defined as

$$\mathcal{LDV}_n^2(X,Y|Z;h) = \{\omega_h(Z)\}^{-2} \sum_{k,l=1}^{n} A_{kl}(Z;h)B_{kl}(Z;h)\omega_{h,kl}(Z).$$

We define the empirical local distance correlation as

$$\mathcal{LDC}_n^2(X,Y|Z;h) = \frac{\mathcal{LDV}_n(X,Y|Z;h)}{\sqrt{\mathcal{LDV}_n(X|Z;h)\mathcal{LDV}_n(Y|Z;h)}},$$

where $\mathcal{LDV}_n^2(X|Z;h) = \mathcal{LDV}_n^2(X,X|Z;h)$.

2.3 Inference Procedure

The next question is to make statistical inference based on LDV or LDC. Our inference procedure consists of carrying out hypothesis test and constructing confidence interval.

To test the dependence of X and Y at a fixed location $Z = z$, we formulate it as follows:

$$H_0 : \mathcal{LDV}(X,Y|Z=z) = 0 \quad v.s. \quad H_1 : \mathcal{LDV}(X,Y|Z=z) > 0. \tag{1}$$

We calculate the p-value of $\mathcal{LDV}_n(X,Y|Z;h)$ by using a local bootstrap procedure [18,25,26] as follows:

(i) Generate X_j^* from $\{X_1,\ldots,X_n\}$ with the probability

$$P(X^* = X_j|Z = Z_i) = \frac{\omega_{h,j}(Z_i)}{\sum_{j=1}^n \omega_{h,j}(Z_i)}$$

for $j = 1,\ldots,n$. Then, we compute $\mathcal{LDV}_n^*$ by using the local bootstrap sample $\{(X_i^*,Y_i,Z_i) : i = 1,\ldots,n\}$.

(ii) Select a resampling number S, say 1,000. Repeat Step (i) S times and obtain $\mathcal{LDV}_{ns}^*$ for $s = 1,\ldots,S$. And then the p-value of the test is given by

$$p \approx \frac{\sum_{s=1}^S I(|\mathcal{LDV}_{ns}^*| > |\mathcal{LDV}_n|) + 1}{S+1}.$$

Given a confidence level α, we construct simultaneous confidence bands for $\mathcal{LDC}(X,Y|Z)$ as follows:

$$P(\mathcal{LDC}_n^{L,\alpha}(X,Y|Z;h) < \mathcal{LDC}(X,Y|Z) < \mathcal{LDC}_n^{U,\alpha}(X,Y|Z;h)) = 1 - \alpha,$$

where $\mathcal{LDC}_n^{L,\alpha}(X,Y|Z;h)$ and $\mathcal{LDC}_n^{U,\alpha}(X,Y|Z;h)$ are the lower and upper limits of simultaneous confidence band, respectively. We use a bootstrap method to approximate the bounds:

(I) Resample $(X_i^*,Y_i^*,Z_i^*), i = 1,\ldots,n$ from $\{(X_k,Y_k,Z_k) : k = 1,\ldots,n\}$ with the probability

$$P((X^*,Y^*,Z^*) = (X_j,Y_j,Z_j)|Z = Z_i) = \frac{\omega_{h,j}(Z_i)}{\sum_{j=1}^n \omega_{h,j}(Z_i)}$$

for $j = 1,\ldots,n$, then compute $\mathcal{LDC}_n^*$ by the bootstrap sample $\{(X_i^*,Y_i^*,Z_i^*) : i = 1,\ldots,n\}$.

(II) Repeat Step (I) with resampling number S times and obtain $\mathcal{LDC}^*_{ns}, s = 1, \ldots, S$. And then the simultaneous confidence band is given by the quantiles at α and $1 - \alpha$ of $\mathcal{LDC}^*_{ns}, s = 1, \ldots, S$.

Like many other smoothing-based method, the performance of the proposed method depends upon the bandwidth h. It is widely acknowledged that the optimal h for nonparametric estimation is generally not optimal for testing. Selecting h to achieve optimal statistical power for (1) is an open problem. In practice, h can not be too large, since the conditional local distance covariance tends to the unconditional one. That is, an inappropriately large bandwidth h will yield a much larger false positive rate when X and Y are dependent. For simplicity, we consider the bandwidth h to eliminate the effect of Z on X and Y in the maximum extent. That is, the bandwidth h is chosen to minimize the mean of local distance covariance at every location $Z = z$. The intuition for the choice of h comes from partial correlation, whose aim is to eliminate the effect of Z on X and Y by the regression of Z on X and Y.

3   Numerical Studies

3.1   Simulations

We use two simulation studies to examine the finite sample performance of LDC. We consider the directional data on the unit sphere R^p, which denoted by $S^{p-1} = \{\mathbf{x} \in R^p : \|\mathbf{x}\|_2 = 1\}$, for both X and Y. Under the canonical Riemannian metric on S^{p-1} induced by the canonical inner product on R^p, the geodesic distance between any two points X and X' is equal to $d_X(X, X') = \arccos(X^T X')$. The sample size is set to be $n = 300$ and 400 in order to examine the finite sample performance of local distance estimate. We calculate the rejection rate at the significance level $\alpha = 0.05$ and $S = 200$. Moreover, 200 replications are used for each simulation setting.

Simulation 1. We set $p = 3$ and consider the spherical coordinate of S^2, denoted as (r, θ, ϕ), where $r \in [0, \infty), \theta \in [0, 2\pi]$, and $\phi \in [0, \pi]$, respectively, represent the radial distance, inclination (or elevation), and azimuth. The simulation datasets $\{(X_i, Y_i, Z_i) \in S^2 \times S^2 \times R : i = 1, \ldots, n\}$ were generated as follows:

(I.1) $X_i = (1, \theta_i^x, \phi_i^x)$, $Y_i = (1, \theta_i^y, \phi_i^y)$, and $Z_i \sim U(\frac{\pi}{5}, \frac{4\pi}{5})$;
(I.2) $X_i = (1, \theta_i^x, Z_i + \varepsilon_i^x)$, $Y_i = (1, \theta_i^y, Z_i + \varepsilon_i^y)$, and $Z_i \sim U(\frac{\pi}{5}, \frac{4\pi}{5})$;
(I.3) $X_i = (1, \theta_i, Z_i + \varepsilon_i^x)$, $Y_i = (1, \theta_i + \varepsilon_i, Z_i + \varepsilon_i^y)$, and $Z_i \sim U(\frac{\pi}{5}, \frac{4\pi}{5})$;
(I.4) Half of samples ($Z \sim U(-\pi + 0.5, 0)$) are generated from (I.2) and the other half ($Z \sim U(0, \pi - 0.5)$) are from (I.3);

where $\theta_i^x, \phi_i^x, \theta_i^y$, and ϕ_i^y were independently simulated from the Uniform distribution $U(-\pi, \pi)$ and the $\varepsilon_i, \varepsilon_i^x$, and ε_i^y were independently simulated from the normal distribution $N(0, 0.2)$. Therefore, X and Y are independent in (I.1), whereas they are dependent in (I.2) and (I.3). In contrast, X and Y are conditionally independent given Z in (I.1) and (I.2), whereas they are conditionally

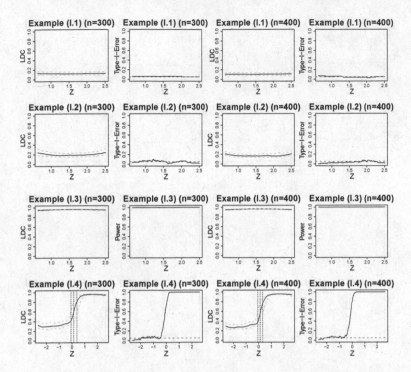

Fig. 1. Figures of local distance correlation (95% confidence bands) and Type-I-Error/Power for $n = 300$ and $n = 400$ in simulation 1.

dependent in (I.3). For (I.4), the first half of samples are conditionally independent and the second half of samples are conditionally dependent given Z.

Figure 1 presents the estimated LDCs between X and Y given Z and their p-values. The Type I error rates based on the local bootstrap procedure are well maintained under the prefixed significance level, while the power of rejecting the null hypothesis is good. As the sample size n increases, simultaneous confidence bands become narrower and the value of local distance correlation is close to zero under the true conditional independence. We use the function *e.cp3o* in R package **ecp** to detect the change point of local distance correlation in (I.4). The estimated change point is very close to the true value of change point.

Simulation 2. We consider the von Mises-Fisher distribution, of which the data can be spherical or hyper-spherical. A p-dimensional unit random vector $x(\|x\|_2 = 1)$ is set to be p-variate von Mises-Fisher distribution $M_p(\boldsymbol{\mu}, \kappa)$. We set $p = 10$ and simulated $\boldsymbol{\mu}$ from the multivariate normal distribution $N(\mathbf{0}, I_{10})$. The simulated datasets were generated as follows:

(II.1) $X_i \sim M_{10}(\boldsymbol{\mu}_x, 15), Y_i \sim M_{10}(\boldsymbol{\mu}_y, 15)$, and $Z_i \sim N(0, 0.5)$;

(II.2) $X_i = X_i^1 + \xi_i$ and $Y_i = Y_i^1 + \xi_i$, where $X_i^1 \sim M_{10}(\boldsymbol{\mu}_x, 15), Y_i^1 \sim M_{10}(\boldsymbol{\mu}_y, 15)$, and $\xi_i = (u_1 Z_i, \ldots, u_{10} Z_i)$, in which $Z_i \sim U(-1, 1)$ and $u_1, \ldots, u_{10} \in \{-\frac{7}{24}, \frac{7}{24}\}$ with equal probability. Then, we project X_i and Y_i to the unit spherical surface;

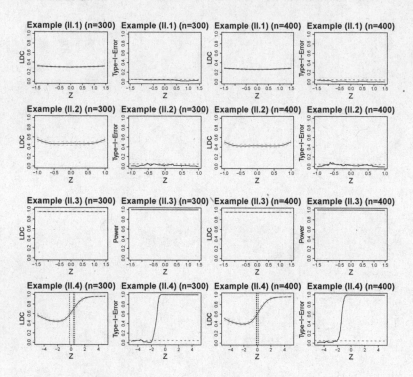

Fig. 2. Figures of local distance correlation (95% confidence bands) and Type-I-Error/Power for $n = 300$ and $n = 400$ in simulation 2.

(II.3) $X_i \sim M_{10}(\boldsymbol{\mu}_x, 15)$, $Y_i = RX_i$, and $Z_i \sim N(0, 0.5)$, where R is a rotation matrix along the direction $\boldsymbol{\mu}_x$ of $\boldsymbol{\mu}_y$;

(II.4) Half of samples $(Z \sim U(-5, 0))$ were generated from (II.1) and the other half $(Z \sim U(0, 5))$ were from (II.3).

Similar to Simulation 1, X and Y are independent in (II.1), whereas they are dependent in (II.2) and (II.3). However, X and Y are conditionally independent given Z in (II.1) and (II.2), while they are conditionally dependent given Z in (II.3). The first half of samples are conditionally independent and the second half of samples are conditionally dependent given Z in (II.4). Inspecting Fig. 2 reveals that the proposed methods work well.

3.2 Real Data Analysis

Alzheimer disease (AD) is a disorder of cognitive and behavioral impairment that markedly interferes with social and occupational functioning. It is an irreversible and progressive brain disease that slowly destroys memory and thinking skills, and eventually even the ability to carry out the simplest tasks. AD affects almost 50% of those over the age of 85 and is the sixth leading cause of death in the United States. The corpus callosum (CC), the largest white matter structure in the brain, has been a structure of high interest in many neuroimaging studies of neuro-developmental pathology. It contains homotopic and heterotopic interhemispheric connections and is essential for communication between the two cerebral hemispheres. Individual differences in CC and their possible implications regarding interhemispheric connectivity have been investigated in last several decades [20, 27].

We consider the CC contour data of the ADNI1 study. We processed the CC shape data for each subject in the ADNI1 study as follows. We used FreeSurfer package [8] to process each T1-weighted MRI, whereas the midsagittal CC area was calculated in the CCseg package.

We are interested in characterizing the change of the CC contour shape and its association with several key covariates of interest, such as age and diagnosis. We focused on $n = 409$ subjects with 223 healthy controls (HCs) and 186 AD patients at baseline of the ADNI1 study. Each subject has a CC planar contour Y_i with 50 landmarks and nine covariates, including gender, age, handedness, marital status (Widowed, Divorced, and Never married), education length, retirement, and diagnosis. The demographic information is shown in Table 1. We treat the CC planar contour Y_i as a manifold-valued response in the Kendall planar shape space and all covariates in the Euclidean space.

The first scientific question of interest is to characterize the relationship between CC shape data and each of the nine covariates. Table 2 presents the distance correlation statistics for correlating CC data with each of the nine covariates. It reveals that the shape of CC planar contour are highly dependent on gender, education length, age and AD diagnosis at the significant level

Table 1. Demographic information for all participants.

Disease status	Number of subjects	Age (years)	Females/males
Healthy control	223	62–90 (76.25)	107/116
AD	186	55–92 (75.42)	88/98

Table 2. The distance correlation (Dcor) statistics for correlating CC contour data and nine covariates. The significance level is 0.05.

Covariates	Dcor	p-value
Gender	0.186	0.001
Handedness	0.094	0.420
Marital status	0.108	0.383
Education length	0.166	0.010
Retirement	0.108	0.165
Age	0.245	0.001
Diagnosis	0.190	0.001

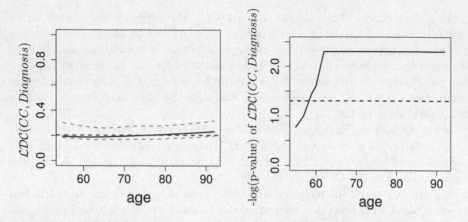

Fig. 3. Figures of estimated local distance correlation and the corresponding negative $\log_{10}$(p-values) between CC planar contour and Diagnosis given Age.

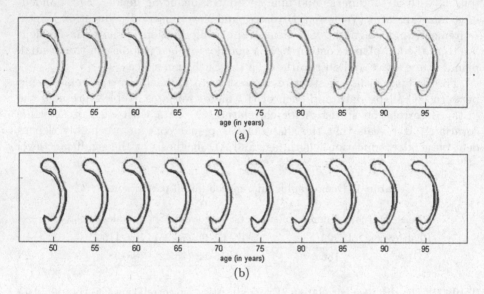

Fig. 4. ADNI data: Mean trajectories within each gender group: (a) female group (blue - normal; magenta - AD); (b) male group (black - normal; red - AD). (Color figure online)

$\alpha = 0.05$. It may indicate that gender, age and AD diagnosis are the most significant influence factors of CC planar contour, which agree with [1,17,22].

The second scientific question of interest is to characterize the relationship between CC shape data and AD diagnosis given age. Figure 3 presents the conditional local distance correlation of CC planar contour and AD diagnosis given age as a function of age. As age increases, the value of the conditional local distance correlation increases. It implies that diagnosis and CC are dependent with each other as age changes. Figure 4 presents the mean age-dependent CC trajectories for healthy controls and AD within each gender group. It can be observed that there is a major difference of the shape between the AD disease and healthy both in male and female groups. The splenium seems to be less thinner and the isthmus is rounded in subjects with AD disease than in healthy controls.

4 Conclusion

We proposed a local distance correlation for modeling data with manifold valued responses and applied this method to a variety of applications, such as the responses restricted to the sphere, shape spaces. The proposed method can detect complex nonlinear relationship and keeps the computational simplicity. In future, we will further investigate the theoretical properties of the new method and other applications in imaging analysis.

References

1. Allen, L.S., Richey, M., Chai, Y.M., Gorski, R.A.: Sex differences in the corpus callosum of the living human being. J. Neurosci. **11**(4), 933–942 (1991)
2. Banerjee, M., Chakraborty, R., Ofori, E., Okun, M.S., Viallancourt, D.E., Vemuri, B.C.: A nonlinear regression technique for manifold valued data with applications to medical image analysis. In: Proceedings of the IEEE Conference on Computer Vision and Pattern Recognition, pp. 4424–4432 (2016)
3. Bhattacharya, A., Dunson, D.B.: Nonparametric Bayesian density estimation on manifolds with applications to planar shapes. Biometrika **97**(4), 851–865 (2010)
4. Bhattacharya, A., Dunson, D.B.: Nonparametric Bayes classification and hypothesis testing on manifolds. J. Multivar. Anal. **111**, 1–19 (2012)
5. Bhattacharya, R., Patrangenaru, V.: Large sample theory of intrinsic and extrinsic sample means on manifolds-i. Ann. Stat. **31**(1), 1–29 (2003)
6. Bhattacharya, R., Patrangenaru, V.: Large sample theory of intrinsic and extrinsic sample means on manifolds-ii. Ann. Stat. **33**(3), 1225–1259 (2005)
7. Cornea, E., Zhu, H., Kim, P.T., Ibrahim, J.G.: Regression models on Riemannian symmetric spaces. J. Roy. Stat. Soc. Ser. B-Stat. Methodol. **79**, 463–482 (2016)
8. Dale, A.M., Fischl, B., Sereno, M.I.: Cortical surface-based analysis I. Segmentation and surface reconstruction. NeuroImage **9**(2), 179–194 (1999)
9. Davis, B.C., Fletcher, P.T., Bullitt, E., Joshi, S.: Population shape regression from random design data. Int. J. Comput. Vis. **90**(2), 255–266 (2010)
10. Fletcher, P.T., Lu, C., Pizer, S.M., Joshi, S.: Principal geodesic analysis for the study of nonlinear statistics of shape. IEEE Trans. Med. Imaging **23**(8), 995–1005 (2004)
11. Grenander, U., Miller, M.I.: Pattern Theory From Representation to Inference. Oxford University Press, Oxford (2007)
12. Huckemann, S., Hotz, T., Munk, A.: Intrinsic manova for Riemannian manifolds with an application to Kendall's space of planar shapes. IEEE Trans. Pattern Anal. Mach. Intell. **32**(4), 593–603 (2010)
13. Kent, J.T.: The Fisher-Bingham distribution on the sphere. J. Roy. Stat. Soc. Ser. B Methodol. **44**, 71–80 (1982)

14. Kim, H.J., Adluru, N., Bendlin, B.B., Johnson, S.C., Vemuri, B.C., Singh, V.: Canonical correlation analysis on Riemannian manifolds and its applications. In: Fleet, D., Pajdla, T., Schiele, B., Tuytelaars, T. (eds.) ECCV 2014. LNCS, vol. 8690, pp. 251–267. Springer, Cham (2014). doi:10.1007/978-3-319-10605-2_17

15. Lyons, R.: Distance covariance in metric spaces. Ann. Probab. **41**(5), 3284–3305 (2013)

16. Machado, L., Leite, F.S., Krakowski, K.: Higher-order smoothing splines versus least squares problems on Riemannian manifolds. J. Dyn. Control Syst. **16**(1), 121–148 (2010)

17. Ota, M., Obata, T., Akine, Y., Ito, H., Ikehira, H., Asada, T., Suhara, T.: Age-related degeneration of corpus callosum measured with diffusion tensor imaging. NeuroImage **31**(4), 1445–1452 (2006)

18. Paparoditis, E., Politis, D.: The local bootstrap for kernel estimators under general dependence conditions. Ann. Inst. Stat. Math. **52**(1), 139–159 (2000)

19. Patrangenaru, V., Ellingson, L.: Nonparametric Statistics on Manifolds and Their Applications to Object Data Analysis. CRC Press, Boca Raton (2015)

20. Paul, L.K., Brown, W.S., Adolphs, R., Tyszka, J.M., Richards, L.J., Mukherjee, P., Sherr, E.H.: Agenesis of the corpus callosum: genetic, developmental and functional aspects of connectivity. Nat. Rev. Neurosci. **8**(4), 287–299 (2007)

21. Pelletier, B.: Kernel density estimation on Riemannian manifolds. Stat. Probab. Lett. **73**(3), 297–304 (2005)

22. Shuyu, L., Fang, P., Xiangqi, H., Li, D., Tianzi, J.: Shape analysis of the corpus callosum in Alzheimer's disease, pp. 1095–1098 (2007)

23. Srivastava, A., Klassen, E.P.: Functional and Shape Data Analysis. Springer, New York (2016)

24. Su, J., Dryden, I.L., Klassen, E., Le, H., Srivastava, A.: Fitting smoothing splines to time-indexed, noisy points on nonlinear manifolds. Image Vis. Comput. **30**(6), 428–442 (2012)

25. Székely, G., Rizzo, M., Bakirov, N.: Measuring and testing dependence by correlation of distances. Ann. Stat. **35**(6), 2769–2794 (2007)

26. Wang, X., Pan, W., Hu, W., Tian, Y., Zhang, H.: Conditional distance correlation. J. Am. Stat. Assoc. **110**(512), 1726 (2016)

27. Witelson, S.F.: Hand and sex differences in the isthmus and genu of the human corpus callosum. A postmortem morphological study. Brain **112**(3), 799–835 (1989)

28. Younes, L.: Shapes and Diffeomorphisms. Springer, Heidelberg (2010)

29. Yuan, Y., Zhu, H., Lin, W., Marron, J.S.: Local polynomial regression for symmetric positive definite matrices. J. Roy. Stat. Soc. Ser. B-Stat. Methodol. **74**(4), 697–719 (2012)

Stochastic Development Regression
on Non-linear Manifolds

Line Kühnel$^{(\boxtimes)}$ and Stefan Sommer

Department of Computer Science, University of Copenhagen, Copenhagen, Denmark
{kuhnel,sommer}@di.ku.dk

Abstract. We introduce a regression model for data on non-linear manifolds. The model describes the relation between a set of manifold valued observations, such as shapes of anatomical objects, and Euclidean explanatory variables. The approach is based on stochastic development of Euclidean diffusion processes to the manifold. Defining the data distribution as the transition distribution of the mapped stochastic process, parameters of the model, the non-linear analogue of design matrix and intercept, are found via maximum likelihood. The model is intrinsically related to the geometry encoded in the connection of the manifold. We propose an estimation procedure which applies the Laplace approximation of the likelihood function. A simulation study of the performance of the model is performed and the model is applied to a real dataset of Corpus Callosum shapes.

Keywords: Regression · Statistics on manifolds · Non-linear statistics · Frame bundle · Stochastic development

1 Introduction

A main focus in computational anatomy is to study the shape of anatomical objects. Performing statistical analysis of anatomical objects is however challenging due to the non-linear nature of shape spaces. The established statistical theory for Euclidean data does not directly allow us to answer questions like: How does a treatment affect the deformation of an organ? or: Is it possible to categorize sick and healthy patients based on the shape of the subject's organs?

Shape spaces are typically non-linear and often equipped with manifold structure. Examples of manifold-valued shape data include landmarks, curves, surfaces, and images with warp variation. The lack of vector space structure for manifold-valued data implies that addition and scalar multiplication are not defined. Several concepts in statistics rely on addition and scalar multiplication, these including mean value, variance, and regression models. Hence, in order to make inference on manifold-valued data, generalization of Euclidean statistical theory is necessary.

This paper focuses on generalization of regression models to manifolds. The aim is to model the relation between Euclidean explanatory variables and a

© Springer International Publishing AG 2017
M. Niethammer et al. (Eds.): IPMI 2017, LNCS 10265, pp. 53–64, 2017.
DOI: 10.1007/978-3-319-59050-9_5

manifold-valued response. The regression model has, as an example, applications in computational anatomy [23]. The proposed model can for example be used to analyze how age affects the shape of Corpus Callosum [7].

Several approaches have previously been proposed for defining normal distributions on manifolds [14,19]. In [19], the distribution is defined based on Brownian motions in $\mathbb{R}^m$ and the fact that normal distributions on $\mathbb{R}^m$ can be defined as transition distributions of Brownian motions. The normal distribution on the manifold is then defined as the transition distribution of the stochastic development of the Euclidean Brownian motion [10]. The proposed regression model will be defined in a similar manner. The construction can be considered intrinsic as it only depends on the connection of the manifold, e.g. the Levi-Civita connection of a Riemannian manifold. It does not rely on linearization of the manifold, and it naturally includes the effect of curvature in the mapping of the stochastic processes.

In Euclidean linear regression, the relation between explanatory variables, X, and a response variable, y, is modeled by an affine function of X,

$$y = a + Xb + \varepsilon. \tag{1}$$

Due to the lack of vector space structure, alternatives for modeling relations between the given variables, X and y, are needed in the non-linear situation. Several ideas have previously been introduced and a selection of these will be described in Sect. 2.

In this paper, the regression model is considered as a transported linear regression defined in $\mathbb{R}^m$. This approach is inspired by the transport of normal distributions defined in [19]. Notice that the linear regression model (1) can be generalized to situations in which several observations are observed over time,

$$y_t = a_t + X_t b + \varepsilon_t, \quad \text{for} \ \ t \in [t_1, t_2]. \tag{2}$$

Our approach suggests to define the regression model by transportation of stochastic processes, $Z_t = a_t + X_t b + \varepsilon_t$, in $\mathbb{R}^m$ on to the manifold in order to obtain the relation to the response variable, y (see Fig. 1).

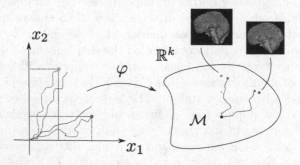

Fig. 1. The idea behind the proposed regression model. Stochastic processes in $\mathbb{R}^m$ is transported to $\mathcal{M}$, by stohcastic development φ, to model the relation between the explanatory variables and the response $y \in \mathcal{M}$.

The paper will be structured as follows. In Sect. 2, we give a discussion on previous methods developed for regression on manifolds. Section 3 presents a short description of development of stochastic paths from a Euclidean space to the manifold. Section 4 introduces the proposed model, followed by a description of the estimation procedure in Sect. 5. In Sects. 6 and 7, illustrative examples are considered for the application and performance of the model. The paper is ended by a discussion of the defined model in Sect. 8.

2   Background

Multiple approaches have been proposed for generalizing regression models to non-linear manifolds. The methods consider the regression problem in different situations. In this paper we will consider the case of Euclidean exaplanatory variables and a manifold-valued response. There have been several works describing regression models for manifold-valued data in other situations [1,4,13,21].

Regression models for describing the relation between a manifold-valued response and Euclidean explanatory variables have also previously been introduced. Examples include [12] in which an extrinsic regression model is introduced, and [15], which defines an intrinsic regression model where the parameter vector is estimated by minimizing the total sum of squares based on the Riemannian manifold distance. Another example is the geodesic regression model introduced in [7], which is a generalization of the linear regression model in Euclidean spaces. The relation is here modeled by a geodesic described by an initial velocity dependent on an explanatory variable and a starting point on the manifold.

In this paper, we will take a different view on how to relate the response and explanatory variables. Instead of considering the relation as being modeled by geodesics on the manifold as in [7], we will describe the relation by stochastic paths transported from the space of explanatory variables to the manifold. By defining the regression model using stochastic paths, we are able to model non-geodesic relations, incorporate several explanatory variables, and consider random effects in the model. Non-geodesic relations have been considered by others before. An example is [17] in which the geodesic regression model from [7] is generalized in order to model more complex shape changes. The regression function is in this case fitted by piecewise cubic splines that describes the variation of one explanatory variable. In [9], a regression model is introduced, in which the non-geodesic relation is obtained by time-warping. Others have proposed to model the non-geodesic relation by either a generalized polynomial regression model or by non-linear kernel-based regression [2,3,6,8,25]. On the contrary, [16] introduces the Hierarchical Geodesic Model which are able to consider several explanatory variables including random variables, but assumes nested observations and does only consider geodesic relations. A regression model, which incorporates both a non-geodesic relation and several explanatory variables, is proposed in [5]. This work defines an intrinsic regression model on Riemannian symmetric spaces, in which the regression function is obtained by minimizing the conditional mean of residuals defined by the log-map.

In addition to describing the proposed model, we perform estimation of model parameters by maximum likelihood using the transition density on the manifold. The model does not linearize the manifold as in many of the local regression models, but instead take into account the curvature of the manifold at each point as encoded in the connection through the mapping of the stochastic process.

3   Stochastic Development

In this section we give a brief description of stochastic development of curves in $\mathbb{R}^m$ to the manifold. The reader is referred to [10,18,20] for a deeper description of this concept.

Let $\mathcal{M}$ be a d-dimensional manifold provided with a connection ∇ and metric g. The connection is necessary for transportation of tangent vectors along curves on the manifold. A frequently used connection is the Levi-Civita connection coming from a Riemannian structure on $\mathcal{M}$. Let ∂_i for $i = 1, \ldots, d$ denote a coordinate frame on $\mathcal{M}$ and let dx^i be the corresponding dual frame. A connection ∇ is given in terms of its Christoffel symbols defined by $\nabla_{\partial_i}\partial_j = \Gamma_{ij}^k \partial_k$. For the Levi-Civita connection, the Christoffel symbols are given by

$$\Gamma_{ij}^k = \frac{1}{2}g^{kl}(\partial_i g_{jl} + \partial_j g_{il} - \partial_l g_{ij}) \tag{3}$$

in which g_{ij} is the components of g in the coordinate basis, i.e. $g = g_{ij}dx^i dx^j$, and g^{ij} is the inverse components.

Consider the frame bundle $\mathcal{FM}$ being the set of tuples (y, ν) in which $y \in \mathcal{M}$ and ν is a frame for the tangent space $T_y\mathcal{M}$. Let $\pi \colon \mathcal{FM} \to \mathcal{M}$ be the projection map given by $\pi(y, \nu) = y$ for $(y, \nu) \in \mathcal{FM}$. A smooth curve U_t on $\mathcal{FM}$ is a smooth selection of frames, i.e. for every $t \in I$, $U_t = (y_t, \nu_t)$ in which $\nu_t \colon \mathbb{R}^d \to T_{\pi(U_t)}\mathcal{M}$ is a frame.

Given a connection ∇, the tangent space of the frame bundle, $T\mathcal{FM}$, splits into a horizontal and a vertical part, $T\mathcal{FM} = H\mathcal{FM} \oplus V\mathcal{FM}$. The horizontal subspace explains infinitesimal changes of the base point on the manifold. On the other hand, tangent vectors in $V\mathcal{FM}$ describe changes of the frame ν keeping the base point fixed. Given a tangent vector $v \in T_y\mathcal{M}$ and a frame ν, a vector in $H_{(y,\nu)}\mathcal{FM}$ can be defined by horizontal lift. The horizontal lift of a tangent vector v is the unique horizontal vector $w \in H_{(y,\nu)}\mathcal{FM}$, satisfying $\pi_\star w = v$, where $\pi_\star \colon H_{(y,\nu)}\mathcal{FM} \to T_y\mathcal{M}$ is induced by the projection π. The horizontal lift of v will be denoted $h_l(v)$.

Consider a probability space $(\Omega, \mathcal{F}, P)$ and a stochastic process $X_t \colon \Omega \to \mathcal{W}(\mathbb{R}^m)$, where $\mathcal{W}(\mathbb{R}^m)$ denotes the path space of $\mathbb{R}^m$. The stochastic development of X_t to $\mathcal{FM}$ can be defined as a solution, U_t, of the Stratonovich stochastic differential equation,

$$dU_t = \sum_{i=1}^d H_i(U_t) \circ dX_t^i, \tag{4}$$

where $\circ$ symbolizes a Stratonovich stochastic differential equation. The vector fields $H_1, \ldots, H_d$ denotes a basis for the horizontal subspace of $T\mathcal{FM}$.

Given a point $u = (y, \nu) \in \mathcal{F}\mathcal{M}$, H_i are defined as $H_i(u) = h_l(\nu(e_i))$, $i = 1, \ldots, d$, where $e_1, \ldots, e_d$ is the canonical basis for $\mathbb{R}^d$. A path Y_t on the manifold $\mathcal{M}$ can then be obtained by the projection of U_t onto $\mathcal{M}$ by the projection map π, i.e. $Y_t = \pi(U_t)$.

Consider two processes X_t^1, X_t^2 in $\mathbb{R}^m$, $t \in [0, T]$ for $T > 0$, for which $X_0^1 = X_0^2 = \boldsymbol{x}_0$ and $X_T^1 = X_T^2$. If Y_t^1, Y_t^2 denotes the stochastic development of X_t^1 and X_t^2 respectively on $\mathcal{M}$, then it does not in general hold that $Y_T^1 = Y_T^2$ on $\mathcal{M}$ due to the curvature of the manifold.

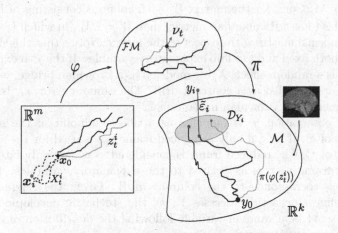

Fig. 2. Illustration of the regression model. Stochastic processes z_t^i, defined in (5), are transported through the frame bundle $\mathcal{F}\mathcal{M}$ to $\mathcal{M}$, with stochastic development, φ. Each observation y_i is then modelled as a noisy member of the endpoint distribution of the transported z_t^i processes. The model supports cases where the endpoint noise $\tilde{\varepsilon}$ perturbes y_i in the ambient space $\mathbb{R}^k$ in which $\mathcal{M}$ is embedded.

4   Model

Let $\mathcal{M}$ be a d-dimensional manifold embedded in the ambient space $\mathbb{R}^k$ for some $k \geq d$ and consider a response variable y in $\mathcal{M}$. Let $\nu_{y_0} : \mathbb{R}^d \to T_{y_0}\mathcal{M}$ be a frame for the tangent space at a reference point $y_0 \in \mathcal{M}$. Assume that $\boldsymbol{y}_1, \ldots, \boldsymbol{y}_n \in \mathbb{R}^k$ are n realizations of $y \in \mathcal{M}$ and let $\boldsymbol{x}_i = (x_i^1, \ldots, x_i^m) \in \mathbb{R}^m$ denote the vector of explanatory variables for the i'th observation. Notice that the realizations of y are assumed to lie in the ambient space $\mathbb{R}^k$ and not required to be in $\mathcal{M}$. This construction allows for observations measured with noise which are not necessarily observed as elements of $\mathcal{M}$.

The strategy of the proposed model is to define stochastic processes according to the generalized linear regression in (2) and transport these to the manifold by stochastic development. All stochastic processes are defined for $t \in [0, T]$ for a

$T > 0$. Consider for each observation i the stochastic process $z_t^i \colon \Omega \to \mathcal{W}(\mathbb{R}^m)$, solution to the stochastic differential equation,

$$dz_t^i = \beta dt + \tilde{W} dX_t^i + d\varepsilon_t. \tag{5}$$

The first term, βdt, is a fixed drift for $\beta \in \mathbb{R}^m$. $\tilde{W} dX_t^i$ is the dependence of the explanatory variables with $X_t^i \colon \Omega \to \mathcal{W}(\mathbb{R}^m)$ being a stochastic process satisfying $X_0^i(\omega) = 0$ and $X_T^i(\omega) = \boldsymbol{x}_i$ for $\omega \in \Omega$. The matrix $\tilde{W}$ is a $m \times m$-dimensional matrix with columns relating to the basis vectors of the frame ν_{y_0} on $\mathcal{M}$. Consider the matrix W with columns consisting of basis vectors of ν_{y_0}. If $\mathcal{M}$ has a Riemannian metric, then $W = U\tilde{W}$, in which U denotes a $d \times m$ orthonormal matrix with respect to the metric. Notice that this model can incorporate both fixed and random explanatory variables. If the j'th explanatory variable, x_i^j, is a random effect, X_t^{ij} is modeled as a Brownian bridge, while it for fixed effects are modeled as a constant drift. The random error, ε_t, is modeled as a multidimensional Brownian motion on $\mathbb{R}^m$.

The i'th observation y_i is modeled as a noisy endpoint of the stochastic development of z_t^i. If $m < d$ only a reduced frame $\tilde{\nu}_{y_0}$ is used for the stochastic development of z_t^i. The reduced frame is considered as we are only interested in the effect of frame vectors associated to the explanatory variables. The basis vectors of $\tilde{\nu}_{y_0}$ corresponds to the columns of W. Given the reference point $y_0 \in \mathcal{M}$, define stochastic processes Y_t^i as the stochastic development of z_t^i. Let $\mathcal{Y}_i^T \colon \Omega \to \mathcal{M}$ be a random variable following the distribution of endpoints of the stochastic development Y_t^i. Then

$$y_i = \mathcal{Y}_i^T + \tilde{\varepsilon}_i, \tag{6}$$

where $\tilde{\varepsilon}_i \sim \mathcal{N}(\boldsymbol{0}, \tau^2 \mathbb{I}_d)$ represents the random measurement error that pulls the realization, y_i, from the manifold. In Fig. 2, the two steps of the model are illustrated. First, the stochastic development of z_t^i are defined on the frame bundle and finally, this stochastic development is projected to the manifold.

Notice that in the case $\mathcal{M} = \mathbb{R}^k$ with the standard connection on $\mathbb{R}^k$, the proposed model reduces to the regular regression model for data in $\mathbb{R}^k$. Assume $y \in \mathbb{R}^k$ and that X_t^i is a vector from 0 to $\boldsymbol{x}_i$. Then β and y_0 relates to the intercept, W is the matrix of regression coefficients and ε_t and $\tilde{\varepsilon}$ the iid. random noise.

5   Estimation

The reference point y_0, the matrix W, the drift β, and the variance parameter τ^2 are the parameters of the model. These parameters can be estimated in several ways. This section describes a Laplace approximation of the marginal likelihood function which are used for finding optimal parameter estimates. We could alternatively use a Monte Carlo EM based procedure using simulations of the missing data, Y_t^i for $t \in [0, T]$, to optimize the complete data likelihood. This will be considered in future works.

Laplace approximation can be used to determine a linear approximation of a non-linear likelihood function [11]. Let θ denote the vector of parameters, and $d\boldsymbol{x}_t$ a discretization of the process X_t at n_s+1 time-points. Hence $d\boldsymbol{x}_t$ is a vector of length $n \cdot m \cdot n_s$, in which n_s denotes the number of time steps, n the number of observations, and m the number of explanatory variables. Let $f(y|\theta)$ be the conditional density of the response $y \in \mathcal{M}$ given θ and $p(d\boldsymbol{x}_t|\theta)$ the density of the discretization of X_t given θ. To find the optimal parameter vector, θ, the following likelihood has to be optimized,

$$L(\theta; \boldsymbol{y}) = f(y|\theta) = \int f(y|d\boldsymbol{x}_t, \theta) p(d\boldsymbol{x}_t|\theta) d(d\boldsymbol{x}_t) = \int e^{-nh(d\boldsymbol{x}_t)} \, d(d\boldsymbol{x}_t), \quad (7)$$

where $h(d\boldsymbol{x}_t) = -\frac{1}{n} \log f(y|d\boldsymbol{x}_t, \theta) - \frac{1}{n} \log p(d\boldsymbol{x}_t|\theta)$. The Laplace approximation of L is then given by

$$L(\theta; \boldsymbol{y}) \approx f(y|d\boldsymbol{x}_t^o, \theta) p(d\boldsymbol{x}_t^o|\theta) (2\pi)^{\frac{mn_s}{2}} |\Sigma|^{\frac{1}{2}} n^{-\frac{mn_s}{2}}, \quad (8)$$

in which $d\boldsymbol{x}_t^o = \operatorname{argmax}_{d\boldsymbol{x}_t} \{-h(d\boldsymbol{x}_t)\}$ and $\Sigma = \left(D^2 h(d\boldsymbol{x}_t)\right)^{-1}$, the inverse of the Hessian of $h(d\boldsymbol{x}_t)$. The approximated likelihood is then optimized wrt. θ to obtain the estimated parameters. In the following simulation study, the Laplace approximation is used for parameter estimation. The code for the estimation algorithm as well as the simulation study below was implemented in Theano [22]. The code is available at https://bitbucket.org/stefansommer/theanodiffgeom.

6 Simulation Study

This section investigates properties of the model on simulated synthetic data. Two setups will be introduced, both considering landmark representations of shapes. The data are assumed to lie in a manifold defined in the LDDMM (Large Deformation Diffeomorphic Metric Mapping) framework [24].

In the LDDMM framework, deformations of shapes are modeled as smooth flows which are solutions to ordinary differential equations defined by vector fields. A point $q \in \mathcal{M}$ is a finite number of landmarks, $q = (x_1^1, x_1^2, \ldots, x_{n_l}^1, x_{n_l}^2)$. The metric on $\mathcal{M}$ is given by $g(v, w) = \sum_{i,j}^{n_l} v K^{-1}(x_i, x_j) w$, where K^{-1} denotes the inverse of a kernel K. In this simulation study K is the Gaussian kernel with standard deviation, $\sigma = 0.5$. Based on this metric the Levi-Civita connection can be obtained by calculating the Christoffel symbols defined in (3).

To begin with, we consider estimation of $\tilde{W}$ and y_0 and investigate the performance of the estimation procedure. The shapes that will be considered consists of 8 landmarks generated from the unit circle with landmarks located at $0, \frac{\pi}{4}, \frac{\pi}{2}, \ldots, \frac{3\pi}{2}, \frac{7\pi}{4}$ radians. The center plot of Fig. 3 shows the unit circle with the chosen frame for each landmark. The number of explanatory variables are set to $m = 2$ and the variables are drawn from a normal distribution with mean 0 and standard deviation 2. The other parameters are set to

$$\tilde{W} = \begin{pmatrix} 0.2 & 0.1 \\ 0.1 & 0.2 \end{pmatrix}, \ \tau = 0.1 \quad (9)$$

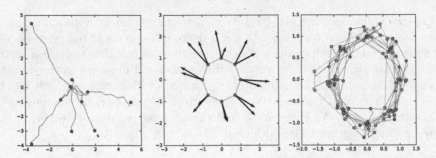

Fig. 3. The figures show the simulation of a dataset. (left) The stochastic paths in $\mathbb{R}^m$ are shown, where the vector of explanatory variables for each observation i is represented by a green dot. (center) The true frame for the simulated data as well as the reference shape are plotted. (right) The simulated observations are shown, with the stochastic developments as the red processes. (Color figure online)

In Fig. 3 is shown an example of simulated observations as well as the sample paths X_t^i. A total of 50 datasets were sampled, in which each consisted of 20 observations. For each simulated dataset, the $\tilde{W}$ matrix was estimated. Each of the estimated distrubtions for the entries of $\tilde{W}$ are shown in Fig. 4. By the results, we conclude that the estimated parameters are fairly stable between the different simulations and that the true values are well centered in each distribution. For this simulation, the estimation procedure is thus able to estimate the true $\tilde{W}$ parameters that were specified in the model.

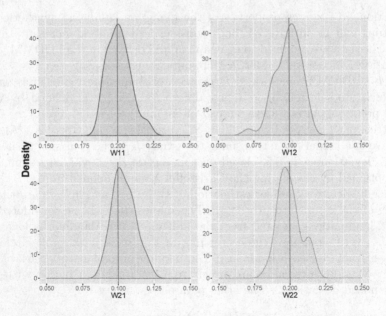

Fig. 4. The distribution of the estimated $\tilde{W}$ parameters. The red horizontal lines show the true parameters given in (9).

Three similar datasets, as explained above, were sampled with different number of observations, 20, 60 and 100 respectively. The matrix $\tilde{W}$ as well as the reference point y_0 were estimated for each of the three datasets. In this case, the estimated $\tilde{W}$ matrix was found to be

$$\hat{W}_{20} = \begin{pmatrix} 0.206 & 0.136 \\ 0.147 & 0.322 \end{pmatrix}, \quad \hat{W}_{60} = \begin{pmatrix} 0.22 & 0.11 \\ 0.11 & 0.21 \end{pmatrix}, \quad \hat{W}_{100} = \begin{pmatrix} 0.205 & 0.104 \\ 0.115 & 0.214 \end{pmatrix} \quad (10)$$

while the estimated reference points are shown in Fig. 5. By increasing the number of observations, we conclude that the estimated parameters $\tilde{W}$ and y_0 converge towards the true parameters.

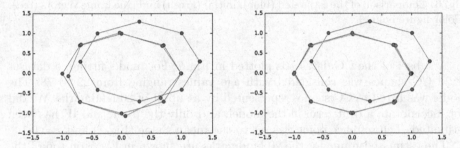

Fig. 5. (left) The estimated reference point y_0 (red) for the dataset with 20 observations. (right) The estimated y_0 for 60 (cyan) and 100 (red) observations. In both plots, the initial (green) and the true reference circle (blue) are shown. (Color figure online)

In the second study, we consider the problem of estimating the frame matrix U. In this case, each observation consists of 3 landmarks that were generated from a setup shown in Fig. 6. We only consider one explanatory variable, meaning that only one frame vector has to be estimated for each landmark. The true frame vectors for each landmark was set to a vertical unit vector. In the estimation procedure, the frame vectors were initialized with the Euclidean linear regression estimate. In Fig. 6 is shown the true (red), the initial (green) and the estimated frame (blue) for each landmark. The estimation procedure converges to a good estimate of the true frame. Estimation of the initial frame was considered for different number of observations, but the estimated frame did not seem to converge for increasing number of observations. The difference in the parameter estimates might therefore be a result of either the linear approximation of the likelihood or that the optimal solution of the initial frame is not unique.

7   Data Example

We now apply the model to a real dataset consisting of landmark representations of Corpus Callosum (CC) shapes. The model is used to describe the effect of age on CC shapes. The manifold considered is the same as that introduced in Sect. 6, but in this case $\sigma = 0.1$. Again the Levi-Civita connection is used.

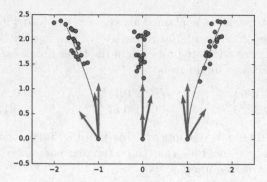

Fig. 6. Comparison of the estimated (blue), initial (green) and true frame vectors (red). (Color figure online)

A subset of the CC dataset is plotted in Fig. 7. For model fitting, a dataset of 20 CC shapes was considered with age values ranging from 22 to 78. The model was fitted to CC shapes represented by a subset of 20 landmarks. We did not incorporate a drift term in the model, and only the frame and $\tilde{W}$ has been estimated. The refrence point was set to the mean shape (Fig. 7) and $\tau = 0.1$.

The estimated frame for the 20 landmarks are shown in Fig. 7 on top of the mean shape. The weight matrix was estimated as $\tilde{W} = -0.0002$. Given the low estimate of $\tilde{W}$ and hence a small frame matrix W, the result of this experiment suggests a low age effect on CC for these data.

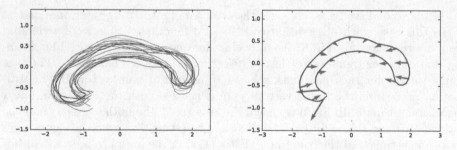

Fig. 7. (left) A subset of the Corpus Callosum data. (right) The mean shape with the estimated frame for the 20 landmarks used in the model fitting.

8   Discussion

A method was proposed for modeling the relation between a manifold-valued response and Euclidean explanatory variables. The relation was modeled by transport of stochastic paths from $\mathbb{R}^m$ to the manifold. The stochastic paths defined on $\mathbb{R}^m$ was given as solutions to a stochastic differential equation with a contribution from a fixed drift, a stochastic process related to the explanatory variables, and a random noise assumed to follow a multidimensional Brownian motion. The response variable was then modeled as a noisy observation of a stochastic variable following the distribution of the endpoints of the transported process. The proposed model is intrinsic and based on a connection on the manifold without making linearization of the non-linear space. Moreover, a likelihood based estimation procedure were described using Laplace approximation of the marginal likelihood. We experimentally illustrated the model and the parameter estimation using a simulation study and a real data example.

Other procedures could be used for estimation of parameters. As an example, the Monte Carlo EM procedure could be used to optimize the complete data likelihood based on simulations of the missing data. Another example is to approximate the distribution of the response by moment matching.

An interesting problem to investigate is how to make variable selection in the model. As the contribution from the explanatory variables is defined in comparison with the frame basis vectors, one idea is to exclude those explanatory variables which corresponds to frame vectors parallel to the curve. These frame vectors will not contribute to the stochastic development and hence will not be important for explaining the relation to the response variable.

An important assumption of the manifold considered, is that the manifold is equipped with a connection. In this paper, the Levi-Civita connection was used, but several other connections could have been chosen. It would be interesting to explore how the choice of connection affects the model.

As it is possible to transport stochastic paths from a manifold to a Euclidean space, the model could be generalized to handle situations in which a Euclidean response variable is compared to manifold-valued explanatory variables. Based on such a model, one might be able to make categorization of individuals based on manifold-valued shapes.

References

1. Aswani, A., Bickel, P., Tomlin, C.: Regression on manifolds: estimation of the exterior derivative. Ann. Stat. **39**(1), 48–81 (2011). arXiv:1103.1457
2. Banerjee, M., Chakraborty, R., Ofori, E., Okun, M.S., Vaillancourt, D.E., Vemuri, B.C.: A nonlinear regression technique for manifold valued data with applications to medical image analysis. In: 2016 IEEE Conference on CVPR, pp. 4424–4432, June 2016
3. Banerjee, M., Chakraborty, R., Ofori, E., Vaillancourt, D., Vemuri, B.C.: Nonlinear regression on Riemannian manifolds and its applications to neuro-image analysis. In: Navab, N., Hornegger, J., Wells, W.M., Frangi, A.F. (eds.) MICCAI 2015. LNCS, vol. 9349, pp. 719–727. Springer, Cham (2015). doi:10.1007/978-3-319-24553-9_88
4. Cheng, M., Wu, H.: Local linear regression on manifolds and its geometric interpretation. J. Am. Stat. Assoc. **108**(504), 1421–1434 (2013)
5. Cornea, E., Zhu, H., Kim, P., Ibrahim, J.G., The Alzheimer's Disease Neuroimaging Initiative: Regression models on Riemannian symmetric spaces. J. Roy. Stat. Soc. B **79**, 463–482 (2017)

6. Davis, B.C., Fletcher, P.T., Bullitt, E., Joshi, S.: Population shape regression from random design data. In: 2007 IEEE 11th International Conference on Computer Vision, pp. 1–7, October 2007

7. Thomas Fletcher, P.: Geodesic regression and the theory of least squares on riemannian manifolds. Int. J. Comput. Vis. **105**(2), 171–185 (2012)

8. Hinkle, J., Muralidharan, P., Fletcher, P.T., Joshi, S.: Polynomial regression on Riemannian manifolds. arXiv:1201.2395, January 2012

9. Hong, Y., Kwitt, R., Singh, N., Vasconcelos, N., Niethammer, M.: Parametric regression on the Grassmannian. IEEE Trans. Pattern Anal. Mach. Intell. **38**(11), 2284–2297 (2016)

10. Hsu, E.P.: Stochastic Analysis on Manifolds. American Mathematical Soc., Providence (2002)

11. Kass, R.E., Steffey, D.: Approximate Bayesian inference in conditionally independent hierarchical models (Parametric Empirical Bayes Models). J. Am. Stat. Assoc. **84**(407), 717–726 (1989)

12. Lin, L., St Thomas, B., Zhu, H., Dunson, D.B.: Extrinsic local regression on manifold-valued data. arXiv:1508.02201, August 2015

13. Loubes, J.-M., Pelletier, B.: A kernel-based classifier on a Riemannian manifold. Stat. Decis. Int. Math. J. Stoch. Methods Models **26**(1), 35–51 (2009)

14. Pennec, X.: Intrinsic statistics on Riemannian manifolds: basic tools for geometric measurements. J. Math. Imaging Vis. **25**, 127 (2006)

15. Shi, X., Styner, M., Lieberman, J., Ibrahim, J.G., Lin, W., Zhu, H.: Intrinsic regression models for manifold-valued data. In: Yang, G.-Z., Hawkes, D., Rueckert, D., Noble, A., Taylor, C. (eds.) MICCAI 2009. LNCS, vol. 5762, pp. 192–199. Springer, Heidelberg (2009). doi:10.1007/978-3-642-04271-3_24

16. Singh, N., Hinkle, J., Joshi, S., Fletcher, P.T.: Hierarchical geodesic models in diffeomorphisms. Int. J. Comput. Vis. **117**, 70–92 (2016)

17. Singh, N., Vialard, F.-X., Niethammer, M.: Splines for diffeomorphisms. Med. Image Anal. **25**(1), 56–71 (2015)

18. Sommer, S.H., Svane, A.M.: Modelling anisotropic covariance using stochastic development and sub-Riemannian frame bundle geometry. J. Geom. Mech. (2016). ISSN: 1941-4889. American Institute of Mathematical Sciences

19. Sommer, S.: Anisotropic distributions on manifolds: template estimation and most probable paths. In: Ourselin, S., Alexander, D.C., Westin, C.-F., Cardoso, M.J. (eds.) IPMI 2015. LNCS, vol. 9123, pp. 193–204. Springer, Cham (2015). doi:10.1007/978-3-319-19992-4_15

20. Sommer, S.: Anisotropically weighted and nonholonomically constrained evolutions on manifolds. Entropy **18**(12), 425 (2016)

21. Steinke, F., Hein, M.: Non-parametric regression between manifolds. In: Advances in Neural Information Processing Systems 21, pp. 1561–1568. Curran Associates, Inc. (2009)

22. Theano Development Team. Theano: a Python framework for fast computation of mathematical expressions. arXiv e-prints, abs/1605.02688, May 2016

23. Younes, L., Arrate, F., Miller, M.I.: Evolutions equations in computational anatomy. NeuroImage **45**(1 Suppl.), S40–S50 (2009)

24. Younes, L.: Shapes and Diffeomorphisms. Springer, Heidelberg (2010)

25. Yuan, Y., Zhu, H., Lin, W., Marron, J.S.: Local polynomial regression for symmetric positive definite matrices. J. Roy. Stat. Soc. Ser. B Stat. Methodol. **74**(4), 697–719 (2012)

Shape Analysis

Spectral Kernels for Probabilistic Analysis and Clustering of Shapes

Loic Le Folgoc$^{(\boxtimes)}$, Aditya V. Nori, and Antonio Criminisi

Microsoft Research, Cambridge, UK
t-lolefo@microsoft.com

Abstract. We propose a framework for probabilistic shape clustering based on kernel-space embeddings derived from spectral signatures. Our root motivation is to investigate practical yet principled clustering schemes that rely on geometrical invariants of shapes rather than explicit registration. To that end we revisit the use of the Laplacian spectrum and introduce a parametric family of reproducing kernels for shapes, extending WESD [12] and shape DNA [20] like metrics. Parameters provide control over the relative importance of local and global shape features and can be adjusted to emphasize a scale of interest. As a result of kernelization, shapes are embedded in an infinite-dimensional inner product space. We leverage this structure to formulate shape clustering via a Bayesian mixture of kernel-space Principal Component Analysers. We derive simple variational Bayes inference schemes in Hilbert space, addressing technicalities stemming from the infinite dimensionality. The proposed approach is validated on tasks of unsupervised clustering of sub-cortical structures, as well as classification of cardiac left ventricles w.r.t. pathological groups.

1 Introduction

This paper introduces a family of spectral kernels for the purpose of probabilistic analysis and clustering of shapes. Statistical shape analysis spans a range of applications in computer vision, medical imaging and computational anatomy: object recognition, segmentation, detection and modelling of pathologies, etc. Many approaches have been developed, including landmark based representations and active shape models [2,4,15], medial representations [11] and Principal Geodesic Analysis [7], deformable registration and diffeomorphometry [5,9,26]. In many applications, the relevant information is invariant to the pose of the object and is encoded instead within its intrinsic geometry. It may then be advantageous to circumvent the challenges of explicit registration, relying on representations that respect these invariants. Spectral shape descriptors [19,20], built from the spectrum of the Laplace(-Beltrami) operator over the object surface or volume, have achieved popularity for object retrieval [3], analysis and classification of anatomical structures [8,16,24], structural or functional inter-subject mapping [14,17,21]. In [12,13], Konukoglu et al. introduce a Weighted

L. Le Folgoc would like to thank the MSR–Inria Joint Centre for their support.

M. Niethammer et al. (Eds.): IPMI 2017, LNCS 10265, pp. 67–79, 2017.
DOI: 10.1007/978-3-319-59050-9_6

Spectral Distance (WESD) on shapes with two appealing properties: a gentle dependency on the finite spectrum truncation, and a parameter p to emphasize finer or coarser scales. For the purpose of shape analysis and clustering, it would be useful to define not merely a metric, but also an inner product structure. This is a prerequisite for many traditional statistical analysis methods *e.g.*, PCA.

Our first contribution is to derive a parametric family of spectral (reproducing) kernels that effectively provide an inner product structure while preserving the multiscale aspect of WESD. As a result, shapes are embedded in an infinite dimensional Hilbert space. Our second contribution is a probabilistic Gaussian mixture model in kernel space, presented within a variational Bayes framework. The kernel space mixture of PCA is of interest in its own right, widely applicable and novel [6]. Together, the two contributions yield a straightforward shape clustering algorithm – a mixture of PCA in spectral kernel space. This approach is validated on tasks of unsupervised and supervised clustering on 69 images from the "Leaf Shapes" database, 240 3D sub-cortical brain structures from the LPBA40 dataset and 45 3D left ventricles from the Sunnybrook cardiac dataset.

2   Background: Laplace Operator, Heat-Trace and WESD

In [12,13], WESD is derived by analyzing the sensitivity of the *heat-trace* to the Laplacian spectrum. Let $\Omega \subset \mathbb{R}^d$ an object (a closed bounded domain) with sufficiently regular boundary $\partial\Omega$, and define its Laplace operator Δ_Ω as

$$[\Delta_\Omega f](\mathbf{x}) \triangleq \sum_{i=1}^{d} \frac{\partial^2}{\partial x_i^2} f(\mathbf{x}), \quad \forall \mathbf{x} \in \Omega \tag{1}$$

for any sufficiently smooth real-valued function f. The Laplacian spectrum is the infinite set $0 \leq \lambda_1 \leq \cdots \leq \lambda_n \cdots$, $\lambda_n \to +\infty$, of eigenvalues for the Dirichlet problem:

$$\begin{cases} \Delta_\Omega f + \lambda f = 0 & \text{in } \Omega \\ f = 0 & \text{on } \partial\Omega. \end{cases} \tag{2}$$

Denoting by ϕ_n the associated $L^2(\Omega)$-orthonormal eigenfunctions, let $K_\Omega(t, \mathbf{x}, \mathbf{y}) \triangleq \sum_{n\geq 1} \exp\{-\lambda_n t\}\phi_n(\mathbf{x})\phi_n(\mathbf{y})$ the heat kernel. The heat kernel is the fundamental solution to the heat equation $\partial_t K_\Omega(t, \mathbf{x}, \mathbf{y}) = \Delta_\Omega K_\Omega(t, \mathbf{x}, \mathbf{y})$ over Ω, with $K_\Omega(0, \mathbf{x}, \mathbf{y}) \equiv \delta_\mathbf{x}(\mathbf{y})$ and Dirichlet boundary conditions. It is at the basis of a variety of point matching techniques in the computer vision and computer graphics literature, as $K_\Omega(t, \mathbf{x}, \mathbf{x})$ encodes information about the local neighbourhood of $\mathbf{x}$ [10]. Similarly the trace of the heat kernel a.k.a. the *heat-trace*, $Z_\Omega(t) \triangleq \int_\Omega K_\Omega(t, \mathbf{x}, \mathbf{x})d\mathbf{x} = \sum_{n=1}^{+\infty} e^{-\lambda_n t}$, summarizes information about local and global invariants of the shape [12]. It provides a convenient link between the intrinsic geometry of the object and the spectrum. For two shapes Ω_λ and Ω_ξ with respective spectrum $\boldsymbol{\lambda}$ and $\boldsymbol{\xi}$, let $\Delta_{\lambda,\xi}^n$ quantify the influence of the change in the nth eigenmode on the heat-trace:

$$\Delta_{\lambda,\xi}^n \triangleq \int_0^{+\infty} \left| e^{-\lambda_n t} - e^{-\xi_n t} \right| dt = \frac{|\lambda_n - \xi_n|}{\lambda_n \xi_n}. \tag{3}$$

The pseudo-metric WESD is obtained by summing all mode contributions:

$$\rho_p(\Omega_\lambda, \Omega_\xi) \triangleq \left[\sum_{n=1}^{+\infty} (\Delta_{\lambda,\xi}^n)^p \right]^{1/p} = \left[\sum_{n=1}^{+\infty} \left(\frac{|\lambda_n - \xi_n|}{\lambda_n \xi_n} \right)^p \right]^{1/p}. \tag{4}$$

Konukoglu et al. show that WESD is well-defined for $p > d/2$. The key element is due to Weyl [10,25], who proved that the eigenvalues λ behave asymptotically as $\lambda_n \sim 4\pi^2 (\frac{n}{B_d V_\Omega})^{2/d} \triangleq \Lambda_n$ when $n \to +\infty$. Here B_d is the volume of the d-dimensional unit ball and V_Ω the volume of Ω. Furthermore from Eq. (2), WESD is made invariant to isotropic rescaling by multiplying the spectrum by $V_\Omega^{2/d}$. Although we refer to objects, shapes and their spectrum interchangeably throughout the article, WESD is a pseudo-metric: objects with different shapes may share the same spectrum. Last but not least, it is multi-scale: its sensitivity to finer scales decreases as p becomes higher. While control over the scale is appealing, the interleaving with the parameter p is somewhat inconvenient. Indeed the metric only defines an inner product structure for $p = 2$. Because this structure is critical for linear statistical analysis, WESD is instead typically used in conjunction with non-linear embedding schemes. We further comment that the choice of measure w.r.t. the time t in the integral of Eq. (3) is arbitrary. This observation turns out to be key for our analysis: the time t is crucial in modulating the sensitivity of the heat-trace $Z_\Omega(t)$ to coarser or finer scales.

3   Shape Spectral Kernels

We now introduce a parametric family of spectral kernels $K_{\alpha,\beta}(\boldsymbol{\lambda}, \cdot)$. These kernels can be interpreted as inner products in some infinite dimensional Hilbert space $\mathcal{H}_{\alpha,\beta}$ and will constitute the basis for the mixture of kernel PCA model of Sect. 4. The parameters α, β control the influence of coarser and finer scales on the metric (Fig. 1). Let us introduce the form of the kernels without further delay, postponing details related to its derivation. For $\alpha, \beta \leq 0$, let

$$K_{\alpha,\beta}(\boldsymbol{\lambda}, \boldsymbol{\xi}) \triangleq \sum_{n=1}^{+\infty} \frac{1}{(\beta + \lambda_n)^\alpha} \frac{1}{(\beta + \xi_n)^\alpha}. \tag{5}$$

The series is shown to converge (electronic appendix) for $\alpha > d/4$, and variants of the kernel for $\alpha > \frac{d}{4} - \frac{1}{2}$. Because it is defined from a convergent series, $K_{\alpha,\beta}(\boldsymbol{\lambda}, \boldsymbol{\xi})$ can be approximated arbitrarily well from a finite term truncation. It shares this property with WESD, unlike shape DNA [20]. Furthermore, invariance to rescaling of the shape can be obtained as for WESD by normalizing the spectrum.

Effect of the Parameters α, β. For the sake of relating the kernel to the literature, let us introduce the corresponding metric via the polarization identity $\rho_{\alpha,\beta}(\Omega_\lambda, \Omega_\xi) \triangleq [K_{\alpha,\beta}(\boldsymbol{\lambda}, \boldsymbol{\lambda}) - 2 \cdot K_{\alpha,\beta}(\boldsymbol{\lambda}, \boldsymbol{\xi}) + K_{\alpha,\beta}(\boldsymbol{\xi}, \boldsymbol{\xi})]^{1/2}$. This leads to:

$$\rho_{\alpha,\beta}(\Omega_\lambda, \Omega_\xi) = \left[\sum_{n=1}^{+\infty} \left(\frac{(\beta + \lambda_n)^\alpha - (\beta + \xi_n)^\alpha}{(\beta + \lambda_n)^\alpha \cdot (\beta + \xi_n)^\alpha} \right)^2 \right]^{1/2}, \tag{6}$$

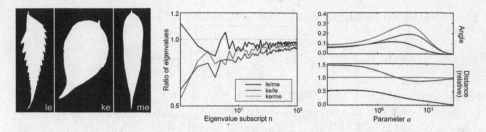

Fig. 1. (Left) Example shapes "ke", "le", "me" from the Leaf Shapes dataset[1]. "ke" is rounder, "me" is elongated, "le" is in-between but its boundary is jagged. (Right) Effect of α on the distance and angle between each pair. Distances are normalized w.r.t. the ke/me pair. Larger (resp. smaller) values of α emphasize coarser (finer) scale features. For instance, the dissimilarity of the pair le/ke relatively to that of the pair le/me shrinks (from 6× to under 3×) at finer scales as the focus shifts, say, from purely the aspect ratio to account for the smooth/jagged boundary. (Middle) Ratio of Laplacian eigenvalues for the three pairs. Small eigenvalues relate to global features (*e.g.* rounder, elongated), thus small eigenvalues of "ke" are even further away from "le", "me".

and may be compared to $\rho_p(\Omega_\lambda, \Omega_\xi)$ of Eq. (4). Firstly, for $\alpha = 1, \beta = 0$ and $p = 2$, WESD and the spectral kernel metric coincide: $\rho_2 = \rho_{1,0}$. In that sense $\rho_{\alpha,0}$ extends the "Euclidean" WESD while providing additional parameters to control the weight of coarser and finer scales. Recall that the larger eigenvalues λ_n relate to finer local details, while the first eigenvalues $\lambda_1, \lambda_2 \ldots$ relate to global invariants (*e.g.* volume, boundary surface). When α increases to large values, global shape features gain overwhelming importance and, in the limit of $\alpha \to +\infty$, only λ_1 matters. Inversely, in the limit of $\alpha \to 0$, the nth term of the series (before squaring) behaves as $\rho_{0,0}^n(\Omega_\lambda, \Omega_\xi) \sim |\log \frac{\lambda_n}{\xi_n}|$, which is sensitive only to the *relative* ratio of eigenvalues, as opposed to the actual values λ_n, ξ_n. In that sense it gives equal weight to all eigenvalues. Most eigenvalues relate to finer scale features, hence smaller α values emphasize these details.

For $\lambda_n, \xi_n \ll \beta$, the nth series term behaves as $|\lambda_n - \xi_n|^2$, which does not penalize the eigenvalue magnitude whatsoever. This is reminiscent of the shape DNA [20, 24] metric $\rho_{\text{DNA}}(\Omega_\lambda, \Omega_\xi) \triangleq \sum_{n=1}^{N_{\max}} |\lambda_n - \xi_n|$. β acts similarly to $N_{\max}$ in selecting a range of relevant eigenvalues for the metric: as it grows, larger eigenvalues are given more importance. Finally, for $\alpha, \beta \to +\infty$ such that $\frac{\alpha}{\beta} = \text{const.} = t_{\alpha,\beta}$, the nth series term (unsquared) behaves as $\rho_{\alpha,\beta}^n(\Omega_\lambda, \Omega_\xi) \sim \exp\{-\lambda_n t_{\alpha,\beta}\} - \exp\{-\xi_n t_{\alpha,\beta}\}$, that is the nth term of $Z_\lambda(t_{\alpha,\beta}) - Z_\xi(t_{\alpha,\beta})$. Hence for large "informative" values of α and β, the ratio α/β selects a heat diffusion time-scale of interest and β the spread around that value. Alternatively, somewhat neutral choices of parameters with a balance between coarser and finer scales are obtained for β small ($\beta = 0$ or $\beta \simeq \Lambda_1$) and α small (*e.g.* $\alpha \leq d/2$).

---

[1] Publicly available from http://imageprocessingplace.com. Developed by Vaibhav E. Waghmare, Govt. College of Engineering Aurangabad, 431 005 MS, INDIA.

The discussion will be clearer from a closer look at the link between the choice of α, β and the corresponding choice of time integration.

Computations in Kernel Space. Before outlining derivations from the heat trace, let us note an attractive computational property of the family of spectral kernels. For the sake of "linear" statistical analysis (*e.g.*, k-means, PCA), weighted sums of kernel representers $K_{\alpha,\beta}(\lambda, \cdot)$ of shapes λ are typically involved. Usually such sums cannot be explicitly computed, but their projections on a given element $K_{\alpha,\beta}(\xi, \cdot)$ can, since $(K_{\alpha,\beta}(\lambda, \cdot)|K_{\alpha,\beta}(\xi, \cdot))_{\mathcal{H}_{\alpha,\beta}} = K_{\alpha,\beta}(\lambda, \xi)$. This is known as the kernel trick. As a drawback many kernel extensions of widespread linear statistical schemes have a complexity tied to (say, the cube of) the number of observations, instead of the *dimensionality* of the data. In the present case fortunately, computations can be done explicitly. Let $\Phi_{\alpha,\beta} : \lambda \mapsto (\cdots (\lambda_n + \beta)^{-\alpha} \cdots)$ map shapes to the space I^2 of l_2 sequences. By construction $K_{\alpha,\beta}(\lambda, \xi) = \langle \Phi_{\alpha,\beta}(\lambda)|\Phi_{\alpha,\beta}(\xi)\rangle_{I^2}$. Addition, scalar multiplication and inner product on elements $K_{\alpha,\beta}(\lambda, \cdot)$ of $\mathcal{H}_{\alpha,\beta}$ are equivalent to explicit addition, scalar multiplication and inner product on elements $\Phi_{\alpha,\beta}(\lambda)$ of I^2. For instance, given two shapes λ and ξ, their mean is given by $\Phi_{\alpha,\beta}(\chi)$, defined by $(\chi_n + \beta)^{-\alpha} \triangleq \frac{1}{2}(\lambda_n + \beta)^{-\alpha} + \frac{1}{2}(\xi_n + \beta)^{-\alpha}$. Any finite N-term truncation of the infinite kernel series is equivalent to an N-term truncation of the l^2 sequence, so that the mean of $|\mathcal{D}|$ points $\{K_{\alpha,\beta}(\lambda_i, \cdot)\}_{1 \le i \le |\mathcal{D}|}$ can for instance be stored as an N-tuple. Moreover, the eigenmodes of the Gram matrix $[K_{\alpha,\beta}(\lambda_i, \lambda_j)]_{1 \le i,j \le |\mathcal{D}|}$ can be obtained from the eigenmodes of the $N \times N$ covariance matrix $\sum_i \Phi_{\alpha,\beta}(\lambda_i)\Phi_{\alpha,\beta}(\lambda_i)^\mathsf{T}$ of the truncated $\Phi_{\alpha,\beta}(\lambda_i)$ tuples. Hence the computational complexity depends on the truncated dimensionality rather than the dataset size, whenever advantageous. Truncation error bounds are given in the electronic appendix.

Derivation of the Spectral Kernels. Similarly to WESD, the proposed kernels are derived by quantifying the influence of the change in the nth eigenmode on the heat-trace. However we consider a variety of measures for the integration w.r.t. time. Let $p_{\alpha,\beta}(t) \triangleq \frac{\beta^\alpha}{\Gamma(\alpha)} \exp\{-\beta t\}t^{\alpha-1}$ the probability density function of the gamma distribution with positive shape parameter α and rate parameter β. We extend Eq. (3) by integrating w.r.t. $p_{\alpha,\beta}$:

$$\Delta_{\alpha,\beta}^n(\lambda, \xi) \triangleq \int_0^{+\infty} |e^{-\lambda_n t} - e^{-\xi_n t}| \cdot p_{\alpha,\beta}(t)dt, \tag{7}$$

$$= \beta^\alpha \cdot \left| \frac{(\beta + \lambda_n)^\alpha - (\beta + \xi_n)^\alpha}{(\beta + \lambda_n)^\alpha \cdot (\beta + \xi_n)^\alpha} \right|, \tag{8}$$

$$= \beta^\alpha \cdot \left| \frac{1}{(\beta + \lambda_n)^\alpha} - \frac{1}{(\beta + \xi_n)^\alpha} \right|. \tag{9}$$

We obtain a (pseudo-)metric on shapes and retrieve Eq. (6) by aggregating the contributions of all modes: $\rho_{\alpha,\beta}(\Omega_\lambda, \Omega_\xi)^2 \triangleq \sum_{n=1}^{+\infty} (\Delta_{\alpha,\beta}^n(\lambda, \xi))^2$. $K_{\alpha,\beta}(\lambda, \xi)$ defined as in Eq. (5) is positive definite as a kernel over spectra and, as an inner product, is consistent with the metric $\rho_{\alpha,\beta}$ up to renormalization.

4   Probabilistic Clustering via mixtures of kernel PCA

We now introduce a probabilistic mkPCA model, tackling the inference in a Variational Bayesian (VB) framework. Let $K : (x, y) \in \mathcal{X} \times \mathcal{X} \mapsto K(x, y) = K_x(y) \in \mathbb{R}$ a reproducing kernel with $(L_K f)(x) \triangleq \int_{\mathcal{X}} K(x, y) f(y) dy$ a compact operator over $L_2(\mathcal{X})$. Let $\mathcal{H}$ the associated reproducing kernel Hilbert space. For $f, g \in \mathcal{H}$, $\langle f | g \rangle_{L_2} \triangleq \int_{\mathcal{X}} fg$ or simply $\langle f | g \rangle$ is the L_2 inner-product, whereas $\mathcal{H}$ is endowed with the inner product $(f | g)_{\mathcal{H}} = \langle f | L_K^{-1} g \rangle_{L_2}$ or simply $(f | g)$. $\|f\|_{\mathcal{H}} \triangleq (f | f)^{1/2}$ or $\|f\|$ stands for the norm of $\mathcal{H}$. Finally we use the braket notation, $|f) \triangleq L_K^{-1/2} f$ and $(f| \triangleq |f)^\intercal$. The main technical hurdles stem from the infinite dimensionality of the data: probability density functions are not properly defined, and the full normalization constants cannot be computed. In solving this obstacle, the decomposition of the covariance into isotropic noise and low rank structure is key.

PCA as a Latent Linear Variable Model. Let $\phi_k \in \mathcal{H}$, $k = 1 \cdots r$, a finite set of basis functions. Assume $f = \sum_{1 \leq k \leq r} \phi_k w_k + \sigma \epsilon$ is generated by a linear combination of the ϕ_k's plus some scaled white noise $\epsilon \sim \mathcal{N}(0, L_K)$. Further assume that $w \sim \mathcal{N}(0, \mathrm{I})$ where $w \triangleq (w_1 \cdots w_r)$. Then $f \sim \mathcal{N}(0, \sigma^2 L_K + \Phi \Phi^\intercal)$ follows a Gaussian process, where $\Phi \triangleq (\cdots \phi_k \cdots)$. It is a natural extension of the probabilistic PCA model of [23], conveniently decomposing the variance as the sum of an isotropic part $\sigma^2 L_K$ (w.r.t. $\| \cdot \|$) and of a low-rank part $\Phi \Phi^\intercal$. The first term accounts for noise in the data, while the latter one captures the latent structure. Furthermore $|f) = \sum_{1 \leq k \leq r} |\phi_k) w_k + \sigma |\epsilon)$ also follows a Gaussian distribution $\mathcal{N}(0, \sigma^2 \mathrm{I} + |\Phi)(\Phi|)$. We use this latter form from now on as it most closely resembles finite dimensional linear algebra. By analogy in the finite case, the following linear algebra updates hold: $(\sigma^2 \mathrm{I} + \Phi \Phi^\intercal)^{-1} = \sigma^{-2}[\mathrm{I} - \Phi(\sigma^2 \mathrm{I}_r + \Phi^\intercal \Phi)^{-1} \Phi^\intercal]$ and $|\sigma^2 \mathrm{I} + \Phi \Phi^\intercal| = |\sigma^2 \mathrm{I}| \cdot |\mathrm{I}_r + \sigma^{-2} \Phi^\intercal \Phi|$. The former Woodbury matrix identity and latter matrix determinant lemma express, using only readily computable terms, the resulting change for (resp.) the inverse and determinant under a low rank matrix perturbation. In particular the determinant conveniently factorizes into a constant term $|\sigma^2 \mathrm{I}|$, improper in the infinite dimensional case, and a well-defined term that depends on Φ. This lets us compute normalization constants and other key quantities required for inference and model comparison, up to a constant.

Probabilistic Mixture of Kernel PCA. Let $\mathcal{D} = \{x_i\}_{i=1}^{|\mathcal{D}|}$ a set of observations and K_{x_i} the kernel embedding of the ith point. Assume K_{x_i} is drawn from a mixture of M Gaussian components, depending on the state of a categorical variable $c_i \in \{1 \cdots M\}$. Let z_{im} the binary gate variable that is set to 1 if $c_i = m$ and 0 otherwise. Let $|K_{x_i})_{\mathcal{H}} | z_{im} = 1 \sim \mathcal{N}(\mu_m, C_m)$ i.i.d. according to a Gaussian process, where $C_m \triangleq \sigma^2 \mathrm{I} + |\Phi_m)(\Phi_m|$ and σ^2 is a fixed parameter. $\Phi_m \triangleq (\cdots \phi_{km} \cdots)$ concatenates an arbitrary number of (random) basis functions $\phi_{km} \in \mathcal{H}$. Denoting $z_i \triangleq \{z_{im}\}_{1 \leq m \leq M}$, the z_i's are i.i.d. following a categorical distribution, i.e. $p(z_i | \pi) = \prod_{1 \leq m \leq M} \pi_m^{z_{im}}$, where $\pi \triangleq \{\pi_m\}_{1 \leq m \leq M}$. A conjugate Dirichlet prior is taken over the mixture proportions, $p(\pi | \kappa_0) \propto \prod_{1 \leq m \leq M} \pi_m^{\kappa_0 - 1}$. (μ_m, Φ_m) is endowed (formally) with the improper prior $\mathcal{N}\big(\mu_m\big|\,|\mathrm{m}_0),\eta_0^{-1}\mathrm{C}_m\big)\cdot|\mathrm{C}_m|^{-\gamma_0/2}\exp-\tfrac{1}{2}\mathrm{tr}(s_0\mathrm{C}_m^{-1})$. As a constraint for the optimal Φ_m to have finite rank, $\gamma_0^{-1}s_0\leq\sigma^2$. The model and its fixed hyperparameters $\{\eta_0,\gamma_0,s_0,\kappa_0,\sigma^2\}$ will be shortened as $\mathcal{M}$. In what follows, bolded quantities stand for the concatenation of their normal font counterpart across all values of the missing indices. For instance $\boldsymbol{z}_m\triangleq\{z_{im}\}_{1\leq i\leq|\mathcal{D}|}$ and $\boldsymbol{z}_i\triangleq\{z_{im}\}_{1\leq m\leq M}$.

VB updates can be derived in closed form for the family $q(\boldsymbol{z})\triangleq q_{\boldsymbol{z}}(\boldsymbol{z})q_{\boldsymbol{\theta}}(\boldsymbol{\theta})$ of variational posteriors where the mixture assignment variables z_i's and the model hyperparameters $\boldsymbol{\theta}=\{\boldsymbol{\pi},\boldsymbol{\mu},\boldsymbol{\Phi}\}$ for all mixtures are factorized, provided that $q_{\boldsymbol{\theta}}(\boldsymbol{\theta})\triangleq q_{\boldsymbol{\pi}}(\boldsymbol{\pi}|\boldsymbol{\mu},\boldsymbol{\Phi})\delta_{\hat{\boldsymbol{\mu}}}(\boldsymbol{\mu}|\boldsymbol{\Phi})\delta_{\hat{\boldsymbol{\Phi}}}(\boldsymbol{\Phi})$ is further restrained to a Dirac (point mass) distribution over the Φ_m's and μ_m's. They closely follow their finite dimensional counterpart as in $e.g.$ [1,23]. For all model variables but $\boldsymbol{\Phi},\boldsymbol{\mu}$, model conjugacies can be exploited and variational posteriors have the same functional form as the corresponding priors. Specifically, $q_{\boldsymbol{z}}(\boldsymbol{z})=\prod_{i=1}^{|\mathcal{D}|}q_{z_i}(z_i)$ and $q_{\boldsymbol{\pi}}(\boldsymbol{\pi}|\boldsymbol{\mu},\boldsymbol{\Phi})=q_{\boldsymbol{\pi}}(\boldsymbol{\pi})$, with $q_{z_i}(z_i)=\prod_{m=1}^{M}\rho_{im}^{z_{im}}$ categorical and $q_{\boldsymbol{\pi}}(\boldsymbol{\pi})=\mathcal{D}(\boldsymbol{\pi}|\boldsymbol{\kappa})$ Dirichlet, denoting $\boldsymbol{\kappa}\triangleq\{\kappa_m\}_{m=1}^{M}$. In addition $\hat{\Phi}_m$ maximizes the posterior $p(\Phi_m|\langle\boldsymbol{z}_m\rangle_{q_{\boldsymbol{z}}},\mathcal{D},\mathcal{M})\propto|\mathrm{C}_m|^{-\frac{\gamma_m}{2}}\exp-\tfrac{1}{2}\mathrm{tr}\{\mathrm{S}_m\mathrm{C}_m^{-1}\}$, $\hat{\mu}_m$ is the mode of $p(\mu_m|\Phi_m,\mathcal{D},\mathcal{M})=\mathcal{N}(\mu_m|\,|\mathrm{m}_m),\eta_m^{-1}\mathrm{C}_m)$. The updates are as follows:

$$\kappa_m=|\mathcal{D}|\bar{\pi}_m+\kappa_0,\eta_m=|\mathcal{D}|\bar{\pi}_m+\eta_0,\gamma_m=|\mathcal{D}|\bar{\pi}_m+\gamma_0 \tag{10}$$

$$\mathrm{m}_m=\frac{|\mathcal{D}|\bar{\pi}_m}{\eta_m}\cdot\bar{\mu}_m+\frac{\eta_0}{\eta_m}\cdot\mathrm{m}_0 \tag{11}$$

$$\mathrm{S}_m=\eta_m\bar{\Sigma}_m^{+0}+s_0\mathrm{I} \tag{12}$$

$$|\Phi_m)=\sqrt{\left(\gamma_m^{-1}\mathrm{S}_m-\sigma^2\mathrm{I}\right)_+} \tag{13}$$

$$\rho_{im}\propto\tilde{\pi}_m\cdot\frac{1}{|\mathrm{I}+\sigma^{-2}(\Phi_m|\Phi_m)_{\mathcal{H}}|^{1/2}}\exp\left\{-\frac{1}{2}\chi_{im}^2\right\} \tag{14}$$

where $\sum_{m=1}^{M}\rho_{im}=1$, $(\cdot)_+$ the projection on positive semidefinite matrices and:

$$\bar{\pi}_m\triangleq\frac{1}{|\mathcal{D}|}\sum_{i=1}^{|\mathcal{D}|}\rho_{im} \tag{15}$$

$$\bar{\mu}_m\triangleq\frac{1}{|\mathcal{D}|\bar{\pi}_m}\sum_{i=1}^{|\mathcal{D}|}\rho_{im}K_{x_i} \tag{16}$$

$$\delta_{im}\triangleq K_{x_i}-\mathrm{m}_m,\quad\delta_{0m}\triangleq\mathrm{m}_0-\mathrm{m}_m \tag{17}$$

$$\bar{\Sigma}_m^{+0}\triangleq\frac{1}{\eta_0+|\mathcal{D}|\bar{\pi}_m}\left(\eta_0\,|\delta_{0m})(\delta_{0m}|+\sum_{i=1}^{|\mathcal{D}|}\rho_{im}\,|\delta_{im})\,(\delta_{im}|\right) \tag{18}$$

$$\chi_{im}^2\triangleq\frac{1}{\sigma^2}\left(\|\delta_{im}\|^2-(\delta_{im}|\Phi_\mathrm{m})\left(\sigma^2\mathrm{I}+(\Phi_m|\Phi_m)\right)^{-1}(\Phi_m|\delta_{im})\right) \tag{19}$$

$$\tilde{\pi}_m\triangleq\exp\langle\log\pi_m\rangle_{q_{\pi_m}}=\exp\left\{\psi(\kappa_m)-\psi(\textstyle\sum_{m'=1}^{M}\kappa_{m'})\right\} \tag{20}$$

The derivation of Eq. (13) closely mirrors the one found in [23]. Fortunately, computations of infinite dimensional quantities $\bar{\Sigma}_m^{+0}$ and S_m need not be conducted explicitly, exploiting generic relationships between the eigenmodes of Gram and scatter matrices. Indeed, $|\Phi_m) = |U_m)\Delta_m$ up to right multiplication by an arbitrary rotation, with the following notations. $\Delta_m \triangleq \text{diag}[(\gamma_m^{-1} d_{km} - \sigma^2)^{1/2}]$ is the $r_m \times r_m$ diagonal matrix such that d_{km} is the kth biggest eigenvalue of S_m among those r_m eigenvalues strictly bigger than $\gamma_m \sigma^2$. The kth column $|U_m)_k$ of $|U_m)$ is the kth eigenvector of S_m. Note that S_m can be rewritten as the sum of $s_0 I$ and $|\mathcal{D}| + 1$ rank one terms of the form $|g_{im})(g_{im}|$. Hence the non-zero eigenvalues of S_m are the same as those of the $(|\mathcal{D}|+1) \times (|\mathcal{D}|+1)$ matrix $(G|G) = [\cdots (g_{im}|g_{jm}) \cdots]_{ij}$. The $|U_m)_k = |G) e_k$ are obtained from the eigenvectors e_k of the latter matrix. Moreover, computations in Eqs. (14) and (19) simplify by noting that $\cdot(\Phi_m|\Phi_m) = \Delta_m^2$ is diagonal.

High-Level Overview. Similarly to the finite dimensional case, Eqs. (10)–(14) can be understood as follows, disregarding terms stemming from priors for simplicity. Each data point i is softly assigned to the mth mixture component with a probability ρ_{im} that depends on the mixing proportion π_m and the point likelihood under the mth component model. Then for each component, the mixing proportion is set to the average of the responsibilities ρ_{im}. The mean m_m is updated to the empirical mean, with data points weighted by ρ_{im}. Similarly the covariance $C_m = \sigma^2 I + |\Phi_m)(\Phi_m|$ is (implicitly) set to the empirical covariance, shrinking all eigenvalues by σ^2 (down to a minimum of 0), after which $|\mathcal{D}|$ non-zero directions remain at most. The algorithm iterates until convergence.

Lower Bound. The evidence lower bound can be computed up to a constant and is given formally by $\sum_i \log \left(\sum_m \rho_{im}^u \right) - \text{KL}[q_{\boldsymbol{\theta}} \| p(\boldsymbol{\theta})]$, where ρ_{im}^u is the unnormalized soft assignment of point i to cluster m (Eq. (14), right-hand side).

Initialization, Choice of σ^2. The mkPCA algorithm is initialized via k-means clustering. In the proposed model σ^2 controls the level of noise in the data. The more noise, the more data variability it accounts for, and the lesser variability attributed to latent structure. Bayesian inference of σ^2 is difficult in infinite dimension, hence not pursued here. If applicable, cross-validation is sound. As an alternative heuristic, let d_i the distance of the ith data point to the centroid of its assigned k-means cluster. $\sum_{1 \le i}^{|D|} d_i^2 / |D|$ gives an estimate of the average variability in the dataset due to both noise and structure. σ^2 is set to a small fraction of that value. A posteriori analysis of the clusters (*e.g.* number of eigenmodes, eigenvalue magnitudes) helps verify the soundness of the setting.

5   Experiments and Results

The proposed framework is implemented in MATLAB, based on the publicly available implementation of WESD[2]. Unless otherwise specified, the scale invariant kernel is used and truncated at $N = 200$ eigenvalues; and σ^2 is set to $0.05 \times$ the k-means average square error. We experiment with values of $\alpha \ge d/2$, and $\beta = 0$ or $\equiv \lambda_1$ and otherwise uninformative values: $\kappa_0 = \gamma_0 = 10^{-6}$, $\eta_0 = 10^{-15}$,

---

[2] http://www.nmr.mgh.harvard.edu/~enderk/software.html.

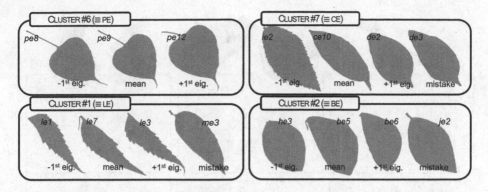

Fig. 2. Inferred leaf clusters. 4 clusters out of 7 are shown, with representative examples for the mean and ±2std. along the first eigenmode. An example mistake is shown if available. For each leaf, the database index is a 3-character code. The cluster assignment of the leaf is deemed wrong whenever the letter prefix differs from that of the cluster.

$s_0 = \gamma_0 \sigma^2 / 10$ and m_0 to the data mean. The best (based on the lower bound) of 10 mkPCA runs (100 iterations) with k-mean initialization is typically selected.

"Leaf Shapes" Dataset: Unsupervised Mining of Leaf Species. The dataset consists of 69 binary images of leaves of 10 different subtypes (*e.g.* "ce", "je"). Each type contains 3 to 12 examples. We aim at retrieving these subtypes using *unsupervised* clustering. 7 clusters are identified. Figure 2 displays 4 of the 7 clusters. For quantitative analysis a label is assigned to each cluster by majority voting, and points are given the label of the maximum a posteriori cluster. The retrieval accuracy for $\alpha = 0.5$, $\beta = 100$ is 71% ± 1%. It is robust w.r.t. α, β ($\geq 68\%$ over 20 runs with chosen values $\alpha \in [0.5, 5]$, $\beta \in [0, 500]$, 67.5% ± 3% over 100 runs with random values in that range). Mislabelling is mostly caused by smaller subtypes with 3 to 4 images not having their own cluster.

LPBA40 Dataset: Clustering Sub-cortical Structures. We proceed with unsupervised clustering of 40×6 volumes of left and right caudates, hippocampuses and putamens from the public LPBA40 dataset [22], using 10 clusters maximum. For qualitative assessment, the data is projected on the 2 largest eigenmodes of each cluster (Fig. 3 for the 6 main clusters). As an indicator of class separation in the learned model, we quantify here again the agreement between the true labels and those assigned by MAP, with 16% average misclassification rate for $\alpha = 1$, $\beta = 0$ (<23% across a wide parameter range).

Learning Left Ventricle Anomalies. The Sunnybrook cardiac dataset [18] (SCD) consists of 45 left ventricle (LV) volumes: a heart failure (HF) group (24 cases), an hypertrophy (HYP) group (12) and a healthy (N) group (9). We evaluate the proposed framework for classification, modelling each group as a 1 (HYP, N) or 2 (HF) component mkPCA. Figure 5 (Left) reports the test accuracy for various hyperparameters. For each setting, mean and std. are computed over 50 runs, training on a random fold of 2/3 of the dataset and testing on the comple-

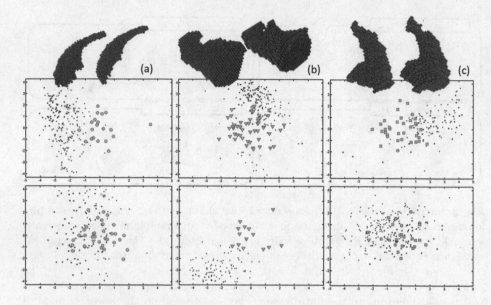

Fig. 3. Unsupervised clustering of subcortical structures. Example (a) caudate nuclei, (b) hippocampi (c) putamina. Below each sub-structure, 2 clusters widely associated with it are shown (projection onto the two first eigenmodes of each cluster, range ±5 std.). Large blue data points belong to the displayed cluster, black dots do not (overlap due to projection). Circle ≡ caudate, triangle ≡ hippocampus, square ≡ putamen. (Color figure online)

ment. The baseline of 53.3% accuracy corresponds to systematically predicting HF. Blood/muscle LV volumes are highly correlated to HF/HYP pathologies and constitute natural predictors that are expected to perform well. The spectrum based mkPCA model classifies better on average ($\sim 75\% \pm 8\%$ across many settings) than a volume based mkPCA ($65\% \pm 9\%$) despite the small training set and low-resolution of the raw data. Figure 4 shows typical (often sensible) classification mistakes. Finally, Fig. 5 evidences strong correlations between eigenmodes of HF/HYP clusters and the cavity/muscle volumes.

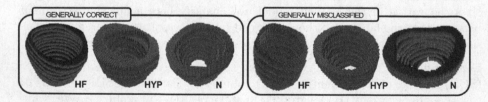

Fig. 4. Example LVs with test misclassification rate >25% (right) or <2% (left).

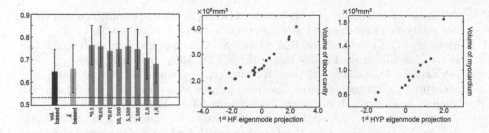

Fig. 5. SCD supervised clustering analysis. (Left) Classification accuracy under various settings (mean and ±std.). Black: volume-based baseline. Yellow: normalized spectrum-based classification. Blue: non-normalized spectrum-based, for various α, β, σ^2 triplets. Default when not specified is $\alpha = 10$, $\beta = 10^3$ and σ^2 set to $0.05\times$ the k-means average error. The last five bars correspond to various α, β pairs, the previous 3 to other σ^2 settings. (Middle) Blood volume as a function of the 1st eigenmode projection for HF cases. (Right) Myocardium volume as a function of 1st eigen. projection for HYP cases. (Color figure online)

6   Conclusion

We proposed a framework for probabilistic clustering of shapes. It couples ideas from the fields of spectral shape analysis and Bayesian modelling to circumvent both the challenges of explicit registration and the recourse to non-linear embeddings. Firstly, a multiscale family of spectral kernels for shapes is introduced. It goes beyond existing work on the Laplace spectrum (shape DNA, WESD) by endowing the space of objects with an inner product structure. This is required for many widespread statistical analysis algorithms. Secondly a probabilistic mixture of kernel space PCA is designed, working out technicalities stemming from the infinite dimensionality. We experimented with supervised and unsupervised clustering tasks on the Leaf Shapes data, on sub-cortical brain structures and left ventricles from the LPBA40 and Sunnybrook cardiac datasets respectively.

References

1. Archambeau, C., Verleysen, M.: Robust Bayesian clustering. Neural Netw. **20**(1), 129–138 (2007)
2. Belongie, S., Malik, J., Puzicha, J.: Shape matching and object recognition using shape contexts. IEEE Trans. Pattern. Anal. Mach. Intell. **24**(4), 509–522 (2002)
3. Bronstein, A.M., Bronstein, M.M., Guibas, L.J., Ovsjanikov, M.: Shape google: geometric words and expressions for invariant shape retrieval. ACM Trans. Graph. **30**(1), 1 (2011)
4. Cootes, T.F., Taylor, C.J., Cooper, D.H., Graham, J.: Active shape models - their training and application. Comput. Vis. Image Underst **61**(1), 38–59 (1995)
5. Durrleman, S., Prastawa, M., Charon, N., Korenberg, J.R., Joshi, S., Gerig, G., Trouvé, A.: Morphometry of anatomical shape complexes with dense deformations and sparse parameters. Neuroimage **101**, 35–49 (2014)

6. Filippone, M., Camastra, F., Masulli, F., Rovetta, S.: A survey of kernel and spectral methods for clustering. Pattern Recognit. **41**(1), 176–190 (2008)
7. Fletcher, P.T., Lu, C., Pizer, S.M., Joshi, S.: Principal geodesic analysis for the study of nonlinear statistics of shape. IEEE TMI **23**(8), 995–1005 (2004)
8. Germanaud, D., Lefèvre, J., Toro, R., Fischer, C., Dubois, J., Hertz-Pannier, L., Mangin, J.F.: Larger is twistier: spectral analysis of gyrification (spangy) applied to adult brain size polymorphism. Neuroimage **63**(3), 1257–1272 (2012)
9. Gori, P., Colliot, O., Marrakchi-Kacem, L., Worbe, Y., Poupon, C., Hartmann, A., Ayache, N., Durrleman, S.: A Bayesian framework for joint morphometry of surface and curve meshes in multi-object complexes. Med. Image Anal. **35**, 458–474 (2017)
10. Grebenkov, D.S., Nguyen, B.T.: Geometrical structure of Laplacian eigenfunctions. SIAM Rev. **55**(4), 601–667 (2013)
11. Joshi, S., Pizer, S., Fletcher, P.T., Yushkevich, P., Thall, A., Marron, J.S.: Multiscale deformable model segmentation and statistical shape analysis using medial descriptions. IEEE Trans. Med. Imaging **21**(5), 538–550 (2002)
12. Konukoglu, E., Glocker, B., Criminisi, A., Pohl, K.M.: WESD-Weighted Spectral Distance for measuring shape dissimilarity. IEEE Trans. Pattern Anal. Mach. Intell. **35**(9), 2284–2297 (2013)
13. Konukoglu, E., Glocker, B., Ye, D.H., Criminisi, A., Pohl, K.M.: Discriminative segmentation based evaluation through shape dissimilarity. IEEE Trans. Med. Imaging **31**(12), 2278–2289 (2012)
14. Lombaert, H., Arcaro, M., Ayache, N.: Brain transfer: spectral analysis of cortical surfaces and functional maps. In: Ourselin, S., Alexander, D.C., Westin, C.-F., Cardoso, M.J. (eds.) IPMI 2015. LNCS, vol. 9123, pp. 474–487. Springer, Cham (2015). doi:10.1007/978-3-319-19992-4_37
15. Myronenko, A., Song, X.: Point set registration: coherent point drift. IEEE Trans. Pattern Anal. Mach. Intell. **32**(12), 2262–2275 (2010)
16. Niethammer, M., Reuter, M., Wolter, F.-E., Bouix, S., Peinecke, N., Koo, M.-S., Shenton, M.E.: Global medical shape analysis using the Laplace-Beltrami spectrum. In: Ayache, N., Ourselin, S., Maeder, A. (eds.) MICCAI 2007. LNCS, vol. 4791, pp. 850–857. Springer, Heidelberg (2007). doi:10.1007/978-3-540-75757-3_103
17. Ovsjanikov, M., Ben-Chen, M., Solomon, J., Butscher, A., Guibas, L.: Functional maps: a flexible representation of maps between shapes. ACM Trans. Graph. **31**(4), 30 (2012)
18. Radau, P., Lu, Y., Connelly, K., Paul, G., Dick, A., Wright, G.: Evaluation framework for algorithms segmenting short axis cardiac MRI. MIDAS **49** (2009)
19. Raviv, D., Bronstein, M.M., Bronstein, A.M., Kimmel, R.: Volumetric heat kernel signatures. In: ACM Workshop on 3D Object Retrieval, pp. 39–44. ACM (2010)
20. Reuter, M., Wolter, F.E., Peinecke, N.: Laplace-Beltrami spectra as Shape-DNA of surfaces and solids. Comput.-Aided Des. **38**(4), 342–366 (2006)
21. Shakeri, M., Lombaert, H., Datta, A.N., Oser, N., Létourneau-Guillon, L., Lapointe, L.V., Martin, F., Malfait, D., Tucholka, A., Lippé, S., Kadoury, S.: Statistical shape analysis of subcortical structures using spectral matching. Comput. Med. Imaging Graph. **52**, 58–71 (2016)
22. Shattuck, D.W., Mirza, M., Adisetiyo, V., Hojatkashani, C., Salamon, G., Narr, K.L., Poldrack, R.A., Bilder, R.M., Toga, A.W.: Construction of a 3D probabilistic atlas of human cortical structures. Neuroimage **39**(3), 1064–1080 (2008)
23. Tipping, M.E., Bishop, C.M.: Mixtures of probabilistic principal component analyzers. Neural Comput. **11**(2), 443–482 (1999)

24. Wachinger, C., Golland, P., Kremen, W., Fischl, B., Reuter, M., ADNI, et al.: Brainprint: a discriminative characterization of brain morphology. Neuroimage **109**, 232–248 (2015)
25. Weyl, H.: Das asymptotische Verteilungsgesetz der Eigenwerte linearer partieller Differentialgleichungen. Math. Ann. **71**(4), 441–479 (1912)
26. Zhang, M., Fletcher, P.T.: Bayesian principal geodesic analysis for estimating intrinsic diffeomorphic image variability. Med. Image Anal. **25**(1), 37–44 (2015)

Optimal Topological Cycles and Their Application in Cardiac Trabeculae Restoration

Pengxiang Wu[1], Chao Chen[2]([⌧]), Yusu Wang[3], Shaoting Zhang[4],
Changhe Yuan[2], Zhen Qian[5], Dimitris Metaxas[1], and Leon Axel[6]

[1] Rutgers University, New Brunswick, NY, USA
[2] CUNY Queens College, Flushing, NY, USA
`chao.chen@qc.cuny.edu`
[3] Ohio State University, Columbus, OH, USA
[4] University of North Carolina at Charlotte, Charlotte, NC, USA
[5] Piedmont Heart Institute, Atlanta, GA, USA
[6] NYU School of Medicine, New York, NY, USA

Abstract. In cardiac image analysis, it is important yet challenging to reconstruct the trabeculae, namely, fine muscle columns whose ends are attached to the ventricular walls. To extract these fine structures, traditional image segmentation methods are insufficient. In this paper, we propose a novel method to jointly detect salient topological handles and compute the optimal representations of them. The detected handles are considered hypothetical trabeculae structures. They are further screened using a classifier and are then included in the final segmentation. We show in experiments the significance of our contribution compared with previous standard segmentation methods without topological priors, as well as with previous topological method in which non-optimal representations of topological handles are used.

Keywords: Topology data analysis · Trabeculae · Cardiac · Segmentation · Homology localization

1 Introduction

The interior of a human cardiac ventricle is filled with fine structures including the papillary muscles and the *trabeculae*, i.e., muscle columns of various width whose both ends are attached to the ventricular wall (Fig. 1). Accurately capturing these fine structures is very important in understanding the functionality of human heart and in the diagnostic of cardiac diseases. These structures compose 23% of left ventricle (LV) end-diastolic volume in average and thus is critical in accurately estimating any volume-based metrics, e.g., ejection fraction (EF) and myocardial mass; these measures are critical in most cardiac disease diagnostics. A detailed interior surface model will also be the basis of a high quality ventricular flow simulation [10], which reveals deeper insight into the cardiac functionality of patients with diseases like hypokinesis and dyssynchrony.

M. Niethammer et al. (Eds.): IPMI 2017, LNCS 10265, pp. 80–92, 2017.
DOI: 10.1007/978-3-319-59050-9_7

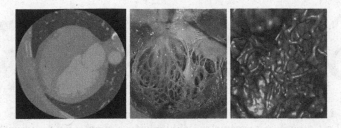

Fig. 1. Left: our input CT image. Middle: interior of LV [8]. Right: our result (a 3D triangle mesh) successfully captures the trabeculae (viewed from the valve).

With modern advanced imaging techniques, e.g., Computed Tomography (CT), we can capture details within cardiac ventricles (Fig. 1(left)). However, most state-of-the-art cardiac analysis methods [16,17], although very efficient, can not accurately capture these complex structures. The challenge is twofold. First, large variation of geometry and intensity of trabeculae makes it difficult to distinguish them from noise. Second, most segmentation models employ global priors, which tend to work against fine structures; the smoothness prior tends to simplify the model and thus remove any fine structures. The shape prior, e.g., the active shape model (ASM), tends to use an average shape and thus remove most fine-scale geometric details.

We exploit novel global information which is more suitable for the extraction of trabeculae, namely, the *topological prior*. A trabeculae is naturally a *topological handle*; both of its ends are attached to the wall, while the intermediate section is freely mobile. Gao *et al.* [9] proposed a topological method that explicitly computes topological handles which are salient compared with their surrounding regions. The saliency is measured based on the theory of *persistent homology* [7] and can be computed efficiently. These handles are further filtered using a classifier and are included in the final segmentation. However, this method fails to provide an ideal description of each detected handle. The generated non-optimal descriptions carry noisy geometric information and will hurt the performance of the classifier and segmentation module down the pipeline.

In this paper, we propose a new topological method that not only detects salient topological handles, but also finds the *ideal description* of each handle. Observe that at the end-diastole state, the heart is maximally relaxed and the trabeculae are maximally stretched out. Therefore, we argue that an ideal description of a topological handle should be geometrically concise; being generally straight rather than wiggling freely. Roughly speaking, a topological handle is an equivalent class of loops that can be continuously deformed into each other (Fig. 2(left)). Any of these loops can be used to represent the handle. We propose to compute the shortest one as it gives us the most concise description. In real data (Fig. 2), we observe that computing optimal loops generates straight trabeculae as desired (Fig. 2(right)), while previous topological method using non-optimal loops generates wiggling trabeculae (Fig. 2(middle-right)).

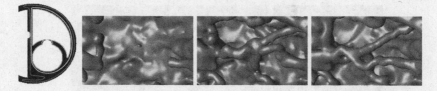

Fig. 2. Left: a topological handle and its representative cycles. The yellow one is the shortest and best describes its geometry. Middle-left: segmentation result without topological prior. Most trabeculae are missed due to the smoothness prior. Middle-right: result with topological prior but without optimal cycles [9]. The reconstructed trabeculae wiggles. Right: our result, using topological prior and optimal cycles generates straight trabeculae. (Color figure online)

Our technical contribution is threefold. First, we formulate a new optimization problem, i.e., for each salient topological handle detected by persistent homology theory, compute its best geometric description (the shortest cycle). Second, we prove a theorem (Theorem 1) as the foundation of the computation of the desired optimal cycles. An algorithm based on homology localization theory [1,2] is proposed accordingly. Third, we propose a new A* search strategy to solve the optimization problem efficiently in practice. The heuristic function of the search strategy is designed based on insights into the problem.

In the last step of our system, accurate geometric features from these optimal loops are used to select correct topological handles as trabeculae and to compute a high quality final segmentation. Figure 3 illustrates the pipeline of our topological method. We validate our method by comparing with segmentation without topological priors and the topological method without geometric optimization [9]. The ground truth of our data is acquired manually. See Sect. 4 for more details.

Contributions. Our contributions, i.e., the formulation and computation of optimal cycles of persistent homology classes, are also novel and important to the topology data analysis community. While many algorithms have been proposed to compute persistent homology [4,6], the computation of optimal cycles representing them have never been tackled. The methodology proposed in this paper will have broad applications in various persistent-homology-based data analytics [3,11,13,14].

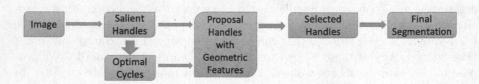

Fig. 3. The flow of our method.

2   Background

Within this paper, we assume the image domain, $\Omega \subseteq \mathbb{R}^3$, is discretized into a cubical complex, K_Ω, i.e., a collection of vertices, edges, squares and cubes. Each vertex corresponds to the center of a voxel. Each edge connects adjacent vertices. Squares are convex hulls of adjacent four vertices. Cubes are convex hulls of adjacent eight vertices. Any portion of the image domain can be approximated by a subcomplex $K \subseteq K_\Omega$. In particular, we are interested in a *sublevel set*, i.e., the part whose image value is no greater than a given threshold, $f_t^{-1} = \{x \in \Omega \mid f(x) \le t\}$, in which $f : \Omega \to \mathbb{R}$ is the image (intensity) function. A sublevel set can be approximated as the complex, $K_t \subseteq K_\Omega$, which includes all elements which fall completely within f_t^{-1}. See Fig. 4(a) for an example complex in 2D and one of its sublevel sets (at threshold 2.0). Different sublevel sets have different topology. Next, we introduce how the topology of a sublevel set K_t is defined. Afterwards, we introduce how topology of different sublevel sets are combined to recover the intrinsic structure of the image.

Homology. We focus on one-dimensional homology over $\mathbb{Z}_2$ field. For a general setting, please refer to a standard algebraic topology textbook [12]. Assume a given complex, K, we call its vertices, edges, squares and cubes the *0-*, *1-*, *2-* and *3-cells*. Any set of p-cells form a *p-chain*. Fixing an index of all p-cells, a p-chain can be written as an n_p dimensional binary vector, in which n_p is the number of p-cells in K. All p-chains constitute an n_p dimensional vector space over modulo-2 addition, called the *chain group*, denoted by $C_p(K)$. The boundary of a p-cell is a $(p{-}1)$-chain comprising all the $(p{-}1)$-cells bounding it. Putting the boundaries of all p-cells together form a $n_{p-1} \times n_p$ matrix called the p-th *boundary matrix*, denoted by ∂_p (Fig. 4(b) and (c)). The boundary of a p-chain, c, is the modulo-2 sum of all the boundaries of c's elements, and can be written as the product $\partial_p c$.

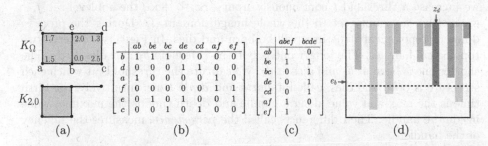

	ab	be	bc	de	cd	af	ef
b	1	1	1	0	0	0	0
d	0	0	0	1	1	0	0
a	1	0	0	0	0	1	0
f	0	0	0	0	0	1	1
e	0	1	0	1	0	0	1
c	0	0	1	0	1	0	0

	abef	bcde
ab	1	0
be	1	1
bc	0	1
de	0	1
cd	0	1
af	1	0
ef	1	0

(a)   (b)   (c)   (d)

Fig. 4. Computation of persistent homology. (a), a 2D cubical complex with given function values on all vertices. We also draw the sublevel set at value 2.0. (b) and (c), the boundary matrices of 1D and 2D, whose columns and rows are sorted according to the function value. (d), A schematic illustration of a reduced boundary matrix. The row and column of each pivot (red cross) give the coordinates of one persistence dot. (Color figure online)

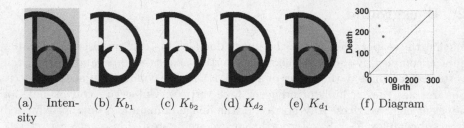

(a) Inten-   (b) K_{b_1} (c) K_{b_2} (d) K_{d_2} (e) K_{d_1} (f) Diagram
sity

Fig. 5. Sublevel sets in persistent homology. (a) Synthetic intensity function. (b)–(e) Sublevel sets at time $b_1 < b_2 < d_2 < d_1$. We also show the intensity inside the sublevel sets. (f) the persistence diagram, with two dots corresponding to the two handles. At time b_1 and b_2, the long handle and the short one are created. At time d_2 and d_1 the short handle and the long one are destroyed.

The set of all p-dimensional boundaries (p-boundaries), called the p-th boundary group, is the image of the $(p+1)$-th boundary operator, $\mathsf{B}_p(K) = \operatorname{im} \partial_{p+1}$.

A p-*cycle* is p-chain with zero boundary. The set of all p-cycles, called the *cycle group*, is the kernel of the boundary operator, $\mathsf{Z}_p(K) = \ker \partial_p$. A boundary is a cycle. But the opposite is not necessarily true. The boundary group is a subspace of the cycle group. The quotient space of the latter over the former is called the *homology group*, $\mathsf{H}_p := \mathsf{Z}_p/\mathsf{B}_p$. Each element in the homology group, called a *homology class*, is an equivalent class of cycles whose differences are boundaries of high-dimensional patches. Picking any element in a class h, $z_h \in h$, we can formally write h as $h := [z_h] = \{z_h + b \mid b \in \mathsf{B}_p\}$. In this case, we call z_h the *representative cycle* of h, and h the homology class of z_h.

Persistent Homology. Given an image function defined over the image domain Ω, simply selecting a single sublevel set and measuring its topology is insufficient. Instead, we need to jointly consider sublevel sets of all different thresholds. If we increase a threshold t continuously from $-\infty$ to $+\infty$, the sublevel set f_t^{-1} grows from an empty set to the whole image domain, Ω. During the process, different topological structures will be born and dies. In Fig. 5, we observe two topological handles. The longer one is born at threshold b_1 and dies at d_1. The shorter one is born at b_2 and dies at d_2. We capture the thresholds at which each structure is born and dies, called its *birth* and *death* time. Intuitively, the birth time is the maximal value along a handle and death time is the maximal value inside the handle. Their difference, called the *persistence*, measures the saliency of the handle.

These structures can be recorded as 2D dots, using their birth and death as the x and y coordinates. The persistence of a dot/structure is its distance from the diagonal ($x = y$). Figure 5(f) shows the point set, called the *persistence diagram*, of the function in Fig. 5(a). The theory of persistent homology [7] provides a principled definition of these topological structures and an efficient algorithm to detect all of them, in spite of their shapes and scales. The detected salient topological structures are provably robust to noise [5], and thus reveal intrinsic structures of the function. In general, a topological structure could be a connected component, a handle, or a void (a thickened sphere). In this paper, we focus on one-dimensional structures, i.e., handles.

Computation. Recall the sublevel sets of different thresholds are approximated by intermediate complexes $K_t \subseteq K_\Omega$. If we sort all rows and columns of the boundary matrices of K_Ω according to the function values of the corresponding cells, these sorted boundary matrices also encode the boundary operators of all intermediate complexes; the boundary matrices of any complex $K_t \subseteq K_\Omega$ are the upper-left submatrices of those of K_Ω. To compute the persistence homology, we reduce all boundary matrices of K_Ω using a column-wise Gaussian elimination with special constraints: no columns can be swapped and we only add columns from left to right. Finally, reading the pivot entries of the *reduced matrices* give us the persistence diagram; the row and column of each pivot entry correspond to the birth and death times of each dot in the persistence diagram. See Fig. 4(d) for an illustration of the reduced matrix. This algorithm has a cubical complexity, but is very efficient in practice.

3   Method

The overall flow of our method is illustrated in Fig. 3. First, we extract salient topological handles from the image based on the theory of persistent homology. Second, we compute optimal loops to represent salient handles. Geometric features are extracted from each optimal loop and are associated to the corresponding topological handle. The combined information is fed to a classifier which selects good handles. Finally, the selected handles are combined with standard image segmentation techniques to generate the final segmentation result.

It remain to solve the optimization problem for each topological handle. In Sect. 3.1, we formalize the problem. In Sect. 3.2, we explain an algorithm to solve the problem. This algorithm, although polynomial, is inefficient in both time and space. To develop a practical system, we propose an efficient A* search algorithm (Sect. 3.3). The heuristic function in the search is based on insights into the topological computation. Due to space constraints, some of the proofs are simplified or omitted. More details will be found in a technical report accompanying this paper.

3.1   Optimal Loops for Persistent Homology

We compute an optimal cycle to represent a topological handle detected by persistent homology, corresponding to a dot in the persistence diagram. Each handle corresponds to a family of homology classes that are created and destroyed at the same birth and death time. At the birth time, several homology classes are created, and only some of them are destroyed at the death time of the handle. We need to identify all these homology classes and find an optimal cycle representing either of them. This is different from a traditional homology localization problem [1,2], in which we compute the optimal cycle of a fixed homology class.

Problem 1 (Optimal Representative Cycle of a Persistence Dot). *Given a persistence dot $p = (b, d)$, compute the shortest element in the set of all cycles of K_b that are created at time b and become boundaries at time d.*

Next, we prove our main theorem (Theorem 1), which provides an algebraic formulation for the space of all representative cycles of a persistence dot, denoted by $RepCycles(p)$. This result is the foundation of the algorithms we propose in the following sections.

Denoted by $\widehat{\partial}_2$ the reduced 2D boundary matrix (Fig. 4(d)). Without loss of generality, we assume only one square has the function value d and one edge has the function value b, denoted as e_b. Let z_d be the corresponding column, whose pivot is at the row of e_b. Let Z_- be the matrix consisting of all columns before column z_d whose pivots are before e_b. Let Z_+ be the matrix consisting of all columns after d whose pivots are before e_b. In Fig. 4(d), we select a fixed dot and its corresponding column z_d (green). All orange columns form Z_- and all purple columns constitute Z_+. We have the following theorem.

Theorem 1 (Main). *The set of representative cycles of $p = (b, d)$ are the sum of z_d and linear combinations of columns in Z_-, formally, $RepCycles(p) = \{z_d + [Z_-]x, \forall x\}$.*

Proof. Since edge e_b is the only new edge in K_b, any new cycle created at b contains this edge. The following lemmas are straightforward.

Lemma 2. *Any cycle in $RepCycles(p)$ contains the edge e_b.*

Lemma 3. *When the image domain Ω is Euclidean and has trivial topology, columns $[Z_-, z_b, Z_+]$ constitute a basis of the cycles in complex K_b.*

Based on these lemmas, we prove our theorem as follows. The set of all columns in $[Z_-, z_d, Z_+]$ form a basis of all cycles of the complex K_b, $Z_1(K_b)$. Since all cycles created at time b has to contain the edge e_b, the space of all cycles of K_b created at time b are in the format of $z_d + [Z_-, Z_+]x$, $\forall x$. However, only columns in Z_- are on the left hand side of z_d, and thus are boundaries in K_d. Therefore, the cycles that are created at b and become boundaries at d are in the format of $z_d + [Z_-]x$, $\forall x$. □

For a more general case, when Ω is not trivial in topology, we can extend the lemma by adding additional columns corresponding to essential cycles, i.e., cycles representing the intrinsic topological handles of Ω.

3.2 OptTopoDij: The First Algorithm

In this section, we introduce our first algorithm to compute the optimal cycle within $RepCycles(p)$. Our algorithm is based on an algebraic annotation technique, which assigns all edges of a given complex different vectors. The annotation satisfies the property that if we walk along any cycle z and add up all the annotations of the edges, the sum immediately certifies whether the cycle belongs to the desired group of cycles $RepCycles(p)$. This technique provides the basis of an efficient algorithm to search through $RepCycles(p)$ for the optimal one despite its exponential size. First, we introduce the annotation technique in details.

Annotation. Let $g' = \text{card}(Z_-)$ and $g = \text{card}(Z_+)$ be the numbers of columns in Z_- and Z_+, respectively. Due to Lemma 3, any cycle of K_b can be written as a linear combination of columns of $Z = [Z_-, z_d, Z_+]$, formally, $z = [Z]\widehat{y_z}$. We call $\widehat{y_z}$ the *coordinate* of z w.r.t. the cycle basis Z. The length of $\widehat{y_z}$ is $g' + g + 1$. We are particularly interested in the coordinate of the cycle z w.r.t. z_d and Z_+. We call the last $g + 1$ entries of $\widehat{y_z}$ z's coordinate w.r.t. $[z_d, Z_+]$, or simply z's *coordinate*. Denote by y_z such coordinate.

Definition 1 (Annotation). *An annotation is a mapping from edges of K_b to $(g + 1)$-dimensional binary vectors, $\alpha : \mathcal{E}_{K_b} \to \mathbb{Z}_2^{g+1}$, satisfying the following property. For any cycle of K_b, z, summing the annotations of its edges gives the coordinate of z, formally, $\sum_{e \in z} \alpha(e) = y_z$. For any one-dimensional chain, whether it is a cycle or not, we say its annotation is the sum of the annotations of its edges, $\alpha(c) = \sum_{e \in c} \alpha(e)$.*

An annotation can be computed by the following algorithm. First, we compute a spanning tree of K_b, T. Any edge that does not belong to T, called a *sentinel edge*, form a unique cycle with the tree. We compute the coordinate of such cycle, z_e, by solving the equation $Zy = z_e$ and keeping the last $g + 1$ entries of the solution. Note that z_e is both a cycle and a binary vector in the reduced matrix $\widehat{\partial}_2$. The coordinate is used as the annotation of the corresponding sentinel edge, e. Any edge in the spanning tree has 0 annotation. Computing the annotations for all edges can be achieved in matrix multiplication time $O(n^\omega)$, in which n is the size of K_b. Now we are ready to introduce the main algorithm.

Algorithm. Our algorithm constructs a new graph $\widehat{\mathcal{G}}$ based on the given complex and the computed annotation, so that the optimal cycle problem is equivalent to the shortest path problem in the new graph $\widehat{\mathcal{G}}$, and thus can be solved using Dijkstra's algorithm.

Denote by $\mathcal{G} = (\mathcal{V}, \mathcal{E})$ the underlying graph of the subcomplex K_b. We construct a new graph, $\widehat{\mathcal{G}} = (\widehat{\mathcal{V}}, \widehat{\mathcal{E}})$ as follows. The vertices of the new graph is 2^{g+1} many copies of the original vertex set, $\widehat{\mathcal{V}} = \mathcal{V} \times \mathbb{Z}_2^{g+1}$. Vertices in each copy correspond to a different possible annotation. Next, we add 2^{g+1} copies of edges into the new graph as follows. For each edge (u, v) with annotation $\alpha(u, v)$ in $\mathcal{G}$, for each vertex $(u, \beta) \in \widehat{\mathcal{V}}$, we add an edge connecting (u, β) and $(v, \beta + \alpha(u, v))$.

Recall the $e_b = (u_b, v_b)$ is the new edge in K_b. By Lemma 2, all cycles in $RepCycles(p)$ contain e_b. The following theorem gives us an algorithm. The proof is omitted due to space constraints.

Theorem 4. *In graph $\widehat{\mathcal{G}}$, assign infinite weight to any copies of the critical edge e_b, $((u_b, *), (v_b, *))$, and weight one to all other edges. Computing the desired shortest cycle is equivalent to computing the shortest path from $(u_b, 0)$ to (v_b, β_0), in which β_0 is the annotation with one at the first entry and zero at the rest entries, $(1, 0, \cdots, 0)^T$.*

In summary, our algorithm is as follows. Compute edge annotations for all edges. Construct the graph $\widehat{\mathcal{G}}$ based on the annotations. In $\widehat{\mathcal{G}}$, compute the shortest path from $(u_b, 0)$ to (v_b, β_0) using Dijkstra's algorithm. The complexity is $O(n^\omega + 2^g g n \log n)$. Under certain mild assumptions, we can show that the algorithm is polynomial as g is upperbounded by a constant c_θ. More details can be found in the technical report.

3.3 OptTopoA*: An Improved Algorithm

Our algorithm, although polynomial, is exponential to the number of salient structures, c_θ. In particular, the constructed graph $\widehat{\mathcal{G}}$ has a size of $O(2^{c_\theta} n)$. The running time of the Dijkstra's algorithm on $\widehat{\mathcal{G}}$ is $O(c_\theta 2^{c_\theta} n \log n)$. In practice, both the time and space complexity can be too large when c_θ is relatively large.

In this section, we propose a heuristic search method to solve the problem more efficiently. We use the A* algorithm so that we do not have to explicitly construct the whole graph, $\widehat{\mathcal{G}}$, and explore all its vertices. Instead, we only exploit a vertex when necessary, based on a heuristic function. Although the worst case complexity is not better, an A* algorithm often leads to better performance in practice, given a well designed heuristic function.

Recall our goal is to find the shortest path from $\widehat{u_b} = (u_b, 0)$ to $\widehat{v_b} = (u_v, \beta_0)$ within the graph $\widehat{\mathcal{G}}$. At any intermediate vertex $\widehat{w}$, we have the cost of the partially completed path from $\widehat{u_b}$ to $\widehat{w}$, $\text{COST}(\widehat{w})$, and a heuristic function estimating the cost from $\widehat{w}$ to $\widehat{v_b}$, $\text{HEU}(\widehat{w})$. At every iteration, a new node with the minimal estimated total cost $\text{COST}(\widehat{w}) + \text{HEU}(\widehat{w})$ is selected and expanded, until the target $\widehat{v_b}$ is reached. A* is guaranteed to find the global optimum.

It remains to define a good heuristic function, $\text{HEU}(\widehat{w})$, which is a lowerbound of the true shortest distance between $\widehat{w}$ and the target $\widehat{v_b}$. Let β be the difference of the annotations of $\widehat{w}$ and $\widehat{v_b}$. The true shortest path from $\widehat{w}$ to $\widehat{v_b}$ is the shortest path connecting w and v_b under the constraint that its annotation is β. Formally, the true shortest distance from $\widehat{w}$ to $\widehat{v_b}$ is $\min_{\gamma \in \Gamma(w,v_b):\alpha(\gamma)=\beta} \text{card}(\gamma)$, in which $\Gamma(w, v_b)$ is the space of all paths connecting w and v_b in the original graph $\mathcal{G}$. Note that we are trying to avoid directly computing such distance. Instead, we approximate it using the following heuristic function.

$$\text{HEU}(\widehat{w}) = \max(\text{HEU}_1(\widehat{w}), \text{HEU}_2(\widehat{w}), \cdots, \text{HEU}_{g+1}(\widehat{w})), \text{ in which}$$
$$\text{HEU}_i(\widehat{w}) = \text{argmin}_{\gamma \in \Gamma(w,v_b):\alpha(\gamma)_i=\beta_i} \text{card}(\gamma).$$

Here $\alpha(\gamma)_i$ and β_i are the i-th entries of the annotation of γ and the difference annotation β, respectively. Intuitively, the cost of $\widehat{w}$ is the optimal length of paths from w to v_b with a fixed annotation β. We construct $g + 1$ heuristic function, $\text{HEU}_i(\widehat{w})$, each of which is the shortest distance with paths whose i-th bit annotation is equal to β_i. Since each such heuristic function is a lowerbound of the cost function, taking their maxima is still a valid heuristic and a tighter lowerbound of the cost function.

Finally, we explain how to compute these heuristic functions. For $\text{HEU}_i(\widehat{w})$, consider the set of all edges in the original graph $\mathcal{G}$ whose i-th bit annotation is one, called $\mathcal{E}_i$. A path, γ, has the i-th bit of its annotation being one if and only if it contains an odd number of edges from $\mathcal{E}_i$. So depending on whether β_i is one or zero, we compute the shortest path from w to v_b with either odd or even number of edges in $\mathcal{E}_i$. This can be achieved by constructing two copies of the original graph, G, and add an edge connecting vertices across copies if it belongs to $\mathcal{E}_i$ and connecting vertices within a same copy if it does not belong to $\mathcal{E}_i$. A Dijkstra's algorithm on this graph gives $\mathrm{HEU}_i(\widehat{w})$ as desired.

4   Experiments

We validate the proposed method on synthetic and real cardiac images. We compare two versions of our methods and two baselines: (1) *RegComp*: a classic segmentation method without topological prior, region competition [18]; (2) *NaiveTopo*: the naive topological method without optimal representative cycle computation [9]; (3) *OptTopoDij*: our topological method which computes the optimal representative cycles by constructing the graph $\widehat{\mathcal{G}}$ explicitly and running Dijkstra's algorithm; (4) *OptTopoA**: our topological method which computes the optimal cycle using A* search. RegComp is implemented in ITK-SNAP [15]. All other three are implemented using C++, and are run on a computer with Intel(R) Xeon(R) CPU E5-1660v3 and 32 GB RAM on Windows 8.1.

Synthetic Experiment 1: Non-optimal vs Optimal Cycles. We compute persistent homology of the synthetic image in Fig. 5(a) and generate cycles to represent the long handle. In Fig. 2(left), we show the cycles generated by the baseline topological method, NaiveTopo (in cyan color), and by our method OptTopoDij (in yellow). This example shows that the quality of generated cycle can be very unsatisfying without the proposed optimization algorithm.

Synthetic Experiment 2: Scalability. Having established the necessity of computing the optimal cycles. We show how important the A* search strategy is in practice. We run our two topological methods, OptTopoDij and OptTopoA*, on synthetic examples with increasing topological complexity, measured by the number of handles. To compute the optimal cycles, we need to construct the graph $\widehat{\mathcal{G}}$, whose size is exponential to the number of handles. In Fig. 6(a) and (b), we show the memory and time consumption of the two methods. See Fig. 6(c)

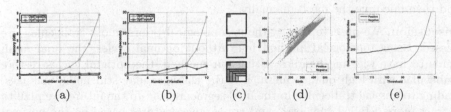

    (a)   (b)   (c)   (d)   (e)

Fig. 6. (a) and (b): memory and time of synthetic data with different numbers of handles. (c): three example input images with different numbers of handles. (d): the persistence diagram of a real heart image. (e): the relationship between the persistence threshold and accuracy.

for example input images (each has 400×400 pixels). While the expense of OptTopoDij increases exponentially as we increase the number of handles in the input image, the expense of OptTopoA* stays linear.

Real Experiments. We validate our method on a real patient dataset consisting of six cardiac CT images at the end-diastolic state ($512 \times 512 \times 320$ voxels with spacial resolution from 0.3 mm to 0.5 mm). For each image, we compute the persistence diagram (Fig. 6(d)) and then compute the optimal cycle for each salient persistence dot (persistence ≥ 80, see Fig. 6(e)). The running time is about seven minutes and the memory is about six to ten GB. This is about the same expense as the topological method without optimal cycle computation, thanks to the high efficiency of the A* search strategy.

After representative cycles of salient handles are extracted, their geometric features, e.g., birth time, death time, relative positions in the ventricle, etc., are used to train a linear SVM classifier, which selects the handles to be included in the final segmentation. We run a six-fold testing; use handles from five images for training and handles from the remaining image for testing, repeat for six times. The prediction accuracy of the classifier is $85.49\% \pm 5.25\%$. The prediction accuracy are similar for both NaiveTopo and OptTopoA*. The reason is the geometric features we are extracting are too simple. Therefore the geometric information of our optimal cycles are not fully leveraged.

However, the optimal cycles do improve our final segmentation quality as they avoid generating wiggling trabeculae. For each handle selected by the classifier, we add the corresponding cycles (thickened) into the standard segmentation result to generate the final mesh. We report the distance error of the result mesh from the ground truth. The performance of RegComp, NaiveTopo and OptTopoA* is reported below. See Figs. 2 and 7 for qualitative comparisons.

	RegComp	NaiveTopo	OptTopoA*
Distance from GT	0.1862 ± 0.7503	0.1258 ± 0.3810	0.0097 ± 0.1701

The ground truth of our data is extremely difficult to obtain. To train the classifier, we visually inspect each topological handle and decide whether it is a trabeculae based on the intensity function in the surrounding area. To obtain the ground truth mesh, we first use selected handles to generate the initial mesh, and then fine-tune the mesh manually.

Discussion. We observe that without topological priors, most trabeculae are missed. Using topological method but without optimal cycles, the final mesh tends to have wiggling handles. Using our method, the optimal cycles restore trabeculae with high quality mesh. But the classifier may still make mistakes, leading to missing trabeculae in the final segmentation. In the future, we plan to extract more detailed geometric and appearance features based on the optimal cycles, in order to further improve the classifier performance. Our ambitious goal is to develop general purpose topological features for the analysis of images of complex systems, e.g., cardiac trabeculae, neurons, cells, etc.

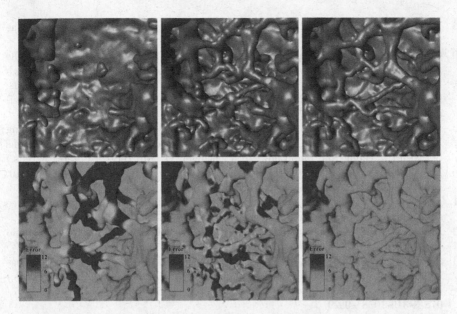

Fig. 7. Qualitative comparison. Top row: segmentation results of three methods, Reg-Comp, NaiveTopo and OptTopoA*. Bottom row: the distance from the ground truth to the segmentation result, rendered on the ground truth mesh. Blue regions are the parts of the ground truth mesh that are not captured by the algorithms. (Color figure online)

Acknowledgment. The research of Chao Chen is partially supported by the grants NSF PSC-CUNY 69844-00 47.

References

1. Busaryev, O., Cabello, S., Chen, C., Dey, T.K., Wang, Y.: Annotating simplices with a homology basis and its applications. In: Fomin, F.V., Kaski, P. (eds.) SWAT 2012. LNCS, vol. 7357, pp. 189–200. Springer, Heidelberg (2012). doi:10.1007/978-3-642-31155-0_17
2. Chen, C., Freedman, D.: Hardness results for homology localization. Discret. Comput. Geom. **45**(3), 425–448 (2011)
3. Chen, C., Freedman, D., Lampert, C.H.: Enforcing topological constraints in random field image segmentation. In: CVPR, pp. 2089–2096 (2011)
4. Chen, C., Kerber, M.: An output-sensitive algorithm for persistent homology. Comput. Geom. **46**(4), 435–447 (2013)
5. Cohen-Steiner, D., Edelsbrunner, H., Harer, J.: Stability of persistence diagrams. Discret. Comput. Geom. **37**(1), 103–120 (2007)
6. Dey, T.K., Fan, F., Wang, Y.: Computing topological persistence for simplicial maps. In: Proceedings of the Thirtieth Annual Symposium on Computational Geometry, p. 345. ACM (2014)
7. Edelsbrunner, H., Harer, J.: Computational Topology: An Introduction. American Mathematical Society, Providence (2010)

8. Ewing Jr., E.P.: Gross pathology of idiopathic cardiomyopathy – Wikipedia, the free encyclopedia (2016). Accessed 09 Dec 2016

9. Gao, M., Chen, C., Zhang, S., Qian, Z., Metaxas, D., Axel, L.: Segmenting the papillary muscles and the trabeculae from high resolution cardiac CT through Restoration of topological handles. In: Gee, J.C., Joshi, S., Pohl, K.M., Wells, W.M., Zöllei, L. (eds.) IPMI 2013. LNCS, vol. 7917, pp. 184–195. Springer, Heidelberg (2013). doi:10.1007/978-3-642-38868-2_16

10. Kulp, S., Gao, M., Zhang, S., Qian, Z., Voros, S., Metaxas, D., Axel, L.: Using high resolution cardiac CT data to model and visualize patient-specific interactions between trabeculae and blood flow. In: Fichtinger, G., Martel, A., Peters, T. (eds.) MICCAI 2011. LNCS, vol. 6891, pp. 468–475. Springer, Heidelberg (2011). doi:10.1007/978-3-642-23623-5_59

11. Li, Y., Ascoli, G., Mitra, P.P., Wang, Y.: Metrics for comparing neuronal tree shapes based on persistent homology. bioRxiv, p. 087551 (2016)

12. Munkres, J.R.: Elements of Algebraic Topology, vol. 2. Addison-Wesley, Menlo Park (1984)

13. Singh, N., Couture, H.D., Marron, J.S., Perou, C., Niethammer, M.: Topological descriptors of histology images. In: Wu, G., Zhang, D., Zhou, L. (eds.) MLMI 2014. LNCS, vol. 8679, pp. 231–239. Springer, Cham (2014). doi:10.1007/978-3-319-10581-9_29

14. Wong, E., Palande, S., Wang, B., Zielinski, B., Anderson, J., Fletcher, P.T.: Kernel partial least squares regression for relating functional brain network topology to clinical measures of behavior. In: 2016 IEEE 13th International Symposium on Biomedical Imaging (ISBI), pp. 1303–1306. IEEE (2016)

15. Yushkevich, P., Piven, J., Hazlett, H., Smith, R., Ho, S., Gee, J., Gerig, G.: User-guided 3D active contour segmentation of anatomical structures: significantly improved efficiency and reliability. Neuroimage 31(3), 1116–1128 (2006)

16. Zhen, X., Zhang, H., Islam, A., Bhaduri, M., Chan, I., Li, S.: Direct and simultaneous estimation of cardiac four chamber volumes by multioutput sparse regression. Med. Image Anal. 36, 184–196 (2017)

17. Zheng, Y., Barbu, A., Georgescu, B., Scheuering, M., Comaniciu, D.: Four-chamber heart modeling and automatic segmentation for 3D cardiac CT volumes using marginal space learning and steerable features. TMI 27(11), 1668–1681 (2008)

18. Zhu, S., Lee, T., Yuille, A.: Region competition: unifying snakes, region growing, energy/Bayes/MDL for multi-band image segmentation. In: ICCV, pp. 416–423, June 1995

From Label Maps to Generative Shape Models: A Variational Bayesian Learning Approach

Shireen Y. Elhabian$^{(\boxtimes)}$ and Ross T. Whitaker

School of Computing, University of Utah, Salt Lake City, UT, USA
{shireen,whitaker}@sci.utah.edu

Abstract. This paper proposes a Bayesian treatment of a latent variable model for learning generative shape models of grid-structured representations, aka *label maps*, that relies on direct probabilistic formulation with a variational approach for deterministic model learning. Spatial coherency and sparsity priors are incorporated to lend stability to the optimization problem, thereby regularizing the solution space while avoiding overfitting in this high-dimensional, low-sample-size scenario. Hyperparameters are estimated in closed-form using type-II maximum likelihood to avoid grid searches. Further, a *mixture* formulation is proposed to capture nonlinear shape variations in a way that balances the model expressiveness with the efficiency of learning and inference. Experiments show that the proposed model outperforms state-of-the-art representations on real datasets w.r.t. generalization to unseen samples.

Keywords: Shape models · Variational inference · Mixture modeling

1 Introduction

Statistical shape modeling has gained wide acceptance in medical imaging applications—*e.g.,* image segmentation [1], hypothesis testing [2], anatomical reconstruction [3], and pathology detection [4]—for representing variability within populations of similar anatomical shapes. Modeling shape variation is often posed as estimating a probability distribution from a set of *i.i.d.* training samples—treated as data points in a high-dimensional *shape space*—drawn from an unknown distribution. This paper focuses on learning generative shape models from grid-structured data that define a binary function over a discrete image domain, aka *label maps*. Learning shape models in the space of label maps is challenging because the space is a *unit hyper-cube* and lacks a vector space structure. Thus, the binary variables entail *non-Gaussian data likelihood*, which leads to intractable marginals and posteriors. The combination of *high-dimensional shape space* and limited training samples presents a risk of overfitting. *Hyperparameters* associated with model complexity often result in computationally expensive grid searches. Furthermore, nonlinear shape variation is often rendered as *multi-modal probability distributions*, which confound the many approaches that rely on

© Springer International Publishing AG 2017
M. Niethammer et al. (Eds.): IPMI 2017, LNCS 10265, pp. 93–105, 2017.
DOI: 10.1007/978-3-319-59050-9_8

Gaussian assumptions (*e.g.*, [5–7]). Nonparametric density estimates (*e.g.*, [8–10]) are promising, but have a ravenous appetite for training samples, posing serious challenges for the estimator robustness and generalization [11].

To handle non-Gaussian data likelihoods associated with label maps, most existing approaches have resorted to learning shape distributions *indirectly*, by representing shapes as level sets, and working in the space of continuous implicit functions, such as blurred label maps (*e.g.*, [6,12]) or signed distance maps (SDMs) (*e.g.*, [6,13]). These ad hoc embeddings lack a statistical interpretation w.r.t. the input label maps, which leads to suboptimal generative models and limits their ability to generalize to unseen data. On the other hand, learning shape variability *directly* on the label map space (*e.g.*, [14]) or a probabilistic label space (*e.g.*, [7]) using, for instance, principal component analysis (PCA) has no underlying generative model, and therefore does not benefit from associated tools for statistical estimation. Moreover, non-Bayesian dimensionality reduction techniques (*e.g.*, linear [5–7] and nonlinear [15]) rely on the maximum-likelihood estimation of the principal subspace, and thus ignore uncertainties associated with the estimated low-dimensional representation and are prone to overfitting in high-dimensional spaces with limited training samples [16]—a typical situation in medical applications. Recently, stochastic neural nets, in particular the shape Boltzmann machine (ShapeBM) [17], have been adopted to learn distributions over binary inputs without relying on any intermediate implicit representation. Nonetheless, these networks do not attempt to model a particular generative process, which requires an exponential number of hidden units and a large amount of training data to approximate an arbitrary binary distribution [18].

To capture nonlinearities or subpopulations, the distribution can be approximated using a finite *mixture* of Gaussians in which model estimation is often made tractable by working with a low-dimensional projection of the data (*e.g.*, [5,8]). Nonetheless, this global projection often collapses or mixes the subpopulations, which derails learning the mixture structure of the underlying shape space [11]. Nonlinearity of shape statistics can also be modeled by lifting training shapes to a higher dimensional feature (aka kernel) space, where the shape distribution is often assumed to be Gaussian (*e.g.*, [15]). However, this approach results in an infinite-dimensional optimization scheme and sacrifices the efficiency of optimizing in low-dimensional subspaces [8]. Further, one is then faced with finding the reverse mapping from feature space to shape space (aka preimage problem), which is often solved approximately.

In addressing the problem of modeling populations of label maps, this paper makes several contributions. *First*, it learns the generative model of a shape population directly in the label map space while not relying on ad hoc, implicit shape representations. *Second*, it proposes a *Bayesian* treatment of a latent variable model – ShapeOdds – as a low-dimensional *shape generating process*. *Third*, it extends recent works in the machine learning literature on variational bounds of logistic-Gaussian integrals designed to circumvent the intractable marginal likelihood and latent posterior leading to *deterministic* learning. *Fourth*, it presents a variational formulation that further reduces the sensitivity to hyperparameters by modeling posterior uncertainties. *Fifth*, it automatically estimates model hyperparameters—with closed-form re-estimation expressions—without the need for discrete searches and cross-validation. *Sixth*, it learns complex shape distributions directly in the high-dimensional shape space as a *mixture* of ShapeOdds models to balance the tradeoff between the model expressiveness with the efficiency of learning and inference without resorting to a global projection of training samples onto a low-dimensional linear subspace. By considering a probabilistic mixture of a latent variable model, we obtain a soft partitioning of the high-dimensional data space that requires only a few parameters for each mixture component and reduces the associated risk of overfitting. Experiments demonstrate that ShapeOdds and its mixture variant compare favorably with several different technologies for state-of-art shape modeling.

2   Latent Gaussian Model for Label Maps

Consider a raster defined over a spatial domain $\Omega \subset \mathbb{R}^d$ $(d = 2, 3)$ containing D pixels. An object $\omega \subset \Omega$ is represented as a *label map* $\mathbf{f} \in \{0, 1\}^D$, where $\mathbf{f}(\mathbf{x}) = 1$, iff $\mathbf{x} \in \omega \;\; \forall \; \mathbf{x} \in \Omega$. In a *generative* sense, $\mathbf{f}$ is a realization of a *spatially correlated* field of D *Bernoulli* random variables defined on Ω with a pixelwise *parameter* $\mathbf{q}(\mathbf{x}) \in [0, 1]$ where $\mathbf{q}(\mathbf{x}) = p(\mathbf{x} \in \omega)$. Spatial regularity on the label maps, typically modeled as Markov random fields (MRFs), helps describe local correlations between nearby label values. The Bernoulli likelihood has an equivalent form in terms of the *exponential family distributions* that is parameterized by a field of real values $\phi(\mathbf{x}) \in \mathbb{R}$, known as *natural parameters* (or LogOdds), where $\phi(\mathbf{x}) = \mathrm{logit}[\mathbf{q}(\mathbf{x})]$ with $\mathbf{q}(\mathbf{x})$ being the first moment of this form and hence denoted as *expectation* parameters. The merit in considering such an equivalence is casting any parameter estimation problem as an *unconstrained* optimization in the natural parameter space. Hence, the *generative model* of a label map includes a pixelwise Bernoulli likelihood and the MRF spatial prior.

$$p(\mathbf{f}|\phi) = \left\{ \prod_{\mathbf{x} \in \Omega} \underbrace{\exp\left[\mathbf{f}(\mathbf{x})\phi(\mathbf{x}) - \mathrm{llp}[\phi(\mathbf{x})]\right]}_{p(\mathbf{f}(\mathbf{x})|\phi(\mathbf{x}))} \right\} \times \frac{1}{Z} \exp\left(-\frac{1}{T} U(\mathbf{f})\right) \qquad (1)$$

where $\mathrm{llp}[\phi] = \log\left(1 + e^{\phi}\right)$ is the *logistic-log-partition* function, $U(\mathbf{f})$ are clique potentials that favor spatially coherent silhouettes, Z is a Gibbs distribution normalization constant, and T is its temperature. Learning a probability distribution over the label map space amounts to estimating the corresponding expectation parameters map $\mathbf{q}$ or equivalently the natural parameters (*i.e.*, LogOdds) map ϕ. Here, we coin the term *ShapeOdds* to refer to a data-driven estimation of *LogOdds* that places label maps in a vector space where global *shape* variation is taken into account in a statistically principled manner.

Consider an unknown *shape distribution* $p(\mathbf{f})$ in the label map space $\mathcal{F}$, of which we have only a finite ensemble $\mathrm{F} = \{\mathbf{f}_n\}_{n=1}^N \subset \mathcal{F}$. In the general case, let

$p(\mathbf{f})$ be a multimodal distribution that is comprised of $K-$mixture components. In latent variable formalism, the distribution of the $k-$th component is governed by a low-dimensional *shape-generating process* – ShapeOdds – of L_k independent latent variables $\mathbf{z}^k \in \mathbb{R}^{L_k}$ where $L_k \ll D$. A label map $\mathbf{f}$ is also associated with a latent binary indicator $\mathbf{y} \in \{0,1\}^K$ that indicates the identity of the mixture component responsible for generating $\mathbf{f}$ where $\mathbf{1}_K^T \mathbf{y} = 1$. Here we consider a class of latent Gaussian models (LGMs). In particular, the $k-$th component is drawn according to the mixing coefficients $p(\mathbf{y}^k = 1) = \pi_k$ where $\boldsymbol{\pi} \in [0,1]^K$ and $\mathbf{1}_K^T \boldsymbol{\pi} = 1$. A point $\mathbf{z}^k$ in the $k-$th *latent factor space* $\mathcal{Z}_k$ is then *generated* according to a Gaussian prior $p(\mathbf{z}^k) = \mathcal{N}(\mathbf{z}^k; \boldsymbol{\mu}_k, \boldsymbol{\Sigma}_k)$, where $\boldsymbol{\mu}_k \in \mathbb{R}^{L_k}$ and $\boldsymbol{\Sigma}_k \in \mathbb{R}^{L_k \times L_k}$, which is mapped to $\boldsymbol{\phi}^k$ in the natural parameter space $\mathcal{P} \subset \mathbb{R}^D$ by a smooth mapping $h_k : \mathcal{Z}_k \to \mathcal{P}$. The logit function further maps $\mathcal{P}$ to the expectation parameter space $\mathcal{Q} \subset [0,1]^D$. A natural parameter map $\boldsymbol{\phi}^k \in \mathbb{R}^D$ is assumed to be confined to a linear subspace in $\mathcal{P}$ parameterized by a component-specific *factor loading* matrix $\mathbf{W}^k \in \mathbb{R}^{D \times L_k}$ and an *offset* vector $\mathbf{w}_0^k \in \mathbb{R}^D$ where $\boldsymbol{\phi}^k = h_k(\mathbf{z}^k) = \mathbf{W}^k \mathbf{z}^k + \mathbf{w}_0^k$. A $\boldsymbol{\phi}^k-$map thus induces a distribution $p(\mathbf{f}|\boldsymbol{\phi}^k)$ of label maps in $\mathcal{F}$. The corresponding $\boldsymbol{\phi}^k-$maps of F, although they lie in a linear subspace in $\mathcal{P}$, typically correspond to a nonlinear manifold in $\mathcal{F}$. To alleviate overfitting and penalize highly irregular mappings h_k, we introduce a Gaussian MRF (GMRF) smoothness prior over loading/offset vectors $\{\mathbf{w}_l^k\}_{l=0}^L$ where the prior on the mapping h_k can be factored out as $p(\mathbf{W}^k, \mathbf{w}_0^k) = \prod_{l=0}^{L_k} p(\mathbf{w}_l^k | \lambda_l^k)$. The smoothness prior over a vector $\mathbf{w}_l^k$ is expressed as a Gibbs distribution, $p(\mathbf{w}_l^k | \lambda_l^k) \propto \exp\{-\lambda_l^k E(\mathbf{w}_l^k)\}$ where $\lambda_l^k > 0$ is a hyperparameter that controls the generalizability aspect of the resultant mapping. We use Laplacian-square energy to favor smooth vectors by penalizing abrupt edges.

The intrinsic dimensionality of the component-specific latent space $\mathcal{Z}_k$ is determined by the choice of $L_k \ \forall k \in \{1, \ldots, K\}$. Nonetheless, an exhaustive grid search over this choice becomes computationally intractable in mixture modeling, because each component would have a different L_k. The probabilistic formulation of LGMs allows this discrete model selection to be handled within the Bayesian paradigm. We make use of the sparsity-inducing automatic relevance determination (ARD) prior to further regularize the solution space via a parameterized data-driven prior distribution that effectively prunes away irrelevant factors of variations [19]. We introduce an ARD prior on the loading vectors $\{\mathbf{w}_l^k\}_{l=1}^{L_k}$ with L_k set to the maximum allowed dimensionality, *i.e.*, $L_k = N - 1$ and $N \ll D$. ARD is a zero-mean isotropic Gaussian prior parameterized by $\beta_l^k \in \mathbb{R}_{>0}$ such that $p(\mathbf{w}_l^k | \beta_l^k) = \mathcal{N}(\mathbf{w}_l^k; \mathbf{0}_D, (\beta_l^k)^{-1} \mathbf{I}_D)$ where $\mathbf{0}_D$ and $\mathbf{I}_D$ are the zero vector and identity matrix in $\mathbb{R}^D$, respectively. During the learning process, $\beta_l^k \to \infty$ for irrelevant factors to remove the unnecessary complexity of the resulting model. Thus, a mixture of *ShapeOdds* refers to the shape-generating process with model parameters $\Theta = \{\Theta_k\}_{k=1}^K$ and priors hyperparameters $\Psi = \{\Psi_k\}_{k=1}^K$. The parameters of the $k-$th ShapeOdds are $\Theta_k = \{\pi_k, \boldsymbol{\mu}_k, \boldsymbol{\Sigma}_k, \mathbf{W}^k, \mathbf{w}_0^k\}$, and its hyperparameters are $\Psi_k = \{\boldsymbol{\lambda}^k, \boldsymbol{\beta}^k\}$ where $\boldsymbol{\lambda}^k \in \mathbb{R}_{>0}^{L_k+1}$ and $\boldsymbol{\beta}^k \in \mathbb{R}_{>0}^{L_k}$. The generative process can be defined as follows where $\mathbf{S}$ is the matrix containing the stencil of the negative bi-Laplacian operator; the first variation of $E(\mathbf{w})$.

$$\mathbf{y}_n|\Theta \sim \text{Cat}[K, \boldsymbol{\pi}], \quad \mathbf{z}_n^k|\Theta_k \sim \mathcal{N}(\boldsymbol{\mu}_k, \boldsymbol{\Sigma}_k), \quad \mathbf{f}_n|\mathbf{z}_n^k, \Theta_k \sim \text{Expon}[\boldsymbol{\phi}_n^k]\,\text{Mrf}[\nu] \tag{2}$$

$$\text{Expon}[\boldsymbol{\phi}_n^k] \doteq \prod_{\mathbf{x}\in\Omega} \text{Expon}[\boldsymbol{\phi}_n^k(\mathbf{x})], \quad \boldsymbol{\phi}_n^k = \mathbf{W}^k\mathbf{z}_n^k + \mathbf{w}_0^k, \tag{3}$$

$$\mathbf{w}_0^k|\lambda_0^k \sim \text{GMrf}[\lambda_0^k], \mathbf{w}_l^k|\lambda_l^k, \beta_l^k \sim \text{GMrf}[\lambda_l^k]\,\text{Ard}[\beta_l^k], \text{GMrf}[\lambda] \doteq \mathcal{N}(\mathbf{0}_D, \lambda^{-1}\mathbf{S}) \tag{4}$$

The MRF prior in (2), whose hyperparameter $\nu > 0$ is related to the temperature in (1), reflects the spatial regularity of the given label maps. Note that the choice of ν does not affect the model learning process. Equation (3) is due to the axiom of local/conditional independence, *i.e.*, the observed variables are conditionally independent given the latent variables, where $\text{Expon}[\boldsymbol{\phi}(\mathbf{x})]$ is given by (1).

3   Model Variational Learning

Consider a set of *i.i.d.* label maps $\mathbf{F} = \{\mathbf{f}_n\}_{n=1}^N$. The corresponding *discrete* latent indicator variables are denoted as $\mathbf{Y} = \{\mathbf{y}_n\}_{n=1}^N$. The component-specific *continuous* latent factor variables $Z_k = \{\mathbf{z}_n^k\}_{n=1}^N$ define the low-dimensional representation w.r.t. the $k-$th generating mixture component. The *marginal likelihood* of $\mathbf{F}$ under the mixture model can be formulated as a marginalization over the latent indicator and factor variables.

$$p(\mathbf{F}|\Theta) = \prod_{n=1}^N \sum_{k=1}^K \int_{\mathcal{Z}_k} p(\mathbf{f}_n|\mathbf{z}_n^k, \Theta_k)p(\mathbf{z}_n^k|\Theta_k)p(\mathbf{y}_n^k = 1|\Theta)d\mathbf{z}_n^k \tag{5}$$

Let $q(\mathbf{y}_n^k = 1, \mathbf{z}_n^k) = q(\mathbf{z}_n^k|\mathbf{y}_n^k = 1)q(\mathbf{y}_n^k = 1)$ be the approximate variational distribution of $k-$th component latent variables. The *lower bound* to the log-marginal likelihood can thus be obtained by dividing and multiplying by the posterior approximate and then applying the Jensen inequality.

$$\mathcal{L}(\Theta) \geq \underline{\mathcal{L}}^J(\Theta) = \sum_{k=1}^K q(\mathbf{y}_n^k = 1)\left\{ \log \frac{p(\mathbf{y}_n^k = 1|\Theta)}{q(\mathbf{y}_n^k = 1)} \right.$$
$$\left. + \sum_{n=1}^N \left(\mathbb{E}_{q(\mathbf{z}_n^k|\mathbf{y}_n^k=1)}\left[\log \frac{p(\mathbf{z}_n^k|\Theta_k)}{q(\mathbf{z}_n^k|\mathbf{y}_n^k = 1)} \right] + \mathbb{E}_{q(\mathbf{z}_n^k|\mathbf{y}_n^k=1)}\left[\log p(\mathbf{f}_n|\mathbf{z}_n, \Theta) \right] \right) \right\} \tag{6}$$

The variational distributions $q(.)$ that would tighten the Jensen lower bound in (6) should satisfy $\partial\underline{\mathcal{L}}^J(\Theta)/\partial q(.) = 0$. Under variational Bayes with exponential family distribution data likelihood, the variational latent factor posterior follows the same family as the factor prior, *i.e.*, Gaussian, leading to a tractable integral. Hence, $q(\mathbf{z}_n^k|\gamma_n^k) = \mathcal{N}(\mathbf{z}_n^k|\mathbf{m}_n^k, \mathbf{V}_n^k)$, where $\gamma_n^k = \{\mathbf{m}_n^k, \mathbf{V}_n^k\}$, is a Gaussian approximate to the factor posterior with mean $\mathbf{m}_n^k \in \mathbb{R}^{L_k}$ and covariance $\mathbf{V}_n^k \in \mathbb{R}^{L_k \times L_k}$. The *first expectation* term in (6) is the negative Kullback-Leibler (KL) divergence that pushes the variational posterior $q(\mathbf{z}_n^k|\mathbf{y}_n^k = 1)$ to the respective Gaussian prior $p(\mathbf{z}_n^k|\Theta_k)$. Its closed form is given by

$$-\text{KL}_{\mathbf{z}_n^k|\mathbf{y}_n^k} = \frac{1}{2}\left\{ \log |\mathbf{V}_n^k\boldsymbol{\Sigma}_k^{-1}| - \text{Tr}[\mathbf{V}_n^k\boldsymbol{\Sigma}_k^{-1}] - (\mathbf{m}_n^k - \boldsymbol{\mu}_k)^T\boldsymbol{\Sigma}_k^{-1}(\mathbf{m}_n^k - \boldsymbol{\mu}_k) + L_k \right\}$$

Taking the functional derivative of $\underline{\mathcal{L}}^J(\Theta)$ w.r.t. $q(\mathbf{y}_n^k = 1)$ and equating to zero, the variational posterior for the latent indicator variables can be written as

$$\log q(\mathbf{y}_n^k = 1) = \log p(\mathbf{y}_n^k = 1|\Theta) + \mathbb{E}_{q(\mathbf{z}_n^k|\mathbf{y}_n^k=1)}\left[\log\left\{p(\mathbf{z}_n^k|\Theta_k)/q(\mathbf{z}_n^k|\mathbf{y}_n^k=1)\right\}\right]$$
$$+ \mathbb{E}_{q(\mathbf{z}_n^k|\mathbf{y}_n^k=1)}\left[\log p(\mathbf{f}_n|\mathbf{z}_n, \Theta)\right] + \text{const} \qquad (7)$$

The distribution in (7) does not admit to a well-known distribution of a closed-form especially with the second intractable term. Nonetheless, we only care about the relative aspect of the indicator variables. Hence, we typically compute $\log q(\mathbf{y}_n^k = 1)$ based on the current model and factor variational parameters and then normalize the distribution such that $\sum_{k=1}^{K} q(\mathbf{y}_n^k = 1) = 1$. The first term in (6) is thus the negative KL divergence that pushes the indicator variational posterior to the respective component prior, $i.e.$, $-\text{KL}_{\mathbf{y}_n^k} = \log \pi_k - \log q(\mathbf{y}_n^k = 1)$ where $p(\mathbf{y}_n^k = 1|\Theta) = \pi_k$. The $second\ expectation$ term in (6) can be expressed in the natural parameter space $\mathcal{P}$ according to the mapping $h_k(\mathbf{z}^k)$ and the conditional independence in (3), in which the Gaussian approximate posterior $q(\mathbf{z}_n^k|\mathbf{y}_n^k = 1)$ in $\mathcal{Z}_k$ induces a per-pixel Gaussian posterior $q(\phi_n^k(\mathbf{x})|\widetilde{\gamma}_n^k(\mathbf{x}))$ in $\mathcal{P}$ with $\widetilde{\gamma}_n^k(\mathbf{x}) = \{\widetilde{\mathbf{m}}_n^k(\mathbf{x}), \widetilde{\mathbf{V}}_n^k(\mathbf{x})\}$ where $\mathbf{w}_0^k(\mathbf{x}) \in \mathbb{R}$ and $\mathbf{W}^k(\mathbf{x}) \in \mathbb{R}^{L_k}$.

$$\widetilde{\mathbf{m}}_n^k(\mathbf{x}) = \mathbf{W}^k(\mathbf{x})\mathbf{m}_n^k + \mathbf{w}_0^k(\mathbf{x}), \quad \widetilde{\mathbf{V}}_n^k(\mathbf{x}) = \mathbf{W}^k(\mathbf{x})\mathbf{V}_n^k[\mathbf{W}^k(\mathbf{x})]^T \qquad (8)$$

Note that the spatial coherency is still promoted through the GMRF prior on the offset and loading vectors. Using the exponential form of the Bernoulli likelihood in (1), the $second\ expectation$ term in (6) can be expressed in $\mathcal{P}$ as

$$\sum_{\mathbf{x}\in\Omega}\left\{\mathbf{f}_n(\mathbf{x})\widetilde{\mathbf{m}}_n^k(\mathbf{x}) - \mathbb{E}_{q(\phi_n^k(\mathbf{x})|\widetilde{\gamma}_n^k(\mathbf{x}))}\left[\text{llp}[\phi_n^k(\mathbf{x})]\right]\right\} \qquad (9)$$
$$\geq \sum_{\mathbf{x}\in\Omega}\underline{\mathcal{B}}_n^k(\mathbf{x}) := \left\{\mathbf{f}_n(\mathbf{x})\widetilde{\mathbf{m}}_n^k(\mathbf{x}) - \overline{\mathcal{B}}(\widetilde{\gamma}_n^k(\mathbf{x}), \alpha_n^k(\mathbf{x}))\right\} \qquad (10)$$

Eq. (9) is intractable due to the llp function and can be lower-bounded in $\mathcal{P}$−space by defining an upper bound $\overline{\mathcal{B}}$ for the expectation of the llp function with $local$, $i.e.$, per-pixel, variational parameters $\alpha_n^k(\mathbf{x})$. To avoid the recomputation of per-pixel/per-component/per-sample $\alpha_n^k(\mathbf{x})$, we use a $fixed$ piecewise quadratic upper bound for the llp function recently proposed in [20] as a proven tight bound compared to other quadratic bounds, where $\alpha_n^k(\mathbf{x}) = \alpha \; \forall \; n, k, \mathbf{x}$ are optimized in advance via a minimax optimization to ensure a tight bound. The upper bound $\overline{\mathcal{B}}$ can thus be expressed in terms of truncated Gaussian moments, due to the approximate Gaussian posterior, whose closed-form expressions along with their gradients are available [20]. The new bound reads as

$$\underline{\mathcal{L}}(\Theta, \gamma, \alpha) = \sum_{n=1}^{N}\sum_{k=1}^{K}\underbrace{q(\mathbf{y}_n^k = 1)\left\{-\text{KL}_{\mathbf{y}_n^k} - \text{KL}_{\mathbf{z}_n^k|\mathbf{y}_n^k} + \sum_{\mathbf{x}\in\Omega}\underline{\mathcal{B}}_n^k(\mathbf{x})\right\}}_{\underline{\mathcal{L}}_n^k(\Theta_k, \gamma_n^k, \alpha)} \qquad (11)$$

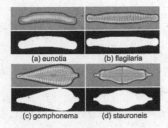

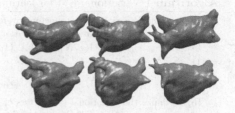

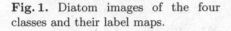

Fig. 1. Diatom images of the four classes and their label maps.

Fig. 2. LA training samples: (top) superior and (bottom) posterior-anterior views.

We propose a variational expectation-maximization (EM) algorithm that optimizes the rigorous lower bound defined in (11). The E-step in (13) optimizes the variational indicator and factor posterior distributions at an iteration i given the current guess of model parameters $\Theta^{(i-1)}$. The M-step chooses the next guess of $\Theta^{(i)}$ to maximize the *regularized* variational bound in (17). Iterating between these two steps involves concave optimizations due to the concavity of the lower bound in (11) [20] and the semipositive definiteness of the bi-Laplacian operator, for which we can use gradient-based optimization (see Algorithm 1 for gradient expressions). The maximum-a-posteriori (MAP) objective of the offset and loading vectors, after removing constant terms, can be written as in (22). The first variation of (22) reads as in (23) and (24): the vectors $\mathbf{g}_n^{\mathbf{m},k}$ and $\mathbf{G}_n^{\mathbf{V},k}$ are bound gradients in (16), $\odot$ refers to a Hadamard product, $\mathbf{m}_{n,l}^k$ is the $l-$th entry of $\mathbf{m}_n^k$, and $\mathbf{V}_{n,l}^k$ is the $l-$th column of $\mathbf{V}_n^k$. To enable large time steps Δt while maintaining stable updates, we use a *semi-implicit scheme* with finite-forward time marching to define iterative updates for $\mathbf{w}_l^k$'s in (26), where spatial convolution $\otimes$ can be efficiently performed as multiplication in the Fourier domain.

Hyperparameters: To complete our Bayesian treatment, we formulate a type-II maximum likelihood estimate, in which we marginalize over Ψ_k for each mixture component. We consider a Jeffrey, *i.e.*, noninformative, prior for λ_l^k and β_l^k where $p(\lambda_l^k) \propto 1/\lambda_l^k$ and $p(\beta_l^k) \propto 1/\beta_l^k$, respectively. The marginalization over the hyperparameters involves λ_l^k-integrals and β_l^k-integrals, each with an analytic form $\frac{\Gamma(D/2)|\mathbf{S}|^{1/2}}{\pi^{D/2}[(\mathbf{w}_l^k)^T\mathbf{S}\mathbf{w}_l^k]^{D/2}}$ and $\frac{\Gamma(D/2)|\mathbf{S}|^{1/2}}{\pi^{D/2}[(\mathbf{w}_l^k)^T\mathbf{w}_l^k]^{D/2}}$, respectively, using a $\Gamma-$function integral form. For a given Ψ_k, the gradient of $\log p(\Theta_k|\Psi_k)$ w.r.t. $\mathbf{w}_l^k$ should coincide with that of the marginal $p(\Theta_k)$ [21]. Hence, the effective values of the hyperparameters in (30) re-estimate Ψ_k after each pair of E- and M-steps to compute the new Ψ_k given the current guess of Θ_k.

Algorithm 1 Variational EM for learning mixture of ShapeOdds

E-Step: Optimize variational parameters given the current model parameters.
(a) Compute the variational distributions of the indicator variables, *i.e.*, $q(\mathbf{y}_n^k = 1)$, $\forall n \in \{1, .., N\}$ and $k \in \{1, ..., K\}$ such that $\sum_{k=1}^{K} q(\mathbf{y}_n^k = 1) = 1$ using $\Theta^{(i-1)}$ and $\gamma_n^{k^{(i-1)}}$ where

$$\log q(\mathbf{y}_n^k = 1) = \pi_k^{(i-1)} - \mathrm{KL}_{\mathbf{z}_n^k | \mathbf{y}_n^k} + \sum_{\mathbf{x} \in \Omega} \underline{\mathcal{B}}_n^k(\mathbf{x}) \quad (12)$$

(b) Optimize the variational parameters of the latent factors approximate posterior, *i.e.*, $q(\mathbf{z}_n^k | \mathbf{y}_n^k = 1)$, $\forall n \in \{1, .., N\}$ and $k \in \{1, ..., K\}$.

$$\gamma_n^{k^{(i)}} = \mathrm{argmax}_{\gamma_n^k} \underline{\mathcal{L}}_n^k(\Theta_k^{(i-1)}, \gamma_n^k, \alpha) \quad (13)$$

$$\frac{\partial \underline{\mathcal{L}}_n^k}{\partial \mathbf{m}_n^k} = q(\mathbf{y}_n^k = 1) \left\{ -\Sigma_k^{-1}(\mathbf{m}_n^k - \mu_k) + \sum_{\mathbf{x} \in \Omega} g_n^{\mathbf{m},k}(\mathbf{x})[\mathbf{W}^k(\mathbf{x})]^T \right\} \quad (14)$$

$$\frac{\partial \underline{\mathcal{L}}_n^k}{\partial \mathbf{V}_n^k} = q(\mathbf{y}_n^k = 1) \left\{ \frac{1}{2} \left[(\mathbf{V}_n^k)^{-1} - \Sigma_k^{-1} \right] + \sum_{\mathbf{x} \in \Omega} G_n^{\mathbf{V},k}(\mathbf{x})[\mathbf{W}^k(\mathbf{x})]^T \mathbf{W}^k(\mathbf{x}) \right\} \quad (15)$$

$$\text{where} \quad g_n^{\mathbf{m},k}(\mathbf{x}) = \frac{\partial \underline{\mathcal{B}}_n^k(\mathbf{x})}{\partial \widetilde{\mathbf{m}}_n^k(\mathbf{x})}, \quad G_n^{\mathbf{V},k}(\mathbf{x}) = \frac{\partial \underline{\mathcal{B}}_n^k(\mathbf{x})}{\partial \widetilde{\mathbf{V}}_n^k(\mathbf{x})} \quad (16)$$

M-Step: Optimize model parameters given the current variational parameters.

$$\Theta^{(i)} = \arg \max_{\Theta} \left\{ \sum_{n=1}^{N} \sum_{k=1}^{K} \underline{\mathcal{L}}_n^k(\Theta_k, \gamma_n^{k^{(i)}}, \alpha) \right\} + \log p(\Theta | \Psi) \quad (17)$$

$$\text{where} \quad p(\Theta | \Psi) = \prod_{k=1}^{K} p(\mathbf{w}_0^k | \lambda_0^k) \prod_{l=1}^{L_k} p(\mathbf{w}_l^k | \lambda_l^k) p(\mathbf{w}_l^k | \beta_l^k) \quad (18)$$

(a) Compute component-specific latent factor prior parameters.

$$\pi_k = \frac{1}{N} \sum_{n=1}^{N} q(\mathbf{y}_n^k = 1) \quad (19)$$

$$\mu_k = \frac{1}{N_k} \sum_{n=1}^{N} q(\mathbf{y}_n^k = 1)\mathbf{m}_n^k \quad \text{where} \quad N_k = \sum_{n=1}^{N} q(\mathbf{y}_n^k = 1) \quad (20)$$

$$\Sigma_k = \frac{1}{N_k} \sum_{n=1}^{N} q(\mathbf{y}_n^k = 1) \left\{ \mathbf{V}_n^k + (\mathbf{m}_n^k - \mu_k)(\mathbf{m}_n^k - \mu_k)^T \right\} \quad (21)$$

(b) Optimize component-specific factor model $\mathbf{W}^k$, $\mathbf{w}_0^k$ $\forall k = \{1, ..., K\}$.

$$\mathcal{E}(\Theta | \gamma, \alpha, \Psi) = -\underline{\mathcal{L}}(\Theta, \gamma, \alpha) + \sum_{k=1}^{K} \left\{ (\lambda_0^k/2)(\mathbf{w}_0^k)^T \mathbf{S} \mathbf{w}_0^k \right.$$
$$\left. + \sum_{l=1}^{L_k} \left[(\lambda_l^k/2)(\mathbf{w}_l^k)^T \mathbf{S} \mathbf{w}_l^k + (\beta_l^k/2)(\mathbf{w}_l^k)^T \mathbf{w}_l^k \right] \right\} \quad (22)$$

$$\frac{d\mathcal{E}}{d\mathbf{w}_0^k} = -\sum_{n=1}^{N} q(\mathbf{y}_n^k = 1) \, \mathbf{g}_n^{\mathbf{m},k} + \lambda_0^k \mathbf{S} \mathbf{w}_0^k, \quad (23)$$

$$\frac{d\mathcal{E}}{d\mathbf{w}_l^k} = -\left\{ \frac{\partial \underline{\mathcal{L}}}{\partial \mathbf{w}_l^k} + \lambda_l^k \mathbf{S} \mathbf{w}_l^k + \beta_l^k \mathbf{w}_l^k \right\} \quad (24)$$

$$\frac{\partial \underline{\mathcal{L}}}{\partial \mathbf{w}_l^k} = \sum_{n=1}^{N} q(\mathbf{y}_n^k = 1) \left[\mathbf{g}_n^{\mathbf{m},k} \mathbf{m}_{n,l}^k + 2\mathbf{G}_n^{\mathbf{V},k} \odot \mathbf{W}^k \mathbf{V}_{n,l}^k \right] \quad (25)$$

$$\mathbf{w}_l^{k^{(t)}} = \left\{ \frac{1}{1 + \Delta t \lambda_l^k \mathbf{S}} \right\} \otimes \left\{ \mathbf{w}_l^{k^{(t-1)}} + \Delta t \left[\frac{\partial \underline{\mathcal{L}}}{\partial \mathbf{w}_l^k} - \delta(l > 0) \beta_l^k \mathbf{w}_l^{k^{(t-1)}} \right] \right\} \quad (26)$$

H-Step:

$$p(\Theta) = \prod_{k=1}^{K} \prod_{l=0}^{L_k} \left\{ \int_0^\infty p(\mathbf{w}_l^k | \lambda_l^k) p(\lambda_l^k) d\lambda_l^k \right\} \times \prod_{k=1}^{K} \prod_{l=1}^{L_k} \left\{ \int_0^\infty p(\mathbf{w}_l^k | \beta_l^k) p(\beta_l^k) d\beta_l^k \right\} \quad (27)$$

$$p(\mathbf{w}_l^k | \lambda_l^k) = \frac{(\lambda_l^k)^{D/2} |\mathbf{S}|^{1/2}}{(2\pi)^{D/2}} \exp \left\{ -\frac{\lambda_l^k}{2} (\mathbf{w}_l^k)^T \mathbf{S} \mathbf{w}_l^k \right\} \quad (28)$$

$$p(\mathbf{w}_l^k | \beta_l^k) = \frac{(\beta_l^k)^{D/2}}{(2\pi)^{D/2}} \exp \left\{ -\frac{\beta_l^k}{2} (\mathbf{w}_l^k)^T \mathbf{w}_l^k \right\} \quad (29)$$

$$\lambda_l^k = \frac{D}{(\mathbf{w}_l^k)^T \mathbf{S} \mathbf{w}_l^k}, \; \beta_l^k = \frac{D}{(\mathbf{w}_l^k)^T \mathbf{w}_l^k} \quad \text{where} \quad (\mathbf{w}_l^k)^T \mathbf{S} \mathbf{w}_l^k = ||\Delta \mathbf{w}_l^k||^2 \quad (30)$$

---

4   Results

We assessed the *generalization* of ShapeOdds and its mixture variant – compared to *baseline* models – w.r.t. modeling unseen shapes, which reflect the ability of a learned density function to spread out between and around the training shapes.

Datasets: We considered two datasets. (1) The *diatoms* dataset[1] contains 360 images from four diatom classes – eunotia, flagilaria, gomphonema, and stauroneis (see Fig. 1) – collected as part of the automatic diatom identification and classification project [22]. This dataset manifests learning ShapeOdds in a high-dimensional shape space that possesses subpopulations with limited training samples compared to significant shape variations across successive generations in a clone, thereby constructing nonlinear shape manifolds. (2) The cardiac *left atrial* (LA) shape dataset[2] contains 60 late-gadolinium enhancement (LGE) MRI volumes with an isotropic resolution of 1.25 mm and expert-delineated binary segmentations for the epicardium. This dataset is an example of 3D anatomical shapes with relatively small training sample size that exhibit high variability, especially within and around the pulmonary veins (see Fig. 2).

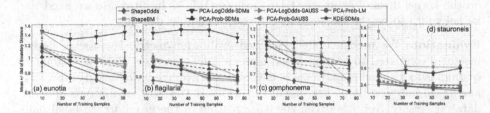

Fig. 3. Statistics of models' generalization on each diatom class. Lower is better.

Baseline Models: For comparison, we considered the state-of-the-art ShapeBM [17], which learns shape models directly in the label map space. For diatoms, we trained ShapeBM with 1×6 receptive fields and an overlap of 20 pixels using pre-training and 1000 epochs. We used 1800 and 200 hidden units for the first and second layers, respectively. We also learned shape models using PCA directly in the label map space (PCA-Prob-LM) as in [14]. We further considered current practices that use intermediate embeddings such as signed distance maps (SDMs) and Gaussian smoothed label maps (GAUSS), where the multiplicative factor for SDMs and the width of the Gaussian kernel were optimized using cross-validation. We learned shape models using PCA in the LogOdds space, similar to [6], and in the expectation parameter space (Prob), similar to [7]. For mixture modeling of diatoms and LA datasets, we used a mixture of probabilistic PCA [23] being learned in the LogOdds space using SDMs- and GAUSS-based

---

[1] Downloaded from the DIADIST project page: rbg-web2.rbge.org.uk/DIADIST/.

[2] Downloaded from the national alliance for medical image computing (NAMIC) project page: https://www.na-mic.org/Wiki/index.php/DBP3:Utah.

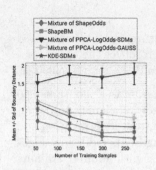

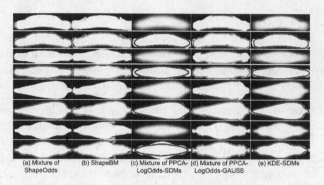

(a) Mixture of   (b) ShapeBM   (c) Mixture of PPCA-   (d) Mixture of PPCA-   (e) KDE-SDMs
ShapeOdds   LogOdds-SDMs   LogOdds-GAUSS

Fig. 4. Generalization of all diatom classes using mixtures of four components.

Fig. 5. Mixture results: (odd rows) samples of estimated $q--$maps and (even rows) $0.5--$levelset of the $q-$map overlayed on the groundtruth label map.

representations in which we parameterized the component-specific covariance matrix through its eigen decomposition. For nonparametric models, we focused on the kernel density estimate (KDE) using SDMs as in [9] where we fixed the kernel width to be the mean squared nearest-neighbor distance.

Evaluation: We used a boundary-based evaluation metric to provide better insight – compared to overlap-based metrics [24] – into how close an estimated $q-$map is to its label map. In particular, we used average boundary distance [24] among all pairwise boundary distances (in pixels and mm for diatoms and LA datasets, respectively) between the $0.5-$crossing of the groundtruth label map and the $0.5-$levelset of the estimated $q-$map.

Proof-of-Concept: We considered each diatom class individually. Figure 3 demonstrates the generalization performance of ShapeOdds compared to baseline models as a function of the training sample size where training subsets of $N = \{15\%, 35\%, 55\%, 75\%\}$ of the full dataset were randomly drawn five times. The poor performance of models that have been learned in the LogOdds space is evident regardless the deployed intermediate representation compared to the expectation parameter space. This reveals that existing ad hoc embeddings are not statistically principled approaches to embed label maps in the natural parameter space. The poorer performance of SDMs-based models indicates that they lead to suboptimal generative models that do not generalize well on unseen data. In particular, signed distance to the shape's boundary is a geometric representation that does not correlate well with the underlying generative process. GAUSS-based models make use of more training samples for better generalization. However, simply blurring the label maps smoothes out shape features in a way that is blind to the underlying shape variability in the input data. KDE-SDMs construct a non-parametric estimate of the expectation parameters based on the similarity of the unseen shape's SDM to each training sample. KDE-SDMs shows a slightly better performance for eunotia and stauroneis classes; however,

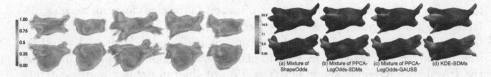

Fig. 6. Volume rendering (top) superior and (bottom) posterior-anterior views of the **q**–maps of ShapeOdds mixture components means.

Fig. 7. Boundary distances as color maps on sample epicardial meshes (superior view). (Color figure online)

it tends to overfit with the other *highly variable* classes. This mode of failure is typical for this model and appears to be an inability to find a good set of weights on training samples to, in turn, recover a good parameter map. ShapeBM advocates an axis-aligned shape space partitioning, in a non-data-driven manner, with a weight-sharing scheme to balance the number of parameters to estimate and the generality of the model. This explains its drastic performance with the stauroneis class where no unique ideal network architecture can be used for all datasets. On the other hand, ShapeOdds compares favorably against all baseline models and shows better generalization performance even with small training sizes compared to the underlying variability.

Mixture Experiment: Here we considered samples from all the diatom classes. Figure 4 depicts the generalization performance as a function of the training sample size. One can note the poor generalization of the SDMs-based mixture model compared to the GAUSS-based one, which emphasizes the inadequacy of a geometric representation to learn a probability distribution over the label maps.

Table 1. Statistics of models generalization on the LA dataset (Lower is better)

Mixture of ShapeOdds	Mixture of PPCA-LogOdds-SDMs	Mixture of PPCA-LogOdds-GAUSS	KDE-SDMs
1.83 ± 0.23 mm	1.94 ± 0.3 mm	2.05 ± 0.45 mm	2.47 ± 0.67 mm

Extending ShapeOdds to mixtures achieves the balance between model capacity and generalizability in a *data-driven* manner and a statistically principled approach – rather than heuristically partitioning the shape space as in ShapeBM – by parameterizing each mixture component by its dominant subspace. Figure 5 demonstrates that the mixture of ShapeOdds generalizes to unseen examples with crisp **q**–maps compared to other baseline models. One can notice the tendency of SDMs-based models (KDE and mixture) to recover over-smoothed q–maps, revealing a failure to learn enough shape variability and leading to parameter maps that do not preserve shape class features such as different shapes of diatom valves. The effect of ShapeBM's space partitioning can be observed where the lack of *enough* receptive field overlap leads to discontinuities in the reconstructed $\mathbf{q}$–map and fails to perserve global shape features. For the LA shapes, training subsets of $N = 75\%$ of the full dataset were randomly drawn three times to train mixture models of five components. Figure 6 visualizes the corresponding expectation parameters of the ShapeOdds mixture means, *i.e.*, $\mathbf{q}_0^k = \mathrm{logit}[\mathbf{w}_0^k]$. The significant LA shape variabilty is evident by having representative parameter maps that pertain to different shape characteristics, especially w.r.t. the elongation and curvature of the pulmonary veins. Table 1 reports the mean and std of the average boundary distance between unseen LA samples and estimated $\mathbf{q}$–maps from different models. Figure 7 shows such a boundary distance on samples of epicardial surfaces where the majority of deviation is concentrated around the pulmonary veins, a highly variable LA shape feature. The mixture of ShapeOdds is able to estimate $\mathbf{q}$–maps with veins that preserve better proximity to the groundtruth shapes compared to other models. Hence, we presented a probabilistic generative shape model that offers a data-driven placement of label maps in a vector space. In the future, we will pursue deep latent models to allow scaling to higher resolution shapes while avoiding overfitting.

References

1. Heimann, T., Meinzer, H.P.: Statistical shape models for 3D medical image segmentation: a review. MedIA **13**(4), 543–563 (2009)
2. Bredbenner, T.L., Eliason, T.D., Potter, R.S., Mason, R.L., Havill, L.M., Nicolella, D.P.: Statistical shape modeling describes variation in tibia and femur surface geometry between control and incidence groups from the osteoarthritis initiative database. J. Biomech. **43**(9), 1780–1786 (2010)
3. Balestra, S., Schumann, S., Heverhagen, J., Nolte, L., Zheng, G.: Articulated statistical shape model-based 2D-3D reconstruction of a hip joint. In: Stoyanov, D., Collins, D.L., Sakuma, I., Abolmaesumi, P., Jannin, P. (eds.) IPCAI 2014. LNCS, vol. 8498, pp. 128–137. Springer, Cham (2014). doi:10.1007/978-3-319-07521-1_14
4. Shen, K.K., Fripp, J., Mériaudeau, F., Chételat, G., Salvado, O., Bourgeat, P.: Detecting global and local hippocampal shape changes in Alzheimers disease using statistical shape models. Neuroimage **59**(3), 2155–2166 (2012)
5. Rousson, M., Paragios, N., Deriche, R.: Implicit active shape models for 3D segmentation in MR imaging. In: Barillot, C., Haynor, D.R., Hellier, P. (eds.) MICCAI 2004. LNCS, vol. 3216, pp. 209–216. Springer, Heidelberg (2004). doi:10.1007/978-3-540-30135-6_26
6. Pohl, K.M., Fisher, J., Bouix, S., Shenton, M., McCarley, R.W., Grimson, W.E.L., Kikinis, R., Wells, W.M.: Using the logarithm of odds to define a vector space on probabilistic atlases. MedIA **11**(5), 465–477 (2007)
7. Cremers, D., Schmidt, F.R., Barthel, F.: Shape priors in variational image segmentation: Convexity, Lipschitz continuity and globally optimal solutions. In: CVPR, pp. 1–6. IEEE (2008)

8. Rousson, M., Cremers, D.: Efficient kernel density estimation of shape and intensity priors for level set segmentation. In: Duncan, J.S., Gerig, G. (eds.) MICCAI 2005. LNCS, vol. 3750, pp. 757–764. Springer, Heidelberg (2005). doi:10.1007/11566489_93

9. Cremers, D., Osher, S.J., Soatto, S.: Kernel density estimation and intrinsic alignment for shape priors in level set segmentation. IJCV **69**(3), 335–351 (2006)

10. Wimmer, A., Soza, G., Hornegger, J.: A generic probabilistic active shape model for organ segmentation. In: Yang, G.-Z., Hawkes, D., Rueckert, D., Noble, A., Taylor, C. (eds.) MICCAI 2009. LNCS, vol. 5762, pp. 26–33. Springer, Heidelberg (2009). doi:10.1007/978-3-642-04271-3_4

11. Dasgupta, S.: Learning mixtures of Gaussians. In: FCS, pp. 634–644. IEEE (1999)

12. Ashburner, J., Friston, K.J.: Computing average shaped tissue probability templates. Neuroimage **45**(2), 333–341 (2009)

13. Sabuncu, M.R., Yeo, B.T., Van Leemput, K., Fischl, B., Golland, P.: A generative model for image segmentation based on label fusion. TMI **29**(10), 1714–1729 (2010)

14. Dambreville, S., Rathi, Y., Tannenbaum, A.: A Shape-based approach to robust image segmentation. In: Campilho, A., Kamel, M.S. (eds.) ICIAR 2006. LNCS, vol. 4141, pp. 173–183. Springer, Heidelberg (2006). doi:10.1007/11867586_17

15. Dambreville, S., Rathi, Y., Tannenbaum, A.: A framework for image segmentation using shape models and kernel space shape priors. TPAMI **30**(8), 1385–1399 (2008)

16. Welling, M., Chemudugunta, C., Sutter, N.: Deterministic latent variable models and their pitfalls. In: SIAM-DM, pp. 196–207 (2008)

17. Eslami, S.A., Heess, N., Williams, C.K., Winn, J.: The shape Boltzmann machine: a strong model of object shape. IJCV **107**(2), 155–176 (2014)

18. Freund, Y., Haussler, D.: Unsupervised learning of distributions on binary vectors using two layer networks. In: NIPS, pp. 912–919 (1992)

19. Wipf, D.P., Nagarajan, S.S.: A new view of automatic relevance determination. In: NIPS, pp. 1625–1632 (2008)

20. Marlin, B.M., Khan, M.E., Murphy, K.P.: Piecewise bounds for estimating Bernoulli-logistic latent Gaussian models. In: ICML, pp. 633–640 (2011)

21. Bishop, C.M.: Neural Networks for Pattern Recognition. Oxford Press, Oxford (1995)

22. Du Buf, H., Bayer, M., Droop, S., Head, R., Juggins, S., Fischer, S., Bunke, H., Wilkinson, M., Roerdink, J., Pech-Pacheco, J., et al.: Diatom identification: a double challenge called ADIAC. In: ICIAP, pp. 734–739. IEEE (1999)

23. Tipping, M.E., Bishop, C.M.: Mixtures of probabilistic principal component analyzers. NECO **11**(2), 443–482 (1999)

24. Taha, A.A., Hanbury, A.: Metrics for evaluating 3D medical image segmentation: analysis, selection, and tool. BMC-MI **15**(1), 29 (2015)

Constructing Shape Spaces
from a Topological Perspective

Christoph Hofer[1,3](✉), Roland Kwitt[1], Marc Niethammer[2],
Yvonne Höller[4,5], Eugen Trinka[3,4,5], Andreas Uhl[1], and for the ADNI

[1] Department of Computer Science, University of Salzburg, Salzburg, Austria
chofer@cosy.sbg.ac.at
[2] UNC Chapel Hill, Chapel Hill, NC, USA
[3] Spinal Cord Injury and Tissue Regeneration Centre (SCI-TReCS) Salzburg,
Paracelsus Medical University, Salzburg, Austria
[4] Department of Neurology, Christian Doppler Medical Centre,
Paracelsus Medical University, Salzburg, Austria
[5] Centre for Cognitive Neuroscience, Paracelsus Medical University,
Salzburg, Austria

Abstract. We consider the task of constructing (metric) shape space(s) from a topological perspective. In particular, we present a generic construction scheme and demonstrate how to apply this scheme when *shape* is interpreted as the *differences that remain after factoring out translation, scaling and rotation*. This is achieved by leveraging a recently proposed injective functional transform of 2D/3D (binary) objects, based on persistent homology. The resulting shape space is then equipped with a similarity measure that is (1) by design robust to noise and (2) fulfills all metric axioms. From a practical point of view, analyses of object shape can then be carried out *directly* on segmented objects obtained from some imaging modality *without* any preprocessing, such as alignment, smoothing, or landmark selection. We demonstrate the utility of the approach on the problem of distinguishing segmented hippocampi from normal controls *vs.* patients with Alzheimer's disease in a challenging setup where volume changes are no longer discriminative.

1   Introduction

Characterization and representation of shapes, cornerstones of human perception of objects, are fundamental and well-studied problems in computer vision and medical image analysis [5,9,14]. Applications range from recognition tasks to the analysis of longitudinal changes. While computer vision mostly focuses on 2D objects, medical image analysis typically studies shape in the context of (binary) 2D/3D segmentations of an anatomical structure (e.g., the hippocampus) that has been extracted from some imaging modality.

Conceptually, to study shapes in a mathematical framework, we need a formalism, a *shape space*, which captures the semantics of the colloquial term 'shape' or 'shape space'. In this work, we present a versatile construction scheme for shape spaces and then follow Kendall [14] who informally defines shape as

© Springer International Publishing AG 2017
M. Niethammer et al. (Eds.): IPMI 2017, LNCS 10265, pp. 106–118, 2017.
DOI: 10.1007/978-3-319-59050-9_9

"what is left when the differences which can be attributed to translations, rotations, and dilations have been quotiented out", to implement a concrete realization of that scheme. Since, a mandatory property of a shape space is not only to separate shapes, but also to assign some sort of similarity measure [21], we equip the shape space with an appropriate metric.

In many applications, where the primary objective is to characterize 2D/3D objects, a *shape space* is often not directly defined, but implicitly generated through the invariances of features extracted from the objects of interest (cf. [27, 28, 30]). In such approaches, the intermediate feature extraction step essentially condenses some discriminative properties (e.g., local curvature) into a compact representation that can be used in a subsequent learning step (e.g., using SVMs). While these approaches work remarkably well for various tasks, it is challenging to study the shape space due to the missing explicit definition.

In contrast, here we are specifically interested in a formal definition of shape. Approaches along this line of research predominantly study landmark-based representations [9, 14] of objects, manifolds (e.g., planar curves and surfaces) [3, 15, 19, 25], and even point clouds [18]. In the seminal work of Kendall [14] for instance, objects are represented via k landmarks in $\mathbb{R}^n$ and shapes are identified by quotienting out rotations, translations and scalings. This strategy has led to various elegant approaches to study shapes, most prominently by introducing a Riemannian structure on the space of landmarks [12, 13, 22]. While this allows to lift many concepts from statistics (e.g., regression) to the shape space, the data needs to be carefully hand-labeled, or landmarks need to be found via optimization. This is a challenging task on its own and typically requires careful preprocessing (e.g., smoothing). In a conceptually different line of research, shapes are considered as equivalence classes of manifolds [19, 25] and then studied by quotienting out reparametrizations. We refer the reader to [3] for a comprehensive review. While these approaches eliminate the need for landmarking, they are mostly theoretical, require considerable preprocessing and are non-trivial to implement. Alternatively, shapes can be represented via point clouds in $\mathbb{R}^n$, and distances can be established via a metric on the isometry classes of compact metric spaces (e.g., Gromov-Hausdorff), cf. [18], where the shape representation is invariant under rigid motions (excluding scalings). While this can be beneficial in certain situations, the Gromov-Hausdorff metric is rather coarse and might not allow to tease-out fine-grained differences. Recently, ideas from topological data analysis [6] have emerged to study 2D/3D objects, either in the form of computing topological invariants of features [16, 23, 24], or by directly analyzing the object of interest [26]. The latter is particularly relevant to our work, as the proposed *persistent homology transform* (1) is injective and (2) it allows to directly analyze the raw data. This idea will enable us to formally define shape space(s).

Contribution. In detail, we develop a construction scheme in which Kendall's notion of shape can be easily translated into the persistent homology transform framework of Turner et al. [26]. A suitable similarity measure with desirable properties such as robustness (to noise) can then be defined and shown to be an actual metric. This has important practical implications, as no preprocessing steps are required to analyze shapes after data has been collected.

2   Theoretical Background

While persistent homology (PH) is fundamental for our proposed shape space construction, one does not need a deep understanding of many parts of this framework to grasp the key ideas. In fact, we refer the interested reader to [10] (and references therein) for a detailed introduction to persistent homology. We only introduce a few necessary key concepts next.

Definition 1 (Filtration of a simplicial complex by a function). *Let K be a finite simplicial complex of dimension n and $f : K^{(0)} \to \mathbb{R}$, where $K^{(0)}$ denotes the 0-skeleton of K. If $\sigma = [v_0, \ldots, v_k]$ is a $k-simplex$ of K, then we naturally expand f to σ by setting $f(\sigma) = \max(\{v_i, 0 \le i \le k\})$. If $f(K) = \{a_1, a_2 \ldots, a_N\}$ with $a_i \le a_{i+1}$, we call the sequence*

$$K_0 \subset K_1 \subset \cdots \subset K_N$$

a filtration of K by f, where $K_0 = \emptyset$, $K_i = f^{-1}((-\infty, a_i])$ for $1 \le i \le N$.

Definition 2 (Persistence diagram). *Let $\Delta = \{(x,x) \in \mathbb{R}^2 : \mathrm{mult}(x) = \infty\}$ be the multiset of the diagonal in $\mathbb{R}^2$, where mult denotes the multiplicity function. A persistence diagram is a multiset of the following form:*

$$\mathcal{D} = \{(b,d) \in \mathbb{R}^2 : d - b > 0 \text{ and } 1 \le \mathrm{mult}((b,d)) < \infty\} \cup \Delta .$$

For a (finite) n-dimensional simplicial complex K and a function f defined on its 0-skeleton, we can interpret persistent homology as a mapping that associates to the filtration of K by f, (K, f), a vector of persistence diagrams, i.e.,

$$(K, f) \xmapsto{\ \mathrm{PH}\ } (\mathcal{D}_0(K, f), \ldots, \mathcal{D}_{n-1}(K, f)) . \tag{1}$$

Each $\mathcal{D}_i$ essentially encodes information about the homology of dimension i of the complexes as the filtration parameter grows, i.e., as we progress from $\emptyset$ to K. For instance, in dimension 0, $\mathcal{D}_0(K, f)$ captures the evolution of *connected components* of (K, f). Hence, $(b, d) \in \mathcal{D}_0(K, f)$ identifies a connected component which first occurs in $f^{-1}((-\infty, b])$ (i.e., it is *born*) and merges into an older one in $f^{-1}((-\infty, d])$ (i.e., it *dies*). To understand why this construction is useful, we briefly review the Bottleneck and Wasserstein distances.

Definition 3 (Bottleneck/Wasserstein distance). *For two persistence diagrams $\mathcal{D}$ and $\mathcal{E}$, we define their Bottleneck and Wasserstein distances by*

$$\mathrm{w}_\infty(\mathcal{D}, \mathcal{E}) = \inf_{\eta} \sup_{x \in \mathcal{D}} \|x - \eta(x)\|_\infty \quad \text{and} \quad \mathrm{w}_p^q(\mathcal{D}, \mathcal{E}) = \inf_{\eta} \left(\sum_{x \in \mathcal{D}} \|x - \eta(x)\|_q^p \right)^{\frac{1}{p}},$$

where $p, q \in \mathbb{N}$ and the infimum is taken over all bijections $\eta : \mathcal{D} \to \mathcal{E}$.

Note that $\mathrm{w}_p^q \to \mathrm{w}_\infty$ for $p \to \infty$. Using the Bottleneck distance, we can equip the space of persistence diagrams with a metric structure [20], and hence with an induced topology. In fact, Chazal et al. showed [7, Theorem 3.2] that (under reasonable constraints) for two filtrated complexes $(K, f_K), (L, f_L)$, the mapping in Eq. (1) is *stable*; for finite complexes this means that $w_\infty(\mathcal{D}_i(K, f_K),$ $\mathcal{D}_i(L, f_L))$ is bounded by the maximum of (1) the Gromov-Hausdorff distance, $d_{GH}(K, L)$, and (2) the $\sup_{(x,y) \in K \times L} |f_K(x) - f_L(y)|$. Further, the Wasserstein distance, w_p^q, inherits those stability properties [8]. Informally, stability reflects the property that small changes in the domain *do not* result in large changes in the co-domain.

Persistent Homology Transform. Our approach is based on the persistent homology transform (PHT), introduced by Turner et al. [26]. It uses the fact that for each direction $v \in \mathbb{S}^{n-1}$ the mapping $x \mapsto \langle x|v \rangle$ induces a filtration on complexes (in $\mathbb{R}^n$). Let $\mathcal{M}_n$ be the set of all subsets of $\mathbb{R}^n$ which can be written as finite simplicial complexes, where we assume two elements of $\mathcal{M}_n$ are equivalent if their linear embeddings[1] are equal. Then, the PHT assigns to each $K \in \mathcal{M}_n$ a mapping, $\text{PHT}(K)$, given by

$$\text{PHT}(K) : \mathbb{S}^{n-1} \to \mathbb{D}^n, \quad v \mapsto (\mathcal{X}_0(K, v), \ldots, \mathcal{X}_{n-1}(K, v)) ,$$

where $\mathcal{X}_k(K, v) = \mathcal{D}_k(K, \langle \cdot | v \rangle)$ and $\mathbb{D}$ denotes the space of persistence diagrams. [26] showed that this mapping is *injective* for $\mathcal{M}_2/\mathcal{M}_3$. With this and the aforementioned stability results, they introduce a *family of metrics* on $\mathcal{M}_2, \mathcal{M}_3$, i.e.,

$$\text{m}(K, L) = \text{m}_{\text{dist},n}(K, L) = \sum_{k=0}^{n-1} \int_{\mathbb{S}^{n-1}} \text{dist}(\mathcal{X}_k(K, v), \mathcal{X}_k(L, v)) \text{d}v , \qquad (2)$$

where $n = 2, 3$ and dist is either w_∞ or w_p^q. When not necessary, we will omit the subscripts (dist, n) for readability. Figure 1 illustrates the PHT for two filtration directions $v_1, v_2 \in \mathbb{S}^1$ and shows the corresponding persistence diagram(s). The metric space $(\mathcal{M}_3, \text{m})$ will be the basis for our shape space construction.

3   Constructing Shape Spaces

To build a *shape space* on top of the metric space $(\mathcal{M}_3, \text{m})$, we follow a group-theoretic construction. In particular, let $(\mathbf{G}, \odot)$ be a group, S be a set and $\triangleright : \mathbf{G} \times S \to S, (g, s) \mapsto g \triangleright s$ a (left) action of $\mathbf{G}$ on S. For $s \in S$ we denote by

$$\mathbf{G} \triangleright s = \{g \triangleright s : g \in \mathbf{G}\} \quad \text{and} \quad \mathbf{G} \triangleright S = \{\mathbf{G} \triangleright s : s \in S\}$$

the *orbit* of s and *the set of orbits* of S, resp., under the action $\triangleright$ of $\mathbf{G}$ on S. The following two lemmas will enable us to (1) obtain a metric on partitions of a metric space (Lemma 1) and (2) to establish a metric on the set of orbits induced by a group action on a metric space (Lemma 2).

Lemma 1 (Selection of representative). *Let (X, d) be a metric space with a partition $\mathcal{P} = \{X_i : i \in I\}$, i.e., $X_i \subset X$, $X_i \cap X_j = \emptyset$ for $i \neq j$ and $\bigcup X_i = X$. If $\iota : \mathcal{P} \to X$ is an injective mapping then*

$$\widetilde{d}(X_i, X_j) = d(\iota(X_i), \iota(X_j)) \quad \text{is a metric on } \mathcal{P}.$$

---

[1] For dimension $k > 0$, we can take the interior of the convex hull of the defining vertices and, for dimension 0, a simplex is mapped to its defining vertex.

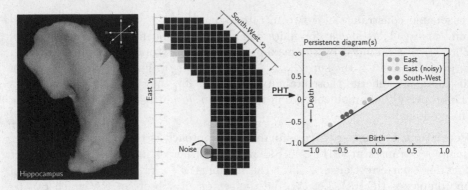

Fig. 1. Illustration of the PHT [26] for a hippocampus slice, represented as a (cubical) simplicial complex K, along two filtration directions v_1 and v_2. The corresponding persistence diagram(s), $\mathcal{X}_0(K, v_1)$ and $\mathcal{X}_0(K, v_2)$, are shown on the *right*. For direction v_1, we artificially added noise to the hippocampus; the corresponding points in the plot are highlighted in red (best-viewed in color).

Proof (Sketch). The identity of indiscernibles follows from the injectivity of ι; the remaining metric axioms follow immediately from d.   □

Lemma 2. *Let (X, d) be a metric space, $(\mathbf{G}, \odot)$ a compact topological group and let $\triangleright : \mathbf{G} \times X \to X$ be a (left) action of $\mathbf{G}$ on X, such that*

(i) $d(x, g \triangleright y)$ is continuous in g, and
(ii) $d(x, y) = d(g \triangleright x, g \triangleright y)$, $\forall x, y \in X, \forall g \in \mathbf{G}$.

Then

$$\widetilde{d}(\mathbf{G} \triangleright x, \mathbf{G} \triangleright y) = \min_{g \in \mathbf{G}} d(x, g \triangleright y)$$

is a metric on $\mathbf{G} \triangleright X$.

Proof. The proof consists of two parts.
Part (1). First, we have to show that $\min_g d(x, g \triangleright y)$ is well-defined, i.e., the minimum exists, and second, it does not depend on the representative of $\mathbf{G} \triangleright x$ and $\mathbf{G} \triangleright y$, respectively. The first property follows directly from condition *(i)* and the extreme value theorem, as d is continuous in g and $\mathbf{G}$ is compact. To show the second property, we choose two representatives $u \triangleright x \in \mathbf{G} \triangleright x$, $v \triangleright y \in \mathbf{G} \triangleright y$, with $u, v \in \mathbf{G}$ and consider

$$
\begin{aligned}
\min_{g \in \mathbf{G}} d(u \triangleright x, g \triangleright (v \triangleright y)) &\overset{(ii)}{=} \min_{g \in \mathbf{G}} d(u^{-1} \triangleright (u \triangleright x), u^{-1} \triangleright (g \triangleright (v \triangleright y))) \\
&= \min_{g \in \mathbf{G}} d(u^{-1} \odot u \triangleright x, u^{-1} \odot g \odot v \triangleright y) \\
&= \min_{g \in \mathbf{G}} d(x, u^{-1} \odot g \odot v \triangleright y) \\
&\overset{(*)}{=} \min_{g \in \mathbf{G}} d(x, g \triangleright y) \ .
\end{aligned}
$$

The last identity $(*)$ follows from the fact that if g runs through all of $\mathbf{G}$, so does $u^{-1} \odot g \odot v$.

Part (2). We will now verify the metric axioms.

Non-negativity. Follows from the non-negativity of d.

Symmetry. This is a consequence of condition *(ii)* as $d(x, g \triangleright y) = d(g \triangleright y, x) = d(g^{-1} \triangleright (g \triangleright y), g^{-1} \triangleright x) = d(\bar{y}, g^{-1} \triangleright x)$ which does not affect the minimum by the same arguments as above, see $(*)$.

Identity of Indiscernibles. First let $\mathbf{G} \triangleright y = \mathbf{G} \triangleright x$. Then $\exists g' \in \mathbf{G}$ such that $y = g' \triangleright x$. Hence,

$$\widetilde{d}(\mathbf{G} \triangleright x, \mathbf{G} \triangleright y) = \min_{g \in \mathbf{G}} d(x, g \triangleright (g' \triangleright x)) = 0 \ ,$$

as $(g')^{-1} \in \mathbf{G}$. Second, let $\widetilde{d}(\mathbf{G} \triangleright x, \mathbf{G} \triangleright y) = 0$, then there exists some g_0 such that $d(x, g_0 \triangleright y) = 0$. Hence, $x = g_0 \triangleright y$ which means that $\mathbf{G} \triangleright x = \mathbf{G} \triangleright y$.

Triangle Inequality. Consider $\mathbf{G} \triangleright x, \mathbf{G} \triangleright y, \mathbf{G} \triangleright z \in \mathbf{G} \triangleright X$. For $g' \in \mathbf{G}$ we get

$$\widetilde{d}(\mathbf{G} \triangleright x, \mathbf{G} \triangleright y) = \min_{g \in \mathbf{G}} d(x, g \triangleright y)$$

$$\overset{(**)}{\leq} \min_{g \in \mathbf{G}} \Big(d(x, g' \triangleright z) + d(g' \triangleright z, g \triangleright y) \Big)$$

$$= d(x, g' \triangleright z) + \min_{g \in \mathbf{G}} d(g' \triangleright z, g \triangleright y)$$

$$\overset{(ii)}{=} d(x, g' \triangleright z) + \min_{g \in \mathbf{G}} d(z, (g')^{-1} \triangleright (g \triangleright y))$$

$$\overset{(*)}{=} d(x, g' \triangleright z) + \widetilde{d}(\mathbf{G} \triangleright z, \mathbf{G} \triangleright y).$$

As g' is arbitrary, this inequality holds also for $g'_0 \in \mathbf{G}$ with $d(x, g'_0 \triangleright z) = \min_{g'} d(x, g' \triangleright z) = \widetilde{d}(\mathbf{G} \triangleright x, \mathbf{G} \triangleright z)$; further, $(**)$ holds due to the triangle inequality of d and $(*)$ holds with the same argumentation as in Part (1). $\square$

4   Practical Implementation

In this section, we show a practical realization of the concepts introduced in Sect. 3. In particular, we (1) construct a shape space in the spirit of Kendall, where translations, scalings and rotations are factored out and (2) show how the metric m can be pushed forward in this construction. At the end of the section, we demonstrate how these ideas translate into an implementation for binary segmentations defined on a pixel/voxel grid.

Remark 1. We follow the convention that if we interpret $K \in \mathcal{M}$ as a simplicial complex, applying $\varphi : \mathbb{R}^n \to \mathbb{R}^n$ to K means to apply φ to each defining vertex, e.g., if $K = (\{[v_1, v_2], [v_1], [v_2]\})$ then $\varphi(K) = \{[\varphi(v_1), \varphi(v_2)], [\varphi(v_1)], [\varphi(v_2)]\}$.

Definition 4. *Let* $\mathbf{S}$ *be a subgroup of the homeomorphism group* $\mathbf{H}$ *of* $\mathbb{R}^n$ *and* $\mathcal{K} \subset \mathcal{M}_n$ *such that* $\mathbf{S}(\mathcal{K}) = \{s(K) : s \in \mathbf{S}, K \in \mathcal{K}\} \subseteq \mathcal{K}$ *for all* $s \in \mathbf{S}$. *Then*

$$\rhd_{\mathbf{S}} : \mathbf{S} \times \mathcal{K} \to \mathcal{K}, \quad (s, K) \mapsto s \rhd_{\mathbf{S}} K = s(K)$$

is well-defined and we call $\mathbf{S}$ *a group of similarity transformations on* $\mathcal{K}$. *We further define by*

$$\mathfrak{S}(\mathbf{S}, \mathcal{K}) = \mathbf{S} \rhd_{\mathbf{S}} \mathcal{K}$$

the (simplicial) shape space of $\mathcal{K}$ *with respect to* $\mathbf{S}$. *If* $\mathfrak{S}(\mathbf{S}, \mathcal{K})$ *is equipped with a metric* d *then we call it a metric (simplicial) shape space.*

If it is clear from the context, we will omit the subscript $\mathbf{S}$ in $\rhd_{\mathbf{S}}$ and simply write $\rhd$. Also, we write $\mathfrak{S}$ instead of $\mathfrak{S}(\mathbf{S}, \mathcal{K})$ if the particular selection of $\mathbf{S}$ and $\mathcal{K}$ is not of specific importance. We now fix $\mathcal{K} = \mathcal{M}_3$ (using metric m) and build a shape space that is invariant under translations $\mathbf{Tr}(\cong \mathbb{R}^n)$, barycentric scalings $\mathbf{Sc}(\cong \mathbb{R}^+)$ and barycentric rotations $\mathbf{Ro}(\cong \mathbf{SO}(3))$.

Remark 2. If $(\mathfrak{S}, d)$ is a metric shape space and ι is a (bijective) isometry to some metric space $(X, \tilde{d})$ then we will identify $\iota(\mathfrak{S})$ with X and d with $\tilde{d}$. This simplifies notation, as we can refer to $(X, \tilde{d})$ as a metric simplicial shape space.

Translations. We start by factoring out *translations*.

Definition 5. *Let, for* $K \in \mathcal{K}$, b_K *be the barycenter of* K. *Then, we set*

$$\iota_{\mathbf{Tr}} : \mathbf{Tr} \rhd \mathcal{K} \to \mathcal{K}, \quad \mathbf{Tr} \rhd K \mapsto K - b_K .$$

Remark 3 ($\iota_{\mathbf{Tr}}$ *is well defined and injective*). Let $t \in \mathbf{Tr}$, then $b_{t \rhd K} = b_{K+t} = b_K + t$. Now let $t \rhd K$ be a representative of $\mathbf{Tr} \rhd K$; then we get $t \rhd K - b_{t \rhd K} = K + t - b_{K+t} = K + t - b_K - t = K - b_K$ which implies that $\iota_{\mathbf{Tr}}$ does not depend on the representative of $\mathbf{Tr} \rhd K$. If $\iota_{\mathbf{Tr}}(\mathbf{Tr} \rhd K) = K - b_K = K - b_L = \iota_{\mathbf{Tr}}(\mathbf{Tr} \rhd L)$, then $L = K - b_k + b_L \in \mathbf{Tr} \rhd K$ which implies $\mathbf{Tr} \rhd K = \mathbf{Tr} \rhd L$, and injectivity follows.

Since $\iota_{\mathbf{Tr}}$ is injective and $\mathbf{Tr} \rhd \mathcal{K}$ is a partition of $\mathcal{K}$ we can invoke Lemma 1 and therefore define a metric $d_{\mathbf{Tr}}$ on $\mathfrak{S}(\mathcal{K}, \mathbf{Tr})$ by setting $d_{\mathbf{Tr}}(\mathbf{Tr} \rhd K, \mathbf{Tr} \rhd L) = \mathrm{m}(\iota_{\mathbf{Tr}}(K), \iota_{\mathbf{Tr}}(L))$. This metric simplicial shape space is isometric to $(\mathcal{K}_{\mathbf{Tr}}, \mathrm{m})$ where $\mathcal{K}_{\mathbf{Tr}} = \iota_{\mathbf{Tr}}(\mathfrak{S}(\mathcal{K}, \mathbf{Tr}))$. After this first step, we have a *subset* of $\mathcal{M}_3$ equipped with m.

Scalings. In order to factor-out *barycentric scalings*, we construct the next shape space $\mathfrak{S}(\mathcal{K}_{\mathbf{Tr}}, \mathbf{Sc})$ from $(\mathcal{K}_{\mathbf{Tr}}, \mathrm{m})$ and equip it with a metric based on m. This is possible, as the barycenter remains unchanged by scalings.

Definition 6. *Let, for* $K \in \mathcal{K}_{\mathbf{Tr}}$, rad_K *be the radius of* K, *i.e.,* $\mathrm{rad}_K = \max_{x \in K} \|x\|_2$. *Then, we set*

$$\iota_{\mathbf{Sc}} : \mathbf{Sc} \rhd \mathcal{K}_{\mathbf{Tr}} \to \mathcal{K}, \quad \mathbf{Sc} \rhd K \mapsto \frac{1}{\mathrm{rad}_K} \cdot K .$$

Remark 4 (ι$_{\mathbf{Sc}}$ is well defined and injective). For $s \in \mathbf{Sc}$ it holds that $\mathrm{rad}_{s \triangleright K} = \mathrm{rad}_{s \cdot K} = s \cdot \mathrm{rad}_K$. Now let $s \triangleright K$ be a representative of $\mathbf{Sc} \triangleright K$, then $\mathrm{rad}_{s \triangleright K}^{-1} \cdot (s \triangleright K) = s^{-1} \cdot \mathrm{rad}_K^{-1} \cdot s \cdot K = \mathrm{rad}_K^{-1} \cdot K$. This implies that $\iota_{\mathbf{Sc}}$ does not depend on the representative in $\mathbf{Sc} \triangleright K$. If $\iota_{\mathbf{Sc}}(\mathbf{Sc} \triangleright K) = \mathrm{rad}_K^{-1} \cdot K = \mathrm{rad}_L^{-1} \cdot L = \iota_{\mathbf{Sc}}(\mathbf{Sc} \triangleright L)$, then $L = \mathrm{rad}_L \cdot \mathrm{rad}_K^{-1} \cdot K \in \mathbf{Sc} \triangleright K$ which implies $\mathbf{Sc} \triangleright K = \mathbf{Sc} \triangleright L$, and injectivity follows.

In the same manner as above, we can invoke Lemma 1. In detail, we set $\mathcal{K}_{\mathbf{Sc}} = \iota_{\mathbf{Sc}}(\mathfrak{S}(\mathcal{K}_{\mathbf{Tr}}, \mathbf{Sc}))$ and get the translation- and barycentric scaling-invariant metric simplicial shape space $(\mathcal{K}_{\mathbf{Sc}}, \mathrm{m})$.

Rotations. In our final step, we factor-out *barycentric rotations*.

Lemma 3. *For $r \in \mathbf{Ro}$ and $K, L \in \mathcal{K}_{\mathbf{Sc}}$, it holds that*

(i) $\mathrm{m}(K, r \triangleright L)$ is continuous in r, and
(ii) $\mathrm{m}(K, L) = \mathrm{m}(r \triangleright K, r \triangleright L)$.

Remark 5. In the following proof, we use two identities: (1) for a metric space (X, d) and $x, y, y' \in X$, we have $|d(x, y) - d(x, y')| \leq d(y, y')$; (2) $\mathcal{X}_k(K, d) = \mathcal{X}_k(r \triangleright K, r \triangleright d)$ for $r \in \mathbf{Ro}$ (as our filtration uses inner products, see Sect. 2).

Proof (of (i)). Consider Eq. (2); it suffices to show that $\mathrm{dist}\big(\mathcal{X}_k(K, d), \mathcal{X}_k(r \triangleright L, d)\big)$ is continuous in r. Let $r, r' \in \mathbf{Ro}$. For $\varepsilon > 0$, we obtain

$$
\begin{aligned}
\big|\mathrm{dist}\big(\mathcal{X}_k(K, d), \mathcal{X}_k(r \triangleright L, d)\big) - \mathrm{dist}\big(\mathcal{X}_k(K, d), \mathcal{X}_k(r' \triangleright L, d)\big)\big| &\overset{\text{Rem. 5 (1)}}{\leq} \\
\mathrm{dist}\big(\mathcal{X}_k(r \triangleright L, d), \mathcal{X}_k(r' \triangleright L, d)\big) &\overset{\text{Rem. 5 (2)}}{=} \\
\mathrm{dist}\big(\mathcal{X}_k(L, r^{-1} \triangleright d), \mathcal{X}_k(L, r'^{-1} \triangleright d)\big) &\overset{\text{[26][Lem. 2.1]}}{\leq} \\
C_L \|(r^{-1} \triangleright d) - (r'^{-1} \triangleright d)\|_2 \leq C_L \|r^{-1} - r'^{-1}\|_F \leq \varepsilon \ ,
\end{aligned}
\tag{3}
$$

where $C_L > 0$ is a constant dependent on L. Since, $\mathbf{Ro}$ is a topological group, the last term in this transformation depends continuously on r and r' and hence, for $\|r - r'\|_F < \delta$ sufficiently small, Eq. (3) is always fulfilled. □

Proof (of (ii)). It was shown in [2] [Proposition 2 (iv)] that for $f : \mathbb{S}^{n-1} \to \mathbb{R}$, the integral over the spherical surface is rotation invariant, i.e., $\int_{\mathbb{S}^{n-1}} f = \int_{\mathbb{S}^{n-1}} f \circ r$ for $r \in \mathbf{Ro}$. In combination with Remark 5 (2), this is sufficient for *(ii)* to hold. □

Most importantly, Lemma 3 now enables us to invoke Lemma 2 with $(X, d) = (\mathcal{K}_{\mathbf{Sc}}, \mathrm{m})$ and $\mathbf{G} = \mathbf{Ro}$. Consequently, we can equip $\mathfrak{S}(\mathcal{K}_{\mathbf{Sr}}, \mathbf{Ro})$ with the metric

$$
\widetilde{\mathrm{m}}(\mathbf{Ro} \triangleright K, \mathbf{Ro} \triangleright L) = \min_{r \in \mathbf{Ro}} \mathrm{m}(K, r \triangleright L) \ .
$$

In summary, we obtain the following *sequence of metric spaces*

$$
\boxed{(\mathcal{K}, \mathrm{m}) \overset{\iota}{\longrightarrow} (\mathcal{K}_{\mathbf{Tr}}, \mathrm{m}) \overset{\iota}{\longrightarrow} (\mathcal{K}_{\mathbf{Sr}}, \mathrm{m}) \overset{\pi}{\longrightarrow} (\mathfrak{S}(\mathcal{K}_{\mathbf{Sr}}, \mathbf{Ro}), \widetilde{\mathrm{m}})}
\tag{4}
$$

where π is the canonical mapping $K \mapsto \mathbf{Ro} \triangleright K$. For $K, L \in \mathcal{K}$ we can thus calculate the distance between K and L as

$$\widetilde{\mathrm{m}}(K, L) = \min_{r \in \mathbf{Ro}} \mathrm{m}\left(\frac{1}{\mathrm{rad}_{K-b_K}}(K - b_K), r \triangleright \left(\frac{1}{\mathrm{rad}_{L-b_L}}(L - b_L)\right)\right) . \tag{5}$$

Implementation. To use the constructed shape space in the context of binary voxel data (e.g., segmentations of some anatomical structure), we need a transition of the binary voxel structure, V, to $K_V \in \mathcal{K}$. In detail, $V \mapsto K_V \in \mathcal{K}$ is achieved by interpreting each voxel as a cube in $\mathbb{R}^3$ and setting the 0-skeleton of K_V, $K_V^{(0)}$, as the union of the centers of those cubes. Then we choose a construction procedure, denoted as `Build`, which iteratively constructs the higher dimensional skeletons from $K_V^{(0)}$, i.e., $K = \mathtt{Build}(K_V^{(0)})$. However, the choice of `Build` is not canonical. In our experiments, we used the algorithm in [29] to compute persistence diagrams for cubical data (implemented in `DIPHA`[2]) from which we obtain the PHTs. Figure 2 (*right*) illustrates this particular choice of `Build`. To calculate the integral in Eq. (2), we decided to use a Lebedev integration scheme with 26 points, which is a quadrature rule optimized for functions defined on a sphere. The key idea is to integrate $f : \mathbb{S}^2 \to \mathbb{R}$ by sampling on a point set which is invariant under the octahedral symmetry group $\mathbf{O}$ (including reflections), i.e., a Lebedev grid. The resulting quadrature formula (see [4] for theoretical details) is invariant under $\mathbf{O}$. To improve efficiency, we calculated the PHT for each object with respect to the 26 directions contained in the Lebedev grid. The minimization in Eq. (5) to calculate $\widetilde{\mathrm{m}}$ can then be approximated by reducing the original minimization domain from $\mathbf{SO}(3)$ to $\mathbf{R}$, where $\mathbf{R} \subset \mathbf{O}$ is the octahedral rotation group. The stability of the Lebedev grid under $\mathbf{O}$ guarantees that the application of each $r \in \mathbf{R}$ just causes a permutation of the 26 directions. Since $\mathbf{R}$ has rank 24, this means each evaluation of $\widetilde{\mathrm{m}}$ results in (less than) $24 \cdot 26$ evaluations of dist. In our experiments, we set dist $= \mathrm{w}_2^2$, but remark that other choices might be better, depending on the specific application. In addition, we map points of the form $(b, \infty) \in \mathcal{X}_k(K, v)$, see Fig. 1, to $(b, \max_{x \in K^{(0)}}(\langle x | v \rangle))$.

5   Experiments

We demonstrate the utility of our approach on (1) a simple toy example and (2) on the problem of separating binary 3D segmentations of the *hippocampus* obtained from healthy controls and patients with Alzheimer's disease (AD). As it is well-known (cf. [1]) that volume changes of the hippocampus are indicative of AD, we construct a particularly challenging setup where we only consider hippocampi from patients that are *close* in volume; in other words, volumetric changes are no longer discriminative in this setup.

Toy Example. Figure 2 presents a toy example of one hippocampus slice, represented as K. The distance plot shows the behavior of the metric $\widetilde{\mathrm{m}}$ when computing $\widetilde{\mathrm{m}}(K, K')$ where K' is obtained by rotating the hippocampus in steps of

---

[2] Available online at https://github.com/DIPHA/dipha.

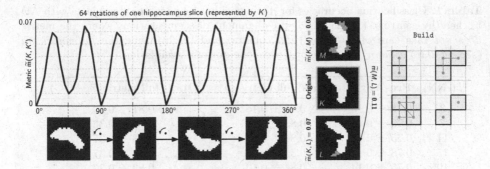

Fig. 2. 2D version of $\widetilde{\mathrm{m}}$, approx. with 8 directions: $(0,1), \frac{1}{\sqrt{2}}(1,1), \ldots, \frac{1}{\sqrt{2}}(1,-1)$ (*left*); Illustration of the construction scheme, Build, of a simplicial complex on a (pixel/voxel) grid in 2D (*right*). Simplices are shown in blue, pixel as squares. (Color figure online)

$(360°/64) \cdot k$, for $0 \leq k \leq 64$ (with nearest-neighbor interpolation). For comparison, we list the distances to two artificially modified versions of the hippocampus (changes in orange). As we can see, the distances $\widetilde{\mathrm{m}}(K, K')$ are *lower* than the distances to the modified hippocampi (i.e., $\widetilde{\mathrm{m}}(K, M), \widetilde{\mathrm{m}}(K, L)$). As the hippocampus is rather small (<500 pixel) this behavior is important, as the interpolation creates artifacts that are similar in size to salient object features.

Real Data. We use segmentations of the *left hippocampus*, obtained from the ADNI dataset via MAPER [11]. All segmentations are publicly available. To focus on actual shape changes, we restrict the data to hippocampi with voxel volumes 1000 ± 50. Under this constraint, we obtain 18 hippocampi associated with AD and 24 hippocampi associated with healthy controls. By design, a Wilcoxon rank-sum test for equality of the median volume does not allow to reject the null-hypothesis at any reasonable significance level (e.g., 0.01, 0.05).

Setup. We consider two setups: *First*, we assess a setup where rigid pre-alignment (implemented via NiftiReg; one healthy control randomly selected as target) is used and minimization of rotations is omitted in the metric. In other words, we work in the shape space $(\mathcal{K}_{\mathbf{Sr}}, \mathrm{m})$, see Eq. (4). In the *second* setup, we invoke the full metric $\widetilde{m}$ (w/o pre-alignment). For classification, we use a simple k-NN classifier and report average classification performance over 1000 balanced cross-validation splits, i.e., 15/15 AD and controls are randomly chosen to configure the k-NN classifier, 3/3 AD and controls are chosen for testing in each run.

Results. Table 1 lists the classification results over a range of k for the k-NN classifier. Several points are worth pointing out. *First*, the results indicate that rigid pre-alignment performs worse than letting the metric take care of rotations. This can be attributed to the fact that the metric does not rely on any registration procedure which, in case of small objects such as the hippocampus, can easily lead to slight misalignment and consequently confound the similarity measure used for classification. *Second*, although volumetric changes cannot

Table 1. Classification accuracies for distinguishing hippocampi of subjects with AD *vs.* healthy controls: (1) via (rigid) pre-alignment of segmentations where the metric *does not* take care of rotations (*first* column) and (2) by using the *full metric* $\tilde{m}$ (*second/third column*). LOO denotes leave-one-out cross-validation.

k(-NN)	Pre-Align	Ours (full metric $\tilde{m}$)	Ours (full metric $\tilde{m}$, LOO)
3	0.78 ± 0.15	0.81 ± 0.15	0.81 ± 0.39
7	0.79 ± 0.16	0.83 ± 0.14	0.88 ± 0.32
11	0.75 ± 0.15	0.84 ± 0.14	0.83 ± 0.37
15	0.78 ± 0.14	0.85 ± 0.13	0.83 ± 0.37
19	0.75 ± 0.14	0.84 ± 0.15	0.83 ± 0.37

separate the groups (as previously shown by the hypothesis test), our metric still allows to distinguish subjects from the AD and control group with performance comparable to what has been previously reported in the literature (although our approach is not specifically-tailored to the problem). *Third*, we highlight that *raw segmentations*, as produced by MAPER, were used in the experiment. While segmentation artifacts might still be present, we argue that it is undesirable to eliminate them during preprocessing, as we cannot reliably distinguish between noise and potentially discriminative/salient features *a-priori*.

6   Discussion

We introduced a versatile construction scheme for shape spaces (equipped with appropriate metrics) on top of a functional transform for objects, based on persistent homology. In a sense this framework (1) is *exact*, as no preprocessing is required and (2) allows to easily refine/coarsen the metric by choosing a higher or lower number of filtration directions, respectively. We argue that avoiding preprocessing is a desirable property, as the data processing theorem [17] specifically advises against reducing information in early stages of a processing chain. While we focused on the construction of a shape space in the sense of Kendall, the principles outlined in Sect. 3 constitute a generic *construction kit* to build all sorts of different shape spaces, with one particular realization shown in Eq. (4). At this stage, it is however unclear if our particular choice of base metric, i.e., the w_2^2 distance, is the most appropriate choice. In fact, a data-driven approach to select the parameters of the metric might be better. Another, conceptually interesting, extension could be to lift the metric to reproducing Kernel Hilbert spaces (cf. [24]), which would readily enable statistical computations.

References

1. Apostolova, L.G., Green, A.E., Babakchanian, S., Hwang, K.S., Chou, Y.Y., Toga, A.W., Thompson, P.M.: Hippocampal atrophy and ventricular enlargement in normal aging, mild cognitive impairment, and Alzheimer disease. Alzheimer Dis. Assoc. Disord. **26**(1), 17–27 (2012)

2. Baker, J.A.: Integration over spheres and the divergence theorem for balls. Am. Math. Mon. **104**(1), 36–47 (1997)
3. Bauer, M., Bruveris, M., Michor, P.W.: Overview of the geometries of shape spaces and diffeomorphism groups. Math. Imaging Vis. **50**(1), 60–97 (2014)
4. Beentjes, C.H.L.: Quadrature on a Spherical Surface (2015). http://people.maths.ox.ac.uk/beentjes/Essays/QuadratureSphere.pdf
5. Bookstein, F.: Size and shape spaces for landmark data in two dimensions. Stat. Sci. **1**(2), 181–242 (1986)
6. Carlsson, G.: Topology and data. Bull. Am. Math. Soc. **46**, 255–308 (2009)
7. Chazal, F., Cohen-Steiner, D., Guibas, L.J., Mémoli, F., Oudot, S.Y.: Gromov-Hausdorff stable signatures for shapes using persistence. Comput. Graph. Forum **28**(5), 1393–1403 (2009)
8. Cohen-Steiner, D., Edelsbrunner, H., Harer, J., Mileyko, Y.: Lipschitz functions have L_p-stable persistence. Found. Comput. Math. **10**(2), 127–139 (2010)
9. Dryden, I.L., Mardia, K.V.: Statistical Shape Analysis. Wiley series in Probability and Statistics. Wiley, New York (1998)
10. Edelsbrunner, H., Harer, J.L., Topology, C.: An Introduction. American Mathematical Society, Providence (2010)
11. Heckemann, R.A., Keihaninejad, S., Aljabar, P., Nielsen, C., Gray, K.R., Rueckert, D., Hajnal, J.V., Hammers, A.: Automatic morphometry in Alzheimer's disease and mild cognitive impairment. Neuroimage **56**(4), 2024–2037 (2011)
12. Hinkle, J., Fletcher, P.T., Joshi, S.: Intrinsic polynomials for regression on Riemannian manifolds. Imaging Vis. **50**, 32–52 (2014)
13. Hinkle, J., Muralidharan, P., Fletcher, P.T., Joshi, S.: Polynomial regression on Riemannian manifolds. In: Fitzgibbon, A., Lazebnik, S., Perona, P., Sato, Y., Schmid, C. (eds.) ECCV 2012. LNCS, vol. 7574, pp. 1–14. Springer, Heidelberg (2012). doi:10.1007/978-3-642-33712-3_1
14. Kendall, D.G.: Shape manifolds, procrustean metrics, and complex projective spaces. Bull. London Math. Soc. **16**(2), 81–121 (1984)
15. Kurtek, S., Klassen, E., Ding, Z., Srivastava, A.: A novel Riemannian framework for shape analysis of 3D objects. In: CVPR (2010)
16. Li, C., Ovsjanikov, M., Chazal, F.: Persistence-based structural recognition. In: CVPR (2014)
17. MacKay, D.: Information Theory, Inference, and Learning Algorithms. Cambridge University Press, Cambridge (2003)
18. Mémoli, F., Sapiro, G.: A theoretical and computational framework for isometry invariant recognition of point cloud data. Found. Comput. Math. **5**(3), 313–347 (2005)
19. Michor, P.W., Mumford, D.B.: Riemannian geometries on spaces of plane curves. J. Eur. Math. Soc. **8**(1), 1–48 (2006)
20. Mileyko, Y., Mukherjee, S., Harer, J.: Probability measures on the space of persistence diagrams. Inverse Probl. **27**(12) (2011)
21. Mumford, D.B.: Mathematical theories of shape: do they model perception? Proc. SPIE **1570**, 2–10 (1991)
22. Fletcher, P.T.: Geodesic regression and the theory of least squares on Riemannian manifolds. Int. J. Comput. Vis. **105**(2), 171–185 (2012)
23. Pachauri, D., Hinrichs, C., Chung, M.K., Johnson, S.C., Singh, V.: Topology-based kernels with application to inference problems in Alzheimer's disease. IEEE Trans. Med. Imaging **30**(10), 1760–1770 (2011)
24. Reininghaus, R., Bauer, U., Huber, S., Kwitt, R.: A stable multi-scale kernel for topological machine learning. In: CVPR (2015)

25. Shah, J.: An H^2 Riemannian metric on the space of planar curves modulo similitudes. Adv. Appl. Math. **51**(4), 483–506 (2013)
26. Turner, K., Mukherjee, S., Boyer, D.M.: Persistent homology transform for modeling shapes and surfaces. Inf. Inference **3**(4), 310–344 (2014)
27. van Kaick, O., Zhang, H., Hamarneh, G., Cohen-Or, D.: A survey on shape correspondence. Comput. Graph. Forum **30**(6), 1681–1707 (2011)
28. Veltkamp, R.C., Hagedoorn, M.: State of the art in shape matching. In: Lew, M.S. (ed.) Principles of Visual Information Retrieval, pp. 87–119. Springer, Heidelberg (2001)
29. Wagner, H., Chen, C., Vuçini, E.: Efficient computation of persistent homology for cubical data. In: Peikert, R., Hauser, H., Carr, H., Fuchs, R. (eds.) Topological Methods in Data Analysis and Visualization II: Theory, Algorithms, and Applications, pp. 91–106. Springer, Heidelberg (2012)
30. Yang, M., Kpalma, K., Ronsin, J.: A survey of shape feature extraction techniques. Pattern Recognit. **15**(7), 43–90 (2008)

Disease Diagnosis/Progression

A Discriminative Event Based Model for Alzheimer's Disease Progression Modeling

Vikram Venkatraghavan[1]([⊠]), Esther E. Bron[1], Wiro J. Niessen[1,2], and Stefan Klein[1]

[1] Biomedical Imaging Group Rotterdam,
Departments of Medical Informatics and Radiology,
Erasmus MC, Rotterdam, The Netherlands
v.venkatraghavan@erasmusmc.nl
[2] Faculty of Applied Sciences, Delft University of Technology,
Delft, The Netherlands

Abstract. The event-based model (EBM) for data-driven disease progression modeling estimates the sequence in which biomarkers for a disease become abnormal. This helps in understanding the dynamics of disease progression and facilitates early diagnosis by staging patients on a disease progression timeline. Existing EBM methods are all generative in nature. In this work we propose a novel discriminative approach to EBM, which is shown to be more accurate as well as computationally more efficient than existing state-of-the art EBM methods. The method first estimates for each subject an approximate ordering of events, by ranking the posterior probabilities of individual biomarkers being abnormal. Subsequently, the central ordering over all subjects is estimated by fitting a generalized Mallows model to these approximate subject-specific orderings based on a novel probabilistic Kendall's Tau distance. To evaluate the accuracy, we performed extensive experiments on synthetic data simulating the progression of Alzheimer's disease. Subsequently, the method was applied to the Alzheimer's Disease Neuroimaging Initiative (ADNI) data to estimate the central event ordering in the dataset. The experiments benchmark the accuracy of the new model under various conditions and compare it with existing state-of-the-art EBM methods. The results indicate that discriminative EBM could be a simple and elegant approach to disease progression modeling.

1 Introduction

Alzheimer's Disease (AD) is characterized by a cascade of biomarkers becoming abnormal, the pathophysiology of which is very complex and largely unknown. However, understanding the progression of several imaging and clinical biomarkers after disease onset is extremely important for both early diagnosis and patient staging. Conventional models of disease progression reconstruct biomarker trajectories in individual subjects using longitudinal data. This is done to get insight into disease progression mechanism [9,10]. However, the utility of such models are restricted by the fact that longitudinal data in large groups of patients is

© Springer International Publishing AG 2017
M. Niethammer et al. (Eds.): IPMI 2017, LNCS 10265, pp. 121–133, 2017.
DOI: 10.1007/978-3-319-59050-9_10

scarce. To circumvent this problem, methods to infer the order in which biomarkers for a disease become abnormal based on cross-sectional data have been proposed [2,5]. Some of these models [5,6] rely on stratification of patients into several subgroups based on symptomatic staging, for inferring the aforementioned ordering. However, the problem with using symptomatic staging is that it is very coarse and qualitative.

Event based modeling (EBM) [2,4,12] is a data-driven approach to disease progression modeling. EBM algorithms neither rely on symptomatic staging nor on the presence of longitudinal data for inferring the temporal ordering of events, where an event is defined by a biomarker becoming abnormal. All the variants of EBM developed so far are generative in nature. The existing state-of-the-art EBM methods are either not very robust in handling disease heterogeneity or scalable to large number of biomarkers, as will be demonstrated in this paper.

In this work, we propose a novel discriminative approach to EBM (DEBM) to address these issues. We assume that the event orderings for each subject in the dataset need not be unique, but form a cluster around a single central ordering. We first compute a noisy estimate of event ordering for each subject by ranking the posterior probabilities of individual biomarkers being abnormal. Subsequently, we introduce a novel probabilistic Kendall's Tau distance to reliably aggregate such noisy subject-specific event orderings to estimate a central ordering over all subjects.

2   Event Based Models

The EBM considers disease progression as a series of events, where each event corresponds to a new biomarker becoming abnormal. Fonteijn's EBM [2] finds the ordering of events (σ_0) such that the likelihood that a dataset was generated from subjects following this event ordering is maximized. This event ordering (σ_0) consists of a discrete set of events $\{E_{\sigma_0(1)}, E_{\sigma_0(2)}, \ldots, E_{\sigma_0(N)}\}$, where N is the number of biomarkers per subject in the dataset.

Given a cross-sectional dataset of M subjects, if X_j denotes a measurement of biomarkers for each subject at a certain timepoint, with each measurement X_j consisting of N biomarker values $\mathbf{x}_{j,i}$, the likelihood of the dataset being generated by σ_0 as defined by [2] is given by:

$$p\left(X|\sigma_0\right) = \prod_{j=1}^{M} \sum_{k=0}^{N} p(k) \left(\prod_{i=1}^{k} p\left(x_{j,\sigma_0(i)}|E_{\sigma_0(i)}\right) \prod_{i=k+1}^{N} p\left(x_{j,\sigma_0(i)}|\neg E_{\sigma_0(i)}\right) \right) \quad (1)$$

where $p(k)$ is the prior probability of a subject being at position k of the event ordering, which is assumed to be equal for each position. With the assumption that all the biomarkers in the control population are normal and that the biomarker values follow a Gaussian distribution, $p\left(x_{j,\sigma_0(i)}|\neg E_{\sigma_0(i)}\right)$ is computed. Abnormal biomarker values in the patient population are assumed to follow a uniform distribution but not all biomarkers of a patient could be assumed to be abnormal. For this reason, the likelihoods were obtained using a mixture model of Gaussian-uniform distributions where only the parameters of the uniform distribution were allowed to be optimized.

This method was slightly modified in [12] to estimate the optimal ordering in a sporadic AD dataset with significant proportions of controls were expected to have presymptomatic AD. A Gaussian distribution was used to describe both the control and patient population, and the mixture model allowed for optimization of parameters for the Gaussians describing both control and patient population. Gaussian mixture model was also used to incorporate more subjects from the dataset with clinical diagnosis of mild cognitive impairment (MCI).

An assumption made in [2] and [12] is the existence of a single ordering common in all the subjects within a cohort. Such as assumption is rather too restrictive for estimating the progression of a complex disease such as AD. This assumption was relaxed in [4], which estimates a distribution of event orderings with a central event ordering and a spread as per a generalized mallows model [8]. Huang's EBM [4] is an expectation maximization algorithm to obtain the central ordering σ_0 and spread ϕ. The E-step estimates the likelihood of a patient's biomarker value measurement following an event order σ_j, given σ_0 and ϕ. In the M-step, σ_0 and ϕ are estimated based on (σ_j) estimated in the E-step. This is done iteratively to maximize the likelihood of generation of patients' data based on σ_0 and ϕ.

While Fonteijn's EBM is computationally inexpensive, the assumptions are very restrictive. The assumptions in Huang's EBM on the other hand are realistic, however the algorithm does not scale well to large number of biomarkers. With these in mind, we propose a discriminative approach to EBM.

3 Discriminative Event Based Model

In this section, we propose our novel method for estimating central ordering of events (σ_0). We postulate that the posterior probability of a biomarker being abnormal signifies the progression of a biomarker. Since this is done for each biomarker measured from a subject, the different amounts of progression for different biomarkers as estimated by their corresponding posterior probabilities signify the event ordering in a subject (σ_j). However, the posterior probability is not only affected by progression of the biomarker to its abnormal state, but also by inherent variability in 'healthy' biomarker values across subjects, and by measurement noise. Since it is not feasible to distinguish between these effects based on a single (cross-sectional) measurement, we expect σ_j to be a noisy estimate. To estimate σ_0 based on noisy estimates of σ_j, we introduce a novel variant of Kendall's Tau distance which takes into account the posterior probability estimates. The proposed framework is discriminative in nature, since we estimate σ_j directly based on the posterior probabilities of individual biomarker becoming abnormal. This is in contrast to the existing EBM models, which estimates the event orderings based on the likelihood of the data being generated by an ordering.

The rest of the section is organized as follows: Given a single cross-sectional measurement of biomarkers from a subject, we present a method to estimate σ_j

in Sect. 3.1. The problem of estimating σ_0, from noisy estimates of σ_j is addressed in Sect. 3.2.

3.1   Biomarker Progression and Subject-Wise Event Ordering

Assuming a paradigm similar to that in previous EBM variants [4,12], the probability density functions (PDF) of normal and abnormal classes in the biomarkers are assumed to be represented by Gaussians. There are two reasons why constructing these PDFs is non-trivial. Firstly, the labels (clinical diagnoses) for the subjects do not necessarily represent the true labels of all the biomarkers extracted from the subject. Not all biomarkers are abnormal for a subject with AD, while some of the controls could have undiagnosed pre-symptomatic conditions. Secondly, the clinical diagnosis is sometimes non-binary and includes classes such as MCI, with significant number of biomarkers in normal and abnormal classes.

In our approach we address these two issues independently. We make an initial estimate of the PDFs using biomarkers from 'easy' controls and 'easy' AD subjects and later refine the estimated PDF using the entire dataset.

A Bayesian classifier is trained for each biomarker using controls and AD subjects, based on the assumption that there are no wrongly-labeled biomarker in either class. This classifier is subsequently applied to the training data, and the predicted labels are compared with the clinical labels. The misclassified data in the training dataset could either be outliers in each class resulting from using untrustworthy labels or could genuinely belong to their respective classes and represent the tails of the true PDFs. Irrespective of the reason of misclassification, we remove them for initial estimation of the PDFs. This procedure thus results, for each biomarker, in a set of 'easy' controls (whose biomarker values represent normal values) and 'easy' AD subjects (whose biomarker values represent abnormal values).

As we use Gaussians to represent the PDFs, we have initial estimates for mean and standard deviation for both normal and abnormal classes for each biomarker. We refine these estimates using a Gaussian mixture model (GMM) and include all the available data, including MCI subjects and previously misclassified cases. The objective function for optimization for biomarker $x_{:,i}$ is:

$$C_i = \sum_j \log \left[(\theta_i \times p(x_{j,i}|E_{j,i})) + ((1 - \theta_i) \times p(x_{j,i}|\neg E_{j,i})) \right] \qquad (2)$$

Where θ_i is the mixing parameter which determines the proportion of abnormal biomarker data in the dataset and lies between $[0, 1]$. To obtain a robust GMM fit, a constrained optimization method is used, putting bounds on the mean and standard deviation parameters. These bounds are set to the 95% confidence interval limits of the initial estimates of means and standard deviation.

The PDF thus obtained is used for classification of the biomarkers using a Bayesian classifier where the mixing parameter θ_i is used as the prior probability when estimating posterior probabilities for each biomarker. We assume these posterior probabilities to be a measure of progression of a biomarker. Thus, sorting these biomarkers based on decreasing estimates of posterior probabilities results in a noisy estimate for σ_j.

3.2   Estimating the Central Ordering

Since the event orderings for each subject are estimated independent of each other, any heterogeneity in disease progression is captured in these estimates of σ_j. The central event ordering (σ_0) is the mean of the subject-specific estimates of σ_j. To describe the distribution of σ_j, we make use of a generalized Mallows model. The generalized Mallows model is parameterized by a central ('mean') ordering as well as spread parameters (analogous to the standard deviation in a normal distribution). The central ordering is defined as the ordering that minimizes the sum of distances to all subject-wise orderings σ_j. To measure distance between orderings, an often used measure is Kendall's Tau distance [4]. Kendall's Tau distance between a subject specific event ordering (σ_j) and central ordering (σ_0) can be defined as:

$$K(\sigma_0, \sigma_j) = \sum_{i=1}^{N-1} V_i(\sigma_0, \sigma_j) \tag{3}$$

where $V_i(\sigma_0, \sigma_j)$ is the number of adjacent swaps needed so that event at position i is the same in σ_j and σ_0.

Since the estimates of σ_j are based on rankings of posterior probabilities, it would be desirable to penalize certain swaps more than others, based on how close the posterior probabilities were to each other. To this end, we introduce a probabilistic Kendall's Tau distance, which penalizes each swap based on the difference in posterior probabilities of the corresponding events. The probabilistic Kendall's Tau is computed sequentially using the following algorithm:

Algorithm 1. Probabilistic Kendall Tau distance between Event Orderings

---
1: **for** $i \in \{1, N-1\}$ **do**
2:     $k \leftarrow \sigma_j^{-1}(\sigma_0(i))$
3:     **if** $k > i$ **then**
4:         $V_i(\sigma_0, \sigma_j) \leftarrow p\left(E_{j,\sigma_0(k)}|x_{j,\sigma_0(k)}\right) - p\left(E_{j,\sigma_0(i)}|x_{j,\sigma_0(i)}\right)$
5:         Move $\sigma_j(k)$ to position i and update σ_j
6:     **else**
7:         $V_i(\sigma_0, \sigma_j) \leftarrow 0$

This variant of Kendall's Tau distance is quite close to the weighted Kendall's Tau distance defined in the permutation space introduced in [7]. The difference stems from the fact that since the probabilistic Kendall's Tau distance is between individual estimates and a central-ordering, the penalization of each swap is weighted asymmetrically as $V_i(\sigma_0, \sigma_j) \neq V_i(\sigma_j, \sigma_0)$. This asymmetrical weighing can be formulated as a special case of the aforementioned weighted Kendall's Tau distance.

Computing a global optimum for the central ordering based on subject-wise orderings is NP-hard. The optimization algorithm used in our implementation is based on algorithm introduced by Fligner and Verducci [8] to make an unbiased estimate of the central ordering.

4   Experiments

This section describes the experiments performed to benchmark the accuracy of the proposed DEBM algorithm and compare it with state-of-the-art EBM methods. We begin with the details of the experiments performed on ADNI data to estimate the event ordering in Sect. 4.1. Such an event ordering serves as a timeline for disease progression and is used for patient staging. Since the groundtruth event ordering is unknown for clinical datasets, we resort to using accuracy of patient staging as an indirect way of measuring the reliability of the event ordering. We also measure the accuracy of event ordering in a much more direct way by performing extensive experiments on synthetic data simulating the progression of AD. The details of these experiments are given in Sect. 4.2.

4.1   ADNI Data

We considered 509 ADNI[1] subjects (162 healthy controls, 210 MCI and 137 AD subjects) who had a 1.5T structural MRI (T1) scan at baseline. The T1w scans were non-uniformity corrected using the N3 algorithm [11]. This was followed by multi-atlas brain extraction using the method described in Bron et al. [1]. Multi-atlas segmentation was performed using the structural MRI scans to obtain a region-labeling for 83 brain regions in each subject using a set of 30 atlases [3]. We calculated the volume of these regions and used the ratio of these volumes with the intra-cranial volume as biomarkers. This is done to compensate for the inter-subject variability in head size. We also downloaded CSF ($A\beta_{1-42}$, tau and p-tau) and cognitive scores (MMSE, ADAS-Cog, RAVLT) biomarker values from the ADNI database. Out of these, volume based biomarkers of 41 regions, 3 CSF and 3 cognitive scores were found to be significant features based on Student's t-test with $p < 0.01$. These biomarker values were used to perform three sets of experiments.

Experiment 1: A subset of 7 biomarkers including the 3 CSF features, MMSE scores, ADAS-Cog scores, volume of the hippocampus and whole brain was created. Event ordering of these 7 biomarkers was inferred using DEBM, Huang's EBM [4] and the variant of Fonteijn's EBM that is suited for AD disease progression modeling [12]. The original Fonteijn's EBM [2] differs from the version in [12] only in the way in which normal and abnormal biomarker distributions are estimated. As an indirect way of measuring the reliability of the estimated

---

[1] http://adni.loni.usc.edu/.

event ordering, we use patient staging based on the estimated event orderings as a way to classify controls and AD subjects in the database. 10-fold cross validation was used for this purpose. AUC measures were used to measure the performance of these classifications and thus indirectly hint at the reliability of the event ordering based on which the corresponding patient staging were performed. We used the patient staging algorithm described in [2] for all three EBMs to ensure that the difference in obtained AUC is strictly because of the obtained event ordering.

Experiment 2: The above experiment was repeated for the entire set of 47 features. This was done to study the scalability of EBM techniques.

Experiment 3: We studied the positional variance of central ordering inferred by DEBM by creating 100 bootstrapped samples of the data with 7 biomarkers followed by computing the central ordering for each of those samples.

4.2 Simulation Data

We use the framework developed by Young *et al.* [13] for simulating cross-sectional data consisting of scalar biomarker values for healthy controls, MCI and AD subjects. In this framework, disease progression in a subject is indicated by a cascade of biomarkers becoming abnormal and individual biomarker trajectories are represented by a sigmoid. The equation for generating biomarker values for different subjects is given below:

$$x_{j,i}(\Psi) = \frac{1}{1 + \exp(-\rho_{j,i}(\Psi - \xi_{j,i}))} + \beta_{j,i} \tag{4}$$

$\rho_{j,i}$ signifies the rate of progression of a biomarker with disease state Ψ. $\xi_{j,i}$ denotes the disease state at which a biomarker becomes abnormal. $\beta_{j,i}$ denotes the value of the biomarker when the subject is normal. We assume $\rho_{j,i}$ to be equal for all the subjects, for all the biomarkers. With this assumption, variability in a population while simulating a cross-sectional dataset could arise because of variation in either β or ξ. Variation in $\xi_{j,i}$ results in variation in ordering. In our experiments, β and ξ are assumed to be Normal random variables N_β and N_ξ respectively. Mean of N_β is equal to the mean value of the corresponding biomarker in the controls of the selected ADNI data. We vary relative standard deviation of N_β (Σ_β) in our experiments, where 1 refers to the expected variation among healthy controls, estimated based on the selected subjects in ADNI data. Mean of N_ξ for various biomarkers were assumed to be equi-spaced on the Ψ scale. Standard deviation of N_ξ (Σ_ξ) is varied in multiples of $\Delta\xi/N$, where $\Delta\xi$ is the difference between mean of N_ξ between adjacent biomarkers.

Using this simulation framework, we study the effect of these two factors in the ability of different variants of EBM algorithms to accurately infer the ground-truth central ordering in the population. Inaccuracy is computed based on the normalized Kendall's Tau distance between the ground truth ordering and most-likely ordering (for Fonteijn's EBM) or central ordering (for DEBM and

Huang's EBM). As the Kendall's Tau distance penalizes pair-wise disagreements between event agreements, a normalization factor for $\binom{N}{2}$, where N is the number of events, was chosen to make the accuracy measure interpretable for different number of biomarkers.

We performed three sets of experiments on simulated data to study the accuracy of the different variants of EBM techniques and several aspects associated with it. For all the experiments, the number of simulated subjects was taken to be equal to the number of subjects in the selected ADNI data.

Experiment 4: The first experiment was based on selecting a subset of 7 biomarkers from the 47 significant biomarkers and study the effect of variation of β and ξ. For each simulation setting, 50 repetitions of simulation data were created and used for benchmarking the accuracies of DEBM, Huang's EBM and Fonteijn's EBM.

Experiment 5: The above experiment was repeated for the entire set of 47 features. This was done to study the scalability of EBM techniques.

Experiment 6: The first experiment was repeated for DEBM and Fonteijn's EBM. In addition to these methods, accuracy of the method using DEBM with normal Kendall's Tau distance and Fonteijn's EBM with the normal and abnormal biomarker distributions estimated based on the method discussed in Sect. 3.1 were computed. This was done to ascertain the contributions of individual novel aspects of the proposed algorithm.

5   Results and Discussions

5.1   ADNI Data

The plots in Fig. 1(a) shows the AUC measures in the 10-folds of cross validation. The different methods mentioned in the plot indicate the method used for obtaining the event ordering based on which patient staging was done. The results on the left and right side of the graph are for the case of 7 biomarkers and 47 biomarkers respectively. It must be noted that, in the absence of groundtruth event ordering, results using clinical data only provide circumstantial evidence about the reliability of the method and do not unambiguously prove that one method is better than the other. It can be observed that DEBM based patient staging outperforms both Fonteijn's EBM and Huang's EBM based staging, when used as a classifier. The reduction in AUC while using 47 biomarkers as compared to 7 biomarkers indicates that the set of 47 biomarkers is not optimum for the purpose of classification and an optimum subset selection might be required if this is indeed meant to be used as a classifier. However, as the purpose here is to understand the disease progression mechanism, the decrease in AUC values is not of much significance. The decrease in AUC measure for Huang's EBM is much more than the other two EBMs, when the number of biomarkers increases. This indicates that Huang's EBM might not be scalable.

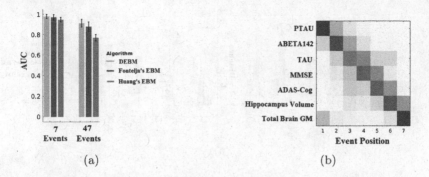

Fig. 1. (a) AUC measures in the 10-folds of cross validation for 7 events and 47 events. (b) Positional variance diagram of the central ordering

The plots in Fig. 1(b) shows the positional variance diagram of the central ordering while using 100 sets of bootstrapped samples. Uncertainty in the estimation of central ordering can be observed in this diagram.

5.2 Simulation Data

Figure 2 shows the variation of mean inaccuracies of DEBM, Fonteijn's EBM and Huang's EBM while varying Σ_β and Σ_ξ of biomarkers. Figures 3(a) and (b) depicts the variation of inaccuracies for 50 repetitions of simulated data for the case of 7 biomarkers and 47 biomarkers respectively. In Fig. 3(a) for the graph on the left, Σ_ξ was fixed to a value of 2/7, while varying Σ_β. For the graph on the right, Σ_β was fixed to be 1 and Σ_ξ was varied from 0 to 4/7 in steps of 1/7. Similarly, in Fig. 3(b) for the graph on the left, Σ_ξ was fixed to a value of 12/47, while varying Σ_β. For the graph on the right, Σ_β was fixed to be 1 and Σ_ξ was varied from 0 to 24/47 in steps of 6/47. Figures 2 and 3(a), (b) show that DEBM outperforms the state-of-the-art EBM techniques in recovering the order in which biomarkers become abnormal. It can also be seen

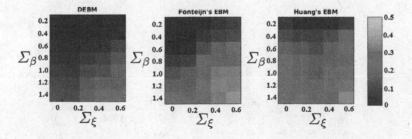

Fig. 2. Effect of Σ_β and Σ_ξ in the mean inaccuracies of DEBM, Fonteijn's EBM and Huang's EBM. Inaccuracies are measured by the distance of estimated event ordering from the groundtruth ordering. These distances are represented based on the shown colormap. (Color figure online)

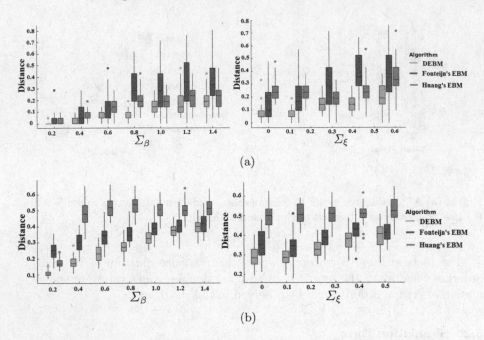

(a)

(b)

Fig. 3. Variation in inaccuracies of DEBM, Fonteijn's EBM and Huang's EBM for 50 repetitions of simulations. The number of events is 7 in (a) and 47 in (b).

that, while the performance of DEBM and Fonteijn's EBM was similar for 7 and 47 biomarkers, the performance of Huang's EBM degrades with increasing number of biomarkers.

Figure 4 shows the results for Experiment 6 detailed in Sect. 4.2. It can be seen that DEBM with probabilistic Kendall's Tau distance outperforms DEBM with normal Kendall's Tau distance. Fonteijn's EBM using normal and abnormal biomarker distributions computed using the technique proposed in Sect. 3.1 outperforms conventional Fonteijn's EBM. It is also interesting to note that

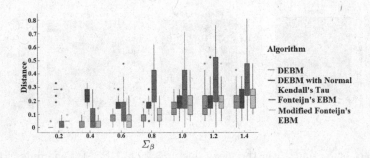

Fig. 4. Variation in inaccuracies of DEBM, DEBM with Kendall's Tau, Fonteijn's EBM and Modified Fonteijn's EBM with respect to Σ_β, with $\Sigma_\xi = 2/7$.

DEBM outperforms the modified Fonteijn's EBM as well, which uses the same biomarker distribution estimation algorithm as DEBM.

Figure 5 shows the mean computation time (in seconds) for the three methods in logarithmic scale. The implementation for all the methods were done in Python and measured in the same computer. DEBM is several orders of magnitude faster than Huang's EBM and comparable to Fonteijn's EBM.

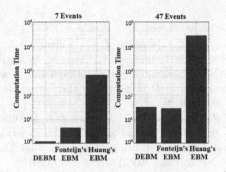

Fig. 5. Computation Time (in seconds)

6 Conclusion and Future Work

We proposed a novel discriminative EBM framework to estimate the ordering in which biomarkers become abnormal during disease progression, based on a cross-sectional dataset. The proposed framework outperforms state-of-the-art EBM techniques in estimating the event ordering and is computationally very efficient as well. In addition to the framework, we also proposed a novel probabilistic Kendall's Tau distance metric and a biomarker distribution estimation algorithm. Each aspect of the proposed algorithm was ascertained to contribute positively in improving the accuracy of estimation.

Fonteijn's EBM assumes a unique event ordering that is common to all the subjects in the database. When this assumption fails, the performance of the algorithm degrades. Huang's EBM and DEBM account for this variation. However, Huang's EBM estimates a lot of parameters through optimization for inferring the central ordering, whereas DEBM is much more direct in estimating the central ordering. This might be one of the reasons why DEBM outperforms Huang's EBM consistently. Moreover, the simplicity of the DEBM algorithm is crucial for its scalability to large number of biomarkers.

Many possible extensions of the work are interesting to consider. Huang's EBM was extended to estimating clusters of central orderings in [13] using Dirichlet process mixtures of generalized Mallows models. Such an extension is also possible using DEBM. Subject-specific event orderings estimated based on cross-sectional data are very noisy. Incorporating longitudinal data to get better estimates of subject-specific event orderings in DEBM is also worth considering.

Acknowledgement. This work is part of the EuroPOND initiative, which is funded by the European Union's Horizon 2020 research and innovation programme under grant agreement No. 666992. The authors also thank Dr. Jonathan Huang for sharing the implementation of Huang's EBM and Dr. Alexandra Young for the useful discussions on estimation of biomarker distributions as well as for sharing the implementation of the simulation system for biomarker evolution.

References

1. Bron, E.E., Steketee, R.M., Houston, G.C., Oliver, R.A., Achterberg, H.C., Loog, M., van Swieten, J.C., Hammers, A., Niessen, W.J., Smits, M., Klein, S., Alzheimer's Disease Neuroimaging Initiative: Diagnostic classification of arterial spin labeling and structural MRI in presenile early stage dementia. Hum. Brain Mapp. **35**(9), 4916–4931 (2014)
2. Fonteijn, H.M., Modat, M., Clarkson, M.J., Barnes, J., Lehmann, M., Hobbs, N.Z., Scahill, R.I., Tabrizi, S.J., Ourselin, S., Fox, N.C., Alexander, D.C.: An event-based model for disease progression and its application in familial Alzheimer's disease and huntington's disease. NeuroImage **60**(3), 1880–1889 (2012)
3. Hammers, A., Allom, R., Koepp, M.J., Free, S.L., Myers, R., Lemieux, L., Mitchell, T.N., Brooks, D.J., Duncan, J.S.: Three-dimensional maximum probability atlas of the human brain, with particular reference to the temporal lobe. Hum. Brain Mapp. **19**(4), 224–247 (2003)
4. Huang, J., Alexander, D.: Probabilistic event cascades for Alzheimer's disease. In: Pereira, F., Burges, C.J.C., Bottou, L., Weinberger, K.Q. (eds.) Advances in Neural Information Processing Systems 25, pp. 3095–3103. Curran Associates, Inc., Red Hook (2012)
5. Iturria-Medina, Y., Sotero, R.C., Toussaint, P.J., Mateos-Prez, J.M., Evans, A.C., Alzheimer's Disease Neuroimaging Initiative: Early role of vascular dysregulation on late-onset Alzheimer's disease based on multifactorial data-driven analysis. Nat. Commun. **7**, 11934 (2016)
6. Jack, C.R., Knopman, D.S., Jagust, W.J., Petersen, R.C., Weiner, M.W., Aisen, P.S., Shaw, L.M., Vemuri, P., Wiste, H.J., Weigand, S.D., Lesnick, T.G., Pankratz, V.S., Donohue, M.C., Trojanowski, J.Q.: Tracking pathophysiological processes in Alzheimer's disease an updated hypothetical model of dynamic biomarkers. Lancet Neurol. **12**(2), 207–216 (2013)
7. Kumar, R., Vassilvitskii, S.: Generalized distances between rankings. In: Proceedings of the 19th International Conference on World Wide Web, WWW 2010, pp. 571–580. ACM, New York (2010)
8. Fligner, M.A., Verducci, S.V.: Multistage ranking models. J. Am. Stat. Assoc. **83**(403), 892–901 (1988)
9. Sabuncu, M.R., Bernal-Rusiel, J.L., Reuter, M., Greve, D.N., Fischl, B.: Event time analysis of longitudinal neuroimage data. NeuroImage **97**, 9–18 (2014)
10. Schmidt-Richberg, A., Ledig, C., Guerrero, R., Molina-Abril, H., Frangi, A., Rueckert, D., Alzheimers Disease Neuroimaging Initiative: Learning biomarker models for progression estimation of Alzheimers disease. PLoS One **11**(04), 1–27 (2016)
11. Tustison, N.J., Avants, B.B., Cook, P.A., Zheng, Y., Egan, A., Yushkevich, P.A., Gee, J.C.: N4ITK: improved N3 bias correction. IEEE Trans. Med. Imaging **29**(6), 1310–1320 (2010)

12. Young, A.L., Oxtoby, N.P., Daga, P., Cash, D.M., Fox, N.C., Ourselin, S., Schott, J.M., Alexander, D.C.: A data-driven model of biomarker changes in sporadic Alzheimer's disease. Brain **137**(9), 2564–2577 (2014)
13. Young, A.L., et al.: Multiple orderings of events in disease progression. In: Ourselin, S., Alexander, D.C., Westin, C.-F., Cardoso, M.J. (eds.) IPMI 2015. LNCS, vol. 9123, pp. 711–722. Springer, Cham (2015). doi:10.1007/978-3-319-19992-4_56

A Vertex Clustering Model for Disease Progression: Application to Cortical Thickness Images

Răzvan Valentin Marinescu[1]([✉]), Arman Eshaghi[1,2], Marco Lorenzi[1,4],
Alexandra L. Young[1], Neil P. Oxtoby[1], Sara Garbarino[1],
Timothy J. Shakespeare[3], Sebastian J. Crutch[3], Daniel C. Alexander[1],
and for the Alzheimer's Disease Neuroimaging Initiative

[1] Centre for Medical Image Computing, Computer Science Department,
University College London, London, UK
razvan.marinescu.14@ucl.ac.uk
[2] Queen Square MS Centre, UCL Institute of Neurology, London, UK
[3] Dementia Research Centre, UCL Institute of Neurology,
University College London, London, UK
[4] University of Côte d'Azur, Inria Sophia Antipolis,
Asclepios Research Project, Biot, France

Abstract. We present a disease progression model with single vertex resolution that we apply to cortical thickness data. Our model works by clustering together vertices on the cortex that have similar temporal dynamics and building a common trajectory for vertices in the same cluster. The model estimates optimal stages and progression speeds for every subject. Simulated data show that it is able to accurately recover the vertex clusters and the underlying parameters. Moreover, our clustering model finds similar patterns of atrophy for typical Alzheimer's disease (tAD) subjects on two independent datasets: the Alzheimer's Disease Neuroimaging Initiative (ADNI) and a cohort from the Dementia Research Centre (DRC), UK. Using a separate set of subjects with Posterior Cortical Atrophy (PCA) from the DRC dataset, we also show that the model finds different patterns of atrophy in PCA compared to tAD. Finally, our model provides a novel way to parcellate the brain based on disease dynamics.

Keywords: Disease progression model · Cortical thickness · Vertex-wise measures · Alzheimer's disease · Posterior Cortical Atrophy

Data used in preparation of this article were obtained from the Alzheimer's Disease Neuroimaging Initiative (ADNI) database (adni.loni.usc.edu). As such, the investigators within the ADNI contributed to the design and implementation of ADNI and/or provided data but did not participate in analysis or writing of this report. A complete listing of ADNI investigators can be found at: http://adni.loni.usc.edu/wp-content/uploads/how_to_apply/ADNI_Acknowledgement_List.pdf.

© Springer International Publishing AG 2017
M. Niethammer et al. (Eds.): IPMI 2017, LNCS 10265, pp. 134–145, 2017.
DOI: 10.1007/978-3-319-59050-9_11

1   Introduction

During the progression of Alzheimer's disease, many biomarkers based on Magnetic Resonance Imaging (MRI) such as cortical thickness become abnormal at different points in the progression. Finding out the precise temporal evolution of these biomarkers facilitates patient staging in clinical trials. However, the analysis of disease progression is limited by several factors: short number of follow-up visits available, different disease onset and progression speed for every subject and cohort heterogeneity.

A hypothetical model of disease progression has been proposed by [1], describing the trajectory of key biomarkers along the progression of Alzheimer's disease. The model suggests that amyloid-beta and tau biomarkers become abnormal long before symptoms appear, followed by brain atrophy measures and cognitive decline. Motivated by this idea, several models such as [2] or [3] have been proposed that reconstruct biomarker trajectories and can be used to stage subjects. However, these models make use of *a priori* clinical categories, which are noisy, biased and can limit the temporal resolution of the model. This motivates the use of fully data-driven approaches that do not use *a priori* clinical stages.

Various data-driven disease progression modelling techniques have been proposed in recent years. One such model is the Event-Based Model [4], which models the progression of disease as a sequence of discrete events, representing underlying biomarkers switching from a normal to abnormal state. Other models such as the Disease Progression Score (DPS) [5] or self-modelling regression approaches [6] have been developed, that build continuous trajectories by "stitching" together short-term follow-up data. Models estimating linear or logistic trajectories by means of Riemannian manifold techniques have also been recently shown [7].

The main limitation of these data-driven models is that they use a small set of biomarkers that are obtained by averaging MRI or PET measures across all voxels or vertices in a Region of Interest (ROI). This can be problematic, especially if different parts of the ROI, say the hippocampus, are affected at different speeds or timepoints in the disease process. Therefore, moving to a voxel-wise approach would allow one to estimate the fine-grained spatial distribution of atrophy, which could give new insights into the disease process and potentially enable more precise staging. A voxel-wise disease progression model [8] has been recently proposed to mitigate this problem, that uses amyloid measures in each voxel as its input data. However, the model by [8] has two limitations: (1) the biomarker trajectories are assumed to be linear, so cannot capture the plateau effect observed in amyloid-beta or tau and (2) the model uses a spatial correlation function for modelling correlation between voxels; while this is necessary, due to the nature of the imaging data, it has been shown that in different types of dementia atrophy patterns match functional networks, which are not spatially connected [9].

In this work, we present a new disease progression model with single vertex resolution that avoids assumptions on spatial correlation. We combine unsupervised learning and disease progression modelling to identify clusters of vertices on the cortical surface, with no spatial constraints, that show a similar trajectory of atrophy over a particular patient cohort. This formulation enables us to gain new insights into the spatial structure of atrophy in different diseases and also provides a novel parcellation of the brain based on temporal change. Moreover, each cluster of vertices has a corresponding sigmoidal trajectory, which avoids the limitation of linear trajectories in [8].

We first show using simulated data that our model is able to recover known underlying clusters, trajectory parameters and subject stages. We then apply our model to cortical thickness vertex-wise measures using ADNI and the DRC dataset and highlight the new insights the model can give. Finally, we validate our model using cross-validation and by correlating the subject stages with cognitive measures.

2   Methods

2.1   Model

We seek to identify groups of image vertices that show a common trajectory during the disease course, while simultaneously placing each visit from each subject within that disease course. In a similar way to [5–7], we estimate a time shift and speed (or rate) of progression for each subject. We relate these time shifts and progression speeds by assigning each subject a disease stage which we will refer to as the Disease Progression Score (DPS). In contrast to [5–7], which model temporal trajectories for a small set of biomarker measures based on *a priori* defined ROIs, we model temporal trajectories for each vertex on the cortical surface. Each trajectory is a function of the disease progression score (i.e. disease stage) of a subject. We estimate each subjects' time shift, progression speed and trajectory parameters from the data. The disease progression score s_{ij} for subject i at visit j is defined as a linear transformation of age t_{ij}:

$$s_{ij} = \alpha_i t_{ij} + \beta_i \tag{1}$$

where α_i and β_i represent the speed of progression and time shift (i.e. disease onset) of subject i.

Our model assumes that the cortical thickness at each vertex on the cortical surface follows a sigmoidal trajectory $f(s)$ given the disease progression score s. We also assume that vertices are grouped into K clusters and we model a unique trajectory for each cluster $k \in [1, \ldots, K]$, which will be referred to as cluster trajectories. The sigmoidal function for cluster k is parametrised as $\theta_k = [a_k, b_k, c_k, d_k]$ where

$$f(s; \theta_k) = \frac{a_k}{1 + exp(-b_k(s - c_k))} + d_k \tag{2}$$

For a given subject i at visit j, the value V_l^{ij} of its cortical thickness at vertex l is a random variable that has an associated discrete latent variable

$Z_l \in [1, \ldots, K]$ denoting the cluster it was generated from. The value of V_l^{ij} given that it was generated from cluster Z_l can be modelled as:

$$p(V_l^{ij}|\alpha_i, \beta_i, \theta_{Z_l}, \sigma_{Z_l}, Z_l) = N(V_l^{ij}|f(\alpha_i t_{ij} + \beta_i|\theta_{Z_l}), \sigma_{Z_l}) \qquad (3)$$

where $N(V_l^{ij}|f(\alpha_i t_{ij} + \beta_i|\theta_{Z_l}), \sigma_{Z_l})$ represents the pdf of the normal distribution that models the measurement noise along the sigmoidal trajectory of cluster Z_l, having variance σ_{Z_l}. Next, we assume the measurements from different subjects are independent, while the measurements from the same subject i at different visits j are linked using the disease progression score from Eq. 1, because we estimate only two parameters (α_i and β_i) using the data from all visits j. Moreover, we also assume a uniform prior on Z_l. This gives the following model:

$$p(V_l, Z_l|\alpha, \beta, \theta, \sigma) = \prod_{(i,j)\in I} N(V_l^{ij}|f(\alpha_i t_{ij} + \beta_i|\theta_{Z_l}), \sigma_{Z_l}) \qquad (4)$$

where $I = (i, j)$ represents the set of all the subjects i and their corresponding visits j. Furthermore, $V_l = [V_l^{ij}|(i, j) \in I]$ is the 1D array of all the values for vertex l across every subject and corresponding visit. Vectors $\alpha = [\alpha_1, \ldots, \alpha_S]$ and $\beta = [\beta_1, \ldots, \beta_S]$, where S is the number of subjects, denote the stacked parameters for the subject shifts. Vectors $\theta = [\theta_1, \ldots, \theta_K]$ and $\sigma = [\sigma_1, \ldots, \sigma_K]$, with K being the number of clusters, represent the stacked parameters for the sigmoidal trajectories and measurement noise specific to each cluster.

We further assume all vertex measurements to be spatially independent, giving the complete data likelihood:

$$p(V, Z|\alpha, \beta, \theta, \sigma) = \prod_l \prod_{(i,j)\in I} N(V_l^{ij}|f(\alpha_i t_{ij} + \beta_i|\theta_{Z_l}), \sigma_{Z_l}) \qquad (5)$$

where $V = [V_1, \ldots, V_L]$, $Z = [Z_1, \ldots, Z_L]$, L being the total number of vertices on the cortical surface. We recall that we don't want to enforce spatial correlation between vertices as we are interested to see if vertices from distinct areas of the brain are grouped together in the same cluster. Our assumption is also justified by the fact that we smoothed the cortical thickness images in the preprocessing steps. We get the final model log likelihood for incomplete data by marginalising over the latent variables Z:

$$p(V|\alpha, \beta, \theta, \sigma) = \prod_{l=1}^{L} \sum_{k=1}^{K} p(Z_l = k) \prod_{(i,j)\in I} N(V_l^{ij}|f(\alpha_i t_{ij} + \beta_i|\theta_k), \sigma_k) \qquad (6)$$

Therefore, the parameters that need to be estimated are $\Theta = [\alpha, \beta, \theta, \sigma]$ where α and β are the subject specific shifting parameters while θ and σ are the cluster specific trajectory and noise parameters.

2.2 Fitting the Model Using EM

Due to the summing over the latent variables Z, it is not possible to find a closed form solution to the maximum likelihood. Therefore, we fit our model using Expectation-Maximisation, which is suitable given the large number of data points and parameters that need to be estimated.

E-Step. In the Expectation step we seek to estimate which cluster has generated each of the L vertices, given the current estimates of the cluster parameters $\theta_k^{old}, \sigma_k^{old}$ as well as the subject specific shift parameters $\alpha_i^{old}, \beta_i^{old}$. More formally, we seek to find $p(Z|V, \Theta^{old}) = \prod_l^L p(Z_l|V_l, \Theta^{old})$, given our independence assumption between vertices. Let us denote by $z_{lk} = p(Z_l = k|V_l, \Theta^{old})$. We then have:

$$z_{lk} = \frac{\prod_{(i,j)\in I} N(V_l^{ij}|f(\alpha_i^{old}t_{ij} + \beta_i^{old}|\theta_k^{old}), \sigma_k^{old})}{\sum_{m=1}^K \prod_{i,j\in I} N(V_l^{ij}|f(\alpha_i^{old}t_{ij} + \beta_i^{old}|\theta_m^{old}), \sigma_m^{old})} \tag{7}$$

Ignoring the normalisation factor, we perform a log transformation and expand the pdfs of the normal distributions. This results in the following update equation for the E-step:

$$log \ z_{lk} \propto -\frac{1}{2} log \left(2\pi \left(\sigma_k^{old}\right)^2\right)|I| - \frac{1}{2\left(\sigma_k^{old}\right)^2} \sum_{(i,j)\in I} (V_l^{ij} - f(\alpha_i^{old}t_{ij} + \beta_i^{old}|\theta_k^{old}))^2$$
$$\tag{8}$$

The original probabilities can be easily recovered by exponentiating them and then normalising with respect to their sum.

M-Step. In the Maximisation step we try to find $\Theta = (\alpha, \beta, \theta, \sigma)$ that maximise $E_{Z|V,\Theta^{old}}[log \ p(V, Z|\Theta)]$. Since there is no closed-form solution, we perform successive refinements of θ_k for each cluster k and α_i, β_i for each subject i until convergence.

In order to get the update rule for the trajectory parameters θ_k corresponding to cluster k we need to maximise the expected log likelihood with respect to θ_k. We get the following simplified optimisation problem:

$$\theta_k = \arg\min_{\theta_k} \left[\sum_{l=1}^L z_{lk} \sum_{(i,j)\in I} (V_l^{ij} - f(\alpha_i t_{ij} + \beta_i|\theta_k))^2 \right] - log \ p(\theta_k) \tag{9}$$

A similar equation is also obtained for σ_k. After estimating θ and σ for every cluster, we use the new values to estimate the subject specific parameters α and β. Let S be the number of subjects and α_i, β_i be the rate and shift for subject $i \in S$. We again maximise the expected log likelihood with respect to α_i, β_i independently, and after simplifications we obtain the following problem:

$$\alpha_i, \beta_i = \arg\min_{\alpha_i,\beta_i} \left[\sum_{l=1}^L \sum_{k=1}^K z_{lk} \frac{1}{2\sigma_k^2} \sum_{j\in I_i} (V_l^{ij} - f(\alpha_i t_{ij} + \beta_i|\theta_k))^2 \right] - log \ p(\alpha_i, \beta_i) \tag{10}$$

In summary, at every single M-step, we iterate between solving for θ, σ and solving for α, β using numerical optimisation until convergence. Due to the use of numerical optimisation, we are not guaranteed to find the global maxima for the expected log likelihood, but EM still works if we only find an increase in the log-likelihood. This approach that involves a partial M-step is called Generalised EM.

2.3   Initialisation and Implementation

Before starting the fitting process, we need to initialise α, β and the clustering probabilities z_{lk}. We set α_i and β_i to be 1 and 0 respectively for each subject. We initialise z_{lk} using k-means clustering using vectors V_l having $|I|$ number of samples and L features. Furthermore, as already explained in [5], the scale of the DPS is arbitrary so we standardise the scores at each EM iteration such that the DPS of controls have a mean μ_N of zero and a standard deviation σ_N of 1. This also requires a rescaling of the cluster parameters θ_k.

In our implementation, we run the main EM loop until convergence of the clustering probabilities z_{lk}. At each M-step we perform numerical optimisation using the Broyden-Fletcher-Goldfarb-Shanno (BFGS) algorithm that makes use of the first derivative of the objective function. In all datasets analysed, the method converges after maximum 25 EM iterations.

3   Simulation Results

We first tested the model in a toy scenario using synthetic data, which we generated as follows: (1) sampled age and shift parameters from 300 subjects with 4 timepoints (each timepoint 1 year apart), with $t_{i1} \sim U(40, 80)$, $\alpha_i \sim N(1, 0.05)$, $\beta_i \sim N(0, 10)$ (2) generated three sigmoids with different center points and slopes (Fig. 1(a), red lines) (3) generated a random cluster assignment for $L = 1,000$ vertices, i.e. every vertex l was assigned to a cluster $a[l] \in \{1, 2, 3\}$ (4) sampled a set of L perturbed trajectories θ_l from each of the original trajectories, one for each vertex (Fig. 1(b), gray lines) and (5) sampled subject data for every vertex l from its corresponding perturbed trajectory θ_l with $\sigma_l = 0.5$

To fit the data we used a uniform prior on the parameters θ and σ and an informative prior on α and β, with $p(\alpha_i) \sim \Gamma(49, 70)$ and $\beta_i \sim N(0, 1)$. We also normalised age to have a mean of 0 and standard deviation of 1 and rescaled the DPS and cluster trajectories accordingly. After convergence, we calculated the agreement between the final clustering probabilities and the true clustering assignments as $A = \frac{1}{L} \sum_{l=1}^{L} p(Z_l = a[l])$. The method also requires us to set the number of clusters a priori, so we optimised the number of clusters using the Bayesian Information Criterion (BIC).

The BIC analysis correctly predicted three clusters for this synthetic experiment. Using three clusters, we also obtained a clustering agreement of $A = 1.0$. Figure 1(a) shows the original trajectories and the recovered trajectories using our model, plotted against the disease progression score on the x-axis and the vertex value on the y-axis. Moreover, in Fig. 1(b) we plotted the recovered DPS of each subject along with the true DPS.

The results show that the model accurately estimated which clusters generated each vertex. Moreover, the recovered trajectories are close to the true trajectories, with some errors for the trajectories corresponding to clusters 1 and 2. The recovered DPS also shows good agreement with the true DPS, with the exception of a few subjects with DPS greater than 2.5. This is explained by the fact that there is not enough signal in that DPS range in terms of trajectory dynamics (i.e. trajectories are mostly flat). The simulation confirms that our model is able to recover the hidden clusters, trajectory parameters and the subject specific parameters. However, more realistic simulations with varying noise levels and numbers of clusters are required to understand the limitations of the model and find out when it fails to recover the true parameters.

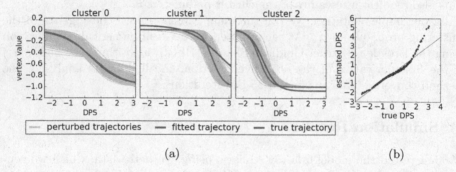

(a)   (b)

Fig. 1. (a) Reconstructed temporal trajectories (blue) from the synthetic data along with the true trajectories (red). The data was generated from the perturbed trajectories, which in turn were generated from the true trajectories. (b) Estimated subject-specific disease progression scores compared to the true scores. (Color figure online)

4   Experimental Results

4.1   Data Acquisition and Preprocessing

Data used in this work were obtained from the Alzheimer's Disease Neuroimaging Initiative (ADNI) database (adni.loni.usc.edu) and from the Dementia Research Centre, UK. For ADNI, we downloaded all T1 MRI images that have undergone gradwarping, intensity correction and scaling for gradient drift. We included subjects that had at least 4 scans, in order to ensure we get a robust estimate of the subject specific parameters. This resulted in 328 subjects with an average number of 4.95 scans each. The DRC dataset consisted of T1 MRI scans from 31 healthy controls, 32 PCA and 23 typical typical AD subjects with at least 3 scans each and an average of 5.26 scans per subject.

On both datasets, in order to extract reliable cortical thickness measures we ran the Freesurfer longitudinal pipeline [10], which first registers the MRI images to an unbiased within-subject template space using inverse-consistent registration. The longitudinally registered images were then registered to the average

Freesurfer template and smoothed at a full-width/half-max (FWHM) level of zero. For each vertex we averaged the thickness levels from both hemispheres. Finally, we standardised the data from each vertex with respect to the values of that vertex in the control population. Each of the final images had a resolution of 163,842 vertices on the cortical surface.

4.2   ADNI and DRC Results

Using ADNI and DRC datasets, we were interested to find out the spatial distribution of cortical atrophy, as well as the rate and timing of this atrophy process. In particular, we wanted to find out: (1) if we get similar results using our model on two independent tAD datasets: ADNI and DRC and (2) if we get different patterns of atrophy on distinct diseases (tAD and PCA) that match previous studies.

BIC analysis predicted that the optimal number of clusters is two for the ADNI cohort and three for both tAD and PCA subjects from the DRC cohort. In order to make the results easily comparable across the different datasets, we ran all experiments using 3 clusters. Figure 2(a) shows the results of our model using all ADNI subjects, where we coloured points on the cortical surface according to the cluster they most likely belong to. We assigned a colour to each cluster according to the slope of its corresponding trajectory, ranging from red (high slope suggesting a fast rate of atrophy) to blue (low slope suggesting a slow rate of atrophy). In Fig. 2(d) we also show the resulting cluster trajectories with samples from the posterior distribution of each θ_k. We repeated the same analysis on the DRC cohort, separately for the tAD subjects (Fig. 2(b) and (e)) and PCA subjects (Fig. 2(c) and (f)).

We notice that in tAD subjects using both ADNI and DRC datasets (Fig. 2), there is widespread atrophy in most temporal, parietal and frontal areas (red cluster), with the notable exception of the motor cortex and the occipital lobe. These patterns of atrophy are similar across the two different datasets. Moreover, the spatial distribution of cortical thinning found with our technique resembles results from previous longitudinal studies such as [11]. However, in contrast to these approaches, our model gives insight into the timing, rate and extent of atrophy and is also able to stage subjects across the disease timecourse.

In the PCA subjects (Fig. 2(c)), we find that the atrophy is more focused on the posterior part of the brain, mostly the posterior parietal and occipital, with more limited spread in the superior temporal and inferior frontal. This is in contrast with the tAD patterns in the other datasets, that lacks the focus on posterior parietal and occipital regions. This posterior pattern of atrophy also matches previous findings in the literature [12]. For all datasets, we find that the cluster trajectories differ less in timing and more in the slope and minima/maxima values at which they plateau (Fig. 2(d), (e) and (f). Our model therefore predicts that regions on the cortical surface are all affected roughly at the same time, but the rate and extent to which they are affected is different.

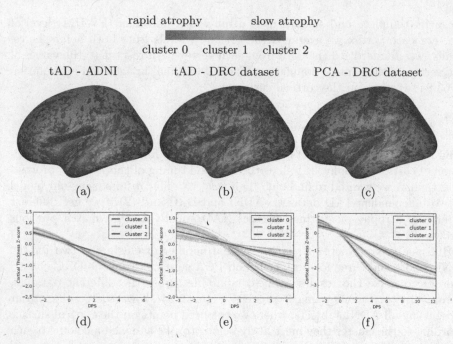

Fig. 2. (a) Clustering results on the ADNI data using our model, where each cluster is coloured according to the slope of its corresponding trajectory, from red (high slope suggesting very affected areas) to blue (low slope suggesting less affected areas). (d) The corresponding trajectories and samples from the posterior distribution of the trajectory parameters for the three clusters in ADNI. The same analysis is shown also for (b, e) tAD subjects from the DRC cohort and (c, f) PCA subjects from the DRC cohort. (Color figure online)

4.3   Model Validation

We tested robustness of the model by performing 10-fold cross validation (CV) on ADNI. Our motivation was to test the following: (1) if similar spatial clustering is estimated at each fold, as quantified by Dice score overlap, (2) if the stages of the test subjects were consistent (i.e. were increasing for follow-up visits) and (3) if the stages of test subjects are clinically meaningful, by correlating them with cognitive tests such as Clinical Dementia Rating Scale - Sum of Boxes (CDRSOB), Alzheimer's Disease Assessment Scale - Cognitive (ADAS-COG), Mini-Mental State Examination (MMSE) and Rey Auditory and Verbal Learning Test (RAVLT).

Figure 3 shows the clusters that were estimated at each fold from the training data only. Moreover, in Fig. 4 we plot the estimated DPS (i.e. disease stage) of each subject from the test set against their age.

The results in Fig. 3 prove that the model is robust in cross-validation, as the estimated clusters are all very similar across folds. The average Dice scores we obtained across all pairs of folds were 0.89, 0.89 and 0.90 for clusters 0, 1 and 2 respectively. Furthermore, 84% of the subjects analysed show increased stages across their follow-up visits, proving that the estimated stages are mostly consistent. Finally, the stages of test subject correlate with clinical measures such as CDRSOB ($\rho = 0.41$, $p < 1e-66$), ADAS-COG ($\rho = 0.40$, $p < 1e-62$), MMSE ($\rho = 0.39$, $p < 1e-58$) and RAVLT ($\rho = 0.35$, $p < 1e-46$), demonstrating that the stages have clinical validity.

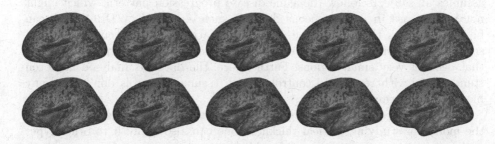

Fig. 3. Clusters estimated for each of the 10 cross-validation folds in ADNI. As before, each cluster is coloured according to the slope of its corresponding trajectory, from red (high rate of atrophy) to blue (low rate of atrophy). (Color figure online)

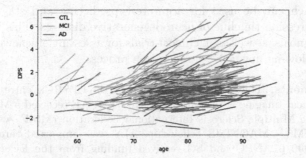

Fig. 4. The disease progression score for each subject from the ADNI dataset estimated during 10-fold cross validation. Each line represents an individual i with different visits j. Later visits generally have a higher corresponding stage.

5   Discussion

We presented a model of disease progression that clusters vertex-wise measures of cortical thickness based on similar temporal dynamics. The model highlights, for the first time, groups of cortical vertices that exhibit a similar temporal trajectory over the population. This provides a new way to parcellate the brain that is specific to the temporal trajectory of a particular disease. The model also finds the optimal temporal shift and progression speed for every subject.

We applied the model to cortical thickness vertex-wise data from the ADNI and DRC cohorts. Our model found similar patterns of atrophy dynamics in the tAD subjects using the two independent datasets. Moreover, it also found different patterns of atrophy dynamics on two distinct diseases: tAD and PCA.

The model has some limitations. First of all, we assumed that cluster trajectories follow sigmoidal shapes, which might not be the case for many types of biomarkers such as cortical thickness. Another limitation of the model is that it assumes all subjects follow the same disease progression pattern, which might not be the case in heterogeneous datasets such as ADNI or DRC. This can be a concern, as there might be a pattern of atrophy that occurs in a small set of subjects. Moreover, our cluster-based model might miss atrophy patterns that occur is very small regions. Furthermore, the data we analysed has been standardised with respect to controls, which assumes controls don't show any biomarker abnormalities.

There are several potential avenues of future research. While we only used the model for studying cortical thickness, one can also apply it to other types of data such as amyloid images or Jacobian compression maps. On the methodological side, the assumption of sigmoidal trajectories can be avoided using nonparametric curves such as Gaussian Processes. Another extension is to model different progression dynamics for distinct subgroups using unsupervised learning methods like the approach of [13], or incorporate subject-specific deviations from the standard pattern of atrophy using a mixed-effects model.

Our approach can be used for accurately predicting and staging patients across the progression timeline of neurodegenerative diseases. This is promising for patient prognosis, as well as in clinical-trials for assessing efficacy of a putative treatment for slowing down the degeneration process.

Acknowledgements. This work was supported by the EPSRC Centre For Doctoral Training in Medical Imaging with grant EP/L016478/1. AE received a McDonald Fellowship from the Multiple Sclerosis International Federation (MSIF, www.msif.org), and the ECTRIMS - MAGNIMS Fellowship. ALY was supported through EPSRC grant EP/J020990/01. NPO and SG received funding from the EU Horizon 2020 research and innovation programme under grant agreement No. 666992. SJC was supported by an Alzheimer's Research UK Senior Research Fellowship and ESRC/NIHR (ES/L001810/1) and EPSRC (EP/M006093/1) grants. DCA's work on this topic has funding from the EU Horizon 2020 research and innovation programme under grant agreement No. 666992, as well as EPSRC grants J020990, M006093 and M020533. Data collection and sharing for this project was funded by the Alzheimer's Disease Neuroimaging Initiative (ADNI) (National Institutes of Health Grant U01 AG024904) and DOD ADNI (Department of Defense award number W81XWH-12-2-0012). The Dementia Research Centre is an ARUK coordination center.

References

1. Jack, C.R., Knopman, D.S., Jagust, W.J., Shaw, L.M., Aisen, P.S., Weiner, M.W., Petersen, R.C., Trojanowski, J.Q.: Hypothetical model of dynamic biomarkers of the Alzheimer's pathological cascade. Lancet Neurol. **9**(1), 119–128 (2010)

2. Bateman, R.J., Xiong, C., Benzinger, T.L., Fagan, A.M., Goate, A., Fox, N.C., Marcus, D.S., Cairns, N.J., Xie, X., Blazey, T.M., Holtzman, D.M.: Clinical and biomarker changes in dominantly inherited Alzheimer's disease. N. Engl. J. Med. **367**(9), 795–804 (2012)

3. Schmidt-Richberg, A., Guerrero, R., Ledig, C., Molina-Abril, H., Frangi, A.F., Rueckert, D.: Multi-stage biomarker models for progression estimation in Alzheimer's disease. In: Ourselin, S., Alexander, D.C., Westin, C.-F., Cardoso, M.J. (eds.) IPMI 2015. LNCS, vol. 9123, pp. 387–398. Springer, Cham (2015). doi:10.1007/978-3-319-19992-4_30

4. Fonteijn, H.M., Modat, M., Clarkson, M.J., Barnes, J., Lehmann, M., Hobbs, N.Z., Scahill, R.I., Tabrizi, S.J., Ourselin, S., Fox, N.C., Alexander, D.C.: An event-based model for disease progression and its application in familial Alzheimer's disease and Huntington's disease. NeuroImage **60**(3), 1880–1889 (2012)

5. Jedynak, B.M., Lang, A., Liu, B., Katz, E., Zhang, Y., Wyman, B.T., Raunig, D., Jedynak, C.P., Caffo, B., Prince, J.L., Initiative, A.D.N.: A computational neurodegenerative disease progression score: method and results with the Alzheimer's Disease Neuroimaging Initiative cohort. Neuroimage **63**(3), 1478–1486 (2012)

6. Donohue, M.C., Jacqmin-Gadda, H., Le Goff, M., Thomas, R.G., Raman, R., Gamst, A.C., Beckett, L.A., Jack, C.R., Weiner, M.W., Dartigues, J.F., Aisen, P.S.: Estimating long-term multivariate progression from short-term data. Alzheimer's & Dementia **10**(5), S400–S410 (2014)

7. Schiratti, J.-B., Allassonnière, S., Routier, A., Colliot, O., Durrleman, S.: A mixed-effects model with time reparametrization for longitudinal univariate manifold-valued data. In: Ourselin, S., Alexander, D.C., Westin, C.-F., Cardoso, M.J. (eds.) IPMI 2015. LNCS, vol. 9123, pp. 564–575. Springer, Cham (2015). doi:10.1007/978-3-319-19992-4_44

8. Bilgel, M., Prince, J.L., Wong, D.F., Resnick, S.M., Jedynak, B.M.: A multivariate nonlinear mixed effects model for longitudinal image analysis: application to amyloid imaging. NeuroImage **134**, 658–670 (2016)

9. Seeley, W.W., Crawford, R.K., Zhou, J., Miller, B.L., Greicius, M.D.: Neurodegenerative diseases target large-scale human brain networks. Neuron **62**(1), 42–52 (2009)

10. Reuter, M., Schmansky, N.J., Rosas, H.D., Fischl, B.: Within-subject template estimation for unbiased longitudinal image analysis. Neuroimage **61**(4), 1402–1418 (2012)

11. Dickerson, B.C., Bakkour, A., Salat, D.H., Feczko, E., Pacheco, J., Greve, D.N., Grodstein, F., Wright, C.I., Blacker, D., Rosas, H.D., Sperling, R.A.: The cortical signature of Alzheimer's disease: regionally specific cortical thinning relates to symptom severity in very mild to mild AD dementia and is detectable in asymptomatic amyloid-positive individuals. Cereb. Cortex **19**(3), 497–510 (2009)

12. Crutch, S.J., Lehmann, M., Schott, J.M., Rabinovici, G.D., Rossor, M.N., Fox, N.C.: Posterior cortical atrophy. Lancet Neurol. **11**(2), 170–178 (2012)

13. Young, A.L., Oxtoby, N.P., Huang, J., Marinescu, R.V., Daga, P., Cash, D.M., Fox, N.C., Ourselin, S., Schott, J.M., Alexander, D.C.: Multiple orderings of events in disease progression. In: Ourselin, S., Alexander, D.C., Westin, C.-F., Cardoso, M.J. (eds.) IPMI 2015. LNCS, vol. 9123, pp. 711–722. Springer, Cham (2015). doi:10.1007/978-3-319-19992-4_56

Unsupervised Anomaly Detection with Generative Adversarial Networks to Guide Marker Discovery

Thomas Schlegl[1,2]([✉]), Philipp Seeböck[1,2], Sebastian M. Waldstein[2], Ursula Schmidt-Erfurth[2], and Georg Langs[1]

[1] Computational Imaging Research Lab,
Department of Biomedical Imaging and Image-guided Therapy,
Medical University Vienna, Vienna, Austria
thomas.schlegl@meduniwien.ac.at
[2] Christian Doppler Laboratory for Ophthalmic Image Analysis,
Department of Ophthalmology and Optometry,
Medical University Vienna, Vienna, Austria

Abstract. Obtaining models that capture imaging markers relevant for disease progression and treatment monitoring is challenging. Models are typically based on large amounts of data with annotated examples of known markers aiming at automating detection. High annotation effort and the limitation to a vocabulary of known markers limit the power of such approaches. Here, we perform unsupervised learning to identify anomalies in imaging data as candidates for markers. We propose *AnoGAN*, a deep convolutional generative adversarial network to learn a manifold of normal anatomical variability, accompanying a novel anomaly scoring scheme based on the mapping from image space to a latent space. Applied to new data, the model labels anomalies, and scores image patches indicating their fit into the learned distribution. Results on optical coherence tomography images of the retina demonstrate that the approach correctly identifies anomalous images, such as images containing retinal fluid or hyperreflective foci.

1 Introduction

The detection and quantification of disease markers in imaging data is critical during diagnosis, and monitoring of disease progression, or treatment response. Relying on the vocabulary of known markers limits the use of imaging data containing far richer relevant information. Here, we demonstrate that relevant *anomalies* can be identified by unsupervised learning on large-scale imaging data.

Medical imaging enables the observation of markers correlating with disease status, and treatment response. While there is a wide range of known markers

---

T. Schlegl—This work has received funding from IBM, FWF (I2714-B31), OeNB (15356, 15929), the Austrian Federal Ministry of Science, Research and Economy (CDL OPTIMA).

M. Niethammer et al. (Eds.): IPMI 2017, LNCS 10265, pp. 146–157, 2017.
DOI: 10.1007/978-3-319-59050-9_12

(e.g., characteristic image appearance of brain tumors or calcification patterns in breast screening), many diseases lack a sufficiently broad set, while in others the predictive power of markers is limited. Furthermore, even if predictive markers are known, their computational detection in imaging data typically requires extensive supervised training using large amounts of annotated data such as labeled lesions. This limits our ability to exploit imaging data for treatment decisions.

Here, we propose unsupervised learning to create a rich generative model of healthy local anatomical appearance. We show how generative adversarial networks (GANs) can solve the central problem of creating a sufficiently representative model of appearance, while at the same time learning a generative and discriminative component. We propose an improved technique for mapping from image space to latent space. We use both components to differentiate between observations that conform to the training data and such data that does not fit.

Related Work. Anomaly detection is the task of identifying test data not fitting the *normal* data distribution seen during training. Approaches for anomaly detection exist in various domains, ranging from video analysis [1] to remote sensing [2]. They typically either use an explicit representation of the distribution of normal data in a feature space, and determine outliers based on the local density at the observations' position in the feature space. Carrera et al. [3] utilized convolutional sparse models to learn a dictionary of filters to detect anomalous regions in texture images. Erfani et al. [4] proposed a hybrid model for unsupervised anomaly detection that uses a one-class support vector machine (SVM). The SVM was trained from features that were learned by a deep belief network (DBN). The experiments in the aforementioned works were performed on real-life-datasets comprising 1D inputs, synthetic data or texture images, which have lower dimensionality or different data characteristics compared to medical images. An investigation of anomaly detection research papers can be found in [5]. In clinical optical coherence tomography (OCT) scan analysis, Venhuizen et al. [6] used bag-of-word features as a basis for supervised random forest classifier training to distinguish diseased patients from healthy subjects. Schlegl et al. [7] utilized convolutional neural networks to segment retinal fluid regions in OCT data via weakly supervised learning based on semantic descriptions of pathology-location pairs extracted from medical reports. In contrast to our approach, both works used some form of supervision for classifier training. Seeböck et al. [8] identified anomalous regions in OCT images through unsupervised learning on healthy examples, using a convolutional autoencoder and a one-class SVM, and explored different classes of anomalies. In contrast to this work, the SVM in [8] involved the need to choose a hyper-parameter that defined the amount of training points covered by the estimated healthy region.

GANs enable to learn generative models generating detailed realistic images [9–11]. Radford et al. [12] introduced deep convolutional generative adversarial networks (DCGANs) and showed that GANs are capable of capturing semantic image content enabling vector arithmetic for visual concepts. Yeh et al. [13] trained GANs on natural images and applied the trained model for semantic image inpainting. Compared to Yeh et al. [13], we implement two

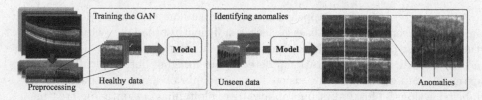

Fig. 1. Anomaly detection framework. The preprocessing step includes extraction and flattening of the retinal area, patch extraction and intensity normalization. Generative adversarial training is performed on healthy data and testing is performed on both, unseen healthy cases and anomalous data. (Color figure online)

adaptations for an improved mapping from images to the latent space. We condition the search in the latent space on the whole query image, and propose a novel variant to guide the search in the latent space (inspired by feature matching [14]). In addition, we define an anomaly score, which is not needed in an inpainting task. The main difference of this paper to aforementioned anomaly detection work is the representative power of the generative model and the coupled mapping schema, which utilizes a trained DCGAN and enables accurate discrimination between normal anatomy, and local anomalous appearance. This renders the detection of subtle anomalies at scale feasible.

Contribution. In this paper, we propose adversarial training of a generative model of normal appearance (see blue block in Fig. 1), described in Sect. 2.1, and a coupled mapping schema, described in Sect. 2.2, that enables the evaluation of novel data (Sect. 2.3) to identify anomalous images and segment anomalous regions within imaging data (see red block in Fig. 1). Experiments on labeled test data, extracted from spectral-domain OCT (SD-OCT) scans, show that this approach identifies known anomalies with high accuracy, and at the same time detects other anomalies for which no voxel-level annotations are available. To the best of our knowledge, this is the first work, where GANs are used for anomaly or novelty detection. Additionally, we propose a novel mapping approach, wherewith the pre-image problem can be tackled.

2 Generative Adversarial Representation Learning to Identify Anomalies

To identify anomalies, we learn a model representing normal anatomical variability based on GANs [13]. This method trains a generative model, and a discriminator to distinguish between generated and real data simultaneously (see Fig. 2(a)). Instead of a single cost function optimization, it aims at the Nash equilibrium of costs, increasing the representative power and specificity of the generative model, while at the same time becoming more accurate in classifying real- from generated data and improving the corresponding feature mapping. In the following we explain how to build this model (Sect. 2.1), and how to use it to identify appearance not present in the training data (Sects. 2.2 and 2.3).

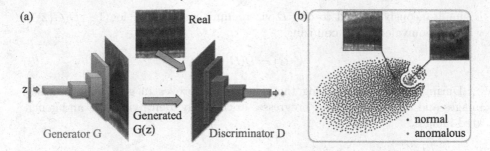

Fig. 2. (a) Deep convolutional generative adversarial network. (b) t-SNE embedding of normal (blue) and anomalous (red) images on the feature representation of the last convolution layer (orange in (a)) of the discriminator. (Color figure online)

2.1 Unsupervised Manifold Learning of Normal Anatomical Variability

We are given a set of M medical images $\mathbf{I}_m$ showing healthy anatomy, with $m = 1, 2, \ldots, M$, where $\mathbf{I}_m \in \mathbb{R}^{a \times b}$ is an intensity image of size $a \times b$. From each image $\mathbf{I}_m$, we extract K 2D image patches $x_{k,m}$ of size $c \times c$ from randomly sampled positions resulting in data $\mathbf{x} = x_{k,m} \in \mathcal{X}$, with $k = 1, 2, \ldots, K$. During training we are only given $\langle \mathbf{I}_m \rangle$ and train a generative adversarial model to learn the manifold $\mathcal{X}$ (blue region in Fig. 2(b)), which represents the variability of the training images, in an unsupervised fashion. For testing, we are given $\langle \mathbf{y}_n, l_n \rangle$, where $\mathbf{y}_n$ are unseen images of size $c \times c$ extracted from new testing data $\mathbf{J}$ and $l_n \in \{0, 1\}$ is an array of binary image-wise ground-truth labels, with $n = 1, 2, \ldots, N$. These labels are only given during testing, to evaluate the anomaly detection performance based on a given pathology.

Encoding Anatomical Variability with a Generative Adversarial Network. A GAN consists of two adversarial modules, a generator G and a discriminator D. The generator G learns a distribution p_g over data $\mathbf{x}$ via a mapping $G(\mathbf{z})$ of samples $\mathbf{z}$, 1D vectors of uniformly distributed input noise sampled from latent space $\mathcal{Z}$, to 2D images in the image space manifold $\mathcal{X}$, which is populated by healthy examples. In this setting, the network architecture of the generator G is equivalent to a convolutional decoder that utilizes a stack of strided convolutions. The discriminator D is a standard CNN that maps a 2D image to a single scalar value $D(\cdot)$. The discriminator output $D(\cdot)$ can be interpreted as probability that the given input to the discriminator D was a real image $\mathbf{x}$ sampled from training data $\mathcal{X}$ or generated $G(\mathbf{z})$ by the generator G. D and G are simultaneously optimized through the following two-player minimax game with value function $V(G, D)$ [9]:

$$\min_{G} \max_{D} V(D, G) = \mathbb{E}_{\mathbf{x} \sim p_{data}(\mathbf{x})} \left[\log D(\mathbf{x}) \right] + \mathbb{E}_{\mathbf{z} \sim p_{\mathbf{z}}(\mathbf{z})} \left[\log(1 - D(G(\mathbf{z}))) \right]. \quad (1)$$

The discriminator is trained to maximize the probability of assigning real training examples the *"real"* and samples from p_g the *"fake"* label. The generator G

is simultaneously trained to fool D via minimizing $V(G) = \log(1 - D(G(\mathbf{z})))$, which is equivalent to maximizing

$$V(G) = D(G(\mathbf{z})). \tag{2}$$

During adversarial training the generator improves in generating realistic images and the discriminator progresses in correctly identifying real and generated images.

2.2   Mapping New Images to the Latent Space

When adversarial training is completed, the generator has learned the mapping $G(\mathbf{z}) = \mathbf{z} \mapsto \mathbf{x}$ from latent space representations $\mathbf{z}$ to realistic (normal) images $\mathbf{x}$. But GANs do not automatically yield the inverse mapping $\mu(\mathbf{x}) = \mathbf{x} \mapsto \mathbf{z}$ for free. The latent space has smooth transitions [12], so sampling from two points close in the latent space generates two visually similar images. Given a query image $\mathbf{x}$, we aim to find a point $\mathbf{z}$ in the latent space that corresponds to an image $G(\mathbf{z})$ that is visually most similar to query image $\mathbf{x}$ and that is located on the manifold $\mathcal{X}$. The degree of similarity of $\mathbf{x}$ and $G(\mathbf{z})$ depends on to which extent the query image follows the data distribution p_g that was used for training of the generator. To find the best $\mathbf{z}$, we start with randomly sampling $\mathbf{z}_1$ from the latent space distribution $\mathcal{Z}$ and feed it into the trained generator to get a generated image $G(\mathbf{z}_1)$. Based on the generated image $G(\mathbf{z}_1)$ we define a loss function, which provides gradients for the update of the coefficients of $\mathbf{z}_1$ resulting in an updated position in the latent space, $\mathbf{z}_2$. In order to find the most similar image $G(\mathbf{z}_\Gamma)$, the location of $\mathbf{z}$ in the latent space $\mathcal{Z}$ is optimized in an iterative process via $\gamma = 1, 2, \ldots, \Gamma$ backpropagation steps.

In the spirit of [13], we define a loss function for the mapping of new images to the latent space that comprises two components, a *residual loss* and a *discrimination loss*. The *residual loss* enforces the visual similarity between the generated image $G(\mathbf{z}_\gamma)$ and query image $\mathbf{x}$. The *discrimination loss* enforces the generated image $G(\mathbf{z}_\gamma)$ to lie on the learned manifold $\mathcal{X}$. Therefore, both components of the trained GAN, the discriminator D and the generator G, are utilized to adapt the coefficients of $\mathbf{z}$ via backpropagation. In the following, we give a detailed description of both components of the loss function.

Residual Loss. The *residual loss* measures the visual dissimilarity between query image $\mathbf{x}$ and generated image $G(\mathbf{z}_\gamma)$ in the image space and is defined by

$$\mathcal{L}_R(\mathbf{z}_\gamma) = \sum |\mathbf{x} - G(\mathbf{z}_\gamma)|. \tag{3}$$

Under the assumption of a perfect generator G and a perfect mapping to latent space, for an ideal normal query case, images $\mathbf{x}$ and $G(\mathbf{z}_\gamma)$ are identical. In this case, the *residual loss* is zero.

Discrimination Loss. For image inpainting, Yeh et al. [13] based the computation of the *discrimination loss* $\mathcal{L}_{\hat{D}}(\mathbf{z}_\gamma)$ on the discriminator output by feeding the generated image $G(\mathbf{z}_\gamma)$ into the discriminator $\mathcal{L}_{\hat{D}}(\mathbf{z}_\gamma) = \sigma(D(G(\mathbf{z}_\gamma)), \alpha)$, where σ is the sigmoid cross entropy, which defined the discriminator loss of real images during adversarial training, with logits $D(G(\mathbf{z}_\gamma))$ and targets $\alpha = 1$.

An Improved Discrimination Loss Based on Feature Matching. In contrast to the work of Yeh et al. [13], where $\mathbf{z}_\gamma$ is updated to fool D, we define an alternative discrimination loss $\mathcal{L}_D(\mathbf{z}_\gamma)$, where $\mathbf{z}_\gamma$ is updated to match $G(\mathbf{z}_\gamma)$ with the learned distribution of normal images. This is inspired by the recently proposed feature matching technique [14].

Feature matching addresses the instability of GANs due to over-training on the discriminator response [14]. In the feature matching technique, the objective function for optimizing the generator is adapted to improve GAN training. Instead of optimizing the parameters of the generator via maximizing the discriminator's output on generated examples (Eq. (2)), the generator is forced to generate data that has similar statistics as the training data, i.e. whose intermediate feature representation is similar to those of real images. Salimans et al. [14] found that feature matching is especially helpful when classification is the target task. Since we do not use any labeled data during adversarial training, we do not aim for learning class-specific discriminative features but we aim for learning good representations. Thus, we do not adapt the training objective of the generator during adversarial training, but instead use the idea of feature matching to improve the mapping to the latent space. Instead of using the scalar output of the discriminator for computing the *discrimination loss*, we propose to use a richer intermediate feature representation of the discriminator and define the *discrimination loss* as follows:

$$\mathcal{L}_D(\mathbf{z}_\gamma) = \sum |\mathbf{f}(\mathbf{x}) - \mathbf{f}(G(\mathbf{z}_\gamma))|, \tag{4}$$

where the output of an intermediate layer $f(\cdot)$ of the discriminator is used to specify the statistics of an input image. Based on this new loss term, the adaptation of the coordinates of $\mathbf{z}$ does not only rely on a hard decision of the trained discriminator, whether or not a generated image $G(\mathbf{z}_\gamma)$ fits the learned distribution of normal images, but instead takes the rich information of the feature representation, which is learned by the discriminator during adversarial training, into account. In this sense, our approach utilizes the trained discriminator not as classifier but as a feature extractor.

For the mapping to the latent space, we define the overall loss as weighted sum of both components:

$$\mathcal{L}(\mathbf{z}_\gamma) = (1 - \lambda) \cdot \mathcal{L}_R(\mathbf{z}_\gamma) + \lambda \cdot \mathcal{L}_D(\mathbf{z}_\gamma). \tag{5}$$

Only the coefficients of $\mathbf{z}$ are adapted via backpropagation. The trained parameters of the generator and discriminator are kept fixed.

2.3 Detection of Anomalies

During anomaly identification in new data we evaluate the new query image $\mathbf{x}$ as being a normal or anomalous image. Our loss function (Eq. (5)), used for mapping to the latent space, evaluates in every update iteration γ the compatibility of generated images $G(\mathbf{z}_\gamma)$ with images, seen during adversarial training. Thus, an *anomaly score*, which expresses the fit of a query image $\mathbf{x}$ to the model of normal images, can be directly derived from the mapping loss function (Eq. (5)):

$$A(\mathbf{x}) = (1 - \lambda) \cdot R(\mathbf{x}) + \lambda \cdot D(\mathbf{x}), \tag{6}$$

where the *residual score* $R(x)$ and the *discrimination score* $D(x)$ are defined by the *residual loss* $\mathcal{L}_R(\mathbf{z}_\Gamma)$ and the *discrimination loss* $\mathcal{L}_D(\mathbf{z}_\Gamma)$ at the last (Γ^{th}) update iteration of the mapping procedure to the latent space, respectively. The model yields a large *anomaly score* $A(\mathbf{x})$ for anomalous images, whereas a small *anomaly score* means that a very similar image was already seen during training. We use the *anomaly score* $A(\mathbf{x})$ for image based anomaly detection. Additionally, the residual image $\mathbf{x}_R = |\mathbf{x} - G(\mathbf{z}_\Gamma)|$ is used for the identification of anomalous regions within an image. For purposes of comparison, we additionally define a *reference anomaly score* $\hat{A}(\mathbf{x}) = (1 - \lambda) \cdot R(\mathbf{x}) + \lambda \cdot \hat{D}(\mathbf{x})$, where $\hat{D}(\mathbf{x}) = \mathcal{L}_{\hat{D}}(\mathbf{z}_\Gamma)$ is the *reference discrimination score* used by Yeh et al. [13].

3 Experiments

Data, Data Selection and Preprocessing. We evaluated the method on clinical high resolution SD-OCT volumes of the retina with 49 B-scans (representing an image slice in zx-plane) per volume and total volume resolutions of $496 \times 512 \times 49$ voxels in z-, x-, and y direction, respectively. The GAN was trained on 2D image patches extracted from 270 clinical OCT volumes of healthy subjects, which were chosen based on the criterion that the OCT volumes do not contain fluid regions. For testing, patches were extracted from 10 additional healthy cases and 10 pathological cases, which contained retinal fluid. The OCT volumes were preprocessed in the following way. The gray values were normalized to range from -1 to 1. The volumes were resized in x-direction to a size of $22\,\mu m$ resulting in approximately 256 columns. The retinal area was extracted and flattened to adjust for variations in orientation, shape and thickness. We used an automatic layer segmentation algorithm following [15] to find the top and bottom layer of the retina that define the border of the retina in z-direction. From these normalized and flattened volumes, we extracted in total 1.000.000 2D training patches with an image resolution of 64×64 pixels at randomly sampled positions. Raw data and preprocessed image representation are shown in Fig. 1. The test set in total consisted of 8192 image patches and comprised normal and pathological samples from cases not included in the training set. For pathological OCT scans, voxel-wise annotations of fluid and non-fluid regions from clinical retina experts were available. These annotations were only used for statistical evaluation but were never fed to the network, neither during training nor in the evaluation phase. For the evaluation of the detection performance, we assigned a positive label to an image, if it contained at least a single pixel annotated as retinal fluid.

Evaluation. The manifold of normal images was solely learned on image data of healthy cases with the aim to model the variety of healthy appearance. For performance evaluation in anomaly detection we ran the following experiments.

(1) We explored qualitatively whether the model can generate realistic images. This assessment was performed on image patches of healthy cases extracted from the training set or test set and on images of diseased cases extracted from the test set.

(2) We evaluated quantitatively the anomaly detection accuracy of our approach on images extracted from the annotated test set. We based the anomaly detection on the *anomaly score* $A(\mathbf{x})$ or only on one of both components, on the *residual score* $R(\mathbf{x})$ or on the *discrimination score* $D(\mathbf{x})$ and report receiver operating characteristic (ROC) curves of the corresponding anomaly detection performance on image level.

Based on our proposed *anomaly score* $A(\mathbf{x})$, we evaluated qualitatively the segmentation performance and if additional anomalies were identified.

(3) To provide more details of individual components' roles, and the gain by the proposed approach, we evaluated the effect on the anomaly detection performance, when for manifold learning the adversarial training is not performed with a DCGAN but with an adversarial convolutional autoencoder (aCAE) [16], while leaving the definition of the *anomaly score* unchanged. An *aCAE* also implements a discriminator but replaces the generator by an encoder-decoder pipeline. The depth of the components of the trained *aCAE* was comparable to the depth of our adversarial model. As a second alternative approach, denoted as GAN_R, we evaluated the anomaly detection performance, when the *reference anomaly score* $\hat{A}(\mathbf{x})$, or the *reference discrimination score* $\hat{D}(\mathbf{x})$ were utilized for anomaly scoring and the corresponding losses were used for the mapping from image space to latent space, while the pre-trained GAN parameters of the *AnoGAN* were used. We report ROC curves for both alternative approaches. Furthermore, we calculated sensitivity, specificity, precision, and recall at the optimal cut-off point on the ROC curves, identified through the Youden's index and report results for the *AnoGAN* and for both alternative approaches.

Implementation Details. As opposed to historical attempts, Radford et al. [12] identified a DCGAN architecture that resulted in stable GAN training on images of sizes 64×64 pixels. Hence, we ran our experiments on image patches of the same size and used widley the same DCGAN architecture for GAN training (Sect. 2.1) as proposed by Radford et al. [12][1]. We used four fractionally-strided convolution layers in the generator, and four convolution layers in the discriminator, all filters of sizes 5×5. Since we processed gray-scale images, we utilized intermediate representations with $512 - 256 - 128 - 64$ channels (instead of $1024 - 512 - 256 - 128$ used in [12]). DCGAN training was performed for 20 epochs utilizing Adam [17], a stochastic optimizer. We ran 500 backpropagation steps for the mapping (Sect. 2.2) of new images to the latent space. We

---

[1] We adapted: https://github.com/bamos/dcgan-completion.tensorflow.

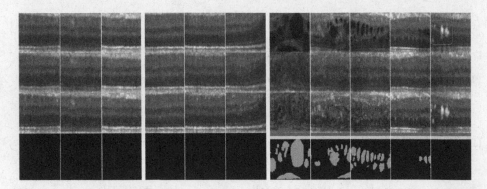

Fig. 3. Pixel-level identification of anomalies on exemplary images. First row: Real input images. Second row: Corresponding images generated by the model triggered by our proposed mapping approach. Third row: Residual overlay. Red bar: Anomaly identification by *residual score*. Yellow bar: Anomaly identification by *discrimination score*. Bottom row: Pixel-level annotations of retinal fluid. First block and second block: Normal images extracted from OCT volumes of healthy cases in the training set and test set, respectively. Third block: Images extracted from diseased cases in the test set. Last column: Hyperreflective foci (within green box). (Best viewed in color)

used $\lambda = 0.1$ in Eqs. (5) and (6), which was found empirically due to preceding experiments on a face detection dataset. All experiments were performed using Python 2.7 with the TensorFlow [18] library and run on a Titan X graphics processing unit using CUDA 8.0.

3.1   Results

Results demonstrate the generative capability of the DCGAN and the appropriateness of our proposed mapping and scoring approach for anomaly detection. We report qualitative and quantitative results on segmentation performance and detection performance of our approach, respectively.

Can the Model Generate Realistic Images? The trained model generates realistic looking medical images (second row in Fig. 3) that are conditioned by sampling from latent representations $\mathbf{z}$, which are found through our mapping approach, described in Sect. 2.2. In the case of normal image patches (see first and second block in Fig. 3), our model is able to generate images that are visually similar to the query images (first row in Fig. 3). But in the case of anomalous images, the pairs of input images and generated images show obvious intensity or textural differences (see third block in Fig. 3). The t-SNE embedding (Fig. 2(b)) of normal and anomalous images in the feature representation of the last convolution layer of the discriminator that is utilized in the *discrimination loss*, illustrates the usability of the discriminator's features for anomaly detection and suggests that our AnoGAN learns a meaningful manifold of normal anatomical variability.

Can the Model Detect Anomalies? Figure 4 shows the ROC curves for image level anomaly detection based on the *anomaly score* $A(\mathbf{x})$, or on one

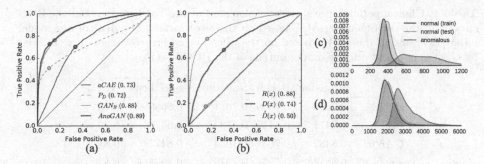

Fig. 4. Image level anomaly detection performance and suitability evaluation. (a) Model comparison: ROC curves based on *aCAE* (blue), *GAN$_R$* (red), the proposed *AnoGAN* (black), or on the output P_D of the trained discriminator (green). (b) Anomaly score components: ROC curves based on the *residual score* $R(\mathbf{x})$ (green), the *discrimination score* $D(\mathbf{x})$ (black), or the *reference discrimination score* $\hat{D}(\mathbf{x})$ (red). (c) Distribution of the *residual score* and (d) of the *discrimination score*, evaluated on normal images of the training set (blue) or test set (green), and on images extracted from diseased cases (red). (Color figure online)

of both components, on the *residual score* $R(\mathbf{x})$, or on the *discrimination score* $D(\mathbf{x})$. The corresponding area under the ROC curve (AUC) is specified in parentheses. In addition, the distributions of the *residual score* $R(\mathbf{x})$ (Fig. 4(c)) and of the *discrimination score* $D(\mathbf{x})$ (Fig. 4(d)) over normal images from the training set and test set or over images extracted from diseased cases show that both components of the proposed *adversarial score* are suitable for the classification of normal and anomalous samples. Figure 3 shows pixel-level identification of anomalies in conjunction with pixel-level annotations of retinal fluid, which demonstrate high accuracy. Last column in Fig. 3 demonstrates that the model successfully identifies additional retinal lesions, which in this case correspond to hyperreflective foci (HRF). On image level, the red and yellow bars in Fig. 3 demonstrate that our model successfully identifies every example image from diseased cases of the test set as beeing anomalous based on the *residual score* and the *discrimination score*, respectively.

How Does the Model Compare to Other Approaches? We evaluated the anomaly detection performance of the GAN_R, the $aCAE$ and the $AnoGAN$ on image-level labels. The results are summarized in Table 1 and the corresponding ROC curves are shown in Fig. 4(a). Although $aCAEs$ simultaneously yield a generative model and a direct mapping to the latent space, which is advantageous in terms of runtimes during testing, this model showed worse performance on the anomaly detection task compared to the $AnoGAN$. It turned out that $aCAEs$ tend to over-adapt on anomalous images. Figure 4(b) demonstrates that anomaly detection based on our proposed *discrimination score* $D(\mathbf{x})$ outperforms the *reference discrimination score* $\hat{D}(\mathbf{x})$. Because the scores for the detection of anomalies are directly related to the losses for the mapping to latent space, these results give evidence that our proposed *discrimination loss* $\mathcal{L}_D(\mathbf{z})$ is

Table 1. Clinical performance statistics calculated at the Youden's index of the ROC curve and the corresponding AUC based on the *adversarial score* $A(\mathbf{x})$ of our model (*AnoGAN*) and of the *aCAE*, based on the *reference adversarial score* $\hat{A}(\mathbf{x})$ utilized by GAN_R, or based directly on the output of the DCGAN (P_D).

	Precision	Recall	Sensitivity	Specificity	AUC
aCAE	0.7005	0.7009	0.7011	0.6659	0.73
P_D	0.8471	0.5119	0.5124	0.8970	0.72
GAN_R	0.8482	0.7631	0.7634	0.8477	0.88
AnoGAN	0.8834	0.7277	0.7279	0.8928	0.89

advantageous compared to the discrimination loss $\mathcal{L}_{\hat{D}}(\mathbf{z})$. Nevertheless, according to the AUC, computed based on the *anomaly score*, the *AnoGAN* and the GAN_R show comparable results (Fig. 4(a)). This has to be attributed to the good performance of the *residual score* $R(\mathbf{x})$. A good anomaly detection performance (cf. P_D in Fig. 4(a) and Table 1) can be obtained when the mapping to the latent space is skipped and a binary decision is derived from the discriminator output, conditioned directly on the query image.

4   Conclusion

We propose anomaly detection based on deep generative adversarial networks. By concurrently training a generative model and a discriminator, we enable the identification of anomalies on unseen data based on unsupervised training of a model on healthy data. Results show that our approach is able to detect different known anomalies, such as retinal fluid and HRF, which have never been seen during training. Therefore, the model is expected to be capable to discover novel anomalies. While quantitative evaluation based on a subset of anomaly classes is limited, since false positives do not take novel anomalies into account, results demonstrate good sensitivity and the capability to segment anomalies. Discovering anomalies at scale enables the mining of data for marker candidates subject to future verification. In contrast to prior work, we show that the utilization of the residual loss alone yields good results for the mapping from image to latent space, and a slight improvement of the results can be achieved with the proposed adaptations.

References

1. Del Giorno, A., Bagnell, J.A., Hebert, M.: A discriminative framework for anomaly detection in large videos. In: Leibe, B., Matas, J., Sebe, N., Welling, M. (eds.) ECCV 2016. LNCS, vol. 9909, pp. 334–349. Springer, Cham (2016). doi:10.1007/978-3-319-46454-1_21
2. Matteoli, S., Diani, M., Theiler, J.: An overview of background modeling for detection of targets and anomalies in hyperspectral remotely sensed imagery. IEEE J. Selected Top. Appl. Earth Obs. Remote Sens. **7**(6), 2317–2336 (2014)

3. Carrera, D., Boracchi, G., Foi, A., Wohlberg, B.: Detecting anomalous structures by convolutional sparse models. In: 2015 International Joint Conference on Neural Networks (IJCNN), IEEE, pp. 1–8 (2015)
4. Erfani, S.M., Rajasegarar, S., Karunasekera, S., Leckie, C.: High-dimensional and large-scale anomaly detection using a linear one-class SVM with deep learning. Pattern Recognit. **58**, 121–134 (2016)
5. Pimentel, M.A., Clifton, D.A., Clifton, L., Tarassenko, L.: A review of novelty detection. Signal Process. **99**, 215–249 (2014)
6. Venhuizen, F.G., van Ginneken, B., Bloemen, B., van Grinsven, M.J., Philipsen, R., Hoyng, C., Theelen, T., Sánchez, C.I.: Automated age-related macular degeneration classification in OCT using unsupervised feature learning. In: SPIE Medical Imaging, International Society for Optics and Photonics, p. 94141I (2015)
7. Schlegl, T., Waldstein, S.M., Vogl, W.-D., Schmidt-Erfurth, U., Langs, G.: Predicting semantic descriptions from medical images with convolutional neural networks. In: Ourselin, S., Alexander, D.C., Westin, C.-F., Cardoso, M.J. (eds.) IPMI 2015. LNCS, vol. 9123, pp. 437–448. Springer, Cham (2015). doi:10.1007/978-3-319-19992-4_34
8. Seeböck, P., Waldstein, S., Klimscha, S., Gerendas, B.S., Donner, R., Schlegl, T., Schmidt-Erfurth, U., Langs, G.: Identifying and categorizing anomalies in retinal imaging data. In: NIPS 2016 MLHC Workshop. Preprint arXiv:1612.00686 (2016)
9. Goodfellow, I., Pouget-Abadie, J., Mirza, M., Xu, B., Warde-Farley, D., Ozair, S., Courville, A., Bengio, Y.: Generative adversarial nets. In: Advances in Neural Information Processing Systems, pp. 2672–2680 (2014)
10. Denton, E.L., Chintala, S., Fergus, R., et al.: Deep generative image models using a Laplacian pyramid of adversarial networks. In: Advances in Neural Information Processing Systems, pp. 1486–1494 (2015)
11. Donahue, J., Krähenbühl, P., Darrell, T.: Adversarial feature learning. arXiv:1605.09782 (2016)
12. Radford, A., Metz, L., Chintala, S.: Unsupervised representation learning with deep convolutional generative adversarial networks. arXiv:1511.06434 (2015)
13. Yeh, R., Chen, C., Lim, T.Y., Hasegawa-Johnson, M., Do, M.N.: Semantic image inpainting with perceptual and contextual losses. arXiv:1607.07539 (2016)
14. Salimans, T., Goodfellow, I., Zaremba, W., Cheung, V., Radford, A., Chen, X.: Improved techniques for training GANs. In: Advances in Neural Information Processing Systems, pp. 2226–2234 (2016)
15. Garvin, M.K., Abràmoff, M.D., Wu, X., Russell, S.R., Burns, T.L., Sonka, M.: Automated 3-D intraretinal layer segmentation of macular spectral-domain optical coherence tomography images. IEEE Trans. Med. Imaging **28**(9), 1436–1447 (2009)
16. Pathak, D., Krähenbühl, P., Donahue, J., Darrell, T., Efros, A.A.: Context encoders: Feature learning by inpainting. CoRR abs/1604.07379 (2016)
17. Kingma, D., Ba, J.: Adam: A method for stochastic optimization. arXiv:1412.6980 (2014)
18. Abadi, M., Agarwal, A., Barham, P., Brevdo, E., Chen, Z., Citro, C., Corrado, G.S., Davis, A., Dean, J., Devin, M., Ghemawat, S., Goodfellow, I., Harp, A., Irving, G., Isard, M., Jia, Y., Jozefowicz, R., Kaiser, L., Kudlur, M., Levenberg, J., Mané, D., Monga, R., Moore, S., Murray, D., Olah, C., Schuster, M., Shlens, J., Steiner, B., Sutskever, I., Talwar, K., Tucker, P., Vanhoucke, V., Vasudevan, V., Viégas, F., Vinyals, O., Warden, P., Wattenberg, M., Wicke, M., Yu, Y., Zheng, X.: TensorFlow: large-scale machine learning on heterogeneous systems (2015). Software available from http://www.tensorflow.org

A Novel Dynamic Hyper-graph Inference Framework for Computer Assisted Diagnosis of Neuro-Diseases

Yingying Zhu[1(✉)], Xiaofeng Zhu[1], Minjeong Kim[1], Daniel Kaufer[2], and Guorong Wu[1]

[1] Department of Radiology and BRIC,
University of North Carolina at Chapel Hill, Chapel Hill, NC 27599, USA
zyy@med.unc.edu, zhuyingying2@gmail.com
[2] Department of Neurology, University of North Carolina at Chapel Hill, Chapel Hill, NC 27599, USA

Abstract. Recently hyper-graph learning gains increasing attention in medical imaging area since the hyper-graph, a generalization of a graph, opts to characterize the complex subject-wise relationship behind multi-modal neuroimaging data. However, current hyper-graph methods mainly have two limitations: (1) The data representation encoded in the hyper-graph is learned only from the observed imaging features for each modality separately. Therefore, the learned subject-wise relationships are neither consistent across modalities nor fully consensus with the clinical labels or clinical scores. (2) The learning procedure of data representation is completely independent to the subsequent classification step. Since the data representation optimized in the feature domain is not exactly aligned with the clinical labels, such independent step-by-step workflow might result in sub-optimal classification. To address these limitations, we propose a novel dynamic hyper-graph inference framework, working in a semi-supervised manner, which iteratively estimates and adjusts the subject-wise relationship from multi-modal neuroimaging data until the learned data representation (encoded in the hyper-graph) achieves largest consensus with the observed clinical labels and scores. It is worth noting our inference framework is also flexible to integrate classification (identifying individuals with neuro-disease) and regression (predicting the clinical scores). We have demonstrated the performance of our proposed dynamic hyper-graph inference framework in identifying MCI (Mild Cognition Impairment) subjects and the fine-grained recognition of different progression stage of MCI, where we achieve more accurate diagnosis result than conventional counterpart methods.

1 Introduction

There is overwhelming consensus that the morphological patterns from neuroimaging data, either structural image (e.g., MRI) or functional image (e.g., PET/SPECT), are highly correlated with neuro-diseases, such as Alzheimer's disease (AD). Large inter-subject variations and complex disease pathology make it challenging to develop imaging-based diagnosis system that can identify individual patient or high risk subjects, in vivo, with high sensitivity and specificity.

© Springer International Publishing AG 2017
M. Niethammer et al. (Eds.): IPMI 2017, LNCS 10265, pp. 158–169, 2017.
DOI: 10.1007/978-3-319-59050-9_13

Since different imaging modalities convey complementary information, many state-of-the-art machine learning approaches have been proposed to improve the diagnosis accuracy using multi-modal imaging. To name a few works, multi-task learning by ensemble SVM and SVR are used for AD and Mild Cognitive Impairment (MCI) classification and regression in [1], Deep Boltzmann machine is used to fuse multiple modality imaging data into a high-level representation for classification [2], etc. Showing the advantage of integrating multi-modal imaging information in assisting diagnosis, those learn models have deficiency in the generality and accuracy due to the limited number of training samples with both multi-modal imaging data and clinical labels. Hence, semi-supervised learning approaches come to the stage which leverage the data distribution of entire population (regardless with or without label) to overcome the lack of labeled subjects. In general, most semi-supervised methods represent data distribution using graph techniques.

Due to large inter-subject variations, pairwise relationship encoded in simple graph is not sufficient to characterize such complex and diverse subject-to-subject relationship. The emerging hyper-graph technique shows potential to solve this problem as it has been successfully applied in various medical imaging applications including image segmentation [3] and classification [4]. Particularly, hyper-graph has been used to combine multi-modal neuroimaging information for the identification of MCI subjects in [4]. The main idea is to construct several hyper-graphs, with each measuring the relevance among a group of subjects based on one modality. Compared to conventional simple graph technique, hyper-graph allows to connect more than two nodes (subjects) in each hyper-edge. Thus, hyper-graph intuitively conveys more information than conventional simple graph through a set of hyper-edges, which makes it more powerful in capturing high-order relationship among different subjects. Given the hyper-graph, the MCI classification is eventually a label propagation procedure to disseminate the clinical labels throughout the hyper-graph structure, following the principle that subjects falling in the same hyper-edge should bear similar clinical labels.

Although promising results have been achieved in [4], there are still several issues. First, the hyper-graph is built for each modality independently. For example, there are two hyper-graphs separately built from morphological features extracted from MR and PET images, as shown by blue and purple solid ellipses in the middle of Fig. 1. The final classification result is the linear combination of label likelihood scores by different hyper-graphs. Although the weights for combination can be learned from training data, the learned prior weights cannot guaranteed to be optimal for each testing subject. Second, the construction of hyper-graphs is exclusively driven by morphological feature representations and completely independent to the subsequent classification and regression task with the morphological patterns already aligned with clinical labels. More critically, the hyper-graphs are fixed once built upon the observed morphological feature only. Due to the possible noisy and redundant patterns existing in the observed high-dimensional imaging features, the learned hyper-graph might be sub-optimal for label propagation, and thus misguide the propagation of clinical labels to each individual testing subject.

To address these issues, we propose a novel dynamic hyper-graph inference framework for multi-modal diagnosis of neuro-diseases. Instead of constructing separate hyper-graphs for different modal imaging data, we propose to learn an unified

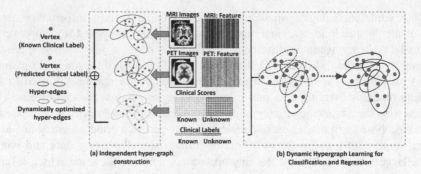

Fig. 1. The comparison between conventional hyper-graph learning (left) and our joint hyper-graph learning, classification and regression method (right) using multiple modal imaging data. The main improvement in our method are (1) hyper-graph across multiple modalities and clinical scores, (2) refinement of hyper-edges dynamically among labelled subjects and unlabeled subjects (designated by the dash ellipses, instead of solid ellipses in the left). (Color figure online)

dynamic hype-graph for all modal imaging data aligned with phenotype data (e.g., clinical labels scores), as shown in the right of Fig. 1. The insight of our work is that all subjects share a common hyper-graph disregard of various appearances of morphological patterns across different modalities. The dynamic hyper-graph is designated to (1) respect the subject-wise relationship measured by the observed multi-modal imaging data (2) automatically learn the optimal weights for dynamical hyper-graph on multi-modal imaging data (3) bring minimal discrepancy after the verification between the estimated data labels and clinical labels assigned in the training dataset. To achieve these goals, we present an iterative solution which alternatively estimates and adjusts the subject-wise relationship from multi-modal neuroimaging data until the learned data representation (encoded in the hyper-graph) achieves largest consensus with the observed clinical labels. Meanwhile, we notice that the clinical scores such as MMSE and CDR scores in AD are widely used in current learning-based diagnosis methods since these phenotype data has higher correlation with the clinical labels compared to imaging data. To that end, we further extend our hyper-graph inference framework to integrate both classification (identifying individuals with neuro-disease) and regression (predicting the clinical scores). We apply our proposed hyper-graph based diagnosis method to identify MCI subjects and classify MCI subjects at different progression stages. The experiments results demonstrated that our method outperforms conventional hyper-graph methods about 1.8% increase in identifying MCI subjects from NC and AD cohorts and 3.1% increase in fine grained recognition of recognizing different stage of MCI respectively.

2   Methods

We will first briefly review the standard hyper-graph learning techniques and then introduce the proposed dynamic hyper-graph learning framework.

2.1   Conventional Hyper-Graph Learning

Conventional Hyper-Graph for One Modality: A hyper-graph is denoted as $\mathcal{G} = (\mathcal{V}, \mathcal{E})$, where $\mathcal{V}$ is the vertex set and each vertex represent one subject here, $\mathcal{E}$ is the hyper-edge set. In a conventional graph, one edge connects a pair of vertex, however, in a hyper-graph, one hyper-edge connects a set of vertexes. Given n subjects with imaging features, we first compute a subject-wise distance matrix $\mathbf{S} \in \Re^{n \times n}$ using imaging features, then, we construct the hyper-graph incidence distance matrix $\mathbf{H} = \{0, 1\} \in \Re^{|\mathcal{V}| \times |\mathcal{E}|}$ to model the relationship among different vertices and edges as,

$$\mathbf{H}(v, e) = \mathbf{1}, \ \mathbf{S}(v, e) < \theta, \ \mathbf{H}(v, e) = \mathbf{0}, \text{ otherwise} \tag{1}$$

where θ is the predefined threshold. The $(v, e) -$ th entry of the incidence matrix indices whether the vertex is connected via the hyper-edge e to other vertices (1 represent connected and 0 represent un-connected). Two diagonal matrices $\mathbf{D}_v$ and $\mathbf{D}_e$ to represent the vertex degrees and hyper-edge degrees are also constructed from the incidence matrix $\mathbf{H}$. The vertex degree and edge degree are computed as,

$$\mathbf{D}_v(v, v) = \sum\nolimits_{e \in \mathcal{E}} \mathbf{H}(v, e), \ \mathbf{D}_e(e, e) = \sum\nolimits_{v \in \mathcal{V}} \mathbf{H}(v, e),$$

After constructed the incidence matrix, vertexes degree matrix and hyper-edge degree matrix, denote $\mathbf{I}$ as the identity matrix, one can compute the hyper-graph Laplacian matrix $\mathbf{L}$ as,

$$\mathbf{L} = \mathbf{I} - \mathbf{D}_v^{-\frac{1}{2}} \mathbf{H} \mathbf{D}_e^{-1} \mathbf{D}_v^{-\frac{1}{2}}, \tag{2}$$

Given known data clinical labels $\mathbf{Y}$ and learned hyper-graph Laplacian matrix, conventional methods solve the following function for classification labels propagation on the hyper-graph,

$$\begin{aligned} \arg \min_{\mathbf{F}} \ \text{tr} \left(\mathbf{F}^{\mathrm{T}} \mathbf{L} \mathbf{F} \right) \\ \text{s.t.} \ \mathbf{A} \mathbf{F} = \mathbf{Y}, \end{aligned} \tag{3}$$

where $\mathbf{F} = [\mathbf{f}_1, \cdots, \mathbf{f}_n]$ are the labels for all subjects, $\mathbf{Y} = [\mathbf{y}_1, \cdots, \mathbf{y}_q]$ are the known clinical labels, $\mathbf{A} \in \Re^{q \times n}$ is a selection matrix to select the known label subjects from all subjects. Equation (3) can be solved using Augmented Lagrange Methods (ALMs) [6].

Multiple Hyper-Graphs for Multiple Modalities: Equation (2) only considers one modality imaging data, in order to apply hyper-graph for multiple modality imaging data, Gao et al. [5] proposed to combine multiple hyper-graph models by a linear model and estimating the unknown data labels on the combined multiple hyper-graph structure. Suppose there are M modalities data, they construct M different hyper-graph Laplacian matrixes $\mathbf{L}_m, \mathbf{m} = \mathbf{1}, \cdots, \mathbf{M}$. A weight matrix $\mathbf{u} = [\mathbf{u}_1, \cdots, \mathbf{u}_M]$ for different modalities is learned to combine M hyper-graphs Laplacian matrixes. The labels are propagated on the combined hyper-graph by solving

$$\arg\min_{u,F} \text{tr}\left(\mathbf{F}^T \sum u_m \mathbf{L}_m)\mathbf{F}\right)$$
$$\text{s.t. } \mathbf{AF} = \mathbf{Y}, \mathbf{u} > 0, \mathbf{u}^T \mathbf{1} = 1. \tag{4}$$

Equation (4) also can be solved using Augmented Lagrange Methods (ALMs) [6] efficiently.

Conventional Hyper-Graph Issues: The hyper-graph construction is only based on the imaging morphological features, which is independent from the clinical label and score propagation process as shown in Fig. 1. There is no guarantee that the learned hyper-graph is optimal to model subject-wise relationship among clinical labels. Therefore, this learned sub-optimal hyper-graph structure can lead to sub-optimal solution in the process of propagating clinical labels and clinical scores from known subjects to unknown subjects.

2.2   Joint Data Representation Learning and Classification on Dynamic Hyper Graph

To address these above issues in the conventional hyper-graph learning, we propose a novel method to solve the hyper-graph learning and classification problems simultaneously. Here, we define an intrinsic subject-wise distance matrix $\mathbf{S}$, where s_{ij} is the similarity between subjects i and j. We learn a dynamic hyper-graph Laplacian matrix $\mathbf{L}$ from the subject-wise similarity matrix $\mathbf{S}$ by: (1) construct incidence matrix, vertex degree and hyper-edge degree matrixes $\mathbf{H}, \mathbf{D}_v, \mathbf{D}_e$ from the estimated similarity matrix $\mathbf{S}$ (2) compute different hyper-graph Laplacian matrix using Eq. (2). We then propose a dynamic hyper-graph classification framework which learns the similarity matrix $\mathbf{S}$ on clinical label domain and feature domain, then update the data clinical labels on the hyper-graph simultaneously,

$$\arg\min_{S,F,L,\alpha} \frac{1}{2}\sum_{ij}^{n}\left(\left\|\mathbf{f}_i - \mathbf{f}_j\right\|_2^2 s_{ij} + \sum_{m=1}^{M}\alpha_m\left\|\mathbf{x}_i^m - \mathbf{x}_j^m\right\|_2^2 s_{ij}\right) + \gamma\text{tr}\left(\mathbf{F}^T\mathbf{L}\mathbf{F}\right) + \|\alpha\|_2^2,$$
$$\text{s.t. } \forall i, m, \mathbf{AF} = \mathbf{Y}, \mathbf{s}_i^T\mathbf{1} = 1, \mathbf{s}_i \geq 0, \alpha^T\mathbf{1} = 1, \alpha \geq 0, \tag{5}$$

where $\mathbf{x}_i^m$ is the feature vector of subject i from modality m, $\mathbf{f}_i$ is the class label for subject i, $\mathbf{F} = [\mathbf{f}_1, \cdots, \mathbf{f}_n], \mathbf{s}_i = [s_{i1}, \cdots, s_{in}]^T \in \mathfrak{R}^{n \times 1}$, $\alpha = [\alpha_1, \cdots, \alpha_m]^T \in \mathfrak{R}^{M \times 1}$ is the weights for each modality. An intrinsic subject distance matrix $\mathbf{S}$ is learned using clinical labels and different modality imaging features from both training and testing subject in this model. Furthermore, the data labels propagation on hyper-graph is performed simultaneously in Eq. (5). Equation (5) is can be considered to be convex problem with respect to each parameter: $\mathbf{S}, \mathbf{F}, \mathbf{L}, \alpha$, so we can break Eq. (5) into several convex problems and solve each sub-convex problem iteratively until converge.

2.3 Joint Classification and Regression on Dynamic Hyper-Graph

The above dynamic hyper-graph model is able to learn hyper-graph representation on imaging data and clinical labels, however, the clinical score are not used yet. Convergent evidence shows that, clinical score (such as cognitive score) prediction can be reliably used to evaluate and analysis the progression of the disease clinically. Furthermore, the clinical score is an additional useful information for disease identification. Therefore, it is straightforward to integrate the clinical score for disease diagnosis. We proposed to adopt a joint clinical score regression model into the dynamic hyper-graph model using conventional graph regression model.

The basic idea of conventional graph regression model is to estimate the value of each vertex on a graph as a linear combination of other vertexes in this graph. Let $C \in \Re^{n \times d}$ denote the clinical score of all subjects on a graph, the clinical score c_i of subject i can be simply computed as, $c_i = w_i^T C$, where $w_i \in \Re^{n \times 1}$ is the linear regression weights for subject i [7]. Denote the regression weight matrix for all subjects as $W = [w_1, \cdots, w_n]$, Q as the known clinical score for training subjects, C as the clinical score for all subjects, A is the selection matrix which select the training subjects from all subjects, we have $Q = AC$. We propose a dynamic hyper-graph which learns the hyper-graph from the imaging features, clinical labels and clinical scores, which jointly perform clinical label and score estimation as,

$$\arg \min_{S,F,L,C,W,\alpha} \frac{1}{2} \sum_{ij}^{n} \left(\|f_i - f_j\|_2^2 s_{ij} + \sum_{m=1}^{M} \alpha_m \|x_i^m - x_j^m\|_2^2 s_{ij} + \beta \|w_i^T C - w_j^T C\|_2^2 s_{ij} \right)$$
$$+ \gamma \mathrm{tr}(F^T L F) + \|\alpha\|_2^2, \tag{6}$$
$$\text{s.t. } \forall i, m, \ AF = Y, \ AC = Q, \ s_i^T 1 = 1, \ s_i \geq 0, \ \alpha^T 1 = 1, \ \alpha \geq 0.$$

where β is the weight for clinical score term. In Eq. (6), the subject-wise distance matrix S is learned on clinical label domain, imaging feature domain and clinical score domain in order to better represent the subject-wise relationship. The similarity matrix S, the regression matrix W and the clinical labels and scores are optimized simultaneously in Eq. (6). Equation (6) can be solved similarly to Eq. (5) with respect to each parameter iteratively [6, 8–10].

Discussion: Recall the conventional hyper-graph methods, they learns a *fixed hypergraph model* on imaging data only, then propagates the subject clinical labels on the pre-learned hyper-graph model as shown in Fig. 2 right. The hyper-graph model is fixed during the label propagation process. Our model learns an *optimal dynamical hyper-graph* representation for multiple modality imaging features, clinical labels and clinical scores as shown in Fig. 2 left. The learned hyper-graph is based on the imaging features, the subject labels and the clinical score information. Furthermore, the learned hyper-graph is optimized on both the training subjects with known clinical data and the testing subjects which only have imaging data. There are three major contributions in the proposed dynamical hyper-graph model as shown in Fig. 2 right, (1) imaging features of both training and testing subjects are used to construct the hyper-graph, which is especially helpful for real clinical practice with sufficient imaging data but

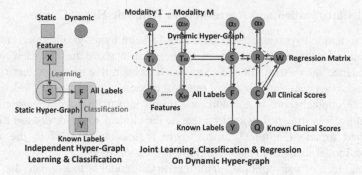

Fig. 2. Comparison of conventional hyper-graph and our method. The conventional hyper-graph is learned using the image feature only and the classification process is performed by propagating the clinical labels on the fixed hyper-graph in conventional hyper-graph method (shown in the left). Our method optimizes both the hyper-graph structure, the subject labels and the subject clinical score dynamically and simultaneously (shown in the right).

very limited clinical labels; (2) Beside multiple modality imaging features, the clinical labels and scores are also employed in hyper-graph construction in order to make the learned hyper-graph structure in census with not only imaging features but also clinical labels and scores; (3) hyper-graph structure learning, clinical label propagation and clinical score prediction are solved in a joint framework with a global optimal solution.

3   Experiments

We apply our method for Alzheimer's Disease diagnosis, which is one of the most common neuro-degenerative disease with memory loss, cognition defects, altered behavior, and as AD progresses, it can lead to ultimate death [11, 12]. A high risk stage before AD is called MCI with noticeable and measurable cognitive ability changes [5, 13, 14]. MCI is a very important stage in the development of Alzheimer's disease (AD). Convergent evidence shows that MCI subjects have high risk to progress towards a prodromal stage of AD, although some subjects can remain steady at the MCI stage for a long time or even goes to the reverse direction [13, 15], which are referred as MCI Non-Converters (MCI-NC). Other MCI subjects eventually developed to AD finally are referred as MCI Converters (MCI-C). Thus, identifying the heterogeneous subtypes such as AD, MCI-C, MCI-NC and predicting the clinical score in the potential AD patients is of high impact in clinical practice. We evaluate the performance of model on identifying the heterogeneous subtypes in AD and also predict the clinical score using multiple modality imaging data.

3.1   Image Processing

In our experiments, we use the baseline MRI, PET images from the ADNI dataset (www.adni-info.org) including 81 AD subjects and 90 NC (Normal Control). In the MCI subjects, there are 50 MCI Converter (MCI Convert) and 60 MCI Non-Converter

(MCI Non-Convert). For each subject, we first register its MR image to the PET image. Then, we apply skull strip, bias correction, and segmentation [16]. After that, we obtain the parcellation of 90 anatomical structures by warping the template to the underlying subject. We use AAL template which has manually labeled 90 regions of interest (ROI). We use hammer for registration (http://www.nitrc.org/projects/hammer/). The volume percentile of gray matter and the average intensity of PET image in each ROI are used as the morphological features.

3.2 Experimental Setting

We have evaluated the performance of our method on two multiple class classification problems: AD/MCI/NC classification and AD/MCI-C/MCI-NC/NC classification tasks. We use a 10-fold cross validation strategy. We randomly partition the subjects into 10 non-overlapping approximately equal size subsets. Each time one subset is used for testing and all rest subsets are used for training. The optimal parameters are learned by grid search strategy in the training set using five-fold inner cross-validation. The search range for parameters γ and β is 10^{-5}–10^5. This procedure is repeated 10 times to compute the overall cross-validation classification performance. Three statistical measures are used for classification performance evaluation, including accuracy (ACC), sensitivity (SEN) and specificity (SPEC). We also evaluate the regression performance of our model for clinical score prediction. The Root Mean Square Error (RMSE) and Correlation Coefficients (CC) are used here to evaluate the regression performance.

Performance Evaluation: We compare our method with the recent static hyper-graph method [5] for multi-modality data classification, which combines several hyper-graphs learned on different modalities linearly for the challenging MCI detection (Denoted as static hyper-graph (Gao et al.)). We also compare our method with the ensemble SVM [2], which is the state of art methods for multiple modality data fusion and classification. The recent work on the counterpart method: transductive graph learning in [17] is also included in our comparison. This model learns a conventional graph model on different modalities and clinical labels for AD diagnosis. Our model is different to transductive graph learning models in several aspects: first, we employ a hyper-graph model which is able to model more complex relationship; secondly, our model is for multiple-class problem; third, we learned the weights among different modalities automatically; last, both the clinical score and labels are jointly optimized in our model. In order to make the static hyper-graph method and transductive graph learning method suitable for regression task, we add graph based regression term and jointly optimize the label propagation and regression on the conventional static hyper-graph model and transductive graph learning model in our experiments.

3.3 Classification Results

Figure 3 shows the MCI classification results of all compared methods using multiple modality imaging data. Our method outperforms all competing state-of-the-art methods. Specifically, by using all modality imaging data, our method achieves an

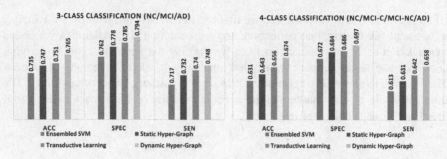

Fig. 3. Multiple class (NC/MCI-C/MCI-NC/AD) classification performance using multiple modality imaging data by ensemble SVM, Static Hyper-Graph and Our Dynamic Hyper-Graph model.

improvement of **1.8%** for the NC/MCI/AD classification problem compared to static hyper-graph model and **1.6%** for the NC/MCI-C/MCI-NC/AD classification problem in terms of accuracy.

Different Sizes of Training Data for Classification: To evaluate the performance of our method on different training data sizes, we vary the size of training data (the data with known clinical labels and clinical scores) and compare the classification performance of our method with static hyper-graph (Gao et al.) method. Figure 5 right shows the accuracy of the competing methods on different data size for three class classification (AD/MCI/NC). Figure 4 left shows the accuracy of competing methods on different data size for four class classification problem (AD/MCI-C/MCI-NC/NC). The performance of our method decreases gracefully when the training dataset size decreases. However, the competing method performance decrease more than our method when training dataset decreases. This result suggests that our method is able to learn a more optimal hyper-graph model than the conventional method (Gao et al.) after using the label information in the hyper-graph learning process.

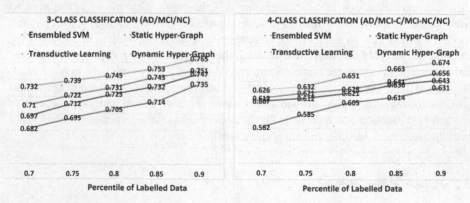

Fig. 4. Classification performance of our method vs. Gao et al.'s method on various sizes of training data. Our method is able to achieve high performance using small amount of labeling data in a semi-supervised manner.

3.4   Regression Results

Figure 5 shows the clinical score regression results of all compared methods using multiple modality imaging data. Our method outperforms all competing state-of-the-art methods. Specifically, as shown in left of Fig. 5, by using all modality imaging data, our method achieves an improvement of **1.8%** for the ADAS-COG regression problem and **2.8%** for the MMSE clinical score regression problem compared to the modified static hyper-graph regression model in terms of accuracy. We furthermore show the performance of competing methods by measuring the Regression Root Mean Square (RMSE) in the right Fig. 5. Our method achieves error decrease at **0.8** on ADAS-COG score and **0.9** on MMSE score compared to the static hyper-graph regression model.

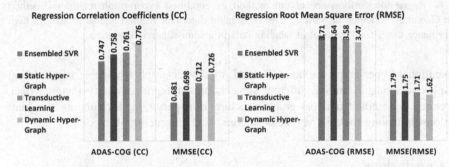

Fig. 5. Clinical score regression performance using multiple modality imaging data by ensemble SVR, Static Hyper-Graph and Our Dynamic Hyper-Graph model. We measure the regression error by the Correlation Coefficients (CC) and Root Mean Square Error (RMSE) term.

Different Sizes of Training Data for Regression: We also evaluate the performance of our method on different training data sizes for clinical score regression task. We change the size of training data (the data with known clinical labels and clinical scores) and compare the classification performance of our method with the modified static hyper-graph method from Gao et al.'s method. Figure 6 right shows the ADAS-COG clinical score errors measured by the Correlation Coefficients (CC) by all competing methods on different data size. Figure 6 left shows the MMSE clinical score regression error in terms of Correlation Coefficients (CC) by all competing methods on different data size. The performance of our method decreases gracefully when the training dataset size decreases. However, the competing method decrease dramatically with training dataset decreases. This result suggests that our method is able to learn a more optimal hyper-graph model than the conventional method (Gao et al.) after using the label and clinical score information in the hyper-graph learning and regression process.

Discussion: The better performance can be dedicated to the following reasons. First, different from conventional hyper-graph methods with learning fixed hyper-graph from imaging data independently of the classification process, our method uses both imaging and clinical data to learn a dynamic hyper-graph to explore the intrinsic relationship among multiple modality data in a semi-supervised way. Thus, the solution space for our method is more optimized on clinical data and imaging data compared to

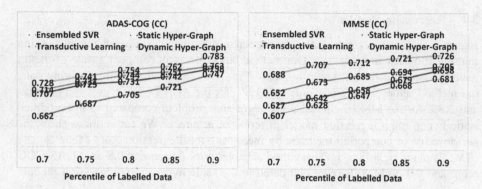

Fig. 6. Regression performance of our method vs. modified hyper-graph regression method from Gao et al.'s method on various sizes of training data. Our method is able to achieve high performance using small amount of labeling data in a semi-supervised manner.

conventional hyper-graph methods. Second, the hyper-graph is capable of modeling complex relationship among different subjects and different modality imaging data, therefore, the employed hyper-graph structure is superior on formulating the joint relationship among multiple vertices compared with simple graph model.

4   Conclusions

In this work, we proposed a dynamic hyper-graph method for joint learning, classification and regression on multiple classification problem (MCI/NC/AD) using multiple modal imaging data. To guide classification on new subjects, our dynamic hyper-graph is constructed by learning from multi-modal imaging data, the clinical labels and clinical scores on both training dataset and testing dataset. We evaluated our method on MCI-C/MCI-NC/NC/AD diagnosis and clinical score prediction. The results demonstrated that our method could improve the performance significantly compared to the conventional multi-modality static hyper-graph learning method on both diagnosis and clinical score prediction.

References

1. Zhu, X., Suk, H.-I., Thung, K.-H., Zhu, Y., Wu, G., Shen, D.: Joint discriminative and representative feature selection for Alzheimer's disease diagnosis. In: Wang, L., Adeli, E., Wang, Q., Shi, Y., Suk, H.-I. (eds.) MLMI 2016. LNCS, vol. 10019, pp. 77–85. Springer, Cham (2016). doi:10.1007/978-3-319-47157-0_10
2. Zhang, D.: Multi-modal multi-task learning for joint feature prediction of multiple regression and classification variables in Alzheimer's disease. Neuroimage **59**, 895–907 (2012)
3. Suk, H., Shen, D.: Hierarchical feature representation and multimodal fusion with deep learning for AD/MCI diagnosis. Neuroimage **1** (2015)

4. Dong, P., Guo, Y., Shen, D., Wu, G.: Multi-atlas and multi-modal hippocampus segmentation for infant MR brain images by propagating anatomical labels on hypergraph. In: Wu, G., Coupé, P., Zhan, Y., Munsell, B., Rueckert, D. (eds.) Patch-MI 2015. LNCS, vol. 9467, pp. 188–196. Springer, Cham (2015). doi:10.1007/978-3-319-28194-0_23
5. Gao, Y., Wee, C.-Y., Kim, M., Giannakopoulos, P., Montandon, M.-L., Haller, S., Shen, D.: MCI identification by joint learning on multiple MRI data. In: Navab, N., Hornegger, J., Wells, W.M., Frangi, A.F. (eds.) MICCAI 2015. LNCS, vol. 9350, pp. 78–85. Springer, Cham (2015). doi:10.1007/978-3-319-24571-3_10
6. Boyd, S., et al.: Distributed optimization and statistical learning via the alternating direction method of multipliers. Found. Trends® Mach. Learn. **3**, 1–122 (2011)
7. Smith, A.: Nonparametric regression on a graph. J. Comput. Graph. Stat. **20** (2011)
8. Zhu, Y.: Convolutional sparse coding for trajectory reconstruction. TPAMI **37**, 529–540 (2015)
9. Zhu, Y., Cox, M., Lucey, S.: 3D motion reconstruction for real-world camera motion. In: CVPR, pp. 1–8 (2011)
10. Zhu, Y., Huang, D., Torre, F.D.L., Lucey, S.: Complex non-rigid motion 3D reconstruction by union of subspaces. In: CVPR, pp. 23–34 (2014)
11. Thompson, P., et al.: Tracking Alzheimer's disease. Ann. N. Y. Acad. Sci. **1097**, 183–214 (2007)
12. Risacher, S., Saykin, A.: Neuroimaging biomarkers of neurodegenerative diseases and dementia. Semin. Neurol. **33**, 386–416 (2013)
13. Reisberg, B., Ferris, S., Kluger, A., Franssen, E., Wegiel, J., De Leon, M.J.: Mild cognitive impairment (MCI): a historical perspective. Int. Psychogeriatr. **20**, 18–31 (2008)
14. Zhang, D., Wang, Y., Zhou, L., Yuan, H., Shen, D.: Alzheimer's Disease Neuroimaging Initiative: Multimodal classification of Alzheimer's disease and mild cognitive impairment. NeuroImage, **55**, 856–867 (2011)
15. Ganguli, M., Dodge, H., Shen, C., DeKosky, S.T.: Mild cognitive impairment, amnestic type an epidemiologic study. Neurology **63**, 115–121 (2004)
16. Guo, X., Wang, Z., Li, K., Li, Z., Qi, Z., Jin, Z., et al.: Voxel-based assessment of gray and white matter volumes in Alzheimer's disease. Neurosci. Lett. **468**, 146–150 (2010)
17. Wang, Z., Zhu, X., Adeli, E., Zhu, Y., Zu, C., Nie, F., Shen, D., Wu, G.: Progressive graph-based transductive learning for multi-modal classification of brain disorder disease. In: Ourselin, S., Joskowicz, L., Sabuncu, M.R., Unal, G., Wells, W. (eds.) MICCAI 2016. LNCS, vol. 9900, pp. 291–299. Springer, Cham (2016). doi:10.1007/978-3-319-46720-7_34

A Likelihood-Free Approach for Characterizing Heterogeneous Diseases in Large-Scale Studies

Jenna Schabdach[1], William M. Wells III[3], Michael Cho[3],
and Kayhan N. Batmanghelich[1,2(✉)]

[1] Department of Biomedical Informatics, University of Pittsburgh, Pittsburgh, USA
{jmschabdach,kayhan}@pitt.edu
[2] Intelligence Systems Program, University of Pittsburgh, Pittsburgh, USA
[3] Brigham and Women's Hospital, Harvard Medical School, Boston, USA
sw@bwh.harvard.edu, remhc@channing.harvard.edu

Abstract. We propose a non-parametric approach for characterizing heterogeneous diseases in large-scale studies. We target diseases where multiple types of pathology present simultaneously in each subject and a more severe disease manifests as a higher level of tissue destruction. For each subject, we model the *collection* of local image descriptors as samples generated by an unknown subject-specific probability density. Instead of approximating the probability density via a parametric family, we propose to side step the parametric inference by directly estimating the divergence between subject densities. Our method maps the collection of local image descriptors to a signature *vector* that is used to predict a clinical measurement. We are able to interpret the prediction of the clinical variable in the population and individual levels by carefully studying the divergences. We illustrate an application this method on simulated data as well as on a large-scale lung CT study of Chronic Obstructive Pulmonary Disease (COPD). Our approach outperforms classical methods on both simulated and COPD data and demonstrates the state-of-the-art prediction on an important physiologic measure of airflow (the forced respiratory volume in one second, FEV1).

1 Introduction

We propose a method that exploits large-scale sample sizes to study heterogeneous diseases. More specifically, we target diseases where each patient can be thought as a superposition of different processes, or subtypes, and where the pathology is not always located in the same place. Our goal is to provide a scalable algorithm that quickly evaluates the statistical power of various feature extraction methods for prediction of a clinical measurement. Scalability and interpretability are at the core of our algorithm. Our motivation comes from a study of Chronic Obstructive Pulmonary Disease (COPD), but the resulting model is applicable to a wide range of heterogeneous disorders.

Emphysema, or destruction of air sacs, is an important phenotype in COPD. Emphysema itself has multiple subtypes with distinct pathological and radiological appearances [17]. Understanding the differences between the subtypes

© Springer International Publishing AG 2017
M. Niethammer et al. (Eds.): IPMI 2017, LNCS 10265, pp. 170–183, 2017.
DOI: 10.1007/978-3-319-59050-9_14

is important since each subtype is associated with different risk factors [19].
Various local image descriptors (e.g., intensity and texture features) have been
proposed to describe disease subtypes using lung CT images [12,21]. To model
the local image descriptors, one can view a patient in a dataset as a mixture of
multiple processes and can then statistically estimate the image representation
of the patient's subtypes from image data [2,3]. However, each image descriptor
has its own statistical properties, and to model a descriptor statistically requires
careful selection of a likelihood function and the noise distribution. For example,
while histogram-based methods often result in non-negative features (e.g., [18]),
features extracted using a wavelet approach (e.g., [5]) usually have no sign restriction. While the multivariate Gaussian distribution might be appropriate for the
latter, it may not be a good choice for the former.

The goal of our method is to quickly screen different feature extraction methods without an explicit likelihood assumption. We use the predictive power of a
clinical variable as a quantitative evaluation measure. The premise of a large sample size is that, as the dataset grows, the chance of observing more phenotypically
similar patients increases. We leverage this idea and non-parametrically estimate divergences between the densities (which correspond to individual patients)
from image data instead of directly parametrizing the probability densities. Our
estimator is based on a nearest neighbor graph that can be constructed efficiently [13]. The graph enables us to map the predictions of the clinical measurements back to the anatomical domain. The mapping delineates a few anatomical
regions which can be used for clinical interpretation. The proposed approach is
highly parallelizable which makes it appropriate for large-scale studies.

We evaluate the performance of our method on a simulated dataset as well
as a large-scale COPD lung CT dataset. In both experiments, our method outperforms the classical parametric bag-of-words model (BOW). We also study
two different divergences. Our experiments demonstrate the importance of the
choice of the divergence on the performance the method.

2   Method

We assume that the image domain of each subject in a dataset is divided into
relatively homogeneous spatially contiguous regions. The number of regions may
vary amongst subjects. To simplify the explanation of our method, we assume
the spatially contiguous regions are patches of image regions; the method is
applicable for superpixels with no modification.

Each subject is represented by a collection of features extracted from the
regions. We let $\psi(v) \in \mathbb{R}^d$ denote the $d-$dimensional image signature of the
patch v. We assume that the image descriptors are randomly generated from K
prototypical tissue types shared across subjects in the population. Let $p^I(\cdot; \theta_k)$
denote the distribution for the image signature of the tissue type k which is parametrized by θ_k. While $\theta_1, \cdots, \theta_K$ are shared across the population, the mixture
proportion may vary amongst subjects. Hence, the distribution of image signa-
tures for subject i (i.e., p_i) is:

$$\psi(v) \sim p_i, \quad p_i(\cdot) = \sum_{k=1}^{K} \pi_k^i p^I(\cdot; \theta_k), \quad \sum_{k=1}^{K} \pi_k^i = 1 \tag{1}$$

where $\pi^i = \left[\pi_1^i, \cdots, \pi_K^i\right]$ is the mixture proportion for subject i. In the literature, this type of model is referred to as an admixture [1] or a topic model [4]. It generalizes the mixture model by allowing subject data to have subject-specific membership to population-level image signatures of the disease subtypes. The π^i characterizes each subject in the spectrum of the disease. It is common to assume a specific form of $p^I(\cdot)$. Such assumptions are mostly made to ensure inference of the parameters is computationally convenient. For example [2,3] assumed p^I to be a multivariate Gaussian density with a conjugate prior. However, a computationally convenient assumption is not necessarily the best choice for the likelihood. By contrast, in this paper we propose to side step inference of θ_k, π^i by avoiding an explicit assumption on p^I. Instead, we estimate the divergences between p_i's and embed them in a lower dimensional manifold, which results in an *implicit* characterization of the subjects. We trade the interpretability of a parametric model with a flexibility of a non-parametric model. We will show in Sect. 2.3 that how some of the interpretability can be retrieved via a careful inspection of the divergence computation. Finally, it is worth mentioning that our method does not replace explicit probabilistic modeling (e.g., topic modeling) but it provides an objective approach to screen different local image descriptors for probabilistic methods such as [2,3].

In the following sections, we first introduce the notion of a k-nearest neighbor graph (Sect. 2.1), which is used in the estimator (Sect. 2.2) and enables us to interpret the predictions (Sect. 2.3).

2.1 $k-$Nearest Neighbor Graph

First, we formally define the directed k-nearest neighbor ($k-$NN) graph which will be used in the following sections. Let $\mathcal{G}_k = (\mathcal{V}, \psi, \mathcal{D})$ denote the directed $k-$NN graph. Let S_i represent the collection of patches from subject i. We define the collection of nodes in the graph as $\mathcal{V} = \cup_i S_i$. For a patch v in the dataset (i.e., $v \in \mathcal{V}$), $\psi(v)$ denotes the corresponding d-dimensional local image descriptor (i.e., $\psi : \mathcal{V} \to \mathbb{R}^d$) and $\mathcal{D}(\cdot, \cdot)$ represents a Euclidean distance in the d-dimensional space. For a given collection S_i, we define a function $\iota_{k,S_i} : \mathcal{V} \to S_i$ that returns the index of the k'th nearest neighbor node of v in the collection S_i based on the distance $\mathcal{D}$ in the feature space defined by ψ. We call ι_{k,S_i} an *index function*. Hence, for $v_1 \in S_i$ and $v_2 \in S_j$, there is a edge $v_2 \to v_1$ if $\iota_{k,S_i}(v_2) = v_1$. We assume that the graph $\mathcal{G}$ does not have self-loops, i.e., if $v \in S_i$, $\iota_{k,S_i}(v)$ returns the k-nearest neighbor not counting v itself.

For brevity of the notation, we introduce a few short-hand notations: $\rho_{k,S_i}(v)$ denotes $\mathcal{D}(\psi(\iota_{k,S_i}(v)), \psi(v))$ which is the $k-$NN distance of v from the closest local descriptor in S_i (see Fig. 1a). For each node in the graph, we define the notion of the *popularity* of a node with respect to another subject (see Fig. 1b). The popularity of node $v \in S_i$ with respect to subject j is defined as the degree of

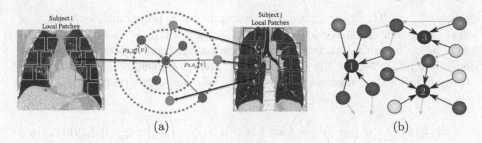

(a)   (b)

Fig. 1. A schematic showing a few nodes of the k−NN graph. (a) The filled blue and green circles represent image features from subjects i and j respectively. The blue and green dashed lines indicate $\rho_{3,S_i}(v)$ and $\rho_{3,S_j}(v)$. (b) Part of the k−NN graph for subject blue is highlighted. The colors indicate different subjects. While the node 2 is more popular amongst the green subjects, node 1 is more popular amongst the red subjects. (Color figure online)

incoming edges from the collection S_j normalized by the total number of patches in the subject j, namely

$$\forall v \in S_i, \quad [\varphi_{S_i}(S_j)]_v = \frac{1}{|S_j|} \sum_{t \in S_j | t \to v} 1 \tag{2}$$

We view $\varphi_{S_i}(S_j) \in \mathbb{R}^{|S_i|}$ as a *popularity vector* where the entry v is defined by Eq. 2. It is straightforward to see that entries of φ_{S_i} sums to one. In the following sections, we use the k−NN graph to define similarity between subjects and to interpret the results.

2.2   Non-parametric Estimation of the Similarity

Subject Dissimilarity: We model subject i as a bag of local image descriptors generated by an unknown density, i.e., $\forall v \in \mathcal{V}, \psi(v) \sim p_i$. We use two well-known divergences to compute the dissimilarity between densities: the Kullback-Leibler (KL) divergence and the Hellinger (HE) distance:

$$\text{KL:} \quad \text{KL}(p_i \| p_j) = \int_{\mathbb{R}^d} \log \frac{p_i(x)}{p_j(x)} p_i(x) dx,$$

$$\text{HE:} \quad \text{HE}(p_i \| p_j) = 1 - \int_{\mathbb{R}^d} p_i^{\frac{1}{2}}(x) p_j^{\frac{1}{2}}(x) dx. \tag{3}$$

While HE is a real distance, KL is not symmetric and does not satisfy the triangle inequality. We will address this issue later in this section. We would like to estimate the divergences without assuming a parametric form for the probability densities.

With mild assumptions on the probability density, p_i can be represented as $p_i(x) = f_i(x)/Z_{f_i}$, where $f_i(x)$ is an unknown positive function and and Z_{f_i} is the corresponding normalizer (i.e., $Z_{f_i} = \int f_i(x)dx$; if $f_i(x)$ is a probability density, $Z_{f_i} = 1$). To estimate $f(x)$, we consider a polynomial expansion of $\log f(x)$ around x, namely $\log f(u)|_x \approx a_0 + (u-x)^T a_1 + (u-x)^T a_2 (u-x)$ where a_0, a_1, a_2 are scalar, vector and matrix parameters, respectively, and vary depending on x. We use the state-of-the-art *local* log-likelihood method [11] to estimate the local parameters. The local log-likelihood of the function f_i at point x is:

$$\mathcal{L}_x(f_i) = \sum_{v \in S_i} w\left(\frac{x - \psi(v)}{h}\right) \log f_i(\psi(v)) - |S_i| \int w\left(\frac{y - x}{h}\right) f_i(y)dy, \quad (4)$$

where $|S_i|$ is the cardinality of collection S_i and $w(x)$ is a window function with bandwidth h. Since the approximation of $\log f_i(x)$ is locally valid, it is reasonable to keep h small; if h goes to infinity, Eq. 4 amounts to the ordinary likelihood estimation and the last term converges to $|S_i|Z_f$.

For certain choices of the window function, f_i has a closed-form solution [11]. For computational reasons, we use the step function: $w(x) = \mathbb{I}(\|x\| \leq 1)$ (see the Appendix A for other choices and the corresponding computational costs). Choosing a data-independent bandwidth is one of the impediments of the non-parametric density estimation. However, we are not interested in density estimation, but rather in estimating a functional of a pair of densities, namely the divergences. In this case, we consider a choice of bandwidth that is local and adaptive, i.e., h is a function of x [7]. We set the h to the k−NN distance from x; $h \equiv \rho_{k,S_i}(x)$ similar to [7,15]. Optimizing Eq. 4, we get the following form for f [11],

$$\hat{f}_i(x) = \frac{1}{|S_i|h \int w(x)dx} \sum_{v \in S_i} w(\psi(v)) = \frac{k}{|S_i|C_d \rho_{k,S_i}^d(x)}, \quad (5)$$

where $C_d \equiv \frac{\pi^{d/2}}{\Gamma(d/2+1)}$, $C_d \rho_{k,S_i}^d(x)$ are the volumes of d-dimensional balls with radius of one and $\rho_{k,S_i}(x)$ respectively, and $\Gamma(\cdot)$ is the Gamma function. An illustration of this concept can be seen in Fig. 1a. Using the re-substitution, we estimate the HE and KL divergences as (See the Appendix A for detail):

KL : $\quad \widehat{KL(p_i\|p_j)} = \frac{d}{|S_i|} \sum_{v \in S_i} \log \frac{\rho_{k,S_i}(v)}{\rho_{k,S_j}(v)} + \log \frac{|S_j|}{|S_i| - 1}$,

HE : $\quad \widehat{HE(p_i, p_j)} = 1 - \frac{(|S_i| - 1)^{\frac{1}{2}} \Gamma(k)^2}{|S_i||S_j|^{\frac{1}{2}} \Gamma(k + \frac{1}{2})\Gamma(k - \frac{1}{2})} \sum_{v \in S_i} \left(\frac{\rho_{k,S_i}(v)}{\rho_{k,S_j}(v)}\right)^d$. (6)

The estimators are unbiased and consistent. In other words, as the number of patches (S_i, S_j) increases, the estimations converge to the true value (See the Appendix A for details).

Subject Similarity: Our aim is to derive a Positive Semi-Definite (PSD) similarity kernel between subjects. In other words, if the entries of a matrix K represent the pairwise similarities between subjects, K should be a PSD matrix. One way of defining a kernel is by exponentiating the negative of the distance between two elements. However, the KL divergence is neither symmetric nor does it satisfy the triangle inequality. Hence, defining a kernel based on KL may not result in a PSD kernel. To ensure positive definiteness, we exponentiate the symmetric KL and project the resulting matrix onto a PSD cone. Namely, we define $\tilde{L}_{ij} = \exp\left(-\text{KL}_{\text{sym}}(p_i, p_j)/\sigma^2\right)$, where the σ is a parameter of the kernel and $\text{KL}_{\text{sym}}(p_i, p_j) = \hat{\text{KL}}(p_i \| p_j) + \hat{\text{KL}}(p_j \| p_i)$. We define the similarity between subjects i and j $(k(S_i, S_j))$ as the ij-th element of the similarity matrix,

$$k(S_i, S_j) = [K_\sigma]_{ij}, \quad K_\sigma = \text{Proj}_{\text{PSD}}(\tilde{L}_\sigma), \quad K_\sigma = BB^T, \tag{7}$$

where B is the Cholesky decomposition of the similarity matrix. The columns of B can be viewed as new representation for the subjects in the N-dimensional space (N is the number of subjects). $\text{Proj}_{\text{PSD}}(\cdot)$ denotes the projection onto the PSD cone. For the projection, we set all negative eigenvalues to zero. We adopt the so-called median trick [20] in the kernel machine and set σ to the median of the divergence.

We explained how to compute the similarity kernel given collections of local image descriptors. In the next section, we explain how to interpret the similarities between subjects on the population and individual levels.

2.3 Can We Trust the Prediction?

To trust the prediction, we would like to be able to *interpret* the predicted values. We perform interpretation on the population and individual levels.

Population-Level: To interpret the similarities on the population level, we observe that parametric mixtures of densities reside on a low-dimensional statistical manifold [9]. Therefore, we use the new representation of the subject-specific distribution (i.e., Eq. 7) and apply the Locally Linear Embedding (LLE) algorithm [24] to empirically chart individuals on a lower dimensional space. We use the coordinates of subjects in the embedding space to predict the clinical measurement.

Individual-Level: To interpret the results on the individual level, we map the predicted value to the image domain to present it to a clinician. Similar ideas have been explored in the machine learning context [23]. The prediction model estimates the clinical measurement from the image data through a complicated chain: computation of the divergences and the kernel, projection onto the PSD, and finally regression or classification. In clinical settings, it is important to identify regions of anatomy that are the most relevant to a model's predictions. We use the notation $g_{\text{cplx}}(S_i)$ to denote the chain of operations resulting in the prediction. For the individual-level interpretation, our aim is to identify a few patches in the lung image of each subject that are the most relevant to the prediction (i.e., $g_{\text{cplx}}(S_i)$). We construct N sparse linear regressions that are good *local* approximations of g_{cplx} around each subject. Let us consider subject i; we use the popularity vector of subject i with respect to other subjects (i.e., $\varphi_{S_i}(\cdot)$ defined in Eq. 2) as the input features to the local sparse linear

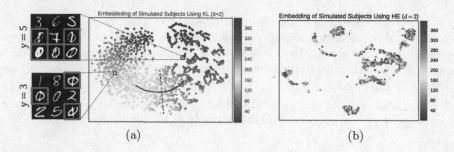

Fig. 2. Embedding of simulated data in 2D using KL and HE. (a) Embedding for KL. Dots denote simulated subjects and colors correspond to the severity, y. The embedding using KL captures the disease severity with the arrow indicating increasing severity. Sample slices from two different subjects are shown. (b) Embedding for HE. Unlike KL, it fails to capture the structure of the population. (Color figure online)

regression. To account for the notion of locality, we use the similarity kernel (Eq. 7) to weight the error term in the regression. Finally, we add a ℓ_1-norm regularization term to the cost function to encourage a parsimonious number of patches. More specifically, for subject i, we solve the following optimization problem:

$$\min_\omega \ell(S_i; \omega) := \min_\omega \sum_{n=1}^N k(S_i, S_n)(\underbrace{g_{\mathrm{cplx}}(S_n) - \langle \omega, \varphi_{S_i}(S_n) \rangle}_{g_{\mathrm{loc}}(S_i, S_n; \omega)})^2 + \lambda\|\omega\|_1 \qquad (8)$$

where $\langle \cdot, \cdot \rangle$ denotes the inner product, g_{loc} and g_{cplx} are the local and the complex predictors, respectively, and $\varphi_{S_i}(S_n) \in \mathbb{R}^{|S_i|}$ is the popularity vector of patches in subject i with respect to subject n (defined in Eq. 2). Using the popularity, we investigate the patches whose popularities (i.e., resemblance to each other in terms of local image features) amongst other subjects is *locally* predictive of g_{cplx}. Note that we use the prediction of the clinical measurement and not the measurement itself because we are interested in locally interpreting g_{cplx}. We use a cross-validated LARS algorithm [6] to find the optimal λ on the regularization path.

2.4　Computational Cost

Computing the divergences for each subject (i.e., rows of $\tilde{L}_\sigma$ matrix) can be done independently, hence it is parallelizable (one task per row). Estimating the divergences requires the construction of a $k-$NN graph. We use an approximate nearest neighbor approach [13] to construct the graph. For subject i, the cost is approximately linear with both $|S_i|$ and d. Computing all pairs of divergences from the graph is quadratic in the number of subjects (N). It is also parallelizable per subject. A naïve computational cost of the embedding is $O(N^3)$, but there are approximate approaches that are not explored in this paper. Finally, the interpretation step can be done independently for each subject, so it, too, is easily parallelizable. The computational cost of the LARS algorithm for subject i is $O(|S_i|^3 + |S_i|^2 N)$, which is a few minutes for each subject in our dataset.

3 Experiments

In this section, we evaluate our algorithm on simulated and clinical datasets. We compare our method with the popular parametric bag-of-words model (k-means algorithm). We also investigate the importance of choosing the correct divergence.

3.1 Simulation

To evaluate our method on simulated data, we start by generating 2000 subjects, where each subject has a different level of disease severity and a set of 400 image patches. We sample the level of severity (y) from a Gaussian distribution clipped to the range of 0 to 400 with a mean of 200 and a standard deviation of 175. Each subject has $(400 - floor(y))$ "normal" patches drawn randomly from the MNIST dataset and y "abnormal" patches. The abnormal patches are novel digits synthesized by overlaying random pairs of 0 and 1 images from the MNIST dataset. Two samples of simulated subjects with different degrees of severity are shown in the left half of Fig. 2a. To reduce the dimensionality of the patches from 28×28, we train a three layer feed-forward neural network on a held out dataset (not used for data generation) to classify 0-9 (the novel digits not included). We pass all normal and abnormal patches through the network and use a 20-dimensional output of the layer before the last layer as features.

We compute the new representation of the features using KL and HE (Eq. 7) and apply LLE to assign a set of low-dimensional coordinates for each subject. Then, we use the low-dimensional representation as the features for a linear ridge regression to predict y. Figure 2 visualizes the 2D embedding for the simulated

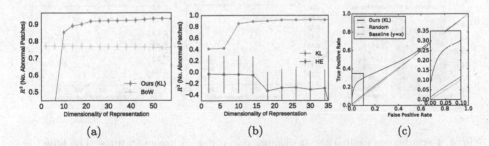

(a)   (b)   (c)

Fig. 3. Performance of our method. (a) compares KL to BOW while (b) illustrates the importance of the divergence choice. While KL outperforms BOW, the HE divergence has a negative R^2, indicating that LLE is not able to accurately approximate the structure of the latent space. (c) The ROC curve indicates the ability of our subject level interpretation method to detect abnormal patches in comparison with random selection. The box in the right shows the zoomed in area of the curve for $FPR < 10\%$.

subjects using KL (Fig. 2a) and HE (Fig. 2b). Each dot represents one subject and the color of the dot indicates the simulated disease severity y. While there is a clear trend in disease severity from left to right using KL divergence, the 2D embedding using HE does not show any trend. Figure 3 demonstrates that this effect is not caused by the dimensionality of the embedding. Figure 3a compares the performance of embedding using KL and BOW in predicting y while Fig. 3b compares the performance of the two divergences. The y-axis is R^2 and the x-axis is the dimensionality of the representation. The performance is measured as the R^2 value for 50-fold cross validation against the dimensionality of the representation. While KL significantly outperforms BOW, HE has negative a R^2 suggesting LLE cannot accurately approximate the manifold structure induced by the HE divergence. The Eq. 8 is designed to detection just a few patches that are sufficiently informative in prediction of y in similar subjects. Since it does not detect all abnormal patches, it is not optimal for detection purpose. Nevertheless, we can compute the false positive rate of the selected patches to evaluate the individual-level interpretation on the simulated data. Figure 3c shows the ROC curve comparing our method with random selection. The interpretation method requires the popularity vector, hence BOW is not included in this evaluation. For real data, a gold standard evaluation of the individual-level interpretation requires human observation and rating.

3.2 COPD Study

We apply our method to lung CT images of 6,253 subjects from the COPDGene study [16]. First, we evaluate various image signatures in term of predicting the severity of disease as measured by a lung function: the Forced Expiratory Volume in one second (FEV$_1$). Second, we show how our method can characterize a patient in the spectrum of COPD present in the population. Third, we compare the performance of the non-parametric approach with a threshold-based

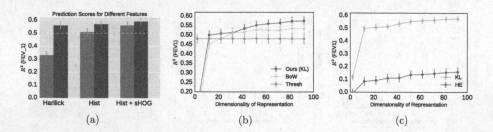

(a)   (b)   (c)

Fig. 4. Performance evaluation: (a) Comparing different image features. The blue bar is our method (KL divergence) and the green is BOW. The y-axis is R^2 of predicting FEV$_1$. The horizontal red line is the image threshold-based baseline. KL outperforms both methods. The combination of sHOG and histogram features results in the best performance. (b) Comparing R^2 versus dimensionality of the representation for KL. (c) Comparing KL and HE (purple line). The graph shows the choice of divergence is crucial. (Color figure online)

image measurement commonly used by clinicians, as well as the classical BOW method, which uses $k-$means clustering. The threshold-based method measures the percentage of voxels with intensity values less than -950 Hounsfield Unit (HU) computed from the inspiratory and expiratory images. Those measurements reflect what is clinically used to quantify emphysema and the degree of gas trapping. Note that our method has access to the inspiratory images only.

We first segment the lung area. Then, instead of patches, we apply an oversegmentation method [8] to divide the lung area into spatially homogeneous superpixels. The superpixels follow the boundaries of anatomy better than the patches; the method explained in Sect. 2 is readily applicable for superpixels without any modification. We extract both histogram and texture features from each superpixel as they have been shown to be important in characterizing emphysema [18,21]. For the histogram features, we divide the intensity histogram of each superpixel into 32 bins following Sorensen *et al.* [21]. We follow the pipeline introduced in [22] and extract the Harilick features from the Gray-Level Cooccurance Matrix (GLCM); the Harilick features already incorporate the intensity information. We use a rotationally invariant image feature proposed by Liu *et al.* [10] as the texture feature. The method views the histogram of the gradient as a continuous angular signal and uses spherical harmonics to extract features from it (referred to as sHOG).

Figure 4a reports the performance of various image signatures for a 100 dimensional embedding for KL density. The y-axis is the average R^2 using 50-fold cross validation for predicting FEV_1, while the horizontal line denotes the prediction using the threshold-based baseline. The error bar shows the 95% confidence interval computed using the bootstrapping method. The combination of sHOG and histogram features yields the best performance. In the rest of the experiments, we report the results using the sHOG and the histogram features.

Figure 4b, c reports the performance of the embedding approach using KL, HE, and BOW against the dimensionality of the representation (i.e., the cluster size of $k-$means and the embedding dimensionality). While our KL-based method outperforms k-means, HE is significantly worse than both approaches. This plot emphasizes the importance of the choice of the right divergence and is consistent with the results from the simulation. Although $R^2 = 0.55$ for KL may seem low, it is significantly higher than the traditional measurements of emphysema based on a single threshold. Furthermore, our local image descriptors are more sensitive to emphysema while FEV_1 is spirometry measurement affected by emphysema, airway disease and many other factors.

In Fig. 5a, we use 2D embedding to visualize only one-third of the population (to avoid visual clutter). Each dot in the scatter plot represents a patient, and its color denotes FEV_1. As the temperature of the color increases, so does the COPD severity. Even 2D embedding captures the structure of the disease; subjects on the bottom right are healthier than subjects on the top left of the embedding space. The results in Fig. 4b confirms this observation in higher dimensional embedding. Figure 5b, c show parts of the anatomy selected by the interpretation algorithm to be the most relevant to the prediction. The figures show one slice

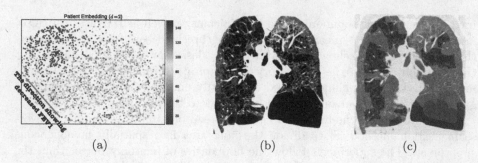

(a)   (b)   (c)

Fig. 5. Interpretation on the population and the individual levels. (a) Embedding COPD subjects in 2D space. A dot denotes a subject and the color represent the disease severity (FEV_1). The hotter the color, the more severe the disease. (b), (c) Individual level interpretation, showing a slice of lung CT image before (b) and after overlaying (c) the regions selected by our algorithm; the color indicates the sign of ω. (Color figure online)

of a subject's lung CT. The colored patches are the regions selected by the interpretation algorithm (Sect. 2.3). For example, regions on the bottom right are obviously abnormal.

4   Conclusion

We proposed a non-parametric approach for characterizing heterogeneous diseases such as COPD. Our method summarizes the image data of each subject from a collection of local image descriptors to one signature vector per subject. The vector represents the coordinates of the subject in a latent low-dimensional space, which can be used for prediction of a clinical variable or visualization of the entire population. The scalable and non-parametric nature of the method enabled us to evaluate various image features quickly. Our method is readily applicable to more sophisticated feature extraction schemes such as deep learning for each patch. We showed that our approach outperforms the parametric bag-of-words (k-means) method. We experimented with two well-known divergences (KL and HE), and the results demonstrated the importance of the choice of divergence.

Acknowledgements. This work was supported by in part by NLM Training grant T15LM007059, NIH NIBIB NAMIC U54-EB005149, NIH NCRR NAC P41-RR13218 and NIH NIBIB NAC P41-EB015902, NHLBI R01HL089856, R01HL089897, K08HL097029, R01HL113264, 5K25HL104085, 5R01HL116931, and 5R01HL116473. The COPDGene study (NCT00608764) is also supported by the COPD Foundation through contributions made to an Industry Advisory Board comprised of AstraZeneca, Boehringer Ingelheim, Novartis, Pfizer, Siemens, GlaxoSmithKline and Sunovion.

A   Appendix: Non-parametric Inference

In this section, we first show that the unnormalized density $f(x)$ has a closed-form using locally constant approximation. Then, we show why the second-order approximation is computationally expensive for our problem. Finally, we provide more detail on the approximation of the KL and HE divergences.

Assuming a locally constant function for $f(x) = \exp(a_0)$, we can compute a closed-form solution for a_0 by differentiating Eq. 4 with respect to a_0:

$$\frac{d\mathcal{L}_x(f_i)}{da_0} = \sum_{v \in S_i} w\left(\frac{x - \psi(v)}{h}\right) - |S_i| \int w\left(\frac{y - x}{h}\right) e^{a_0} dy = 0$$

If we set $h \equiv \rho_{k,S_i}(x)$ and use the step window function ($w(x) = \mathbb{I}(\|x\| \leq 1)$), the first term in the right hand-side becomes exactly k and the second term is the volume of a d-dimensional hyper-sphere with radius h which is $C_d h^d$, and we arrive at Eq. 5. For the Gaussian window function, the first term becomes a weighted sum k points in the vicinity of x and the second term has the same closed-form as the normalizer of the Gaussian distribution.

If we set h to a constant and use the Gaussian window function and the second-order polynomial, i.e., $\log f(u)|_x \approx a_0 + (u - x)^T a_1 + (u - x)^T a_2 (u - x)$, the local parameters have closed-forms [7, 11]:

$$a_0 = \log(A_0) - \frac{\|A_1\|^2}{A_0^2} - (d \log \sqrt{2\pi} + (d+1) \log n), a_1 = \frac{1}{hA_0} A_1,$$

$$a_2 = \frac{1}{2h^2} I_{d \times d} - \frac{A_0}{2h^2} \left(A_2 - A_1 A_1^T\right)^{-1}$$

where $A_0 \equiv \sum_{v \in S_i} \alpha_v(x)$ and $\alpha_v(x) \equiv \exp\left(-\frac{\|\psi(v) - x\|^2}{2h^2}\right)$, for $D(x, v) \equiv \frac{1}{h}(\psi(v) - x)$, $A_1 \equiv \sum_{v \in S_i} \alpha_v(x) D(x, v)$, and $A_2 \equiv \sum_{v \in S_i} \alpha_v(x) D(x, v) D(x, v)^T$. It is straightforward to see computing a_2 demands inversion of a $d \times d$ matrix ($O(d^3)$) which needs to be done for every patch hence it is computationally prohibitive.

The KL divergence is a straightforward substitution of Eq. 5. Our estimator for HE is proposed by Poczos et al. [14]. The HE estimator is also based on substitution. The minor adjustment (the term behind the summation in Eq. 6) makes sure that the estimator is unbiased.

References

1. Alexander, D.H., Novembre, J., Lange, K.: Fast model-based estimation of ancestry in unrelated individuals. Genome Res. **19**(9), 1655–1664 (2009)
2. Batmanghelich, N.K., Saeedi, A., Cho, M., Estepar, R.S.J., Golland, P.: Generative method to discover genetically driven image biomarkers. Int. Conf. Inf. Process. Med. Imaging **17**(1), 30–42 (2015)
3. Binder, P., Batmanghelich, N.K., Estepar, R.S.J., Golland, P.: Unsupervised discovery of emphysema subtypes in a large clinical cohort. In: Wang, L., Adeli, E., Wang, Q., Shi, Y., Suk, H.-I. (eds.) MLMI 2016. LNCS, vol. 10019, pp. 180–187. Springer, Cham (2016). doi:10.1007/978-3-319-47157-0_22

4. Blei, D.M., Ng, A.Y., Jordan, M.I.: Latent dirichlet allocation. J. Mach. Learn. Res. **3**, 993–1022 (2003)
5. Depeursinge, A., Chin, A.S., Leung, A.N., Terrone, D., Bristow, M., Rosen, G., Rubin, D.L.: Automated classification of usual interstitial pneumonia using regional volumetric texture analysis in high-resolution computed tomography. Invest. Radiol. **50**(4), 261–267 (2015)
6. Efron, B., Hastie, T., Johnstone, I., Tibshirani, R., Ishwaran, H., Knight, K., Loubes, J.M., Massart, P., Madigan, D., Ridgeway, G., Rosset, S., Zhu, J.I., Stine, R.A., Turlach, B.A., Weisberg, S., Hastie, T., Johnstone, I., Tibshirani, R.: Least angle regression. Ann. Stat. **32**(2), 407–499 (2004)
7. Gao, W., Oh, S., Viswanath, P.: Breaking the bandwidth barrier: geometrical adaptive entropy estimation (2016). http://arxiv.org/abs/1609.02208
8. Holzer, M., Donner, R.: Over-segmentation of 3D medical image volumes based on monogenic cues. In: CVWW, pp. 35–42 (2014). http://citeseerx.ist.psu.edu/viewdoc/download?doi=10.1.1.707.2473&rep=rep1&type=pdf
9. Lauritzen, S.L., Barndorff-Nielsen, O.E., Kass, R.E., Lauritzen, S.L., Rao, C.R.: Chapter 4: Statistical Manifolds, pp. 163–216. Institute of Mathematical Statistics (1987). http://projecteuclid.org/euclid.lnms/1215467061
10. Liu, K., Skibbe, H., Schmidt, T., Blein, T., Palme, K., Brox, T., Ronneberger, O.: Rotation-invariant HOG descriptors using fourier analysis in polar and spherical coordinates. Int. J. Comput. Vis. **106**(3), 342–364 (2014)
11. Loader, C.R.: Local likelihood density estimation. Ann. Stat. **24**(4), 1602–1618 (1996)
12. Mendoza, C.S., et al.: Emphysema quantification in a multi-scanner HRCT cohort using local intensity distributions. In: 2012 9th IEEE International Symposium on Biomedical Imaging (ISBI), pp. 474–477. IEEE (2012)
13. Muja, M., Lowe, D.G.: Scalable nearest neighbour algorithms for high dimensional data. IEEE Trans. Pattern Anal. Mach. Intell. **36**(11), 2227–2240 (2014)
14. Póczos, B., Schneider, J.G.: On the estimation of alpha-divergences. In: AISTATS, pp. 609–617 (2011)
15. Poczos, B., Xiong, L., Schneider, J.: Nonparametric divergence estimation with applications to machine learning on distributions. Uncertainty in Artificial Intelligence (2011)
16. Regan, E.A., Hokanson, J.E., Murphy, J.R., Make, B., Lynch, D.A., Beaty, T.H., Curran-Everett, D., Silverman, E.K., Crapo, J.D.: Genetic epidemiology of COPD (COPDGene) study design. COPD: J. Chronic Obstructive Pulm. Dis. **7**(1), 32–43 (2011)
17. Satoh, K., Kobayashi, T., Misao, T., Hitani, Y., Yamamoto, Y., Nishiyama, Y., Ohkawa, M.: CT assessment of subtypes of pulmonary emphysema in smokers. CHEST J. **120**(3), 725–729 (2001)
18. Shaker, S.B., Bruijne, M.D., Sorensen, L., Shaker, S.B., De Bruijne, M.: Quantitative analysis of pulmonary emphysema using local binary patterns. IEEE Trans. Med. Imaging **29**(2), 559–569 (2010)
19. Shapiro, S.D.: Evolving concepts in the pathogenesis of chronic obstructive pulmonary disease. Clin. Chest Med. **21**(4), 621–632 (2000)
20. Song, L., Siddiqi, S.M., Gordon, G., Smola, A.: Hilbert space embeddings of hidden Markov models. In: The 27th International Conference on Machine Learning (ICML2010), pp. 991–998 (2010)
21. Sorensen, L., Nielsen, M., Lo, P., Ashraf, H., Pedersen, J.H., De Bruijne, M.: Texture-based analysis of COPD: a data-driven approach. IEEE Trans. Med. Imaging **31**(1), 70–78 (2012)

22. Vogl, W.-D., Prosch, H., Müller-Mang, C., Schmidt-Erfurth, U., Langs, G.: Longitudinal alignment of disease progression in fibrosing interstitial lung disease. In: Golland, P., Hata, N., Barillot, C., Hornegger, J., Howe, R. (eds.) MICCAI 2014. LNCS, vol. 8674, pp. 97–104. Springer, Cham (2014). doi:10.1007/978-3-319-10470-6_13
23. Zhang, Q., Goncalves, B.: Why should I trust you? Explaining the predictions of any classifier, p. 4503. ACM (2015)
24. Zhang, Z., Wang, J.: MLLE: modified locally linear embedding using multiple weights. In: Advances in Neural Information Processing Systems, pp. 1593–1600 (2006)

Multi-source Multi-target Dictionary Learning for Prediction of Cognitive Decline

Jie Zhang[1], Qingyang Li[1], Richard J. Caselli[2], Paul M. Thompson[3], Jieping Ye[4], and Yalin Wang[1(✉)]

[1] School of Computing, Informatics, and Decision Systems Engineering, Arizona State University, Tempe, AZ, USA
Yalin.Wang@asu.edu
[2] Department of Neurology, Mayo Clinic Arizona, Scottsdale, USA
[3] Imaging Genetics Center, Institute for Neuroimaging and Informatics, University of Southern California, Marina del Rey, CA, USA
[4] Department of Computational Medicine and Bioinformatics, University of Michigan, Ann Arbor, MI, USA

Abstract. Alzheimer's Disease (AD) is the most common type of dementia. Identifying correct biomarkers may determine presymptomatic AD subjects and enable early intervention. Recently, Multi-task sparse feature learning has been successfully applied to many computer vision and biomedical informatics researches. It aims to improve the generalization performance by exploiting the shared features among different tasks. However, most of the existing algorithms are formulated as a supervised learning scheme. Its drawback is with either insufficient feature numbers or missing label information. To address these challenges, we formulate an unsupervised framework for multi-task sparse feature learning based on a novel dictionary learning algorithm. To solve the unsupervised learning problem, we propose a two-stage Multi-Source Multi-Target Dictionary Learning (MMDL) algorithm. In stage 1, we propose a multi-source dictionary learning method to utilize the common and individual sparse features in different time slots. In stage 2, supported by a rigorous theoretical analysis, we develop a multi-task learning method to solve the missing label problem. Empirical studies on an $N = 3970$ longitudinal brain image data set, which involves 2 sources and 5 targets, demonstrate the improved prediction accuracy and speed efficiency of MMDL in comparison with other state-of-the-art algorithms.

Keywords: Multi-task · Alzheimer's disease · Dictionary learning

1 Introduction

Alzheimer's disease (AD) is known as the most common type of dementia. It is a slow progressive neurodegenerative disorder leading to a loss of memory

---

J. Zhang and Q. Li—These two authors contributed equally to this work.

© Springer International Publishing AG 2017
M. Niethammer et al. (Eds.): IPMI 2017, LNCS 10265, pp. 184–197, 2017.
DOI: 10.1007/978-3-319-59050-9_15

and reduction of cognitive function. Many clinical/cognitive measures such as Mini Mental State Examination (MMSE) and Alzheimer's Disease Assessment Scale cognitive subscale (ADAS-Cog) have been designed to evaluate a subject's cognitive decline. Subjects are commonly divided into three different groups: AD, Mild Cognitive Impairment (MCI) and Cognitively Unimpaired (CU), defined clinically based on behavioral and above assessments. It is crucial to predict AD related cognitive decline so an early intervention or prevention becomes possible. Prior research have shown that measures from brain magnetic resonance (MR) images correlate closely with cognitive changes and have great potentials to provide early diagnostic markers to predict cognitive decline presymptomatically in a sufficiently rapid and rigorous manner.

The main challenge in AD diagnosis or prognosis with neuroimaging arises from the fact that the data dimensionality is intrinsically high while only a small number of samples are available. In this regard, machine learning has been playing a pivotal role to overcome this so-called "large p, small n" problem. A dictionary that allows us to represent original features as superposition of a small number of its elements so that we can reduce high dimensional image to a small number of features. Dictionary learning [8] has been proposed to use a small number of basis vectors to represent local features effectively and concisely and help image content analysis. However, most existing works on dictionary learning focused on the prediction of target at a single time point [19] or some region-of-interest [18]. In general, a joint analysis of tasks from multiple sources is expected to improve the performance but remains a challenging problem.

Multi-Task Learning (MTL) has been successfully explored for regression with different time slots. The idea of multi-task learning is to utilize the intrinsic relationships among multiple related tasks in order to improve the prediction performance. One way of modeling multi-task relationship is to assume all tasks are related and the task models are connected to each other [6], or the tasks are clustered into groups [21]. Alternatively, one can assume that tasks share a common subspace [4], or a common set of features [1]. Recently, Maurer et al. [12] proposed a sparse coding model for MTL problems based on the generative methods. In this paper, we proposed a novel unsupervised multi-source dictionary learning method to learn the different tasks simultaneously which utilizes shared and individual dictionaries to encode both consistent and individual imaging features for longitudinal image data analysis.

Although a general unsupervised dictionary learning may overcome the missing label problem to obtain the sparse features, we still need to consider the prediction labels at different time points after we learn the sparse features. A forthright method is to perform linear regression at each time point and determine weighted matrix W separately. However, even when we have the common dictionary which models the relationship among different tasks, if prediction is purely based on linear regression which treats all tasks independently and ignores the useful information reserved in the change along the time continuum, there still exists strong bias to predict future multiple targets clinical scores.

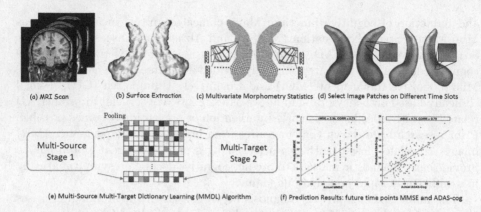

(a) MRI Scan   (b) Surface Extraction   (c) Multivariate Morphometry Statistics   (d) Select Image Patches on Different Time Slots

(e) Multi-Source Multi-Target Dictionary Learning (MMDL) Algorithm   (f) Prediction Results: future time points MMSE and ADAS-cog

Fig. 1. The pipeline of our method. We extracted hippocampi from MRI scans (a), then we registered hippocampal surfaces (b) and computed surface multivariate morphometry statistics (c). Image patches were extracted from the surface maps to initialize the dictionary (d) for Multi-Source Multi-Target Dictionary Learning (e). We used features from two time points to predict five future time points MMSE and ADAS-cog (f).

To excavate the correlations among the cognitive scores, several multi-task models were put forward. Wang *et al.* [14] proposed a sparse multi-task regression and feature selection method to jointly analyze the neuroimaging and clinical data in prediction of the memory performance. Zhang and Shen [17] exploited a $l_{2,1}$-norm based group sparse regression method to select features that could be used to jointly represent the different clinical status and two clinical scores (MMSE and ADAS-cog). Xiang *et al.* [16] proposed a sparse regression-based feature selection method for AD/MCI diagnosis to maximally utilize features from multiple sources by focusing on a missing modality problem. However, the clinical scores for many patients are missing at some time points, i.e., the target vector y_i may be incomplete and the above methods all failed to model this issue. A simple strategy is to remove all patients with missing target values. It, however, significantly reduces the number of samples. Zhou *et al.* [21] considered multi-task with missing target values in the training process, but the algorithm did not incorporate multiple sources data.

In this paper, we propose a novel integrated unsupervised framework, termed Multi-Source Multi-Target Dictionary Learning (MMDL) algorithm, we utilize shared and individual dictionaries to encode both consistent and changing imaging features along longitudinal time points. Meanwhile, we also formulate different time point clinical score predictions as multi-task learning and overcome the missing target values in the training process. The pipeline of our method is illustrated in Fig. 1. We evaluate the proposed framework on the $N = 3970$ longitudinal images from Alzheimer's Disease Neuroimaging Initiative (ADNI) database and use longitudinal hippocampal surface features to predict future cognitive scores. Our experimental results outperform some other state-of-the-art methods and demonstrate the effectiveness of the proposed algorithm.

Our main contributions can be summarized into threefold. Firstly, we considered the variance of subjects from different time points (Multi-Source) and proposed an unsupervised dictionary learning method in stage 1 of the MMDL algorithm, in which not only does a patient share features between different time slots but different patients share some common features within the same time point. We also explore the relationship between the shared and individual dictionary in stage 1. Secondly, we use sparse features learned from dictionary learning as an input and multiple future clinical scores as corresponding labels (Multi-Target) to train the multi-task prediction model in stage 2 of the MMDL Algorithm. To the best of our knowledge, it is the first learning model which unifies both multiple source inputs and multiple target outputs with dictionary learning research for brain imaging analysis. Lastly, we also take into account the incomplete label problem. We deal with the missing label problem during the regression process and theoretically prove the correctness of the regression model. Our extensive experimental results on the ADNI dataset show the proposed MMDL achieves faster running speed and lower estimation errors, as well as reasonable prediction scores when comparing with other state-of-the-art algorithms.

2   Multi-source Multi-target Dictionary Learning

2.1   Stage 1: Multi-source Dictionary Learning Stage

Given subjects from T time points: $\{X_1, X_2, \ldots, X_T\}$, our goal is to learn a set of sparse codes $\{Z_1, Z_2, \ldots, Z_T\}$ for each time point where $X_t \in \mathbb{R}^{p \times n_t}$, $Z_t \in \mathbb{R}^{l_t \times n_t}$ and $t \in \{1, \ldots, T\}$. p is the feature dimension of each subject, n_t is the number of subjects for X_t and l_t is the dimension of each sparse code in Z_t. When employing the online dictionary learning (ODL) method [11] to learn the sparse codes Z_t by X_t individually, we obtain a set of dictionary $\{D_1, \ldots, D_T\}$ but there is no correlation between learnt dictionaries. Another solution is to construct the subjects $\{X_1, \ldots, X_T\}$ into one data matrix X to obtain the dictionary D. However, only one dictionary D is not sufficient to model the variations among subjects from different time points. To address this problem, we integrate the idea of multi-task learning into the ODL method. We propose a novel online dictionary learning algorithm, called Multi-Source Multi-Target Dictionary Learning (MMDL), to learn the subjects from different time points.

For the subject matrix X_t of a particular time point, MMDL learns a dictionary D_t and sparse codes Z_t. D_t is composed of two parts: $D_t = [\hat{D}_t, \bar{D}_t]$ where $\hat{D}_t \in \mathbb{R}^{p \times \hat{l}}$, $\bar{D}_t \in \mathbb{R}^{p \times \bar{l}_t}$ and $\hat{l} + \bar{l}_t = l_t$. $\hat{D}_t$ is the common dictionary among all the learnt dictionaries $\{D_1, \ldots, D_T\}$ while $\bar{D}_t$ is different from each other and only learnt from the corresponding matrix X_t. Therefore, objective function of MMDL can be reformulated as follows:

$$\min_{\substack{D_1, \cdots, D_T \in \Psi_t \\ Z_1, \cdots, Z_T}} \sum_{t=1}^{T} \frac{1}{2} \|X_t - [\hat{D}_t, \bar{D}_t] Z_t\|_F^2 + \lambda \sum_{t=1}^{T} \|Z_t\|_1, \text{ subjects to: } \hat{D}_1 = \cdots = \hat{D}_T$$

$$(1)$$

where $\Psi_t = \{D_t \in \mathbb{R}^{p \times l_t} : \forall j \in 1, \dots, l_t, \|[D_t]_j\|_2 \leq 1\}$ $(t = 1, 2, \cdots, T)$ and $[D_t]_j$ is the jth column of D_t.

Figure 2 illustrates the framework of MMDL with subjects of ADNI from three different time points which represents as X_1, X_2 and X_3, respectively. Through the multi-source dictionary learning stage of MMDL, we obtain the dictionary and sparse codes for subjects from each time point t: D_t and Z_t. In Stage 1, a dictionary D_t is composed by a shared part $\hat{D}_t$ and an individual part $\bar{D}_t$. In this example, $\hat{D}_1$, $\hat{D}_2$ and $\hat{D}_3$ are the same. For the individual part of dictionaries, MMDL learns different $\bar{D}_t$ only from the corresponding matrix X_t. We vary the number of columns $\bar{l}_t$ in $\bar{D}_t$ to introduce the variant in the learnt sparse codes Z_t. As a result, the feature dimensions of learnt sparse codes matrix Z_t are different from each other. Then we employ the max-pooling [2] method to extract the features and use extracted features to perform the regression across different time points.

The initialization of dictionaries in MMDL is critical to the whole learning process. We propose a random patch method to initialize the dictionaries from different time points. The main idea of the random patch method is to randomly select l image patches from n subjects $\{x_1, x_2, \dots, x_n\}$ to construct D where $D \in \mathbb{R}^{p \times l}$. It is a similar way to perform the random patch approach in MMDL. In MMDL, the way we initialize $\hat{D}_t$ is to randomly select $\hat{l}$ subjects from subjects across different time points $\{X_1, \cdots, X_T\}$ to construct it. For the individual part of each dictionary, we randomly select $\bar{l}$ subjects from the corresponding matrix X_t to construct $\bar{D}_t$. After initializing dictionary D_t for each time point, we set all the sparse codes Z_t to be zero at the beginning. For each sample X_t at t-th time point, $X_t \in \mathbb{R}^{p \times n_t}$.

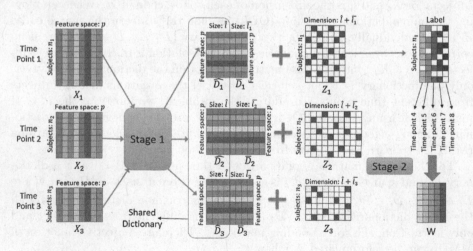

Fig. 2. Illustration of the learning process of MMDL on ADNI datasets from multiple different time points to predict multiple future time points clinical scores.

Algorithm 1. Multi-source Multi-target Dictionary Learning (MMDL)

Input: Samples and corresponding labels from different time points: $\{X_1, X_2, ...X_T\}$
   and $\{Y_1, Y_2, ...Y_T\}$
Output: The model for different time points: $\{W_1, ..., W_T\}$.
  1: **Stage 1:** Multi-Source Dictionary Learning
  2: **for** $k = 1$ to κ **do**
  3:    For each image patch $x_t(i)$ from sample X_t, $i \in \{1, ..., n_t\}$ and $t \in \{1, ..., T\}$.
  4:    Update $\hat{D}_t^k$: $\hat{D}_t^k = \Phi$.
  5:    Update $z_t^{k+1}(i)$ and index set $I_t^{k+1}(i)$ by a few steps of CCD:
  6:       $[z_t^{k+1}(i), I_t^{k+1}(i)] = CCD(\hat{D}_t^k, \bar{D}_t^k, x_t(i), I_t^k(i), z_t^k(i))$.
  7:    Update the $\hat{D}_t$ and $\bar{D}_t$ by one step SGD:
  8:       $[\hat{D}_t^{k+1}, \bar{D}_t^{k+1}] = SGD(\hat{D}_t^k, \bar{D}_t^k, x_t(i), I_t^{k+1}(i), z_t^{k+1}(i))$.
  9:    Normalize $\hat{D}_t^{k+1}$ and $\bar{D}_t^{k+1}$ based on the index set $I_t^{k+1}(i)$.
 10:    Update the shared dictionary Φ: $\Phi = \hat{D}_t^{k+1}$.
 11: **end for**
 12: Obtain the learnt dictionaries and sparse codes: $\{D_1, ..., D_T\}$, $\{Z_1, ..., Z_T\}$.
 13: **Stage 2:** Multi-Target Regression with incomplete label
 14: **for** $t = 1$ to T **do**
 15:    Given the jth column $Y_t(j)$ in Y_t, for the jth model $w_t(j)$ in W_t
 16:    $w_t(j) = (\widetilde{Z}_t \widetilde{Z}_t^T + \xi I)^{-1} \widetilde{Z}_t \widetilde{Y}_t(j)$
 17: **end for**

2.2   Stage 2: Multi-target Learning with Missing Label

In the longitudinal AD study, we measure the cognitive scores of selected patients at multiple time points. Instead of considering the prediction of cognitive scores at a single time point as a regression task, we formulate the prediction of clinical scores at multiple future time points as a multi-task regression problem. We employ multi-task regression formulations in place of solving a set of independent regression problems since the intrinsic temporal smoothness information among different tasks can be incorporated into the model as prior knowledge. However, the clinical scores for many patients are missing at some time points, especially for 36 and 48 months ADNI data. It is necessary to formulate a multi-task regression problem with missing target values to predict clinical scores.

In this paper, we use a matrix $\Theta \in \mathbb{R}^{m_t \times n_t}$ to indicate missing target values, where $\Theta_{i,j} = 0$ if the target value of label $Y_t(i, j)$ is missing and $\Theta_{i,j} = 1$ otherwise. Give the sparse codes $\{Z_1, \ldots, Z_T\}$ and corresponding labels $\{Y_1, \ldots, Y_T\}$ from different times where $Y_t \in \mathbb{R}^{m_t \times n_t}$, we formulate the multi-target learning stage with missing target values as:

$$\min_{W_1, \cdots, W_T} \sum_{t=1}^{T} ||\Theta(Y_t - W_t Z_t)||_F^2 + \xi \sum_{t=1}^{T} ||W_t||_F^2 \tag{2}$$

Although the Eq. 2 is associated with missing values on the labels, we show that it has a close form and present the theoretical analysis of stage 2 as follows:

Theorem. *For the data matrix pair* (Z_t, Y_t), *we denote the* j *th row's labels* $\widetilde{Y}_t(j)$ *in* Y_t. *We use* $\widetilde{Z}_t$ *and* $\widetilde{Y}_t(j)$ *to represent the remaining datasets after removing the missing value in* $Y_t(j)$. *The problem of (Eq. 2) can decomposed as the following equation:*

$$\min_{w_t(j)} ||(\widetilde{Y}_t(j) - w_t(j)\widetilde{Z}_t)||_2^2 + \xi||w_t(j)||_2^2 \tag{3}$$

Proof. Equation (3) is known the Ridge regression [7]. To optimize the problem, we calculate the gradient and set the gradient to be zero. Then we can get the optimal $w_t(j)$ by the following steps:

$$2\widetilde{Z}_t(\widetilde{Z}_t^T w_t(j) - \widetilde{Y}_t(j)) + 2\xi w_t(j) = 0, \widetilde{Z}_t\widetilde{Z}_t^T w_t(j) - \widetilde{Z}_t\widetilde{Y}_t(j) + \xi w_t(j) = 0,$$
$$(\widetilde{Z}_t\widetilde{Z}_t^T + \xi I)w_t(j) = \widetilde{Z}_t\widetilde{Y}_t(j), w_t(j) = (\widetilde{Z}_t\widetilde{Z}_t^T + \xi I)^{-1}\widetilde{Z}_t\widetilde{Y}_t(j) \qquad \square$$

After solving $w_t(j)$ for every time point where $j \in \{1, \ldots, m_t\}$, we can obtain the learnt model $\{W_1, \ldots, W_T\}$ to predict the clinical scores.

Our MMDL algorithm can be summarized into Algorithm 1. k denotes the epoch number where $k \in \{1, \ldots, \kappa\}$. Φ represents the shared part of each dictionary D_t which is initialized by the random patch method. For each image patch $x_t(i)$ extracted from X_t, we learn the i-th sparse code $z_t^{k+1}(i)$ from Z_t by several steps of Cyclic Coordinate Descent (CCD) [3]. Then we use learnt sparse codes $z_t^{k+1}(i)$ to update the dictionary $\hat{D}_t^{k+1}$ and $\bar{D}_t^{k+1}$ by one step Stochastic Gradient Descent (SGD) [20]. Since $z_t^{k+1}(i)$ is very sparse, we use the index set $I_t^{k+1}(i)$ to record the location of non-zero entries in $z_t^{k+1}(i)$ to accelerate the update of sparse codes and dictionaries. Φ is updated by the end of the k-th iteration to ensure $\hat{D}_t^{k+1}$ is the same part among all the dictionaries.

2.3   Updating the Sparse Codes

After we pick an image patch $x_t(i)$ from the sample X_t at the time point t, we fix the dictionary and update the sparse codes by following the ODL method. Then the optimization problem we need to solve becomes the following equation:

$$\min_{z_t(i)} F(z_t(i)) = \frac{1}{2}||x_t(i) - [\hat{D}_t, \bar{D}_t]z_t(i)||_2^2 + \lambda||z_t(i)||_1. \tag{4}$$

It is known as the Lasso problem [13]. Coordinate descent [3] is known as one of the state-of-the-art methods for solving this problem. In this study, we perform the CCD to optimize Eq. (4). Empirically, the iteration may take thousands of steps to converge, which is time-consuming in the optimization process of dictionary learning. However, we observed that after a few steps, the support of the coordinates, i.e., the locations of the non-zero entries in $z_t(i)$, becomes very accurate, usually after less than ten steps. In this study, we perform P steps CCD to generate the non-zero index set I_t^{k+1}, recording the non-zero entry of $z_t^{k+1}(i)$. Then we perform S steps CCD to update the sparse codes only on the non-zero entries of $z_t^{k+1}(i)$, accelerating the learning process significantly. SCC

[9,10] employs a similar strategy to update the sparse codes in a single task. For the multi-task learning, we summarize the updating rules as follows:

(a) Perform P steps CCD to update the locations of the non-zero entries $I_t^{k+1}(i)$ and the model $z_t(i)^{k+1}$.
(b) Perform S steps CCD to update the $z_t(i)^{k+1}$ in the index of $I_t^{k+1}(i)$.

In (a), for each step CCD, we will pick up j-th coordinate to update the model $z_t(i)_j$ and non-zero entries, where $j \in \{1, \ldots, l_t\}$. We perform the update from the 1st coordinate to the l_t-th coordinate. For each coordinate, we calculate the gradient g based on the objective function (4) then update the model $z_t^{k+1}(i)_j$ based on g. The calculation of g and $z_t^{k+1}(i)_j$ follows the equations:

$$g = [\hat{D}_t^k, \bar{D}_t^k]_j^T (\Omega([\hat{D}_t^k, \bar{D}_t^k], z_t^k(i), I_t^k(i)) - x_t(i)), \tag{5}$$

$$z_t^{k+1}(i)_j = \Gamma_\lambda(z_t^k(i)_j - g), \tag{6}$$

where Ω is a sparse matrix multiplication function that has three input parameters. Take $\Omega(A, b, I)$ as an example, A denotes a matrix, b is a vector and I is an index set that records the locations of non-zero entries in b. The returning value of function Ω is defined as: $\Omega(A, b, I) = Ab$. When multiplying A and b, we only manipulate the non-zero entries of b and corresponding columns of A based on the index set I, speeding up the calculation by utilizing the sparsity of b. Γ is the soft thresholding shrinkage function [5] and the definition of Γ is given by:

$$\Gamma_\varphi(x) = sign(x)(|x| - \varphi). \tag{7}$$

In the end of (a), we count the non-zero entries in $z_t^{k+1}(i)$ and store the non-zero index in $I_t^{k+1}(i)$. In (b), we perform S steps CCD by only considering the non-zero entries in $z_t^{k+1}(i)$. As a result, for each index μ in $I_t^{k+1}(i)$, we calculate the gradient g and update the $z_t^{k+1}(i)_\mu$ by:

$$g = [\hat{D}_t^k, \bar{D}_t^k]_\mu^T (\Omega([\hat{D}_t^k, \bar{D}_t^k], z_t^{k+1}(i), I_t^{k+1}(i)) - x_t(i)), \tag{8}$$

$$z_t^{k+1}(i)_\mu = \Gamma_\lambda((z_t^{k+1}(i)_\mu - g). \tag{9}$$

Since we only focus on the non-zero entries of the model and P is less than 10 iteration and S is a much larger number, we accelerate the learning process of sparse codes significantly.

2.4 Updating the Dictionaries

We update the dictionaries by fixing the sparse codes and updating the current dictionaries. Then, the optimization problem becomes as follow:

$$\min_{\hat{D}_t, \bar{D}_t} F(\hat{D}_t, \bar{D}_t) = \frac{1}{2}||x_t(i) - [\hat{D}_t, \bar{D}_t]z_t(i)||_2^2 \tag{10}$$

After we update the sparse codes, we have already known the non-zero entries of $z_t^{k+1}(i)$. Another key insight of MMDL is that we just need to focus on updating the non-zero entries of the dictionaries but not all columns of the dictionaries, and it accelerates the optimization dramatically. For example, when we update the i-th column and j-th row's entry of the dictionary D, the gradient of $D_{j,i}$ is set to be $\nabla D_{j,i} = z_i(D_j^T z - x_j)$. If the i-th entry of z is equal to zero, the gradient would be zero. As a result, we do not need to update the i-th column of the dictionary D. The learning rate is set to be an approximation of the inverse of the Hessian matrix H_t^{k+1}, which is updated by the sparse codes $z_t^{k+1}(i)$ in k-th iteration. In the beginning, we update the Hessian matrix by:

$$H_t^{k+1} = H_t^k + z_t^{k+1}(i)z_t^{k+1}(i)^T. \tag{11}$$

We perform one step SGD to update the dictionaries: $\hat{D}_t^{k+1}$ and $\bar{D}_t^{k+1}$. To speed up the computation, we use a vector to store the information $Dz - x$:

$$R = \Omega([\hat{D}_t^k, \bar{D}_t^k], z_t^{k+1}(i), I_t^{k+1}(i)) - x_t(i). \tag{12}$$

For entry of dictionary in the μ-th column and j-th row, the procedure of learning dictionaries take the form of

$$[\hat{D}_t^{k+1}, \bar{D}_t^{k+1}]_{j,\mu} = [\hat{D}_t^k, \bar{D}_t^k]_{j,\mu} - \frac{1}{H_t^{k+1}(\mu,\mu)} z_t^{k+1}(i)_\mu R_j, \tag{13}$$

where μ is the non-zero entry stored in $I_t^{k+1}(i)$. For the μ-th column of dictionary, we set the learning rate as the inverse of the diagonal element of the Hessian matrix, which is $1/H_t^{k+1}(\mu,\mu)$

Due to $D_t \in \Psi_t$ in Eq. (1), it is necessary to normalize the dictionaries $\hat{D}_t^{k+1}$ and $\bar{D}_t^{k+1}$ after updating them. We can perform the normalization on the corresponding columns of non-zero entries from $z_t^{k+1}(i)$ because the dictionaries updating only occurs on these columns. Utilizing the non-zero information from $I_t^{k+1}(i)$ can accelerate the whole learning process significantly.

3   Experiments

3.1   Experimental Setting

We studied multiple time points structural MR Imaging from ADNI baseline (837) and 6-month (733) datasets. The responses are the MMSE and ADAS-cog coming from 5 different time points: M12, M18, M24, M36 and M48. Thus, we learned a total of 3970 images which combines 2 sources and 5 targets. The sample sizes corresponding to 5 targets are 728, 326, 641, 454 and 251. We used hippocampal surface multivariate statistics [15] as learning features, which is a 4×1 vector on each vertex of 15000 vertices on every hippocampal surface.

We built a prediction model for the above datasets using MMDL algorithm. To train the prediction models, 1102 patches of size 10×10 are extracted from surface mesh structures and each patch dimension is 400. The model was trained on an Intel(R) Core(TM) i7-6700 K CPU with 4.0 GHz processors, 64 GB of globally addressable memory and a single Nvidia GeForce GTX TITAN X GPU. In the experimental setting of Stage 1 in MMDL, the sparsity $\lambda = 0.1$. Also, we selected 10 epochs with a batch size of 1 and 3 iterations of CCD (P is set to be 1 and S is 3). When the dictionaries and sparse codes were learned, Max-Pooling was used to generate features for annotation and get a 1×1000 vector feature for each images. In the Stage 2, 5-fold cross validation is used to select model parameters ξ in the training data (between 10^{-3} and 10^3).

In order to evaluate the model, we randomly split the data into training and testing sets using a 9:1 ratio and used 10-fold cross validation to avoid data bias. Lastly, we evaluated the overall regression performance using weighted correlation coefficient (wR) and root mean square error (rMSE) for task-specific regression performance measures. The two measures are defined as $wR(Y, \hat{Y}) = \sum_{i=1}^{t} Corr(Y_i, \hat{Y}_i) n_i / \sum_{i=1}^{t} n_i$, $rMSE(y, \hat{y}) = \sqrt{||y - \hat{y}||_2^2 / n}$. For wR, Y_i is the ground truth of target of task i and $\hat{Y}_i$ is the corresponding predicted value, $Corr$ is the correlation coefficient between two vectors and n_i is the number of subjects of task i. For each task of rMSE, y and n is the ground truth of target and the number of subjects and $\hat{y}$ is the corresponding prediction. The smaller rMSE, the bigger wR mean the better results. We report the mean and standard deviation based on 50 iterations of experiments on different splits of data.

We compared MMDL (code available on the Github[1]) with multiple state-of-the-art methods, ODL-L: the single-task online dictionary learning [11] followed by Lasso, L21: the multi-task method called $L_{2,1}$ norm regularization with least square loss [1]. TGL: the disease multi-task progression model called Temporal group Lasso [21], as well as Ridge and Lasso. For the parameters selection, we used the same method with the experimental setting in our stage 2.

3.2 Experimental Results

The Size of Common Dictionaries in MMDL. In Stage 1 of MMDL, the common dictionary is assumed to be shared by different tasks. It is necessary to evaluate what is an appropriate size of such common dictionary. Therefore, we set the dictionary size to be 1000 and partitioned the dictionary by different proportions: 125:875, 250:750, 500:500, 750:250 and 875:125, where the left number is the size of common dictionary while the right one is the size of individual dictionary for each task. Figure 3 shows the results of rMSE of MMSE and ADAS-cog prediction. As it shows in Fig. 3, the rMSE of MMSE and ADAS-Cog are lowest when we split the dictionary by half and a half. It means the both of common and individual dictionaries are of equal importance during the multi-task learning. In all experiments, we use the split of 500:500 as the size of common and individual dictionaries, the dimension of each sparse code in MMDL is 1000.

---

[1] https://github.com/liohzhee/Multi-Task-Dictionary-Learning.

Time Efficiency Comparison. We compare the efficiency of our proposed MMDL with the state-of-the-art online dictionary learning (ODL). In this experiment, we focus on the single batch size setting, that is, we process one image patch in each iteration. We vary the dictionary size as: 500, 1000 and 2000. For MMDL, the ratio between the common dictionary and the individual parts is 1:1. We

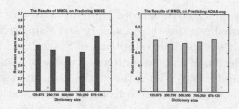

Fig. 3. Comparison of rMSE performance by varying the size of common dictionary.

report the results in Table 1. We observe that the proposed MMDL use less time than ODL. When the size of dictionary are increasing, MMDL is more efficient and has a higher speedup compared to ODL.

Table 1. Time comparisons of MMDL and ODL by varying dictionary size.

Dictionary size	MMDL	ODL
500	1.74 h	8.84 h
1000	3.34 h	21.95 h
2000	6.93 h	49.90 h

Performance Comparison. We report the results of MMDL and other methods on the prediction model of MMSE with ADNI group in Table 2. The proposed approach MMDL outperformed ODL-L, Lasso and Ridge, in terms of both rMSE and correlation coefficient wR on four different time points. The results of Lasso and Ridge are very close while sparse coding methods are superior to them. For sparse coding models, we observe that MMDL obtained a lower rMSE and higher correlation result than traditional sparse coding method ODL-L since we consider the correlation between different time slots for different tasks and the relationship with different time points on the same patient among all tasks. We also notice that the proposed MMDL's significant accuracy improvement for later time points. This may be due to the data sparseness in later time points, as the proposed sparsity-inducing models are expected to achieve better prediction performance in this case.

Table 2. The prediction results of MMSE on whole dataset.

Methods	wR	M12	M18	M24	M36	M48
Lasso	0.40 ± 0.09	4.04 ± 0.77	3.46 ± 0.97	5.53 ± 0.86	4.39 ± 0.74	4.73 ± 1.49
Ridge	0.41 ± 0.07	4.26 ± 0.56	3.56 ± 0.93	5.05 ± 0.54	4.21 ± 0.47	3.62 ± 0.91
L21	0.57 ± 0.01	3.32 ± 0.63	4.75 ± 0.75	4.64 ± 0.88	4.08 ± 1.01	3.11 ± 1.05
ODL-L	0.63 ± 0.08	2.99 ± 0.63	$\mathbf{2.88 \pm 0.68}$	4.29 ± 0.84	3.62 ± 1.45	2.93 ± 1.07
TGL	0.70 ± 0.05	2.73 ± 0.72	4.00 ± 1.31	4.00 ± 0.64	3.19 ± 1.38	2.60 ± 1.42
MMDL	$\mathbf{0.73 \pm 0.02}$	$\mathbf{2.61 \pm 0.55}$	3.37 ± 1.01	$\mathbf{3.66 \pm 0.78}$	$\mathbf{2.73 \pm 1.09}$	$\mathbf{2.52 \pm 1.20}$

Table 3. The prediction results of ADAS-cog on whole dataset.

Methods	wR	M12	M18	M24	M36	M48
Lasso	0.49 ± 0.05	6.81 ± 1.03	6.87 ± 0.74	7.62 ± 0.87	8.08 ± 1.39	6.55 ± 1.34
Ridge	0.46 ± 0.07	7.68 ± 0.96	6.89 ± 1.69	7.84 ± 1.54	8.59 ± 0.62	6.64 ± 1.58
L21	0.53 ± 0.07	6.40 ± 0.51	6.95 ± 0.88	8.07 ± 0.67	8.00 ± 1.04	5.92 ± 0.60
ODL-L	0.53 ± 0.05	5.65 ± 0.73	4.97 ± 0.67	7.30 ± 0.77	7.25 ± 0.69	5.56 ± 1.22
TGL	0.72 ± 0.04	5.52 ± 1.15	5.70 ± 0.53	6.85 ± 1.06	$\mathbf{6.36 \pm 1.22}$	5.73 ± 0.61
MMDL	$\mathbf{0.77 \pm 0.02}$	$\mathbf{5.18 \pm 0.88}$	$\mathbf{4.64 \pm 1.12}$	$\mathbf{6.76 \pm 1.35}$	6.78 ± 1.54	$\mathbf{5.27 \pm 1.76}$

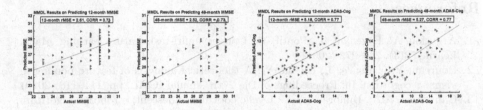

Fig. 4. Scatter plots of actual MMSE and ADAS-Cog versus predicted values on M12 and M48 by using MMDL.

We follow the same experimental procedure in the MMSE study and explore the prediction model by ADAS-cog scores. The prediction performance results are shown in Table 3. We can observe that the best performance of predicting scores of ADAS-Cog is achieved by MMDL for four time points.

Comparing with L21, after MMDL dealing with missing label, the results more linear, reasonable and accurate. Due to the dimension of M36 and M48 is too small, it is hard to learn a complete model. TGL also considered the issue of missing labels, however, MMDL still achieved the better results because MMDL incorporates multiple sources data and uses common and individual dictionaries. Although the result of MMDL had bias, MMDL still achieved the best result compared with the other five methods on predicting both MMSE and ADAS-cog, which shows our method is more efficient about dealing with missing data.

We show the scatter plots for the predicted values versus the actual values for MMSE and ADAS-Cog on the M12 and M48 in Fig. 4. In the scatter plots, we see the predicted values and actual clinical scores have a high correlation. The scatter plots show that the prediction performance for ADAS-Cog is better than that of MMSE.

4   Conclusion and Future Work

In this paper, we propose a novel Multi-Source Multi-Target Dictionary Learning for modeling cognitive decline, which allows simultaneous selections of a common set of biomarkers for multiple time points and specific sets of biomarkers for different time points using dictionary learning. We consider predicting future clinical scores as multi-task and deal with the missing labels problem. The effectiveness of the proposed progression model is supported by extensive experimental studies. The experimental results demonstrate that the proposed progression model is more effective than other state-of-the-art methods. In future, we will extend our algorithm to multi-modality data and propose more completely multiple sources with multiple targets algorithms.

Acknowledgments. The research was supported in part by NIH (R21AG049216, RF1AG051710, U54EB020403) and NSF (DMS-1413417, IIS-1421165).

References

1. Argyriou, A., Evgeniou, T., Pontil, M.: Convex multi-task feature learning. Mach. Learn. **73**(3), 243–272 (2008)
2. Boureau, Y.L., Ponce, J., LeCun, Y.: A theoretical analysis of feature pooling in visual recognition. In: Proceedings of the 27th Annual ICML, pp. 111–118 (2010)
3. Canutescu, A.A., Dunbrack, R.L.: Cyclic coordinate descent: a robotics algorithm for protein loop closure. Protein Sci. **12**(5), 963–972 (2003)
4. Chen, J., et al.: A convex formulation for learning shared structures from multiple tasks. In: Proceedings of the 26th Annual ICML, pp. 137–144. ACM (2009)
5. Combettes, P.L., Wajs, V.R.: Signal recovery by proximal forward-backward splitting. Multiscale Model. Simul. **4**(4), 1168–1200 (2005)
6. Evgeniou, T., Micchelli, C.A., Pontil, M.: Learning multiple tasks with kernel methods. J. Mach. Learn. Res. **6**, 615–637 (2005)
7. Hoerl, A.E., Kennard, R.W.: Ridge regression: biased estimation for nonorthogonal problems. Technometrics **12**(1), 55–67 (1970)
8. Lee, H., Battle, A., Raina, R., Ng, A.Y.: Efficient sparse coding algorithms. In: Advances in Neural Information Processing Systems, pp. 801–808 (2006)
9. Lin, B., et al.: Stochastic coordinate coding and its application for drosophila gene expression pattern annotation. arXiv preprint arXiv:1407.8147 (2014)
10. Lv, J., et al.: Task fMRI data analysis based on supervised stochastic coordinate coding. Med. Image Anal. **38**, 1–16 (2017)
11. Mairal, J., Bach, F., Ponce, J., Sapiro, G.: Online dictionary learning for sparse coding. In: Proceedings of the 26th Annual ICML, pp. 689–696. ACM (2009)
12. Maurer, A., Pontil, M., Romera-Paredes, B.: Sparse coding for multitask and transfer learning. In: Proceedings of the 26th Annual ICML 2013, Atlanta, GA, USA, 16–21 June 2013, pp. 343–351 (2013)
13. Tibshirani, R.: Regression shrinkage and selection via the lasso. J. R. Stat. Soc. Ser. B (Methodol.) **58**(1), 267–288 (1996)
14. Wang, H., et al.: Sparse multi-task regression and feature selection to identify brain imaging predictors for memory performance. In: ICCV, pp. 557–562. IEEE (2011)
15. Wang, Y., et al.: Surface-based TBM boosts power to detect disease effects on the brain: an N = 804 ADNI study. Neuroimage **56**(4), 1993–2010 (2011)
16. Xiang, S., et al.: Bi-level multi-source learning for heterogeneous block-wise missing data. NeuroImage **102**, 192–206 (2014)
17. Zhang, D., Shen, D., Initiative, A.D.N., et al.: Multi-modal multi-task learning for joint prediction of multiple regression and classification variables in Alzheimer's disease. Neuroimage **59**(2), 895–907 (2012)

18. Zhang, J., et al.: Hyperbolic space sparse coding with its application on prediction of Alzheimer's disease in mild cognitive impairment. In: Ourselin, S., Joskowicz, L., Sabuncu, M.R., Unal, G., Wells, W. (eds.) MICCAI 2016. LNCS, vol. 9900, pp. 326–334. Springer, Cham (2016). doi:10.1007/978-3-319-46720-7_38

19. Zhang, J., et al.: Applying sparse coding to surface multivariate tensor-based morphometry to predict future cognitive decline. In: 2016 IEEE 13th International Symposium on Biomedical Imaging (ISBI), pp. 646–650. IEEE (2016)

20. Zhang, T.: Solving large scale linear prediction problems using stochastic gradient descent algorithms. In: Proceedings of the 25th Annual ICML, p. 116. ACM (2004)

21. Zhou, J., Liu, J., Narayan, V.A., Ye, J.: Modeling disease progression via fused sparse group lasso. In: Proceedings of the 18th ACM SIGKDD International Conference on Knowledge Discovery and Data Mining, pp. 1095–1103. ACM (2012)

Predicting Interrelated Alzheimer's Disease Outcomes via New Self-learned Structured Low-Rank Model

Xiaoqian Wang[1], Kefei Liu[2,3], Jingwen Yan[2,3], Shannon L. Risacher[2],
Andrew J. Saykin[2], Li Shen[2], Heng Huang[1(✉)], and for the ADNI

[1] Computer Science and Engineering, University of Texas at Arlington,
Arlington, USA
heng@uta.edu
[2] Radiology and Imaging Sciences, Indiana University School of Medicine,
Indianapolis, USA
[3] BioHealth, Indiana University School of Informatics and Computing,
Indianapolis, USA

Abstract. Alzheimer's disease (AD) is a progressive neurodegenerative disorder. As the prodromal stage of AD, Mild Cognitive Impairment (MCI) maintains a good chance of converting to AD. How to efficaciously detect this conversion from MCI to AD is significant in AD diagnosis. Different from standard classification problems where the distributions of classes are independent, the AD outcomes are usually interrelated (their distributions have certain overlaps). Most of existing methods failed to examine the interrelations among different classes, such as AD, MCI conversion and MCI non-conversion. In this paper, we proposed a novel self-learned low-rank structured learning model to automatically uncover the interrelations among classes and utilized such interrelated structures to enhance classification. We conducted experiments on the ADNI cohort data. Empirical results demonstrated advantages of our model.

1 Introduction

Alzheimer's Disease (AD) usually progresses along a temporal continuum, initially from a preclinical stage, subsequently to mild cognitive impairment (MCI) and ultimately deteriorating to AD [19]. As the transitional step between normal

H. Huang—At UTA, this work was partially supported by NIH R01 AG049371, NSF IIS 1302675, IIS 1344152, DBI 1356628, IIS 1619308, IIS 1633753. At IU, this work was partially supported by NIH R01 EB022574, R01 LM011360, U01 AG024904, P30 AG10133, and R01 AG19771.
Data used in preparation of this article were obtained from the Alzheimer's Disease Neuroimaging Initiative (ADNI) database (adni.loni.usc.edu). As such, the investigators within the ADNI contributed to the design and implementation of ADNI and/or provided data but did not participate in analysis or writing of this report. A complete listing of ADNI investigators can be found at: http://adni.loni.usc.edu/wp-content/uploads/how_to_apply/ADNI_Acknowledgement_List.pdf.

M. Niethammer et al. (Eds.): IPMI 2017, LNCS 10265, pp. 198–209, 2017.
DOI: 10.1007/978-3-319-59050-9_16

aging and dementia, MCI has attracted high attention since it provides promising opportunities for early detection of AD. MCI is recognized as a clinical state of individuals who are memory impaired but functioning well otherwise, which does not meet the clinical criteria for dementia [13]. According to [11], MCI patients preserve a conversion-to-AD rate of approximately 15% per year, thus it is of great importance to distinguish MCI patients with high potential of AD conversion from those not years before dementia.

Recent advances in neuroimaging have offered a helping hand for exploring associations between brain structure and behavior, which have provided effective features for early detection of AD [7,8]. In the past few years, several machine learning techniques have been applied to predict MCI conversion by means of neuroimaging data [12]. Researches utilized various classification models to identify MCI converters from other classes, *e.g.*, health control samples and MCI non-converters by adopting neuroimaging data only in baseline time, which indicated a promising approach of "forecasting" stage changes of MCI patients several years before the conversion happens. As successful early detection of MCI conversion can boost therapeutic intervention of AD to a large extent, studies on this topic have attracted high attention in recent time.

However, most existing models hold a simple and common assumption that the neuroimaging data is drawn from an unimodal distribution [11,12,16–18], which is not applicable for all occasions. In AD research, since MCI converters and AD eventually evolve to AD with certain common biological mechanism, it is reasonable to assume that these subjects share similar distribution patterns, but their distributions are distinct from that of health control samples. That is to say, the brain data may come from multimodal distribution, *e.g.*, mixture of Gaussian. Thus, it is natural to assume latent group structure exists among different classes. Discovery of such subspace structure can enhance MCI conversion prediction and improve image biomarker discovery.

The most straightforward way to discover such groupwise interrelations is to cluster different data into groups before classification. However, since the clustering step is detached with the classification model, the learned interrelation structures are not associated to the prediction results. Such separated steps usually lead to suboptimal result. Here, we propose a novel structured low-rank learning model to simultaneously uncover the interrelations among different diagnostic stages and employ such interrelated structures to enhance the prediction of MCI conversion. We adopt Schatten p-norm to identify the shared low-rank subspace. Our new model is applied to the ADNI cohort for MCI conversion prediction. All empirical results show that the proposed classification model is capable of predicting MCI conversion with better performance.

2   Self-learned Low-Rank Structured Classification Model

Multi-class classification problem with c classes can be seen as a multi-task learning problem with c tasks, where each task is to classify one class from all others via the one-vs-rest technique. Suppose these c tasks come from g groups, where tasks in each group are mutually related. We introduce and optimize a group index matrix set $Q = \{Q_1, Q_2, \ldots Q_g\}$ to discover this group structure. Each Q_i is a diagonal matrix with $Q_i \in \{0,1\}^{c \times c}$ showing the assignment of tasks to the i-th group. For the (k, k)-th element of Q_i, $(Q_i)_{kk} = 1$ means the k-th task belongs to the i-th group while $(Q_i)_{kk} = 0$ means not. To avoid overlap of groups, we have $\sum_{i=1}^{g} Q_i = I$.

Since each group of tasks share correlative dependence, we reasonably assume the latent subspace of each group maintains a low-rank structure. Schatten-p norm [10] can be used as a low-rank regularization for uncovering common subspaces shared by tasks.

For a matrix $A \in \mathbb{R}^{d \times n}$, suppose σ_i is its i-th singular value, then the rank of A can be written as $rank(A) = \sum_{i=1}^{min\{d,n\}} \sigma_i^0$, where $0^0 = 0$. The definition of p-th power Schatten p-norm $(0 < p < \infty)$ is:

$$\|A\|_{S_p}^p = Tr((A^T A)^{\frac{p}{2}}) = \sum_{i=1}^{min\{d,n\}} \sigma_i^p.$$

The well-known trace norm (*a.k.a.* nuclear norm) is a special case of Schatten p-norm with $p = 1$: $\|A\|_* = \|A\|_{S_1} = Tr((A^T A)^{\frac{1}{2}}) = \sum_{i=1}^{min\{d,n\}} \sigma_i$.

Obviously, when $0 < p < 1$, Schatten p-norm makes a better approximation of $rank(A)$ thus a more strict low-rank constraint than trace norm. The more closer p is to 0, the more strict low-rank constraint the regularization term $\|A\|_{S_p}^p$ imposes.

According to the above analysis, we can formulate our novel self-learned structured low-rank classification model as follows:

$$\min_{W, \mathbf{b}, Q_i|_{i=1}^{g} \in \{0,1\}^{c \times c}, \sum_{i=1}^{g} Q_i = I} \mathcal{L}(Y; X, W, \mathbf{b}) + \gamma \sum_{i=1}^{g} (\|W Q_i\|_{S_p}^p)^k, \tag{1}$$

In Problem (1), we use a general classification loss $\mathcal{L}(Y; X, W, \mathbf{b})$, which can be any loss function, *e.g.*, logistic regression, hinge loss, *etc.* $W \in \mathbb{R}^{d \times c}$ is the weight matrix for classification, $\mathbf{b} \in \mathbb{R}^{c \times 1}$ is the bias, and $Y \in \mathbb{R}^{n \times c}$ is the label matrix. Moreover, we add a power parameter k to the Schatten p-norm regularization term for robustness of Problem (1), whose influence will be elaborately discussed in Sect. 4.

When $0 < p < 1$, it is apparent that the new objective is non-convex thus difficult for optimization. In the next section, we adopt an efficient re-weighted optimization algorithm.

3   Optimization Algorithm

Here, we first introduce a re-weighted algorithm to solve a general problem with (1) being a special case, and then discuss the detailed optimization of (1).

3.1   Optimization Algorithm for a General Problem

Lemma 1. *Let $g_i(x)$ denote a general function over x, where x can be a scalar, vector or matrix, $\mathcal{C}$ denotes the constraints on x, then we can claim:*
  When $\delta \to 0$, The optimization problem

$$\min_{x \in \mathcal{C}} f(x) + \sum_i Tr((g_i^T(x)g_i(x))^{\frac{p}{2}}),$$

is equivalent to

$$\min_{x \in \mathcal{C}} f(x) + \sum_i Tr(g_i^T(x)g_i(x)D_i), \quad where \quad D_i = \frac{p}{2}(g_i^T(x)g_i(x) + \delta I)^{\frac{p-2}{2}}.$$

Proof: When $\delta \to 0$, it's apparent that the optimization problem

$$\min_{x \in \mathcal{C}} f(x) + \sum_i Tr((g_i^T(x)g_i(x) + \delta I)^{\frac{p}{2}}), \tag{2}$$

will reduce to

$$\min_{x \in \mathcal{C}} f(x) + \sum_i Tr((g_i^T(x)g_i(x))^{\frac{p}{2}}). \tag{3}$$

So with a fairly small parameter δ, we turn the non-smooth Problem (3) to the smooth Problem (2).

The Lagrangian function of Problem (2) is:

$$f(x) + \sum_i Tr((g_i^T(x)g_i(x) + \delta I)^{\frac{p}{2}}) - \lambda \tilde{I}_C(x),$$

where $\tilde{I}_C(x)$ equals 0 if $x \in C$ and ∞ otherwise [4]. Take derivative w.r.t. x and set it to zero. Based on the chain rule [2], we have:

$$\sum_i \frac{Tr\left(2\frac{p}{2}(g_i^T(x)g_i(x) + \delta I)^{\frac{p-2}{2}} g_i^T(x)\partial g_i(x)\right)}{\partial x} + f'(x) - \lambda \frac{\partial \tilde{I}_C(x)}{\partial x} = 0. \tag{4}$$

According to the Karush-Kuhn-Tucker conditions [4], if we can find a solution x that satisfies Eq. (4), then we usually find a local/global optimal solution to Problem (2). We can derive the x as follows.

If $D_i = \frac{p}{2}(g_i^T(x)g_i(x) + \delta I)^{\frac{p-2}{2}}$ is a given constant, Eq. (4) can be reduced to

$$f'(x) + \sum_i \frac{Tr\left(2D_i g_i^T(x)\partial g_i(x)\right)}{\partial x} - \lambda \frac{\partial \tilde{I}_C(x)}{\partial x} = 0. \tag{5}$$

Based on the chain rule [2], the optimal solution x^* of Eq. (5) is also an optimal solution to the following problem:

$$\min_{x \in \mathcal{C}} f(x) + \sum_i Tr(g_i^T(x)g_i(x)D_i). \tag{6}$$

Based on this observation, we can first guess a solution x, next calculate D_i based on the current solution x, and then update the current solution x by the optimal solution of Problem (6) on the basis of the calculated D_i. We can iteratively perform this procedure until it converges.   □

3.2 Optimization of Problem (1)

It is obvious that Problem (1) can be optimized via Lemma 1. Noticing that $Q_i Q_i^T = Q_i$, our objective becomes:

$$\min_{W,\mathbf{b},\, Q_i|_{i=1}^{g} \in \{0,1\}^{c \times c},\, \sum_{i=1}^{g} Q_i = I} \mathcal{L}(Y; X, W, \mathbf{b}) + \gamma \sum_{i=1}^{g} Tr(WQ_iW^T D_i), \quad (7)$$

where D_i is defined as:

$$D_i = \frac{kp}{2} (\|WQ_i\|_{S_p}^{p})^{k-1} (WQ_iW^T + \delta I)^{\frac{p-2}{2}}, \quad (8)$$

with δ being a fairly small parameter close to zero.

We can solve Problem (7) by means of the alternating optimization method.

The first step is fixing W and solving Q, then Problem (7) becomes:

$$\min_{Q_i|_{i=1}^{g} \in \{0,1\}^{c \times c},\, \sum_{i=1}^{g} Q_i = I} \sum_{i=1}^{g} Tr((W^T D_i W) Q_i), \quad (9)$$

Let $A_i = W^T D_i W$, then the solution of each Q_i is evident as follows:

$$Q_i(l,l) = \begin{cases} 1, i = \arg\min_j A_j(l,l) \\ 0, \text{otherwise} \end{cases} \quad (10)$$

The second step is fixing Q and solving W, $\mathbf{b}$, then Problem (7) becomes:

$$\min_{W,\mathbf{b}} \mathcal{L}(Y; X, W, \mathbf{b}) + \gamma \sum_{i=1}^{g} Tr(WQ_iW^T D_i). \quad (11)$$

Problem (11) can be solved according to the choice of the classification loss $\mathcal{L}(Y; X, W, \mathbf{b})$.

Here, we take an example to illustrate the optimization steps of Problem (11) when we adopt hinge loss for $\mathcal{L}(Y; X, W, \mathbf{b})$. Problem (11) can be written as:

$$\min_{W,\mathbf{b}} C \sum_{i=1}^{n} \sum_{j=1}^{c} h_{ij} \left(1 - y_{ij}(\mathbf{w}_j^T \mathbf{x}_i + b_j)\right) + \frac{1}{2} \|W\|_F^2 + \gamma \sum_{i=1}^{g} Tr(WQ_iW^T D_i). \quad (12)$$

where $H \in \mathbb{R}^{n \times c}$ is a slack variable defined as: $h_{ij} = \begin{cases} 1, y_{ij}(\mathbf{w}_j^T \mathbf{x}_i + b_j) \leq 1 \\ 0, \text{otherwise} \end{cases}$

Taking derivative of (12) *w.r.t.* $\mathbf{b}$ and set it to zero, then we get: $\sum_{i=1}^{n} h_{ij} y_{ij} = 0$.
which indicates that $\mathbf{b}$ can be updated according to the support vectors.

Take derivative of Problem (12) *w.r.t.* $\mathbf{w}_j$ and set it to zero, then we have:
$$\mathbf{w}_j = C(I + 2\gamma(\sum_{i=1}^{g} Q_i(j,j)D_i))^{-1} \sum_{i=1}^{n} h_{ij} y_{ij} \mathbf{x}_i.$$

Algorithm 1. Algorithm to solve problem (7).

Input:
Imaging feature data $X \in \mathbb{R}^{d \times n}$, label matrix $Y \in \mathbb{R}^{n \times c}$, parameter p, k, γ, group number g.

Output:
Weight matrix $W \in \mathbb{R}^{d \times c}$ and g different group matrices $Q_i|_{i=1}^{g} \in \mathbb{R}^{c \times c}$ which groups the c classes into g subspaces.
Initialize W by the optimal solution to the ridge regression problem.
Initialize Q randomly.
while not converge do
    1. Update D according to the definition in Eq. (8)
    2. Update Q according to the solution in Eq. (10)
    3. Update W and $\mathbf{b}$ by solving Problem (11). The solution differs w.r.t. the choice of loss function $\mathcal{L}(Y; X, W, \mathbf{b})$.
end while

We can iteratively update D, Q, W and $\mathbf{b}$ with the alternating steps mentioned above and the algorithm of Problem (7) is summarized in Algorithm 1.

Convergence and Time Analysis: Our algorithm as a whole employs the alternating optimization method to update variables, whose convergence has already been proved in [3]. Our model usually converges in 15 iterations. In our experiments on the ADNI data, the runtime for five-fold cross validation is around 3 s.

4   Discussion of Parameters

We introduced several hyper-parameters to make our model more general and adaptive to various circumstances. Here, we analyze the functionality of each parameter in detail.

In Problem (1), the parameter p is the norm parameter for the low-rank regularization term. It adjusts the stringency of the low-rank penalty. As is analyzed in previous section, Schatten p-norm makes a more strict low-rank constraint than trace norm when $0 < p < 1$. The closer p is to 0, the more rigorous low-rank constraint the regularization term $\|M\|_{S_p}^{p}$ imposes. But empirically we don't set p to a too small value since it makes the model contain too many local-minima thus is sensitive to noise and outliers.

The parameter k in Problem (1) is proposed to guarantee the robustness of our model. When p is small, the number of local solutions becomes more thus lead the model to be more sensitive to outliers. Under this condition, a larger k value will render the model more robust to outliers. According to our pre-experiments, we usually set k value in the range of $[2, 3]$.

Parameter γ is use to balance the role of the low-rank penalty, which can be adjusted to accommodate different cases. γ can be set to any positive value.

In the experiments, we did not spend too much time tuning the parameters. On the contrary, in order to fairly compare all methods, we simply set each parameter to a reasonable value, which is discussed in the next section. While these parameters introduced significant challenges in optimizing our objective, they make our model more flexible and adapt to different situations.

5   Experimental Results

5.1   Experimental Settings

In the classification experiment, we employed hinge loss in Problem (1). We compared with the following methods: Support Vector Machine with ℓ_1-norm loss (L1SVM) as baseline, k-Nearest Neighbors algorithm (KNN), Least Square SVM (LSSVM) [15] and SVM with ℓ_2-norm loss (L2SVM). To apply SVM model to the multi-class classification problem, we adopted 1-vs-all mechanism. Besides, we compared with one state-of-art method conducting structured multi-task learning via trace norm regularization (TMTL) [9]. In TMTL model, we also used hinge loss to conduct classification. It is notable that TMTL makes a special case of our model (1) with $p = 1$ and $k = 1$.

In our experiments, we exploited the LIBSVM toolbox [6] to implement both L1SVM and L2SVM. All participating data were normalized to the range of $[0, 1]$ and randomly divided using 5-fold cross validation. We excavated the classification result in each fold and recorded the average in these 5 times repetition.

The evaluation of different methods was based on the percentage of correctly classified samples, *i.e.*, classification accuracy. For KNN, we set $k = 1$. For all other methods using the hinge loss, we tuned the C parameter in the range of $\{10^{-3}, 10^{-2}, \ldots, 10^3\}$ on training and validation data and recorded the performance on testing data using the best parameter *w.r.t.* each method.

Our model consists of several other parameters such as p, γ, k and δ. In our pre-experiments, we use cross-validation to find a reasonable range for each parameter. We found the performance of our model relatively stable within the reasonable range of parameters (data not shown). Indeed, we can further improve the performance with fine-tuning the parameters. Instead, we simply fix $p = 0.25$, $\gamma = 1$, $k = 3$ and $\delta = 10^{-12}$ in the experiments. Unless specified otherwise, we set the number of groups as $g = 2$. These parameters were determined according to the theoretical reasonable range discussed in Sect. 4 and empirical convention.

5.2   Description of ADNI Data

Data used in this paper was obtained from the ADNI database (https://adni.loni.usc.edu). One goal of ADNI has been to test whether serial MRI, PET, other biological markers, and clinical and neuropsychological assessment can be combined to measure the progression of MCI and early AD. For up-to-date information, we refer interested readers to visit www.adni-info.org. We downloaded baseline 1.5 T MRI scans and demographic information for 818 ADNI-1 participants. For each baseline MRI scan, FreeSurfer [14] was employed for brain segmentation and cortical parcellation, and extracted 90 thickness and volume measures, which were pre-adjusted by intracranial volume (ICV) using the regression weights derived from the healthy control (HC) participants. Besides, we performed voxel-based morphometry (VBM) [14] on the MRI data, and extracted mean gray matter (GM) density measures for 90 target regions of interest (ROIs). All participants with no missing MRI measurements and diagnostic status were involved in this study. We have 516 sample subjects in our study, including 105 AD samples, and 237 MCI samples and 174 health control (HC) samples. Among the 237 MCI samples, 9 of them become HC in M36, 95 become AD in M36 while the rest 133 remain as MCI along this three-year continuum.

5.3   Performance Comparison on ADNI Cohort

We labeled the ADNI data according to a three-year clinical observation to five different classes, which are: 1. health control (HC), 2. MCI(baseline)-HC(M36), 3. MCI(baseline)-MCI(M36), 4. MCI(baseline)-AD(M36) and 5. AD. Classification experiments were performed only on the baseline neuroimaging data so as to compare the "forecasting" ability of different methods. Our goal is to classify these different classes using baseline data, $i.e.$, detect MCI stage changes three years before the clinical diagnosis, which will make a contribution to therapeutic intervention of AD in the most effective stage. The comparison results are summarized in Table 1.

From Table 1, we found that our new method performs better than the counterparts in classifying the different classes using merely baseline data. Besides, we get two other interesting observations: (1) SVM methods outperforms KNN on the ADNI data; (2) L1SVM and L2SVM perform equal or better than LSSVM. The reason may go as follows: For KNN, it is a method focused more on the local data structure, while SVM model is meant to effectively find the separating hyperplanes, which is more suitable for classification. The unilateral loss is more interpretable and robust than bilateral loss for classification, thus we notice that L1SVM and L2SVM perform equal or better than LSSVM method. As for our proposed method, we utilized the unilateral hinge loss to be adaptive for classification and also automatically discovered the groupwise structure among different classes, which strengthened the classification performance. To compare our method with TMTL, even though both methods attempted to detect the groupwise structure among different tasks, our model is more general and robust. The use of Schatten p-norm and the power parameter k make our model better approximate the low-rank structure of the latent subspaces thus perform better.

It is also worth mentioning that in this classification, we only use neuroimaging data but not cognitive test information as previous papers do, $e.g.$, [12]. In [12], the classification accuracy is over 70% by adding the cognitive test information to prediction. However, cognitive assessment is a direct diagnostic criterion of MCI and AD [1]. Predicting MCI with cognitive scores is like classifying with label information, which will definitely boost the performance. But using the cognitive test scores as features, the classification is no longer "forecasing" but just a classification of existing information.

Table 1. Classification accuracy (%) comparison using "FreeSurfer" and "VBM" data

	KNN	L1SVM	LSSVM	L2SVM	TMTL	OURS
VBM	33.21 ± 8.00	43.66 ± 1.73	44.14 ± 5.64	44.15 ± 5.61	42.55 ± 3.37	**44.79 ± 4.46**
FreeSurfer	37.77 ± 3.74	45.78 ± 3.71	44.23 ± 3.60	45.02 ± 4.97	44.83 ± 4.79	**48.48 ± 3.25**

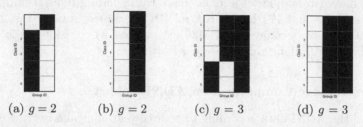

(a) $g = 2$ (b) $g = 2$ (c) $g = 3$ (d) $g = 3$

Fig. 1. Illustration of the detected group structure among different classes in our method ((a) and (c)) and TMTL ((b) and (d)) in the VBM analysis. We set the number of groups to be 2 and 3, respectively. White blocks denote that a class belongs to a certain group while black block denote otherwise. The five classes are: 1. health control (HC), 2. MCI(baseline)-HC(M36), 3. MCI(baseline)-MCI(M36), 4. MCI(baseline)-AD(M36) and 5. AD.

Moreover, we present the detected group structure from TMTL and our method on VBM analysis in Fig. 1. It seems that TMTL fails to detect the appropriate group structure among the five classes, but put them all together in one group. On the contrary, our method successfully finds the intrinsic group information among different classes. Figure 1 shows an interesting phenomenon that no matter what group number g we set, our model always groups the five classes into two clusters. This illustrates that our model is able to find the intrinsic group structure regardless of g settings. Also, according to the detected structure, we know that even though three different types of MCI patients *i.e.,* class 2, 3 and 4, end up with 3 different stages in month 36, they adopt a similar pattern in the baseline. As a subdivision, MCI-AD shows a potential similarity with AD while the other two types of MCI obtain patterns like HC. Such detected group information may help with the diagnosis of MCI and AD.

5.4   Discussion on Top Ranked Features

In this section, let's take an insight into the results. We use heat maps and brain maps to intuitively indicate the degree of influence imposed by each imaging feature, such that important features in classification can be determined.

Shown in Figs. 2 and 3 are the heat maps of sorted neuroimaging feature weights and corresponding brain maps. The figures demonstrate the capture of a small set of features that are predominant for classification. Among the selected features, we found LHippoCampus and LPostCentral on the top, whose impact on AD have already been proved in the previous papers [5, 20]. These

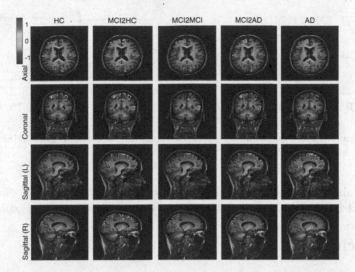

Fig. 2. Neuroimaging features mapped on the brain for the FreeSurfer analysis.

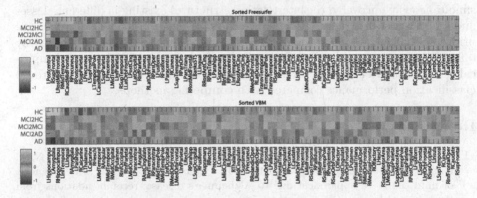

Fig. 3. Heat maps of sorted neuroimaging feature weights in our method in descending order from left to right. The feature weight matrix is learned on the entire data.

identified imaging disease associations warrant further investigation in independent cohorts. If replicated, these findings can potentially contribute to biomarker discovery for diagnosis and drug design.

5.5 Experiments of Convergence Analysis

In this subsection, we empirically analyze the convergence of our algorithm with respect to the two parameters p and k in Eq. (1). We apply our method to the entire data with two different p values (0.25 and 0.75) and two different k values (2 and 3), then record the objective value of our model in each iteration.

We use the results on FreeSurfer as an example. The convergence plots are shown in Fig. 4. We notice that the number of iterations need before convergence

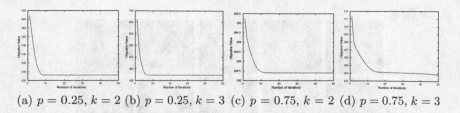

(a) $p = 0.25$, $k = 2$ (b) $p = 0.25$, $k = 3$ (c) $p = 0.75$, $k = 2$ (d) $p = 0.75$, $k = 3$

Fig. 4. Objective function value of Eq. (1) with different k and p parameters in each iteration on the FreeSurfer data.

is fairly stable with respect to the settings of p and k parameters. No matter what p and k values are, our model usually converges within 15 iterations.

6   Conclusions

In this paper, we proposed a novel low-rank structured classification model to predict MCI conversion using neuroimaging data in the baseline time. Our model simultaneously uncovered the interrelation structures existing in different classes and employed such structure to enhance the classification model. Moreover, we utilized Schatten p-norm to extract the common low-rank subspace shared by different patient classes. We conducted experiments on ADNI cohort. Empirical results validated the effectiveness of our model by demonstrating improved classification performance compared with competing methods.

References

1. Albert, M.S., DeKosky, S.T., Dickson, D., Dubois, B., Feldman, H.H., Fox, N.C., Gamst, A., Holtzman, D.M., Jagust, W.J., Petersen, R.C., et al.: The diagnosis of mild cognitive impairment due to Alzheimer's disease: recommendations from the national institute on aging-Alzheimer's association workgroups on diagnostic guidelines for Alzheimer's disease. Alzheimer's Dement. **7**(3), 270–279 (2011)
2. Bentler, P., Lee, S.Y.: Matrix derivatives with chain rule and rules for simple, hadamard, and kronecker products. J. Math. Psychol. **17**(3), 255–262 (1978)
3. Bezdek, J.C., Hathaway, R.J.: Convergence of alternating optimization. Neural Parallel Sci. Comput. **11**(4), 351–368 (2003)
4. Boyd, S., Vandenberghe, L.: Convex Optimization. Cambridge University Press, Cambridge (2004)
5. Cacabelos, R., Yamatodani, A., Niigawa, H., Hariguchi, S., Tada, K., Nishimura, T., Wada, H., Brandeis, L., Pearson, J.: Brain histamine in Alzheimer's disease. Methods Find. Exp. Clin. Pharmacol. **11**(5), 353–360 (1989)
6. Chang, C.C., Lin, C.J.: LIBSVM: a library for support vector machines. ACM Trans. Intell. Syst. Technol. **2**, 27:1–27:27 (2011). Software available at. http://www.csie.ntu.edu.tw/cjlin/libsvm
7. Devanand, D., Pradhaban, G., Liu, X., Khandji, A., De Santi, S., Segal, S., Rusinek, H., Pelton, G., Honig, L., Mayeux, R., et al.: Hippocampal and entorhinal atrophy in mild cognitive impairment prediction of Alzheimer disease. Neurology **68**(11), 828–836 (2007)

8. Hua, X., Leow, A.D., Parikshak, N., Lee, S., Chiang, M.C., Toga, A.W., Jack, C.R., Weiner, M.W., Thompson, P.M., ADNI, et al.: Tensor-based morphometry as a neuroimaging biomarker for Alzheimer's disease: an MRI study of 676 AD, MCI, and normal subjects. Neuroimage **43**(3), 458–469 (2008)

9. Kang, Z., Grauman, K., Sha, F.: Learning with whom to share in multi-task feature learning. In: Proceedings of the 28th International Conference on Machine Learning (ICML 2011), pp. 521–528 (2011)

10. Kittaneh, F.: Inequalities for the schatten p-norm. Glasgow Math. J. **26**(02), 141–143 (1985)

11. Misra, C., Fan, Y., Davatzikos, C.: Baseline and longitudinal patterns of brain atrophy in MCI patients, and their use in prediction of short-term conversion to AD: results from ADNI. Neuroimage **44**(4), 1415–1422 (2009)

12. Moradi, E., Pepe, A., Gaser, C., Huttunen, H., Tohka, J., ADNI, et al.: Machine learning framework for early MRI-based Alzheimer's conversion prediction in MCI subjects. Neuroimage **104**, 398–412 (2015)

13. Petersen, R., Stevens, J., Ganguli, M., Tangalos, E., Cummings, J., DeKosky, S.: Practice parameter: early detection of dementia: mild cognitive impairment (an evidence-based review) report of the quality standards subcommittee of the American academy of neurology. Neurology **56**(9), 1133–1142 (2001)

14. Shen, L., Kim, S., Risacher, S.L., Nho, K., Swaminathan, S., West, J.D., Foroud, T., Pankratz, N., Moore, J.H., Sloan, C.D., et al.: Whole genome association study of brain-wide imaging phenotypes for identifying quantitative trait loci in MCI and AD: a study of the ADNI cohort. Neuroimage **53**(3), 1051–1063 (2010)

15. Suykens, J.A., Van Gestel, T., De Brabanter, J., De Moor, B., Vandewalle, J.: Least Squares Support Vector Machines, vol. 4. World Scientific (2002)

16. Wang, H., Nie, F., Huang, H., Risacher, S., Ding, C., Saykin, A.J., Shen, L., ADNI: Sparse multi-task regression and feature selection to identify brain imaging predictors for memory performance. In: IEEE Conference on Computer Vision, pp. 557–562 (2011)

17. Wang, H., Nie, F., Huang, H., Risacher, S., Saykin, A.J., Shen, L., ADNI: Joint classification and regression for identifying ad-sensitive and cognition-relevant imaging biomarkers. In: The 14th International Conference on Medical Image Computing and Computer Assisted Intervention (MICCAI), pp. 115–123 (2011)

18. Wang, H., Nie, F., Huang, H., Risacher, S.L., Saykin, A.J., Shen, L., ADNI: Identifying disease sensitive and quantitative trait relevant biomarkers from multidimensional heterogeneous imaging genetics data via sparse multi-modal multi-task learning. Bioinformatics **28**(12), i127–i136 (2012)

19. Wenk, G.L., et al.: Neuropathologic changes in Alzheimer's disease. J. Clin. Psychiatry **64**, 7–10 (2003)

20. West, M.J., Coleman, P.D., Flood, D.G., Troncoso, J.C.: Differences in the pattern of hippocampal neuronal loss in normal ageing and Alzheimer's disease. Lancet **344**(8925), 769–772 (1994)

Weakly-Supervised Evidence Pinpointing and Description

Qiang Zhang[1(✉)], Abhir Bhalerao[1], and Charles Hutchinson[2]

[1] Department of Computer Science, University of Warwick, Coventry, UK
q.zhang.13@warwick.ac.uk
[2] University Hospital Coventry and Warwickshire, Coventry, UK

Abstract. We propose a learning method to identify which specific regions and features of images contribute to a certain classification. In the medical imaging context, they can be the evidence regions where the abnormalities are most likely to appear, and the discriminative features of these regions supporting the pathology classification. The learning is weakly-supervised requiring only the pathological labels and no other prior knowledge. The method can also be applied to learn the salient description of an anatomy discriminative from its background, in order to localise the anatomy before a classification step. We formulate evidence pinpointing as a sparse descriptor learning problem. Because of the large computational complexity, the objective function is composed in a stochastic way and is optimised by the Regularised Dual Averaging algorithm. We demonstrate that the learnt feature descriptors contain more specific and better discriminative information than hand-crafted descriptors contributing to superior performance for the tasks of anatomy localisation and pathology classification respectively. We apply our method on the problem of lumbar spinal stenosis for localising and classifying vertebrae in MRI images. Experimental results show that our method when trained with only target labels achieves better or competitive performance on both tasks compared with strongly-supervised methods requiring labels and multiple landmarks. A further improvement is achieved with training on additional weakly annotated data, which gives robust localisation with average error within 2 mm and classification accuracies close to human performance.

1 Introduction

Pathology classification based on radiological images is a key task in medical image computing. A clinician often inspects consistent and salient structures for localising the anatomies, then evaluates the appearance of certain local regions for evidence of pathology. In a computer-aided approach, by learning to identify or *pinpoint* these regions and describing them discriminatively could provide precise information for localising the anatomies and classifying pathology. In this paper, we describe a method to automatically pinpoint the evidence regions as well as learn the discriminative descriptors in a weakly-supervised manner, i.e., only the class labels are used in training, and no other supervisory information

© Springer International Publishing AG 2017
M. Niethammer et al. (Eds.): IPMI 2017, LNCS 10265, pp. 210–222, 2017.
DOI: 10.1007/978-3-319-59050-9_17

is required. For localisation, we learn which features describe the anatomies saliently on a training set of aligned images. For classification, given the images with pathological labels, we learn the local features which provide evidence for discriminating between the normal and abnormal cases. We interpret evidence region pinpointing as a sparse descriptor learning problem [1,2] in which the optimal feature descriptors are selected from a large candidate pool with various locations and sizes. Because of its large scale, the problem is formulated in a stochastic learning manner and the Regularised Dual Averaging algorithm [3,4] is used for the optimisation.

The evidence pinpointing task is reminiscent of the multiple-instance problem as described in [5] in which instances or features responsible for the classification are identified. Here, the learnt descriptors have several advantages over conventional hand-crafted representations, such as shape and appearance models, and local features, e.g., histogram of oriented gradient (HOG) [6] and local binary patterns [7]: (1) The training is weakly-supervised requiring no annotation of key features; (2) The learnt descriptors are more discriminative and informative, and therefore can contribute to better localisation and classification performance; (3) The evidence regions supporting the classification are automatically pinpointed which may be used by clinicians to determine the aetiology.

It is worth noting that the Convolutional Neural Network (CNN) architecture [8–11] learns discriminative features from pathological labels with weak supervision as well, but requires large number of training samples and sufficient training. Instead of learning from raw image pixels, we formulate it as salient feature learning from a higher-level description of the image, which circumvents any need for the low-level feature training. As a result the optimisation is straightforward, consuming much less computing resource, and requiring no massive training data and no parameter tuning. Moreover, our descriptor learning method differs from the recent CNN based evidence pinpointing techniques [12,13] in that we not only localise the evidence regions but at the same time give the description of these regions at optimal feature scales.

We apply our method to lumbar spinal stenosis for localising the vertebrae in axial images and predicting the pathological labels. Two conditions are evaluated, namely central canal stenosis and foraminal stenosis. Descriptors are learnt to classify each condition respectively. The dataset for validation consists of three weakly annotated subsets of 600 L3/4, L4/5, L5/S1 axial images with classification labels, and three densely annotated subsets of 192, 198, 192 images with labels and dense landmarks. We show that compared with supervised methods trained with labels and landmarks, our descriptor learning method gives competitive performance trained on the same subsets with labels only. With further training on the weakly annotated subset, a significant improvement is obtained which validates the learning ability of our method with weak-supervision.

2   Methodology

An anatomy can be localised by certain salient local structures distinctive from the background. Also, a pathological condition in an anatomy is often shown

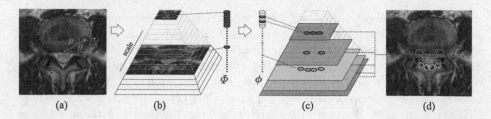

Fig. 1. (a) Region candidate on an image. (b) Region candidates on an image pyramid having multiple region sizes and feature scales. (c) For a certain task, the salient regions are selected by sparse learning. (d) The learnt descriptors.

as changes in intensity or structure in local regions. Learning to identify and describe these discriminative regions accordingly can therefore capture the key information for localisation and classification tasks. We next detail the formulation and optimisation of discriminative region learning.

2.1 Formulation

Assume we have a set of training images classified into a subset $\mathcal{N}$ with negative labels and a subset $\mathcal{P}$ with positive labels. For example, for classification tasks $\mathcal{N}$ and $\mathcal{P}$ consist of normal and pathological images. For localisation tasks, $\mathcal{N}$ refers to the images with the anatomies aligned, and $\mathcal{P}$ the misaligned images.

To learn the local regions and features that lead to the classification, we generate a pool of region candidates having various locations and sizes, and select the most discriminative ones. Specifically, to generate the location candidates, each region is represented by a Gaussian weighted window $g(\rho, \theta, \sigma)$ with ρ and θ being the polar coordinate of the window on the image, and σ the size of the window, see Fig. 1(a). Parameters $\{\rho, \theta\}$ are sampled over the ranges $\rho = [0, \rho_1]$, $\theta = [0, 2\pi]$ such that the regions cover the whole image. To include multiple sizes of local features in the candidate pool, we build an image pyramid with the lower resolution images containing larger scale textures. The region candidates are sampled from each layer with the same size in pixels, which results in larger effective region sizes and feature scales on lower resolution images, see Fig. 1(b).

To represent each region, instead of using raw image features, we decompose the local textures into complementary frequency components for a compact description. This is achieved by designing window functions to partition the spec-

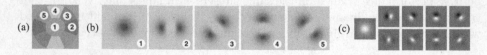

Fig. 2. (a) Spectrum partition. (b) Filter windows in the Fourier domain. (c) Filters in the spatial domain corresponding to intensity, gradient and curvature features respectively.

trum, see Fig. 2(a). The specific form of the windows are shown in Fig. 2(b). The low-pass window is a Gaussian function, and the oriented windows are logarithmic functions along radius in four directions. Each of the 4 oriented windows in Fig. 2(b) corresponds to 2 spatial-domain filters (real and imaginary part separately) and together with the low-pass filter, we obtain 9 filters, see Fig. 2(c). Note that the filters correspond to the intensity, first and second order derivative features respectively. The filters are similar to Haar and discrete wavelet filters but with enhanced smoothness and complementary properties. We calculate the response map of the image to each filter, and accumulate over the i-th region to obtain the region descriptor $\Phi_i \in \mathbb{R}^{1 \times 9}$. The region descriptors from different locations and pyramid levels form a candidate pool $\Phi = \{\Phi_i\}_{i=1}^N \in \mathbb{R}^{N \times 9}$, where N is the total number of the region candidates. Φ gives a redundant (overcomplete) description of the image, see Fig. 1(b).

The task then is to select from the candidate pool Φ a few regions containing the discriminative information, which we formulate as a sparse learning problem. The selection can be described by the operation,

$$\phi = W^{\frac{1}{2}}\Phi. \tag{1}$$

$W \in \mathbb{R}^{N \times N}$ is a diagonal matrix with sparse entries $\boldsymbol{w} = [w_1, w_2, \ldots, w_N]$, in which w_i is the assigned weight of the i-th region Φ_i, and the non-zeros weights corresponding to the regions selected. ϕ represents the selected salient features (Fig. 1(c)).

The objective is to learn $\boldsymbol{w}$ such that the selected descriptors ϕ are consistent within class and discriminative between classes. Let $\phi(p), p \in \mathcal{P}$ and $\phi(n), n \in \mathcal{N}$ be the descriptors of two random examples from the positive and negative image set respectively. The distances between the descriptors can be calculated by,

$$\|\phi(p) - \phi(n)\|_2^2 = \sum_{i=1}^N \|\sqrt{w_i}\Phi_i(p) - \sqrt{w_i}\Phi_i(n)\|^2 = \sum_{i=1}^N w_i\|\Phi_i(p) - \Phi_i(n)\|^2 = \boldsymbol{w}^T \boldsymbol{d}(p,n), \tag{2}$$

where $\boldsymbol{d}(p,n) \in \mathbb{R}^{N \times 1}$ is a vector with each entry $d_i(p,n)$ being the feature difference calculated at a region, i.e., $d_i(p,n) = \|\Phi_i(p) - \Phi_i(n)\|^2$.

Similarly we randomly sample two examples $n_1, n_2 \in \mathcal{N}$ from the negative set and calculate the distance denoted by $\boldsymbol{d}(n_1, n_2)$. To penalise the differences within the negative set and reward the distances between the positive and negative sets, we set a margin-based constraint,

$$\boldsymbol{w}^T \boldsymbol{d}(n_1, n_2) + 1 < \boldsymbol{w}^T \boldsymbol{d}(p,n). \tag{3}$$

We do not penalise the differences within the positive set as it represents the misaligned or pathological images with large variations, see Fig. 3(a).

The objective function enforcing the constraint may be composed in a sparse learning form,

$$\underset{w \geqslant 0}{\arg\min} \sum_{p \in \mathcal{P}; n, n_1, n_2 \in \mathcal{N}} \mathcal{L}(\boldsymbol{w}^T \boldsymbol{d}(n_1, n_2) - \boldsymbol{w}^T \boldsymbol{d}(p,n)) + \mu\|\boldsymbol{w}\|_1, \tag{4}$$

where $\mathcal{L}(z) = \max\{z + 1, 0\}$ is a loss function penalising the non-discriminative entries, and the $\ell 1$-norm $\|\boldsymbol{w}\|_1$ is a sparsity-inducing regulariser which encourages the entries of $\boldsymbol{w}$ to be zero, thus performs region selection. Note that each

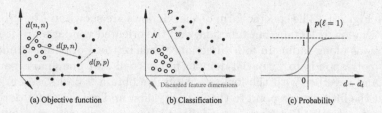

(a) Objective function   (b) Classification   (c) Probability

Fig. 3. (a) The objective function of sparse descriptor learning. (b) The zero entries in the learnt w remove the non-salient feature dimensions (region candidates), the non-zero entries define the hyperplane for classification in the salient feature space. (c) The sigmoid probability function.

n in the function represent an independent random index from the negative set, and p from the positive set. The number of the summands is not fixed, which fits with the stochastic learning and online optimisation procedure, i.e., repetitively drawing random samples $d(n_1, n_2)$, $d(p, n)$ and optimising w until a criterion is met. The random sampling also enables incremental learning which means we can refine the model without re-learning it all over again when new training data become available. We deduce the solution to (4) in the next section.

2.2 Optimisation

Finding the sparse parameter w in (4) is a regularised stochastic learning problem where the objective function is the sum of two convex terms: one is the loss function of the learning task fed recursively by random examples, and the other is a $\ell1$-norm regularisation term for promoting sparsity. It can be solved efficiently by the Regularised Dual Averaging (RDA) algorithm [3,4], which recursively learns and updates w with new examples.

At the t-th iteration, RDA takes in a new observation, which in our case are random pairs $d(p, n)$ and $d(n_1, n_2)$. The loss subgradient g_t is calculated by,

$$g_t = \frac{\partial \mathcal{L}\left(w^T\left(d(n_1, n_2) - d(p, n)\right)\right)}{\partial w} \tag{5}$$

$$= \begin{cases} d(n_1, n_2) - d(p, n), & w^T\left(d(n_1, n_2) - d(p, n)\right) > -1 \\ 0, & otherwise. \end{cases}$$

g_t is used to update the average subgradient, $\bar{g}_t = \frac{1}{t}\sum_{i=1}^{t} g_i$. Updating the parameter w with RDA takes the form,

$$w_{t+1} = \arg\min_{w}(w^T \bar{g}_t + u||w||_1 + \frac{\beta_t}{t} h(w)) \tag{6}$$

in which the last term is an additional strong convex regularisation term. One can set $h(w) = \frac{1}{2}||w||_2^2 = \frac{1}{2}w^T w$, $\beta_t = \gamma\sqrt{t}, \gamma > 0$ for a convergence rate of

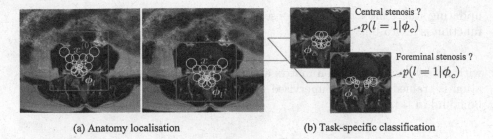

(a) Anatomy localisation   (b) Task-specific classification

Fig. 4. Applying the learnt descriptors for localisation and classification.

$O(1/\sqrt{t})$. By writing $\boldsymbol{u}$ as a N dimension vector with each elements being u, equation (6) becomes,

$$\boldsymbol{w}_{t+1} = \arg\min_{\boldsymbol{w}}(\boldsymbol{w}^T\bar{\boldsymbol{g}}_t + \boldsymbol{w}^T\boldsymbol{u} + \frac{\gamma}{2\sqrt{t}}\boldsymbol{w}^T\boldsymbol{w}), \tag{7}$$

which can be solved by Least Squares method to give,

$$\boldsymbol{w}_{t+1} = -\frac{\sqrt{t}}{r}(\bar{\boldsymbol{g}}_t + \boldsymbol{u}). \tag{8}$$

The discriminative regions and optimal descriptors are obtained by keeping only the candidates with non-zero weights indicated by the learnt $\boldsymbol{w}$. An example is given in Fig. 1(d).

2.3   Localisation and Classification

Denoting $\boldsymbol{\phi}_l$ as the learnt optimal descriptor for localising anatomy, and $\boldsymbol{\phi}_c$ the descriptor for a certain classification task, we show how the optimal descriptors are applied (Fig. 4).

Localisation. The anatomy is described discriminatively by $\boldsymbol{\phi}_l$ which represents the salient structures. Localising the anatomy in the image is conducted by searching for these structures. Given an initial estimation $\boldsymbol{x}^{(0)}$ of the location, which can be set at the centre of the image, the descriptor at the initial location $\boldsymbol{\phi}_l(\boldsymbol{x}^{(0)})$ is observed to deduce the true location $\boldsymbol{x}^*$. The deduction can be expressed as solving the regression $\boldsymbol{\phi}_l(\boldsymbol{x}^{(0)}) \mapsto \boldsymbol{x}^*$. The direct mapping function is non-linear in nature and training such function comes up against the overfitting problem. In practice the mapping can be decomposed into a sequence of linear mapping and updating steps,

$$\begin{cases} \text{Mapping:} & \boldsymbol{\phi}_l(\boldsymbol{x}^{(k)}) \mapsto \Delta\boldsymbol{x}^{(k)}, \\ \text{Updating:} & \boldsymbol{x}^{(k+1)} = \boldsymbol{x}^{(k)} + \Delta\boldsymbol{x}^{(k)}, \end{cases} \tag{9}$$

where in the mapping stage, a prediction for the correction of the location is made, based on the observation $\boldsymbol{\phi}_l(\boldsymbol{x}^{(k)})$ at the current location $\boldsymbol{x}^{(k)}$; and in the updating stage, the location and observation is updated. The learning mapping function is set to be,

$$\Delta x^{(k)} = R^{(k)} \phi_l(x^{(k)}) + b^{(k)},\qquad(10)$$

with $R^{(k)}$ being a projection matrix and $b^{(k)}$ the bias. $\{R^{(k)}, b^{(k)}\}$ in each iteration is trained with the Supervised Descent Method, the details of which can be found in [14].

Classification. Learning w in the objective function (4) can be viewed as a simultaneous feature selection and classification process. The zero entries in w correspond to the non-salient features (or region candidates) to be discarded. In fact, the non-zero entries in w form a vector defining the hyperplane classifying the positive and negative samples in the salient feature space, which is similar to a support vector in Support Vector Machine classifier, see Fig. 3(b).

For a specific pathological condition, the learnt descriptor ϕ_c covers the regions where the abnormalities are most likely to appear, and preserves their discriminative features for classification. To predict the class label ℓ of a test image, we extract the descriptor $\phi_c(x^*)$ at the detected location x^* and calculate the average distance to the normal descriptors,

$$d = \frac{1}{|\mathcal{N}|} \sum_{n \in \mathcal{N}} ||\phi_c(x^*) - \phi_c(n)||_2^2,\qquad(11)$$

where n indexes all the cases in the normal set $\mathcal{N}$.

A larger d indicates a greater probability of the case being abnormal. More formally, the probability of the case being abnormal is modelled by a sigmoid function (Fig. 3(c)),

$$p(\ell = 1|\phi_c(x^*)) = \frac{1}{1 + e^{-(d-d_t)}},\qquad(12)$$

where d_t is a threshold distance. The cases with $p > 0.5$ are classified as abnormal, with confidence p. Conversely, the cases with $p < 0.5$ are classified as normal with the confidence $(1 - p)$.

3   Experiments

3.1   Clinical Background

Lumbar spinal stenosis (LSS) is a common disorder of the spine. The disorder can be observed in radiological studies as morphological abnormalities. Intervertebral disc-level axial images in MRI scans can provide rich information revealing the condition of important anatomies such as the disc, central canal, neural foramen and facet. In most cases the original axial scans are not aligned to the disc planes caused by the curvature of the spine. To obtain the precise intervertebral views, we localise the disc planes in the paired sagittal scans (red line in Fig. 5), and

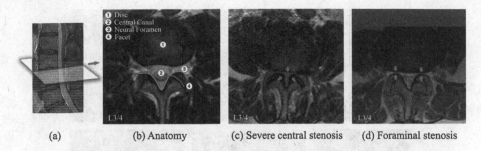

Fig. 5. (a) Mid-sagittal view of a lumbar spine. Grey dashed lines show the raw axial scans. Red lines show the aligned disc-level planes, from which the axial images are extracted. (b) Anatomy of a L3/4 disc-level axial image. (c) A case with severe central stenosis. (d) A case with foraminal stenosis (Color figure online)

map the geometry to the axial scans to calculate the coordinates, where the voxels are sampled to extract the aligned images. On a disc-level image shown in Fig. 5(b), conditions of the posterior disc margins (red line) and the posterior spinal canal (cyan line) are typically inspected for the diagnosis. Degeneration of these structures can constrict the spinal canal (pink area) and the neural foramen (yellow area) causing central and foraminal stenosis.

Data. The data collected from routine clinics consists of T2-weighted MRI scans of 600 patients with varied LSS symptoms. Each patient has paired sagittal-axial scans. The L3/4, L4/5, L5/S1 intervertebral planes are localised in the sagittal scans and the images sampled from the axial scans. We obtain three sets of 600 disc-level axial images for the three intervertebral planes respectively. The images are resampled to have an pixel space of 0.5 mm. All cases are inspected and annotated with classification labels with respect to the central stenosis and foraminal narrowing. In addition, the dense annotations are available for the first 192, 198, 192 images in the three subsets, in which each image is delineated with 37 landmarks outlining the disc, central canal and facet, see Fig. 7(a). In summary the dataset for validation contains three sets of 600 data with classification labels and three subsets of 192, 198, 192 data with dense annotations, which are referred to as weakly and densely annotated datasets respectively.

3.2   Results

Validation Protocols. In each of the three intervertebral subsets we randomly select 100 densely annotated images as the test set, and the remaining densely annotated images as the training set. The additional images with only classification labels are used for further training the weakly supervised methods. The selection of training and test sets is repeated for an unbiased validation. The training sets is used for learning descriptors for both localisation and task-specific classifications. In the testing stage, the localisation and classification tasks are carried out by each method independently, and the performance is evaluated.

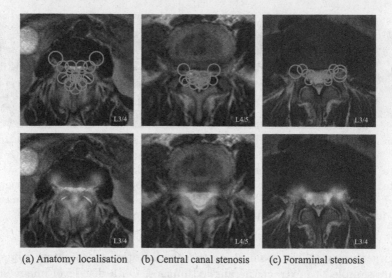

(a) Anatomy localisation   (b) Central canal stenosis   (c) Foraminal stenosis

Fig. 6. The discriminative descriptors (top) and evidence regions (bottom) learnt for the task of (a) anatomy localisation (b) central stenosis classification and (c) foraminal stenosis classification.

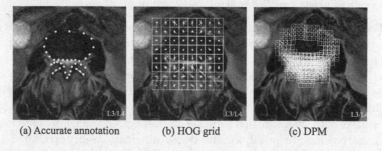

(a) Accurate annotation   (b) HOG grid   (c) DPM

Fig. 7. Comparative descriptors: landmarks, HOG-grid and DPM.

Anatomy Localisation. The learning result of the optimal descriptor for local-ising the vertebrae, L3/4 as an example, is shown in Fig. 6(a). The hot maps of salient regions are visualised by showing the selected region candidates as Gaussian blobs. It is interesting to compare these with the biological anatomy in Fig. 5(b) and the annotations by the clinician in Fig. 7(a). The learnt descriptor highlights the posterior margin of the disc and the posterior arch, which have sharp textures and high contrast. Note that compared with a clinician's annota-tions, the front edge of the disc is not selected. The reason for this may be there being less consistency across images because of the variation in disc size, as well as the ambiguous boundaries to the abdominal structures in some of the cases.

We compare our method with HOG grid [6] and Deformable Part Models (DPM) [7,15]. The HOG grid is a hand-crafted descriptor covering the holistic appearance, see Fig. 7(b). It assumes no prior clinical knowledge and assigns equal weights to the local features of the anatomy. The DPM is a strongly

Table 1. Precision of anatomy localisation in mm ([+] Require landmarks. [*] Trained on additional weakly annotated data).

Data	Initial	HOG grid[*]	DPM[+]	Learnt	Learnt[*]
L3/4	16.41 ± 10.10	2.45 ± 1.69	2.01 ± 1.62	1.95 ± 1.58	$\mathbf{1.22 \pm 1.01}$
L4/5	16.59 ± 10.80	2.37 ± 1.55	1.73 ± 1.30	1.76 ± 1.26	$\mathbf{1.57 \pm 1.36}$
L5/S1	12.86 ± 8.29	2.52 ± 1.71	1.85 ± 1.42	2.09 ± 1.52	$\mathbf{1.24 \pm 0.96}$

supervised method which describes the anatomy by local patches at each of the landmarks as well as the geometry of the landmark locations (Fig. 7(c)). Each patch is described by a SIFT descriptor. In all the methods the initial location is set at the centre of the images and the searching is driven by the SDM algorithm [14]. The experimental results are reported in Table 1. The initial distances to the true locations are also given. We can see that our learnt descriptors give comparable localisation precision with DPM when trained on the same densely annotated subsets, but use no landmark annotation. With further training on additional data, a significant improvement is observed indicating the learning ability of our method on weakly annotated data.

Pathology Classification. The classification follows on from the anatomy localisation step. The learnt discriminative descriptors and evidence regions for the classification of central canal stenosis and foramen stenosis are shown in Fig. 6(b), (c) respectively. We can see that the descriptor learnt on central stenosis labels highlights the spinal canal area. When learnt on foraminal stenosis labels, it pinpoints the neural foramen as the evidence regions. These evidence regions pinpointed automatically by our methods (Fig. 6(b), (c)) show high agreement with the medical definition of the pathologies shown in Fig. 5(c), (d).

The learnt descriptors are extracted at the detected location for classification on test images. The predicted pathological labels as well as the confidences of prediction are given by (12). For comparison, in the HOG grid method, the descriptors are centred at the detected location. In the DPM method, two forms of descriptions are considered, i.e., the geometry represented by the landmarks, and the SIFT descriptors extracted from the aligned landmarks, which are denoted by DPM (Geo) and DPM (SIFT) respectively. The classifiers for the methods compared are trained with the AdaBoost, with decision trees as the weak learners. The performance is evaluated by the agreement with labelling done by a clinician, calculated by $(pp + nn)/M$, in which pp and nn are the number of agreed positive and agreed negative cases, and M is the total number of cases.

The results of the two classification tasks are shown in Table 2. Our descriptor learning method gives better or competitive classification accuracies compared with supervised methods, trained on the same densely annotated subset but requires no landmarks to be identified. A significant improvement is again seen with additional training on weakly annotated data. Note that the performance is

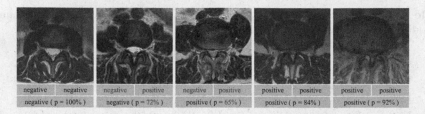

Fig. 8. Example images with different degrees of degeneration. First row: the repeated labels for central stenosis by the same clinician, made at different times. Disagreement is shown in blue. Second row: the labels and probabilities by our classification method. (Color figure online)

Table 2. Agreement (%) of classification. ($^+$ Require landmarks. * Trained on additional weakly annotated data.)

	Human	HOG grid	DPM(Geo)$^+$	DPM(SIFT)$^+$	Learnt	Learnt*
Central canal stenosis						
L3/4	88.5	80.6 ± 4.9	79.5 ± 4.5	81.0 ± 4.9	85.7 ± 3.5	$\mathbf{87.2 \pm 3.2}$
L4/5	87.4	81.3 ± 4.6	78.3 ± 4.1	82.4 ± 4.5	84.2 ± 3.4	$\mathbf{85.1 \pm 3.4}$
L5/S1	89.2	81.8 ± 4.7	81.4 ± 4.5	82.7 ± 4.4	86.0 ± 3.7	$\mathbf{87.5 \pm 3.3}$
Foraminal stenosis						
L3/4	86.5	79.6 ± 4.5	81.2 ± 4.8	83.1 ± 4.7	82.9 ± 4.5	$\mathbf{84.3 \pm 3.9}$
L4/5	87.2	81.5 ± 4.9	82.4 ± 4.6	83.3 ± 4.3	82.5 ± 4.5	$\mathbf{84.0 \pm 4.0}$
L5/S1	89.5	81.7 ± 4.4	81.8 ± 4.7	82.9 ± 4.5	84.1 ± 3.8	$\mathbf{87.1 \pm 3.4}$

affected by the precision of the human labels, as the clinician can only achieve a certain level of agreement between themselves when the labelling step is repeated on same dataset. We report the self-agreement of a clinician in Table 2, denoted as the human performance. The disagreement is generally caused by ambiguous conditions in many cases. We give several example images with different degrees of degenerations, and show the classification labels by the clinician as well as the labels and probabilities by our method in Fig. 8. The probability indicates the confidence of our prediction, which may be helpful for being aware of and understanding errors in the classification results.

4   Conclusions

We propose a method for learning the optimal descriptors for anatomy localisation and classification. The learnt descriptors for localising an anatomy highlights consistent and salient structures across a set of images. The descriptors for classifying a specific condition, learnt with no prior knowledge but the labels, pinpoint the evidence regions where the abnormalities are most likely to appear. The information in the descriptors is highly discriminative leading to more accurate classification results. The training is straightforward with no need of parameter tuning. We have shown that promising results can be achieved when learnt on 600 labelled images. The average training time for one task is about 27 min in MATLAB on a 3.20 GHz GPU with 16 GB RAM. The method can be readily applied to other clinical tasks for rapidly pinpointing and describing evidence of abnormalities directly from expertly labelled data. Further work includes extending the method to 3D where the increased scale might be handled by random candidate sampling. The MATLAB toolbox of the methods described here will be made public available for research purposes.

References

1. Simonyan, K., Vedaldi, A., Zisserman, A.: Descriptor learning using convex optimisation. In: Fitzgibbon, A., Lazebnik, S., Perona, P., Sato, Y., Schmid, C. (eds.) ECCV 2012. LNCS, vol. 7572, pp. 243–256. Springer, Heidelberg (2012). doi:10.1007/978-3-642-33718-5_18
2. Simonyan, K., Vedaldi, A., Zisserman, A.: Learning local feature descriptors using convex optimisation. IEEE Trans. PAMI **36**(8), 1573–1585 (2014)
3. Xiao, L.: Dual averaging method for regularized stochastic learning and online optimization. In: Advances in Neural Information Processing Systems, pp. 2116–2124. Curran Associates, Inc. (2009)
4. Xiao, L.: Dual averaging methods for regularized stochastic learning and online optimization. J. Mach. Learn. Res. **11**(Oct), 2543–2596 (2010)
5. Chen, Y., Bi, J., Wang, J.Z.: MILES: multiple-instance learning via embedded instance selection. IEEE Trans. PAMI **28**(12), 1931–1947 (2006)
6. Lootus, M., Kadir, T., Zisserman, A.: Vertebrae detection and labelling in lumbar MR images. In: Yao, J., Klinder, T., Li, S. (eds.) Computational Methods and Clinical Applications for Spine Imaging. LNCVB, vol. 17, pp. 219–230. Springer, Cham (2014). doi:10.1007/978-3-319-07269-2_19
7. Zhao, Q., Okada, K., Rosenbaum, K., Kehoe, L., Zand, D.J., Sze, R., Summar, M., Linguraru, M.G.: Digital facial dysmorphology for genetic screening: hierarchical constrained local model using ICA. Med. Image Anal. **18**(5), 699–710 (2014)
8. Shen, W., Zhou, M., Yang, F., Yang, C., Tian, J.: Multi-scale convolutional neural networks for lung nodule classification. In: Ourselin, S., Alexander, D.C., Westin, C.-F., Cardoso, M.J. (eds.) IPMI 2015. LNCS, vol. 9123, pp. 588–599. Springer, Cham (2015). doi:10.1007/978-3-319-19992-4_46
9. Shin, H.C., Roth, H.R., Gao, M., Lu, L., Xu, Z., Nogues, I., Yao, J., Mollura, D., Summers, R.M.: Deep convolutional neural networks for computer-aided detection: CNN architectures, dataset characteristics and transfer learning. IEEE Trans. Med. Imaging **35**(5), 1285–1298 (2016)
10. Schlegl, T., Waldstein, S.M., Vogl, W.-D., Schmidt-Erfurth, U., Langs, G.: Predicting semantic descriptions from medical images with convolutional neural networks. In: Ourselin, S., Alexander, D.C., Westin, C.-F., Cardoso, M.J. (eds.) IPMI 2015. LNCS, vol. 9123, pp. 437–448. Springer, Cham (2015). doi:10.1007/978-3-319-19992-4_34
11. Mahapatra, D., Roy, P.K., Sedai, S., Garnavi, R.: Retinal image quality classification using saliency maps and CNNs. In: Wang, L., Adeli, E., Wang, Q., Shi, Y., Suk, H.-I. (eds.) MLMI 2016. LNCS, vol. 10019, pp. 172–179. Springer, Cham (2016). doi:10.1007/978-3-319-47157-0_21

12. Oquab, M., Bottou, L., Laptev, I., Sivic, J.: Is object localization for free? Weakly supervised learning with convolutional neural networks. In: Proceedings of the IEEE Conference on CVPR, pp. 685–694 (2015)
13. Jamaludin, A., Kadir, T., Zisserman, A.: SpineNet: automatically pinpointing classification evidence in spinal MRIs. In: Ourselin, S., Joskowicz, L., Sabuncu, M.R., Unal, G., Wells, W. (eds.) MICCAI 2016. LNCS, vol. 9901, pp. 166–175. Springer, Cham (2016). doi:10.1007/978-3-319-46723-8_20
14. Xiong, X., Torre, F.: Supervised descent method and its applications to face alignment. In: Proceedings of the IEEE Conference on CVPR, pp. 532–539 (2013)
15. Felzenszwalb, P.F., Girshick, R.B., McAllester, D., Ramanan, D.: Object detection with discriminatively trained part-based models. IEEE Trans. PAMI **32**(9), 1627–1645 (2010)

Quantifying the Uncertainty in Model Parameters Using Gaussian Process-Based Markov Chain Monte Carlo: An Application to Cardiac Electrophysiological Models

Jwala Dhamala[1]([✉]), John L. Sapp[2], Milan Horacek[2], and Linwei Wang[1]

[1] Rochester Institute of Technology, Rochester, NY 14623, USA
jd1336@rit.edu
[2] Dalhousie University, Halifax, Canada

Abstract. Estimation of patient-specific model parameters is important for personalized modeling, although sparse and noisy clinical data can introduce significant uncertainty in the estimated parameter values. This importance source of uncertainty, if left unquantified, will lead to unknown variability in model outputs that hinder their reliable adoptions. Probabilistic estimation model parameters, however, remains an unresolved challenge because standard Markov Chain Monte Carlo sampling requires repeated model simulations that are computationally infeasible. A common solution is to replace the simulation model with a computationally-efficient surrogate for a faster sampling. However, by sampling from an approximation of the exact posterior probability density function (pdf) of the parameters, the efficiency is gained at the expense of sampling accuracy. In this paper, we address this issue by integrating surrogate modeling into Metropolis Hasting (MH) sampling of the exact posterior pdfs to improve its acceptance rate. It is done by first quickly constructing a Gaussian process (GP) surrogate of the exact posterior pdfs using deterministic optimization. This efficient surrogate is then used to modify commonly-used proposal distributions in MH sampling such that only proposals accepted by the surrogate will be tested by the exact posterior pdf for acceptance/rejection, reducing unnecessary model simulations at unlikely candidates. Synthetic and real-data experiments using the presented method show a significant gain in computational efficiency without compromising the accuracy. In addition, insights into the non-identifiability and heterogeneity of tissue properties can be gained from the obtained posterior distributions.

Keywords: Probabilistic parameter estimation · Personalized modeling · Markov chain Monte Carlo · Gaussian process

1 Introduction

Patient-specific models are showing increasing promise in personalized medicine [12]. While advancement in medical imaging has made personalized geometrical models a reality, the challenge of obtaining patient-specific tissue properties in

© Springer International Publishing AG 2017
M. Niethammer et al. (Eds.): IPMI 2017, LNCS 10265, pp. 223–235, 2017.
DOI: 10.1007/978-3-319-59050-9_18

the form of model parameters remains unresolved. These model parameters often cannot be directly measured, but have to be inferred from clinical data that are sparse and noisy.

Most existing works on parameter estimation use deterministic methods to find an *optimal* value of the model parameter so that model outputs best fit the measurement data [4,12,15]. However, significant uncertainty can exist in the estimated parameter values due to the uncertainty in available data. This important source of uncertainty will result in unknown variability in model outputs that, if left unquantified, will hinder their reliable adoptions. Additionally, over-parameterization and coupling between parameters may result in many parameter configurations that fit the data equally well. This issue of identifiability cannot be observed when only an *optimal* solution is being sought.

A probabilistic estimation of model parameters can address the above challenges by obtaining the posterior probability density (pdf) of the parameters conditioned on the data [5,6,11]. However, limited progress has been made in this direction because the posterior pdf comprises of a complex simulation model that are analytically intractable and computationally expensive. While Markov Chain Monte Carlo (MCMC) methods are natural choices for drawing samples from an analytically-intractable pdf, they become prohibitive in this context because the evaluation of each sample involves a model simulation that could take hours or even days for a single run. To address this critical challenge, an effective approach is to construct an efficient surrogate for the compute-intensive simulation model using methods such as polynomial chaos [5] and kriging [11]. These surrogate models can then replace the original model in the posterior pdf for substantially faster sampling [5,11]. However, this approach has two major limitations. First, the sampling is carried out on an approximated rather than the exact posterior pdf. Thus the efficiency is gained at the expense of sampling accuracy. Second, the surrogate is built to be accurate in important regions of the simulation model [5,11]. Thus the approximation accuracy can be limited in important regions of the posterior pdf, such as those of high probability.

We propose to overcome these issues by integrating surrogate modeling of the posterior pdf into the classic form of MCMC sampling to improve its acceptance rate. A similar idea was reported in [6], where a Gaussian process (GP) surrogate of the posterior pdf was constructed using hybrid Monte Carlo (HMC), the gradient of which was then used to find better proposals when sampling the exact posterior pdf. However, to construct the GP surrogate by random exploration of the sampling space, the number of model simulations needed increases exponentially with the number of unknown parameters. In addition, although the gradient of the GP surrogate allows a smarter exploration of the sampling space during HMC, the simulation model still needs to be probed at each proposed sample whereas a large portion of such heavy computation is spent at rejecting unwanted proposals. Important challenges remain in order to further reduce the number of model simulations needed in this type of approaches.

In this paper, we address these challenges from both the end of surrogate modeling and MCMC sampling. First, rather than a random exploration, we quickly construct a GP surrogate of the posterior pdf by deterministic optimiza-tion favoring high accuracy in regions of high posterior probability. Second, we modify common proposal distributions in Metropolis Hastings (MH) sampling by first testing the acceptance of each proposal on the far-cheaper-to-evaluate GP surrogate, quickly rejecting a large number of proposals and allowing only those accepted by the surrogate to be tested by the exact pdf. Compared to directly sampling from an approximated pdf [5,11], the presented method ensures a high accuracy by generating the final samples from the exact distribution. Compared to directly sampling the exact pdf, the presented method reduces computation by avoiding expensive model simulations at unlikely proposals.

We evaluate the presented method on estimating tissue excitability of a cardiac electrophysiological model using non-invasive electrocardiogram (ECG) data. In synthetic experiments, we first evaluate the sampling accuracy and computational cost of the presented method against directly sampling the exact posterior pdf. Using the exact posterior pdf as a baseline, we then compare the accuracy of the presented method to an approach that, similar to existing work [11], samples only the surrogate posterior pdf. Finally, in both synthetic and real-data studies, we analyze the uncertainty, identifiability, and heterogeneity of tissue excitability using its posterior pdfs personalized from ECG data.

2   Cardiac Electrophysiological System

Whole-Heart Electrophysiology Model: Simplified electrophysiological models are popular candidates for parameter estimation in personalized model-ing [12]. They can reproduce the general shape of action potential with a small number of parameters and reasonable computation. As a preliminary demon-stration of the presented method, we consider the two-variable *Aliev-Panfilov* (AP) model [2]:

$$\partial u/\partial t = \partial/\partial x_i d_{ij} \partial u/\partial x_j - ku(u-a)(u-1) - uv,$$
$$\partial v/\partial t = \varepsilon(u,v)(-v - ku(u-a-1)), \tag{1}$$

where u is the action potential and v is the recovery current. Parameter d_{ij} is the conductivity, parameter ε controls the coupling between the recovery current and action potential, k controls the repolarization, and a controls the excitability of the myocyte. As a proof of concept, in this study we consider quantifying the uncertainty of parameter a because it is closely associated with the ischemic severity of the myocardial tissue and model output u is sensitive to its value.

The meshfree method as described in [14] is used to discretize and solve the AP model on the 3D myocardium. The direct estimation of parameter a at the resolution of the cardiac mesh is impossible due to non-identifiability and heavy computation. Instead, we consider the estimation of parameter a at a reduced dimension. Any appropriate dimension reduction method can be used. Here, we use a recently reported method that automatically groups spatial nodes of the cardiac mesh into 5–17 regions that are at various resolutions and that are most homogeneous in tissue properties [4].

Measurement Model: Spatio-temporal cardiac action potential produces time-varying ECG signals on the body surface. This relationship can be described by the quasi-static approximation of the electromagnetic theory [7]. Solving the governing equations on a discrete mesh of heart and torso [14], a linear model between ECG data $\mathbf{Y}$ and action potential $\mathbf{U}$ can be obtained as: $\mathbf{Y} = \mathbf{H}\mathbf{U}(\boldsymbol{\theta})$. Here, $\mathbf{H}$ is the transfer matrix unique to each heart and torso geometry, and $\boldsymbol{\theta}$ is the vector of spatially-varying local parameters a at a reduced dimension.

3   Probabilistic Parameter Estimation

The relationship between parameter $\boldsymbol{\theta}$ and ECG data $\mathbf{Y}$ can be expressed as:

$$\mathbf{Y} = F(\boldsymbol{\theta}) + \boldsymbol{\epsilon} \tag{2}$$

where F consists of the whole-heart electrophysiological model and the measurement model as described in Sect. 2. $\boldsymbol{\epsilon}$ accounts for discrepancy between model outputs and measurement data. Using Bayes' theorem, the unnormalized posterior density of the model parameter $\boldsymbol{\theta}$ can be obtained as:

$$\pi(\boldsymbol{\theta}|\mathbf{Y}) \propto \pi(\mathbf{Y}|\boldsymbol{\theta})\pi(\boldsymbol{\theta}) \tag{3}$$

Assuming noise $\boldsymbol{\epsilon}$ to follow a zero mean Gaussian distribution with a diagonal covariance $\boldsymbol{\Sigma}_e = \sigma_e^2\mathbf{I}$, the likelihood $\pi(\mathbf{Y}|\boldsymbol{\theta})$ can be formulated as:

$$\pi(\mathbf{Y}|\boldsymbol{\theta}) \propto \exp(-1/2\sigma_e^2||\mathbf{Y} - F(\boldsymbol{\theta})||^2) \tag{4}$$

The prior distribution $\pi(\boldsymbol{\theta})$ quantifies prior knowledge over the parameter. Here we use a uniform distribution in bounded space $[0, 0.52]$ to include the minimal physiological knowledge about the range of values for this parameter: $a \sim 0.15$ represents normal excitability, while increased value represents increased loss of excitability until $a \sim 0.5$ represents necrotic tissue.

MCMC sampling of the posterior pdf in Eq. (3) is infeasible because the evaluation of each sample requires an expensive model simulation. Below we describe the presented method that accelerates MCMC sampling of (3) via the use of an efficient GP surrogate in the modification of proposal distributions.

GP Surrogate of Posterior Functions: GP is a popular method to model a function that lacks an explicit form or is difficult to evaluate. such as a deep learning model, an experiment to be designed, and a multiscale simulation model [9]. Here, we use it to approximate the exact posterior pdf in Eq. (3).

To initialize, we take a GP with a zero mean function and an anisotropic "Mátern 5/2" co-variance function [9]:

$$\kappa(\boldsymbol{\theta}_1, \boldsymbol{\theta}_2) = \alpha^2\{1 + \sqrt{5d^2(\boldsymbol{\theta}_1, \boldsymbol{\theta}_2)} + 5/3d^2(\boldsymbol{\theta}_1, \boldsymbol{\theta}_2)\exp(-\sqrt{5d^2(\boldsymbol{\theta}_1, \boldsymbol{\theta}_2)}\} \tag{5}$$

where $d^2(\boldsymbol{\theta}_1, \boldsymbol{\theta}_2) = (\boldsymbol{\theta}_1 - \boldsymbol{\theta}_2)^\mathsf{T}\boldsymbol{\Lambda}(\boldsymbol{\theta}_1 - \boldsymbol{\theta}_2)$, the diagonal of $\boldsymbol{\Lambda}$ are length scales, and α^2 is the co-variance amplitude. This kernel relaxes the assumption on the smoothness of the posterior pdf compared to commonly-used squared exponential kernel. The GP is then learnt by an iteration of the following two steps:

1. *Finding optimal points to build the GP:* Sample points used to build the GP are placed so as to: (1) globally approximate the posterior pdf, and (2) concentrate more in regions of high posterior probability. For the former, points are chosen where the predictive uncertainty $\sigma(\boldsymbol{\theta})$ of the current GP is high (to facilitate exploration of uncertain space). For the latter, points are chosen where the predictive mean $\mu(\boldsymbol{\theta})$ of the current GP is high (to exploit current knowledge about the space of high posterior probability). This is done by finding the point that maximizes the upper confidence bound of the GP [9]:

$$\hat{\boldsymbol{\theta}} = \underset{\boldsymbol{\theta}}{\mathrm{argmax}} \left\{ \mu(\boldsymbol{\theta}) + \beta^{1/2}\sigma(\boldsymbol{\theta}) \right\} \tag{6}$$

where $\mu(\boldsymbol{\theta})$ and $\sigma(\boldsymbol{\theta})$ are evaluated by the Sherman-Morrison-Woodbury formula [9]. The parameter β balances between exploitation and exploration of the sample space [9]. Equation (6) is optimized using Bound Optimization BY Quadratic Approximation (BOBYQA) [8].

2. *Updating the GP surrogate:* Once a new point is obtained, the exact posterior pdf (3) is evaluated at this point and the GP is updated. After every a few updates of the GP, we optimize the hyperparameters (length scales $\boldsymbol{\Lambda}$ and covariance amplitude α) by maximizing the marginal likelihood.

These two steps iterate until new points collected change little. In this way, we quickly obtain a surrogate $\pi^*(\boldsymbol{\theta}|\mathbf{Y})$ of the exact posterior pdf (3) that is much cheaper to evaluate and is most accurate in regions of high posterior probability.

MCMC Acceleration Using GP Approximation: Metropolis Hasting (MH) is commonly used for generating a Markov chain of samples from a stationary distribution [1]. Supposing that the nth sample in the Markov chain is $\boldsymbol{\theta}_n$, MH in its native form first draws a random candidate from a proposal distribution $q(\boldsymbol{\theta}|\boldsymbol{\theta}_n)$, and then accepts the candidate with an acceptance probability given as:

$$\rho(\boldsymbol{\theta}_n, \boldsymbol{\theta}) = \min\left(1, \frac{q(\boldsymbol{\theta}_n|\boldsymbol{\theta})\pi(\boldsymbol{\theta}|\mathbf{Y})}{q(\boldsymbol{\theta}|\boldsymbol{\theta}_n)\pi(\boldsymbol{\theta}_n|\mathbf{Y})}\right) \tag{7}$$

which means that the expensive posterior pdf (3) has to be probed — namely, the simulation model to be run — at every proposed sample. Because obtaining a proposal $q(\boldsymbol{\theta}|\boldsymbol{\theta}_n)$ similar to the exact posterior pdf is notoriously difficult [1], the acceptance rate is often low which leads to an infeasible amount of computation that will mainly be spent at rejecting unwanted proposals.

To improve the acceptance rate of MH, we use the much-faster-to-evaluate GP surrogate to modify commonly-used proposal distributions, such as a Gaussian distribution centered at $\boldsymbol{\theta}$ with covariance $\boldsymbol{\Sigma}_p = \sigma_p^2\mathbf{I}$. A candidate sample $\boldsymbol{\theta}$ is first drawn from the proposal distribution as usual. Instead of directly testing the acceptance of this candidate using Eq. (7), we first test the acceptance of this candidate against the surrogate GP $\pi^*(\boldsymbol{\theta}|\mathbf{Y})$ using a probability ρ_A:

$$\rho_A(\boldsymbol{\theta}_n, \boldsymbol{\theta}) = \min\left(1, \frac{q(\boldsymbol{\theta}_n|\boldsymbol{\theta})\pi^*(\boldsymbol{\theta}|\mathbf{Y})}{q(\boldsymbol{\theta}|\boldsymbol{\theta}_n)\pi^*(\boldsymbol{\theta}_n|\mathbf{Y})}\right) \tag{8}$$

which is computationally much cheaper to evaluate compared to (7). Intuitively, this additional stage of acceptance or rejection modifies the proposal distribution by filtering out candidates that have a high probability of being rejected by the exact pdf. Only the candidates accepted by the GP surrogate are then evaluated against the exact posterior pdf for acceptance with a probability ρ_E:

$$\rho_E(\boldsymbol{\theta}_n, \boldsymbol{\theta}) = \min\left(1, \frac{\pi(\boldsymbol{\theta}|\mathbf{Y})\pi^*(\boldsymbol{\theta}_n|\mathbf{Y})}{\pi(\boldsymbol{\theta}_n|\mathbf{Y})\pi^*(\boldsymbol{\theta}|\mathbf{Y})}\right) \tag{9}$$

In this way, the acceptance rate is improved and unnecessary model simulations are avoided at proposals that would have been rejected with high probability. This is achieved without sacrificing sampling accuracy because the final Markov chain is generated via acceptance by the exact posterior pdf. Due to space limit, refer to [3] for discussions on the ergodicity and convergence of the Markov chain to the exact pdf when modifying the proposal using an approximation.

4   Experiments

Synthetic Experiments: On two image-derived human heart-torso models, we include six cases of infarcts of different sizes and locations of the LV. Note that a relatively small number of experiments is considered because it is time consuming to obtain samples on the exact posterior pdf as a baseline. For each synthetic case, parameter a in the AP model is set to be 0.15 for normal tissue and 0.5 for infarct tissue. 120-lead ECG is simulated and corrupted with 20 dB Gaussian noise as measurement data. After dimensionality reduction [4], the number of parameters to be estimated in each case ranges from 9 to 12.

In all MH sampling, we use a four parallel chains with same Gaussian proposal distribution but four different initial points. Because the GP surrogate is efficient to sample, we use it to tune the variance of the proposal distribution and the starting point for each MCMC chain. The former is tuned to attain an acceptance rate of 0.3–0.4. For the latter, a rapid sampling of the GP surrogate is first conducted using slice sampling for 20,000 samples; assuming that these samples come from a mixture of four Gaussian distributions, the mean of each is then used to start each of the four parallel chains. After discarding initial burn-in samples and picking alternate samples to avoid auto-correlation in each chain, the samples from four chains are combined. The convergence of all MCMC chains are tested using trace plots, Geweke statistics, and Gelman-Rubin statistics [1].

Validation Against Exact Posterior Pdf: Figure 1(a)–(b) presents examples of posterior pdfs obtained from two experiments where the dimension of unknown parameters are 9 and 10, respectively. As shown, the presented sampling strategy (green curve) closely reproduces true posterior pdf (red curve). In the mean time, it reduces the computational cost by an average of 53.56% (Fig. 1(c)) despite the overhead of constructing the GP surrogate which, as highlighted in the purple bar in Fig. 1(c), is negligible compared to the computation required for sampling.

Comparison with Directly Sampling the GP Surrogate: Directly sampling the GP posterior pdf in replacement of the exact pdf, as commonly done in existing

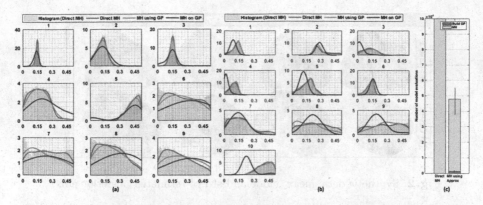

Fig. 1. (a)–(b): Examples of exact posterior pdfs (red) *vs.* those obtained by the presented method (green) and sampling the GP surrogate only (blue). (c): Comparison of efficiency in terms of the number of model simulations between the presented method (right bar) and sampling the exact posterior pdf (left bar). (Color figure online)

Table 1. Absolute errors in mean, mode, and standard deviation against the exact posterior pdf: the presented method *vs.* directly sampling the GP surrogate.

	Mean	Mode	Standard deviation
Presented method	0.0154 ± 0.0186	0.0510 ± 0.0711	0.0059 ± 0.0074
Sampling surrogate	0.0549 ± 0.0532	0.0972 ± 0.1111	0.0309 ± 0.0306

methods [11], requires significantly less computation because no model simulation is needed. However, the sampling accuracy is limited. This is especially evident in Fig. 1(b) where sampling the GP surrogate (blue curve) produces a distribution that is different from the exact pdf not only in general shape but also in locations of the mode. Using the mean, mode, and standard deviation (std) of the exact pdf as a baseline, Table 1 shows that sampling errors of the presented method are significantly lower than those from sampling the surrogate (paired t-test on 60 estimated parameters, $p < 0.0012$).

Analysis of Uncertainty and Identifiability: Figure 2 shows maps of summary statistics obtained by the presented method in two cases with septal infarcts. In case 1, there are 7 regions of the heart to be parameterized. As shown, a strong false positive at the RV lateral wall is present at both the posterior mode and mean of the estimated parameters. The std map indicates that this false positive is associated with a high uncertainty. For a closer look at the reason for such uncertainty, Fig. 3 shows posterior pdfs of the estimated parameters (the region on which each parameter is estimated is shown in the first column, where green indicates a healthy region and red an infarcted region). As shown, the first three regions correspond to healthy regions and their parameters are estimated with a prominent single mode and low uncertainty. Regions 4 and 5 correspond to two small healthy regions close to the infarct. Their parameters are estimated

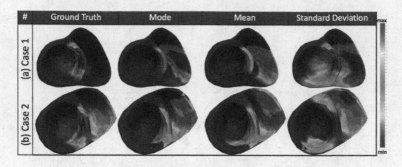

Fig. 2. Synthetic data: mean, mode and std of estimated posterior pdfs.

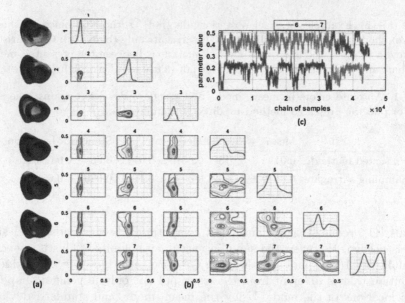

Fig. 3. (a) Regions of heart to be parameterized (red: infarct, green: non-infarct/mixed). (b) Uni-variate and bi-variate marginal pdf plots. (c) Trace plot for parameters of regions 6 and 7 showing switching behavior. (Color figure online)

accurately but with higher uncertainty. The last two regions correspond to the infarcted region and the RV wall. Their parameters show a coupling that results in a bimodal distribution. This also exhibits as a switching behavior in the trace plot of these two parameters (Fig. 3(c)): if the parameter of region 6 is estimated towards a healthier state, the parameter of region 7 would tend towards an infarcted state. Such switching property in Markov chains is associated with non-identifiability [13], *i.e.*, either combination of the two parameter values could fit the measurement data similarly well. Knowledge about this non-identifiability is valuable for placing proper trust in the obtained posterior point estimates.

In case 2, there are 11 regions to be parameterized, five of which along with their estimated parameter pdfs are shown in Fig. 4. As shown, the parameter of the region that contains the true infarct (a) is correctly estimated with a narrow

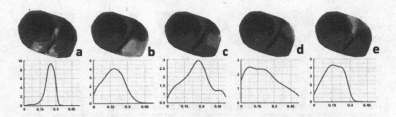

Fig. 4. Uni-variate marginal probability density plots and the corresponding regions of heart to be parameterized for case 2 from Fig. 2.

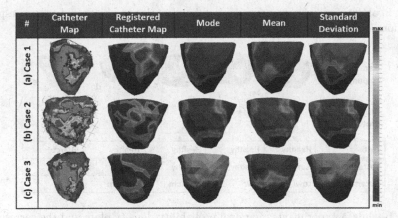

Fig. 5. Real-data experiments: mean, mode and std of posterior pdfs. (Color figure online)

uni-modal distribution. In comparison, several RV regions adjacent to the septal infarct (b–e) have difficulty converging which we suspect could be again caused by non-identifiability. As a result, we obtain a solution where the true septal infarct is estimated with high confidence, whereas the false positives are associated with a higher uncertainty as summarized in Fig. 2. Namely, uncertainty analysis helps differentiate false positives from true positives in this case.

Real-Data Experiments: We conduct real-data studies on three patients who underwent catheter ablation of ventricular tachycardia due to prior infraction [10]. Patient-specific heart-torso geometrical models are obtained from axial CT images. The uncertainty of tissue excitability in the AP model (1) is estimated from 120-lead ECG data. For evaluation of the results, bipolar voltage data from *in-vivo* catheter mapping are used. However, it should be noted that voltage maps are not a direct measure of tissue excitability and thus should be interpreted as a reference but not the validation data. Figure 5 shows the catheter data along with the estimation results, where the first column shows the original voltage maps (red: dense scar ≤ 0.5 mV; purple: healthy tissue > 1.5 mV; green: scar border 0.5–1.5 mV) and the second column shows the same voltage data registered to CT-derived cardiac meshes. As shown, compared to synthetic data, a real infarct is often distributed with higher heterogeneity.

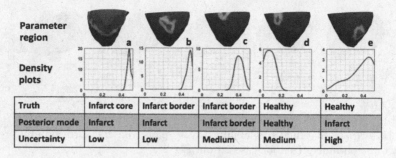

Fig. 6. Real-data experiments: marginal probability density plots and the corresponding regions of heart being parameterized in case 1.

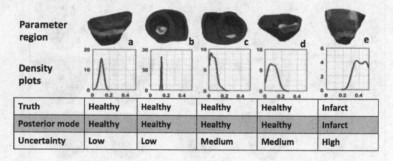

Fig. 7. Real-data experiments: marginal probability density plots and the corresponding regions of heart being parameterized in case 2.

The resolution to which such heterogeneity can be captured is largely limited by the method of dimensionality reduction. Below we show how uncertainties of the lower-resolution estimation are associated with the heterogeneity of the underlying tissue.

Case 1: The voltage data for case 1 (Fig. 5(a)) shows a dense infarct at inferolateral LV with a heterogeneous region extending to lateral LV. Dimensionality reduction generates 12 regions of the heart to be parameterized, five of which are listed in Fig. 6 along with the estimated posterior marginal pdfs for their parameters. As shown, the parameter for the region of infarct core (a) is correctly estimated with low uncertainty. For several regions around the heterogeneous infarct border (b–d), uncertainties of the estimation become higher. A particularly high uncertainty is obtained at a small healthy region by the scar border (e), where the parameter is incorrectly estimated. This produces an estimation with correct posterior mode/mean and low uncertainty at the infarct core, increased uncertainty at the heterogeneous infarct border, and high uncertainty at a region of false-positive near the infarct border as summarized in Fig. 5(a).

Case 2: The voltage data for case 2 (Fig. 5(b)) shows a massive yet quite heterogeneous infarct at lateral LV. Dimensionality reduction generates 8 regions of the heart to be parameterized, five of which are listed in Fig. 7 along with the estimated posterior marginal pdfs for their parameters. As shown, for healthy

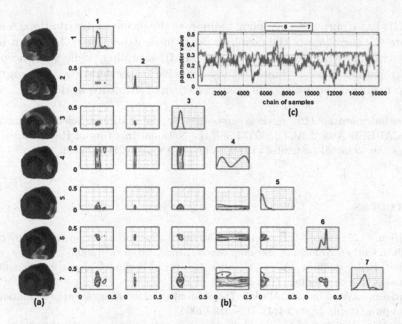

Fig. 8. Real-data experiments for case 3. (a) Regions of heart to be parameterized. (b) Uni-variate and bi-variate marginal pdf plots. (c) Trace plot for parameters of regions 6 and 7.

regions remote from the infarct (a–b), their parameters are correctly estimated with high confidence. For healthy regions close to the infarct (c–d), their parameters are correctly estimated but with lower confidence. For the region that corresponds to the infarct (e), its abnormal parameter is correctly captured but with a high uncertainty – likely reflecting the heterogeneous nature of tissue properties in this region. As summarized in Fig. 5(b), while the estimation correctly reveals the region of infarct as in case 1, it is also associated with a higher uncertainty compared to the less heterogeneous infarct in case 1.

Case 3: The catheter data for case 3 (Fig. 5(c)) shows low voltage at lateral LV and RV, although it was not clear whether the low voltage on lateral RV was due to an infarct or fat layer. As shown in Fig. 8, there are 7 regions of the heart to be parameterized. The abnormal parameter in lateral LV (region 1) is estimated with a narrow uni-modal distribution. In contrast, the marginal distribution for the parameter in lateral RV (region 4) shows a bimodal distribution with one mode in healthy range and the other in infarcted range. Markov chains for the parameters of two nearby regions at RV (regions 6–7) also show a switching behavior (Fig. 8(c)). This produces an estimate of abnormal tissue property with high confidence at lateral LV (Fig. 5(c)), and less confidence at lateral RV.

5   Conclusion

This paper presents a novel approach to efficiently yet accurately sample the distribution of parameters in complex simulation models. This is achieved by using GP-based surrogate modeling to improve the proposal distribution. A more accurate GP surrogate of the posterior pdf is more expensive to build but more effective in improving the acceptance rate of MH sampling, while a less accurate GP surrogate is faster to build but less effective in accelerating MH sampling. How to maintain this balance is to be investigated in future works.

Acknowledgments. This work is supported by the National Science Foundation under CAREER Award ACI-1350374 and the National Institute of Heart, Lung, and Blood of the National Institutes of Health under Award R21Hl125998.

References

1. Adrieu, C., Freitas, N., Doucet, A., Jordan, M.: An introduction to Markov chain Monte Carlo for machine learning. Mach. Learn. **50**, 5–43 (2003)
2. Aliev, R.R., Panfilov, A.V.: A simple two-variable model of cardiac excitation. Chaos, Solitons Fractals **7**(3), 293–301 (1996)
3. Christen, J.A., Fox, C.: Markov chain Monte Carlo using an approximation. J. Comput. Graph. Stat. **14**(4), 795–810 (2005)
4. Dhamala, J., Sapp, J.L., Horacek, M., Wang, L.: Spatially-adaptive multi-scale optimization for local parameter estimation: application in cardiac electrophysiological models. In: Ourselin, S., Joskowicz, L., Sabuncu, M.R., Unal, G., Wells, W. (eds.) MICCAI 2016. LNCS, vol. 9902, pp. 282–290. Springer, Cham (2016). doi:10.1007/978-3-319-46726-9_33
5. Konukoglu, E., et al.: Efficient probabilistic model personalization integrating uncertainty on data and parameters: application to eikonal-diffusion models in cardiac electrophysiology. Prog. Biophys. Mol. Biol. **107**(1), 134–146 (2011)
6. Lê, M., Delingette, H., Kalpathy-Cramer, J., Gerstner, E.R., Batchelor, T., Unkelbach, J., Ayache, N.: Bayesian personalization of brain tumor growth model. In: Navab, N., Hornegger, J., Wells, W.M., Frangi, A.F. (eds.) MICCAI 2015. LNCS, vol. 9350, pp. 424–432. Springer, Cham (2015). doi:10.1007/978-3-319-24571-3_51
7. Plonsey, R.: Bioelectric Phenomena. Wiley Online Library, Hoboken (1969)
8. Powell, M.J.: Developments of NEWUOA for minimization without derivatives. IMA J. Numer. Anal. **28**(4), 649–664 (2008)
9. Rasmussen, C.E.: Gaussian Processes for Machine Learning. MIT Press, Cambridge (2006)
10. Sapp, J., Dawoud, F., Clements, J., Horáček, M.: Inverse solution mapping of epicardial potentials: quantitative comparison to epicardial contact mapping. Circ. Arrhythmia Electrophysiol. **5**(5), 1001–1009 (2012)
11. Schiavazzi, D., Arbia, G., Baker, C., et al.: Uncertainty quantification in virtual surgery hemodynamics predictions for single ventricle palliation. Int. J. Numer. Methods Biomed. Eng. (2015)
12. Sermesant, M., Chabiniok, R., Chinchapatnam, P., et al.: Patient-specific electromechanical models of the heart for the prediction of pacing acute effects in CRT: a preliminary clinical validation. Med. Image Anal. **16**(1), 201–215 (2012)
13. Siekmann, I., Sneyd, J., Crampin, E.J.: MCMC can detect nonidentifiable models. Biophys. J. **103**(11), 2275–2286 (2012)

14. Wang, L., Zhang, H., Wong, K.C., Liu, H., Shi, P.: Physiological-model-constrained noninvasive reconstruction of volumetric myocardial transmembrane potentials. IEEE Trans. Biomed. Eng. **57**(2), 296–315 (2010)
15. Wong, K.C.L., Relan, J., Wang, L., Sermesant, M., Delingette, H., Ayache, N., Shi, P.: Strain-based regional nonlinear cardiac material properties estimation from medical images. In: Ayache, N., Delingette, H., Golland, P., Mori, K. (eds.) MICCAI 2012. LNCS, vol. 7510, pp. 617–624. Springer, Heidelberg (2012). doi:10.1007/978-3-642-33415-3_76

Cancer Metastasis Detection via Spatially Structured Deep Network

Bin Kong[1], Xin Wang[2], Zhongyu Li[1], Qi Song[2(✉)], and Shaoting Zhang[1(✉)]

[1] Department of Computer Science, UNC Charlotte, Charlotte, NC, USA
szhang16@uncc.edu
[2] CuraCloud Corporation, Seattle, WA, USA
song@curacloudcorp.com

Abstract. Metastasis detection of lymph nodes in Whole-slide Images (WSIs) plays a critical role in the diagnosis of breast cancer. Automatic metastasis detection is a challenging issue due to the large variance of their appearances and the size of WSIs. Recently, deep neural networks have been employed to detect cancer metastases by dividing the WSIs into small image patches. However, most existing works simply treat these patches independently and do not consider the structural information among them. In this paper, we propose a novel deep neural network, namely Spatially Structured Network (Spatio-Net) to tackle the metastasis detection problem in WSIs. By integrating the Convolutional Neural Network (CNN) with the 2D Long-Short Term Memory (2D-LSTM), our Spatio-Net is able to learn the appearances and spatial dependencies of image patches effectively. Specifically, the CNN encodes each image patch into a compact feature vector, and the 2D-LSTM layers provide the classification results (i.e., normal or tumor), considering its dependencies on other relevant image patches. Moreover, a new loss function is designed to constrain the structure of the output labels, which further improves the performance. Finally, the metastasis positions are obtained by locating the regions with high tumor probabilities in the resulting accurate probability map. The proposed method is validated on hundreds of WSIs, and the accuracy is significantly improved, in comparison with a state-of-the-art baseline that does not have the spatial dependency constraint.

1 Introduction

Breast cancer is the second most common cancer that can occur in women. Fortunately, early diagnosis and treatment can greatly improve patients' chances of recovery; e.g., the five-year relative survival rate rises from 24% when breast cancer is diagnosed at the distant stage to 99% if it is diagnosed at the localized stage [8]. Metastasis detection in lymph nodes is one of the most important criteria to assist early diagnosis, considering that lymph nodes are the first place where breast cancer is likely to metastasize. In recent years, Whole-slide Images

---

B. Kong and X. Wang—Equal contribution.

© Springer International Publishing AG 2017
M. Niethammer et al. (Eds.): IPMI 2017, LNCS 10265, pp. 236–248, 2017.
DOI: 10.1007/978-3-319-59050-9_19

(WSIs) have been widely adopted for the detection of cancer metastases. However, manual detection of cancer metastases in WSIs requires exhaustive examination and analysis by pathologists, which is labor intensive and time-consuming, and the detection results may be subjective. Therefore, computer-assisted detection is a logical development to offer more reliable and consistent detection of cancer metastasis in WSIs.

Automatic detection of cancer metastases in WSIs is a challenging task for the following reasons: (1) the WSIs are extremely large (e.g., $100,000 \times 200,000$ pixels), which cannot be fed into any existing algorithm directly for detection and analysis, and (2) the malignant tissues/cells have various shapes, textures, etc., and some of them only have subtle differences with benign parts, which are hard to differentiate by traditional methods. In recent years, many attempts have focused on the automatic cancer detection in WSIs. For example, Apou et al. [1] over-segmented the WSIs into superpixels. Each of these superpixels is described by a texture feature based on the quantized color histograms. However, the hand-crafted features are not discriminative enough to represent WSIs. Thus, Geçer [3] proposed a hierarchical scheme to analyze the WSIs based on deep neural networks. They assumed that only a small part of the WSI was crucial to the diagnosis. Therefore, they

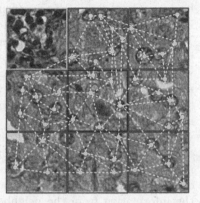

Fig. 1. Illustration of the structure embedded in image patches: the center patch is more likely to have the same properties as its neighbors; i.e., most of them are tumor patches. The nuclei (green dots) in the tumor region indicate underlying spatial structures. (Color figure online)

employed Fully Convolutional Networks [15] to locate the salient tumor regions hierarchically. Finally, the suspicious regions are found by classifying these regions with a CNN. In order to detect cancer metastases in massive WSIs in a fine-grained level, several works have tried to divide WSIs into small patches (e.g., 256×256) and tackle them individually. For example, by setting small image patches as input, Hou et al. [7] combined patch-based CNNs with supervised decision fusion for the analysis of WSIs. More recently, Wang et al. [20] employed CNNs to assign a prediction value to each patch for the final diagnosis decisions. All of the above methods treat the image patches independently. However, image patches and their neighbors usually include spatial patterns that are vital for the inference.

In general, when a patch is in the tumor region, its neighboring patches also have a high probability to be labeled as tumor, since they are co-located in neighboring regions. Figure 1 illustrates a sub-region in a WSI, which includes nine patches. The top left patch is in the normal region, and the other eight patches (except the center) are already labeled as tumor. Accordingly, we can reasonably infer that the center patch is also likely in the tumor region because of its neighboring patches. This prior knowledge reflects the spatial constraint or structure of image patches, which are usually not preserved in previous methods [20]. In fact, by observing the distributions of the nuclei in the tumor region (dots in Fig. 1), we can find that they have certain underlying patterns (e.g., the spatial arrangements of tumor nuclei are totally different from those of the normal nuclei). Indeed, these nuclei form a structure that has been proven to be very useful for diagnosis purposes; e.g., architecture features [2]. However, if only a single patch is considered, such topological information may be lost. To fully explore and model the spatially structured information in WSIs, this paper proposed a novel deep learning-based architecture, named Spatio-Net, which combines CNN and 2D-LSTM to detect the metastasis locations automatically. Different from the previous methods, our system not only considers the appearances of each patch, but also embeds spatial relationships between neighboring patches in the deep architecture. Specifically, our system is motivated by the observation that the neighboring patches have dependencies on each other. Based on this prior knowledge, we use 2D-LSTM layers to explicitly model this spatial constraint in our system. With the information propagation of the nodes in the 2D-LSTM layers, our framework can seamlessly integrate the information from the neighboring patches to make a better prediction. In addition, we also enforce this constraint in the loss function to further improve the performance.

The rest of this paper is organized as follows. Section 2 introduces the methodology details. Section 3 demonstrates the experimental results and comparisons. Sections 4 draws the conclusions and discusses future directions.

2   Methodology

In this section, we first provide an overview of the proposed framework. Then we present the methodology details of the Spatio-Net, including the network architectures and its optimization.

2.1   Overview

The top row of Fig. 2 shows an overview of the proposed framework. First, whole-slide images are divided into small image patches with fixed-size. Unlike previous deep neural network methods that treat each small image patch independently, the proposed framework combines each image patch and its neighbors together for consideration. Particularly, the Spatio-Net not only extracts discriminative features from each patch, but also considers the spatially structured information that is embedded among the image patch and its neighbors. The Spatio-Net then returns a probability map, which indicates the probability of each image patch as a normal or a tumor region. Accordingly, metastases in each WSI can be located by considering the generated probability map.

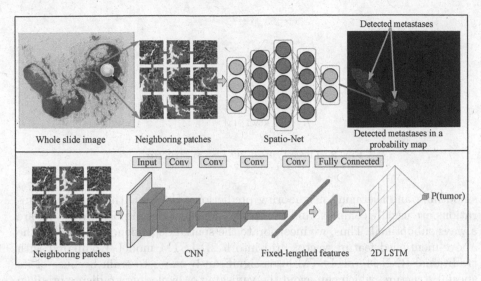

Fig. 2. Overview of the proposed framework and the architectures of our Spatio-Net. The top row is the proposed framework. The WSIs are divided into small patches. Each patch and its neighbors are fed into Spatio-Net with spatial structured constraint, resulting in a probability map, which is further processed to locate the metastases. The bottom row shows the detailed structures of the Spatio-Net. The CNN encodes each patch and its neighbors into a grid of fixed-length vectors. Afterwards, 2D-LSTM layers are employed to further explore the remaining spatially structured information in the grid to give a more accurate prediction. Different from [20], Spatio-Net explicitly models the spatially structured information in 2D-LSTM layers.

2.2 Spatio-Net Architectures

The Spatio-Net architecture (the bottom row of Fig. 2) includes two main modules: CNN and 2D-LSTM. The CNN acts as an effective feature extractor to encode each patch and its neighboring patches into compact fixed-length vectors, resulting in a small grid of vectors. Subsequently, we embed the spatially structured information in this grid, which is further explored in 2D-LSTM.

Patch Encoding with CNN: Hand-crafted features [22,23] are not powerful enough to represent and discriminate the large variances of WSIs. To fully capture the useful information from every image patch, a CNN is employed as a powerful feature extractor. In recent years, we have witnessed numerous kinds of CNN architectures [12,19,21]. In our framework, the deep residual network [5] is employed for feature extraction, since it is highly discriminative to distinguish the subtle differences between normal and tumor patches. Essentially, the deep residual network acts as a feature transformer $\psi(I; U)$ which can map the image patch I to a fixed-length vector $x \in \mathbb{R}^d$, where U is the learned weights.

Accurate Prediction via 2D-LSTM: A straightforward way to incorporate the spatial dependencies among image patches is post-processing, such as

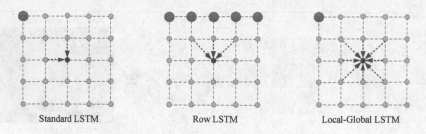

Standard LSTM   Row LSTM   Local-Global LSTM

Fig. 3. Three typical 2D-LSTM structures.

smoothing and averaging neighboring predictions. However, the patch configurations are usually complex, and the spatial dependencies in post-processing are always suboptimal. Thus, we incorporate the spatial dependency by passing the above-mentioned feature vector grid into a 2D-LSTM model. Compared with traditional RNN [4], an LSTM [6] is significantly easier to train because of its special structure, which can avoid the vanishing or exploding gradients problem during back-propagation. Each LSTM unit at current time step t contains a hidden state $\boldsymbol{h}_t$ and a memory cell $\boldsymbol{c}_t$. The memory cell aims to learn when to forget previous memory and when to update it. In addition, it contains four gates to control the flow of the corresponding information; i.e., input gate i_t, forget gate f_t, memory gate m_t, and output gate o_t. Accordingly, the hidden state and the memory cell for the next time step $t + 1$ can be updated as:

$$
\begin{aligned}
i_{t+1} &= \sigma(W_i \boldsymbol{H}_t) \\
f_{t+1} &= \sigma(W_f \boldsymbol{H}_t) \\
o_{t+1} &= \sigma(W_o \boldsymbol{H}_t) \\
m_{t+1} &= \sigma(W_m \boldsymbol{H}_t) \\
c_{t+1} &= f_{t+1} \odot c_t + i_{t+1} \odot m_t \\
h_{t+1} &= \tanh(o_{t+1} \odot \boldsymbol{c}_t)
\end{aligned}
\tag{1}
$$

where $\boldsymbol{H}_t$ is the concatenation of the input x_i and current hidden state $\boldsymbol{h}_t$. W_i, W_f, W_o, and W_m are the weight matrices for the input, forget, output, and memory gates, respectively. Nonlinear function $\sigma(x) = (1 + e^{-x})^{-1}$ squashes its input x to $[-1, 1]$. And $\odot$ denotes element-wise product. Following [17], **LSTM** is used as a shorthand for Eq. 1. Then, it can be simplified as:

$$
(\boldsymbol{m}_{t+1}, \boldsymbol{h}_{t+1}) = \mathbf{LSTM}(\boldsymbol{H}_t, \boldsymbol{m}_t, \boldsymbol{W})
\tag{2}
$$

where $\boldsymbol{W}$ is the concatenation of weight matrices of the four current gates discussed above.

A 2D-LSTM usually does not have an explicit sequential order. To propagate information among the 2D-LSTM units, the propagation order and the starting points have to be manually defined. There are various ways to broadcast the information among 2D-LSTM units (e.g., three examples in Fig. 3). The Standard LSTM [10] starts from the upper-left node, and every node's state is updated by considering its top and left units. The Row LSTM [16] starts from its top row and the information is propagated from the top to the bottom. Local-Global LSTM [13,14] also starts from the upper-left node, but each node's state is updated by considering all its neighbors. Following [13], we use the Local-Global 2D-LSTM to update the nodes' states due to its superior performance.

In order to determine the current hidden states of each location j, we extract the corresponding hidden states from the N neighboring ($N = 8$ in our case) LSTM units in the i-th 2D-LSTM layer and the corresponding hidden states from the previous 2D-LSTM layer. Let $h_{j,i,n}^{s}$ ($n = 1, 2, \ldots, N$) denote the hidden states from the n-th neighboring LSTM unit in the i-th 2D-LSTM layer, and $h_{j,i}^{d}$ indicates the hidden states of the i-th 2D-LSTM layer at location j. Similar to regular 1D-LSTM, for the current LSTM unit j, we use $H_{j,i}$ as the concatenation of the previous hidden states $h_{j,i,n}^{s}$, and the input from the i-th 2D-LSTM layer at the corresponding position $h_{j,i}^{d}$. The memory cells and hidden states of each location j in the $(i + 1)$-th 2D-LSTM layer can be calculated by:

$$
\begin{aligned}
(m_{j,i+1,n}^{s}, \hat{h}_{j,i+1,n}^{s}) &= \mathbf{LSTM}(H_{j,i}, m_{j,i,n}^{s}, W_{i}^{s}) \\
(m_{j,i+1}^{d}, h_{j,i+1}^{d}) &= \mathbf{LSTM}(H_{j,i}, m_{j,i}^{d}, W_{i}^{d})
\end{aligned}
\tag{3}
$$

where $m_{j,i,n}^{s}$ is the memory cell for the n-th neighboring 2D-LSTM node, and $m_{j,i}^{d}$ is the corresponding memory cell from the previous layer. W_{i}^{d} and W_{i}^{s} are the weight matrices for the spatial and depth dimensions, respectively.

The 2D LSTM layers are followed by a fully connected layer and normalized by a softmax function afterwards. The final output can be interpreted as the probabilities of patches being tumorous or normal.

2.3 Optimization with Spatially Structured Constraints

Given an image patch and its neighbors, the proposed Spatio-Net can learn to predict their categories, considering spatially structured information. Aside from the 2D-LSTM layers, we further model this constraint in the loss layer. The deep neural network proposed in this article defines a classifier η. Ideally, given the current patch x_*, its neighbors x_l ($l = 1, 2, \ldots, N$), and their ground truth labels y_* and y_l, the predictions for them should be consistent with their labels; i.e., $|\eta(x_*) - \eta(x_l)|$ should be small if $y_* = y_l$. Otherwise, the difference should be huge for those belonging to different categories; i.e., $|\eta(x_*) - \eta(x_l)|$ should be large if $y_* \neq y_l$. To enforce this constraint in Spatio-Net, a novel loss function, namely spatially structured loss, is defined:

$$
\begin{aligned}
L_{spatio} &= \frac{1}{2}(L_{ind} - L_{dif}) \\
L_{ind} &= \frac{1}{N} \sum_{x_* \in \mathbb{D}} \sum_{l} \{\mathbb{1}(y_* = y_l) \cdot [\eta(x_*) - \eta(x_l)]^2\} \\
L_{dif} &= \frac{1}{N} \sum_{x_* \in \mathbb{D}} \sum_{l} \{\mathbb{1}(y_* \neq y_l) \cdot [\eta(x_*) - \eta(x_l)]^2\}
\end{aligned}
\tag{4}
$$

where $\mathbb{1}(\cdot)$ is the indicator function. $\mathbb{D}$ is the training set. L_{ind} ensures that the predictions for x_* and x_l are similar if they are from the identical category; i.e., $y_* = y_l$. L_{dif} rewards the network to maximally distinguish x_* from x_l if $y_* = y_l$.

Having defined the spatially structured loss, the training criteria for the whole network can be further explored. Given the training set $\mathbb{D}$, the training objective becomes the task of estimating the network weights $\lambda = (U, V)$ (U and V are the parameters for the CNN and 2D LSTM layers, respectively):

$$L_{reg}(\lambda) = \frac{1}{2}(\|U\|_2^2 + \|V\|_2^2)$$
$$L_{cls} = - \sum_{x_* \in \mathbb{D}} log(\eta(x_*)) \tag{5}$$
$$\lambda = \arg\min_{\lambda}\{L_{cls} + \alpha L_{reg}(\lambda) + \beta L_{spatio}\}$$

where L_{reg} is the regularization penalty term, which ensures the learned weights are sparse. L_{cls} is the cross entropy loss function. α and β are hyper-parameters which are cross-validated in our experiments.

2.4   Global State Updating for Long Range Dependencies

The information propagation of the 2D-LSTM grid (3×3 in our case) starts from the upper-left node. Usually, LSTMs' starting states are initialized with zero vectors in the beginning, indicating that the LSTM units do not store any information. In our case, however, if the states of the 2D-LSTM grid are initialized with zero vectors (illustrated in Fig. 4(a)), the entire network will degrade into a slightly larger network, which only considers the locally structured information, since it is isolated from the other patches.

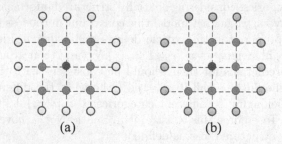

(a)   (b)

Fig. 4. Different initialization methods. (a) The 2D-LSTM's boundary nodes (green) are initialized with zero vectors (white). In this setting, we assume that we know nothing about other patches except the given nine patches. Thus the nine patches are separated from the rest patches. (b) The 2D-LSTM's boundary nodes (green) are initialized with the memory information of the other nodes (blue) which are previously stored. In this setting, the spatial information can expand to a wide scope. (Color figure online)

In order to extract long range dependency information from image patches, we propose to keep a record of memory information from each patch (illustrated in Fig. 4(b)). During the training phase, we randomly select a training patch and find its neighbors. The network retrieves the corresponding memory information from the record. Then, this memory information is employed to initialize the boundary nodes' memory. In the testing phase, our network iterates through the WSI patches in a sliding window manner. We start from the upper-left patch and store its corresponding memory, which is used to initialize the next 2D-LSTM. In addition, as the memory information of the current patch is stored, updated, and employed to initialize the 2D-LSTM of the next position, theoretically, it can be spread to influence the predictions of distant image patches.

After generating the probability map for the WSI, a simple image processing method is employed to locate the metastases, following [20]. It consists of two steps: thresholding and metastasis localization. In the first step, the probability map is thresholded to generate a binary mask image. In the second stage, each of the regions in the binary mask image is labeled as a metastasis region. In the output, the region centers are set as the metastasis locations, and the probability mean in each region is set as the final confidence score.

3 Experiments

3.1 Experimental Settings

In this section, extensive experiments were conducted on the CAMELYON16[1] dataset to evaluate the proposed Spatio-Net for cancer metastasis detection in WSIs. This dataset consists of 160 normal and 110 tumor WSIs, which were labeled by the pathologists. Most of the WSIs are over $60,000 \times 100,000$ pixels, and together they amount to approximately 500 gigabytes. The cancer metastasis regions and locations were carefully delineated by the pathologist in the format of binary mask. The WSIs were stored in a pyramid structure; i.e., they usually contain multiple magnification levels (e.g., $40\times$, $20\times$, $10\times$). Our experiments were conducted on $40\times$ magnification to fully leverage the information in the WSIs. The free-response receiver operating characteristic (FROC) curve, which is the plot of sensitivity against average number of false-positives per image, is employed to quantify the error between the predicted and the ground truth metastasis locations. The accuracy for the metastasis detection system was evaluated by average FROC (Ave. FROC) [18]. The higher numerical values suggest better performances. It is defined as the average sensitivity at 6 predefined false positive (FP) rates: 1/4, 1/2, 1, 2, 4, and 8 FPs per WSI. Five-fold cross-validation was performed on the dataset to obtain quantitative results.

Regarding the implementation, the residual neural network [5] with 101 layers was chosen as the CNN feature extractor, which was followed by four 2D-LSTM layers. The whole system is based on Caffe [9] and the hyper-parameters of the proposed Spatio-Net and other compared systems were all cross-validated

---

[1] https://camelyon16.grand-challenge.org/.

for fair comparison. For every training WSI, 1,500 negative patches with size of 256×256 were randomly extracted. As not all of the WSIs are tumorous, 1,500 positive patches with the size of 256×256 were randomly extracted only from each tumorous WSI. Therefore, there are in total more than a half million image patches used to train the network. In the training stage, these image patches were augmented with random translation, re-scaling, flipping, cropping, deforming, and blurring. The whole network was trained with back propagation. In the testing stage, the WSI tissue regions were evaluated by Spatio-Net in a sliding window fashion, with a stride of 64. After scoring each sliding window by Spatio-Net, the probability map was obtained, with each pixel corresponding to the score of one patch. Global state updating was adopted in both the training and testing stage. The probability map was processed to locate the metastasis regions, following the convention in [20].

3.2   Results and Discussions

We conducted multiple experimental evaluations of the Spatio-Net. In the first experiment, we focused on the effectiveness of the spatially structured constraint for Spatio-Net. We implemented [20] as the baseline system, which is a single net architecture. The only difference is that we use ResNet [5] with 101 layers instead of GoogleNet [19], since it achieved better performance in our experiments[2]. Compared to the baseline, the other methods follow the same network architecture. The difference is that the Baseline+PostPro adds smoothing and averaging as post-processing to the neighboring output labels, which should be similar, and the Spatio-Net integrated the spatially structured constraint in the network. The results of these three algorithms were summarized in Table 1. Although adding post-processing brings certain spatial dependency, it only marginally improves

Table 1. Quantitative comparisons. The baseline system is implemented as the published state-of-the-art framework [20], but using ResNet with 101 layers [5] instead of GoogleNet [19] for better accuracy. Baseline+PostPro means that smoothing and averaging operations are added upon output labels as the post-processing to enforce the spatially structured constraints. Spatio-Net is our proposed method, with this spatially structured constraint seamlessly unified in the network architecture.

Methods	Baseline	Baseline+PostPro	Spatio-Net
Ave. FROC	0.7012	0.7104	**0.7539**
STD	0.012	0.015	**0.008**

---

[2] The published state-of-the-art results for the cancer metastasis detection competition were reported in our chosen baseline [20]. However, the competition was already closed, and the ground truth of the testing data was no longer available, so we were unable to evaluate our method upon the same testing data. Therefore, for fair comparison, we reimplemented the framework of [20] and evaluated all methods with five-fold cross-validation using the same released dataset.

Table 2. Comparisons of different CNN models, with or without the spatially structured (SS) constraint.

Methods	ZFNet	ZFNet (with SS)	GoogleNet	GoogleNet (with SS)	ResNet-101	ResNet-101 (with SS)
Ave. FROC	0.6832	0.7249	0.6932	0.7438	0.7012	0.7539
STD	0.018	0.013	0.011	0.014	0.012	0.008

the result (less than 1%), since the constraint is not integrated into the model. Our Spatio-Net outperforms the method of [20] by more than 5%, benefiting from the fact that it optimizes the problem with the spatially structured information, while the previous network architecture only has local-optimal solutions.

Evaluation of Different CNN Models: To demonstrate that our spatially structured constraint is effective for different CNN models, we also evaluated it upon three different CNN models: ZFNet [21], GoogleNet [19], and ResNet with 101 layers [5]. These three networks were evaluated in the same way with and without the spatially structured constraint. The results were reported in Table 2. First, with more powerful CNN architectures; i.e., from ZFNet [21] to GoogleNet [19] and ResNet-101 [5], the performance improved. In fact, as we divided the whole slide images into small patches, we generated almost millions of training examples, which were sufficient to train a deep neural network from scratch with high capacity. Second, the improvements upon three different CNN architectures are consistent. Without the spatially structured constraint, the ave. FROC is only 0.6832 for ZFnet [21], 0.6932 for GoogleNet [19], and 0.7012 for ResNet-101 [5]. After adding the spatially structured constraint, performance was improved by 4.1%, 5.1%, and 5.3%, respectively. Therefore, the spatially structured constraint can benefit generic CNN models, making it an effective "plug-in" in different network architectures.

Evaluation of Parameters: Although this model has few parameters, the stride of sliding window is an important one. Therefore, we evaluated the proposed method with different values of the stride; i.e., 256, 128, and 64. The results were 0.6787, 0.7358, and 0.7539, respectively. From these results, we can draw the following conclusions: (1) With smaller values of the stride (from 256, then to 128, and finally to 64), the performance improved, and (2) The performance gain becomes marginal when the stride is small; e.g., the Ave. FROC increased by 5.7% from stride 256 to 128, while it is only increased by 1.8% from stride 128 to 64. This means that even if we further reduce the stride, the performance may not improve dramatically, while the computational complexity can grow quadratically with the decreasing of the stride. Therefore, it is necessary to find a trade-off between efficiency and accuracy[3].

---

[3] Note that we do not exhaustively tune these parameters, since our goal is to show improvement when using the spatially structured constraint under the same framework for fair comparison.

Evaluation of the Computational Efficiency: Without optimizing or tuning the implementation, the baseline takes 101 s to process one WSI during testing, while a straightforward implementation of our network takes 718 s, owing to the computational overhead of encoding each patch multiple times (e.g., a specific patch can be the neighbor of multiple patches, so it needs to be encoded when processing neighboring patches each time). However, such overhead can be greatly reduced with the following strategy. Considering that employing the CNN to encode image patches costs most of the computation, we feed all patches into the trained CNN only once and stored the encoded feature vectors in a matrix. Then, each feature vector and its neighbors are fed into the 2D-LSTM layers to generate the final prediction. Accordingly, each patch only goes through the CNN once. With this scheme, our Spatio-Net only needs 105 s to process one WSI, which is comparable to the baseline. To summarize, adding the spatially structured constraint does not significantly sacrifice the computational efficiency, but greatly benefits the accuracy.

4   Conclusion

In this paper, we propose a novel deep neural network, namely Spatio-Net, to detect cancer metastasis in whole-slide images. Particularly, the Spatio-Net integrates the CNN with 2D-LSTM, which not only learns representative features for each small patch divided from WSIs, but also considers the spatial dependencies between neighboring patches. Moreover, we design a novel loss function to embed the spatially structured constraints in Spatio-Net for more accurate detection. Extensive experiments show that the Spatio-Net with spatial structure is effective for cancer metastasis detection, compared with state-of-the-art methods. More importantly, as spatial structures are common in varieties of medical images (e.g., cardiac MRI [11]), we expect that our Spatio-Net is useful to boost performance in a variety of medical image analytical challenges.

References

1. Apou, G., Naegel, B., Forestier, G., Feuerhake, F., Wemmert, C.: Efficient region-based classification for whole slide images. In: Battiato, S., Coquillart, S., Pettré, J., Laramee, R.S., Kerren, A., Braz, J. (eds.) VISIGRAPP 2014. CCIS, vol. 550, pp. 239–256. Springer, Cham (2015). doi:10.1007/978-3-319-25117-2_15
2. Doyle, S., Agner, S., Madabhushi, A., Feldman, M., Tomaszewski, J.: Automated grading of breast cancer histopathology using spectral clustering with textural and architectural image features. In: 2008 5th IEEE International Symposium on Biomedical Imaging: From Nano to Macro, pp. 496–499. IEEE (2008)
3. Geçer, B.: Detection and classification of breast cancer in whole slide histopathology images using deep convolutional networks. Ph.D. thesis, Bilkent University (2016)
4. Goodfellow, I., Bengio, Y., Courville, A.: Deep Learning. MIT Press (2016, in preparation). http://www.deeplearningbook.org

5. He, K., Zhang, X., Ren, S., Sun, J.: Deep residual learning for image recognition. In: Proceedings of the IEEE Conference on Computer Vision and Pattern Recognition, pp. 770–778 (2016)
6. Hochreiter, S., Schmidhuber, J.: Long short-term memory. Neural Comput. **9**(8), 1735–1780 (1997)
7. Hou, L., Samaras, D., Kurc, T.M., Gao, Y., Davis, J.E., Saltz, J.H.: Patch-based convolutional neural network for whole slide tissue image classification. In: Proceedings of the IEEE Conference on Computer Vision and Pattern Recognition, pp. 2424–2433 (2016)
8. Howlader, N., Noone, A., Krapcho, M., Garshell, J., Neyman, N., Altekruse, S., Kosary, C., Yu, M., Ruhl, J., Tatalovich, Z., et al.: SEER Cancer Statistics Review, 1975–2010. National Cancer Institute, Bethesda (2013)
9. Jia, Y., Shelhamer, E., Donahue, J., Karayev, S., Long, J., Girshick, R., Guadarrama, S., Darrell, T.: Caffe: convolutional architecture for fast feature embedding. In: Proceedings of the 22nd ACM International Conference on Multimedia, pp. 675–678. ACM (2014)
10. Kalchbrenner, N., Danihelka, I., Graves, A.: Grid long short-term memory. arXiv preprint arXiv:1507.01526 (2015)
11. Kong, B., Zhan, Y., Shin, M., Denny, T., Zhang, S.: Recognizing end-diastole and end-systole frames via deep temporal regression network. In: Ourselin, S., Joskowicz, L., Sabuncu, M.R., Unal, G., Wells, W. (eds.) MICCAI 2016. LNCS, vol. 9902, pp. 264–272. Springer, Cham (2016). doi:10.1007/978-3-319-46726-9_31
12. Krizhevsky, A., Sutskever, I., Hinton, G.E.: Imagenet classification with deep convolutional neural networks. In: Advances in Neural Information Processing Systems, pp. 1097–1105 (2012)
13. Liang, X., Shen, X., Feng, J., Lin, L., Yan, S.: Semantic object parsing with graph LSTM. In: Leibe, B., Matas, J., Sebe, N., Welling, M. (eds.) ECCV 2016. LNCS, vol. 9905, pp. 125–143. Springer, Cham (2016). doi:10.1007/978-3-319-46448-0_8
14. Liang, X., Shen, X., Xiang, D., Feng, J., Lin, L., Yan, S.: Semantic object parsing with local-global long short-term memory. In: Proceedings of the IEEE Conference on Computer Vision and Pattern Recognition, pp. 3185–3193 (2016)
15. Long, J., Shelhamer, E., Darrell, T.: Fully convolutional networks for semantic segmentation. In: Proceedings of the IEEE Conference on Computer Vision and Pattern Recognition, pp. 3431–3440 (2015)
16. van den Oord, A., Kalchbrenner, N., Kavukcuoglu, K.: Pixel recurrent neural networks. arXiv preprint arXiv:1601.06759 (2016)
17. Peng, Z., Zhang, R., Liang, X., Lin, L.: Geometric scene parsing with hierarchical LSTM. arXiv preprint arXiv:1604.01931 (2016)
18. Shiraishi, J., Li, Q., Suzuki, K., Engelmann, R., Doi, K.: Computer-aided diagnostic scheme for the detection of lung nodules on chest radiographs: localized search method based on anatomical classification. Med. Phys. **33**(7), 2642–2653 (2006)
19. Szegedy, C., Liu, W., Jia, Y., Sermanet, P., Reed, S., Anguelov, D., Erhan, D., Vanhoucke, V., Rabinovich, A.: Going deeper with convolutions. In: Proceedings of the IEEE Conference on Computer Vision and Pattern Recognition, pp. 1–9 (2015)
20. Wang, D., Khosla, A., Gargeya, R., Irshad, H., Beck, A.H.: Deep learning for identifying metastatic breast cancer. arXiv preprint arXiv:1606.05718 (2016)
21. Zeiler, M.D., Fergus, R.: Visualizing and understanding convolutional networks. In: Fleet, D., Pajdla, T., Schiele, B., Tuytelaars, T. (eds.) ECCV 2014. LNCS, vol. 8689, pp. 818–833. Springer, Cham (2014). doi:10.1007/978-3-319-10590-1_53

22. Zhang, X., Liu, W., Dundar, M., Badve, S., Zhang, S.: Towards large-scale histopathological image analysis: hashing-based image retrieval. IEEE Trans. Med. Imaging **34**(2), 496–506 (2015)
23. Zhang, X., Xing, F., Su, H., Yang, L., Zhang, S.: High-throughput histopathological image analysis via robust cell segmentation and hashing. Med. Image Anal. **26**(1), 306–315 (2015)

Risk Stratification of Lung Nodules Using 3D CNN-Based Multi-task Learning

Sarfaraz Hussein[1]($\boxtimes$), Kunlin Cao[2], Qi Song[2], and Ulas Bagci[1]

[1] Center for Research in Computer Vision (CRCV), University of Central Florida, Orlando, FL, USA
shussein@knights.ucf.edu, bagci@crcv.ucf.edu
[2] CuraCloud Corporation, Seattle, WA, USA

Abstract. Risk stratification of lung nodules is a task of primary importance in lung cancer diagnosis. Any improvement in robust and accurate *nodule characterization* can assist in identifying cancer stage, prognosis, and improving treatment planning. In this study, we propose a 3D Convolutional Neural Network (CNN) based nodule characterization strategy. With a completely 3D approach, we utilize the volumetric information from a CT scan which would be otherwise lost in the conventional 2D CNN based approaches. In order to address the need for a large amount of training data for CNN, we resort to *transfer learning* to obtain highly discriminative features. Moreover, we also acquire the task dependent feature representation for six high-level nodule attributes and fuse this complementary information via a Multi-task learning (MTL) framework. Finally, we propose to incorporate potential disagreement among radiologists while scoring different nodule attributes in a graph regularized sparse multi-task learning. We evaluated our proposed approach on one of the largest publicly available lung nodule datasets comprising 1018 scans and obtained state-of-the-art results in regressing the malignancy scores.

Keywords: Computer-Aided Diagnosis (CAD) · Lung nodule characterization · 3D Convolutional Neural Network · Multi-task learning · Transfer learning · Computed Tomography (CT) · Deep learning

1 Introduction

Cancer is the number-one cause of deaths in the world. Out of 8.2 million deaths due to cancer worldwide, lung cancer accounts for the highest number of mortalities i.e. 1.59 million [1]. Risk stratification of lung nodules can aid in identifying cancer stage leading to improved treatment and higher chances of survival. In addition, any significant development to accurately and automatically characterize lung nodules can save significant manual exertion as well as valuable time.

Early diagnosis is one of the ways to reduce deaths related to lung cancer [2]. In this regard, lung screening programs are especially beneficial. Low Dose Computed Tomography (CT) scans are usually used to perform lung nodule diagnosis, including both detection and risk stratification. Although CT imaging

© Springer International Publishing AG 2017
M. Niethammer et al. (Eds.): IPMI 2017, LNCS 10265, pp. 249–260, 2017.
DOI: 10.1007/978-3-319-59050-9_20

remains the gold standard for lung cancer detection and diagnosis, Computer-Aided Diagnosis (CAD) and quantification tools are often necessary. Moreover, research in developing CAD algorithms can help explore the domain of imaging features and biomarkers which can be then studied by radiologists to further improve clinical decision making.

The development of a fast, robust and accurate system to perform risk stratification of lung nodules is therefore of significant importance. Specially the availability of large publicly available datasets such as LIDC-IDRI from Lung Image Database Consortium [3] has helped accelerate the research in this regard. However, the variability in nodule characteristics, including shape, size, intensity, location and uncertainty among radiologists' interpretation have made this problem particularly challenging. The advancement in machine learning methods, including the development of novel classification and feature learning techniques, has increased the efficacy of this task. However, there remains a substantial progress to be done in order to develop a CAD system attractive enough to be used in routine clinical evaluations of lung nodules.

In this work, we address the challenge of risk-stratification of lung nodules in low-dose CT scans. Capitalizing on the significant progress of deep learning technologies for image classification and their potential applications in radiology [4], we propose a 3D Convolutional Neural Network (CNN) based approach for rich feature representation of lung nodules. We argue that the use of 3D CNN is paramount in the classification of lung nodules in low-dose CT scans which are 3D by nature. By using the conventional CNN methods, however, we implicitly lose the important volumetric information which can be very significant for accurate risk stratification. The superior performance of 3D CNN over 2D networks is well studied in [5]. We also avoid hand-crafted feature extraction, painstaking feature engineering, and parameter tuning. Moreover, any information about six high-level nodule attributes such as calcification, sphericity, margin, lobulation, spiculation and texture (Fig. 1) can help in improving the benign-malignant risk assessment of the nodules. Taking forward this idea, we identify features corresponding to these high-level nodule attributes and fuse them in a multi-task learning framework to obtain the final risk assessment scores. An overview of the proposed approach is presented in Fig. 2. Overall, our main contributions in this work can be summarized as follows:

- We propose a 3D CNN based method to utilize the volumetric information from a CT scan which would be otherwise lost in the conventional 2D CNN based approaches. Moreover, we also circumvent the need for a large amount of volumetric training data to train the 3D network by transfer learning. We use the CT data to fine-tune a network which is trained on 1 million videos. To the best of our knowledge, our work is the first to empirically validate the success of transfer learning of a 3D network for lung nodules.
- We perform experimental evaluations on one of the largest publicly available datasets comprising lung nodules from more than 1000 low-dose CT scans.
- We employ graph regularized sparse multi-task learning to fuse the complementary feature information from high-level nodule attributes for malignancy determination. We also propose a scoring function to measure the inconsistency in risk assessment among different experts (radiologists).

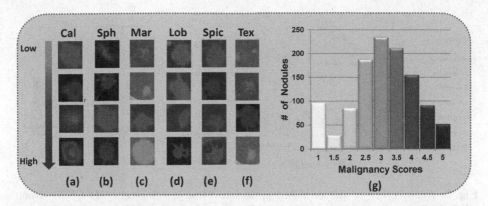

Fig. 1. Lung nodule attributes with different scores. As we move from the top (attribute missing) to the bottom (attribute with the highest prominence), the prominence of the attributes increases. Column (a) and (b) show calcified and spherical nodules; (c) represents margin where the top row is for poorly defined nodules and the bottom row shows well-defined nodules. Column (d) and (e) show lobulated and spiculated nodules whereas (f) represents nodules with different textures. The top row in (f) represents non-solid nodule and the bottom row shows solid nodule. The graph in (g) shows the number of nodules with different malignancy scores

2 Related Work

Conventionally, the characterization of lung nodules comprised nodule segmentation, extraction of hand-crafted imaging features, followed by the application of an off-the-shelf classifier/regressor. The method by Uchiyama et al. [6] was based on the extraction of various physical measures, including intensity statistics and then classification using Artificial Neural Networks. El-Baz et al. [7] first segmented the lung nodules using appearance-based models and used spherical harmonic analysis to perform shape analysis. The final step was the classification using k-nearest neighbor. Proposing a study based on texture analysis, Han et al. [8] extracted 2D texture features such as Haralick, Gabor and Local Binary Patterns (LBP) and extended them to 3D. Support Vector Machine (SVM) was employed to perform the classification. In another classical work by Way et al. [9], segmentation is performed using 3D active contours followed by the extraction of texture features from the rubber band straightening transform of the surrounding voxels. The classification was performed using Linear Discriminant Analysis (LDA) classifier. In another study, Lee et al. [10] proposed a feature selection based approach using both imaging and clinical data. An ensemble classifier, combining genetic algorithm (GA) and random subspace method (RSM) was then used to gauge feature relevance and information content. Finally, LDA was employed to perform classification on the reduced feature set.

Following up on the success of deep learning, the medical imaging community has moved from feature engineering to feature learning. In those frameworks, CNN had been used for feature extraction and an off-the-shelf classifier

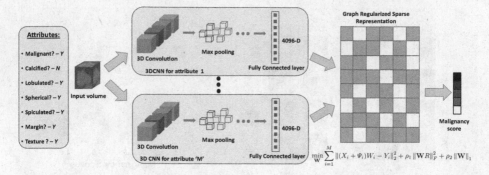

Fig. 2. An overview of the proposed approach. First, we fine-tune 3D CNNs using labels for malignancy and six attributes. Given the input volume, we pass it through different 3D CNNs each corresponding to an attribute (task). The network comprises 5 convolution, 5 max pooling, and 2 fully connected layers. We use the output from the first fully connected layer as the feature representation. The features from different CNNs are fused together using graph regularized sparse least square optimization function to obtain coefficient vectors corresponding to each task. During the testing phase, we multiply the feature representation of the testing image with the coefficient vector to obtain the malignancy score.

such as Random Forest (RF) was employed for classification [11,12]. Recently, Buty et al. [12] combined spherical harmonics along with deep CNN features and then classified them using RF. However, the use of CNN for lung nodule classification has been confined to 2D image analysis [13], thus falling short of utilizing the important volumetric and contextual information.

Moreover, the use of high-level image attributes had been found to be instrumental in the risk assessment and classification of lung nodules. In an effort to study the relationship between nodules attributes and malignancy, Furuya et al. [14] found that in a particular dataset, 82% of the lobulated, 97% of the densely spiculated, 93% of the ragged and 100% of the halo nodules were malignant. Moreover, 66% of the round nodules were found to be benign. Inspired by this study, in this work we utilize 3D CNN to learn discriminative feature set corresponding to each of the 6 attributes. We then fuse these feature representations via MTL to determine the malignancy likelihood.

3 Method

3.1 Problem Formulation

Let $X = [x_1, x_2 \ldots x_n] \in \mathbb{R}^{n \times d}$ be the data matrix comprising features from n data points in $\mathbb{R}^d$. Each sample corresponds with a regression score given by $Y = [y_1, y_2 \ldots y_n]$ where $Y \in \mathbb{R}^{n \times 1}$. Here the objective is to learn the coefficient vector or the regression estimator W from the training data. In this case, the ℓ_1 regularized least square regressor is defined as:

$$\min_{W} \|XW - Y\|_2^2 + \lambda \|W\|_1, \tag{1}$$

where λ controls the sparsity level for coefficient vector $W = [w_1, w_2 \dots w_d]$. The problem in Eq. 1 is an *unconstrained convex optimization* problem, and it remains non-differentiable when $w_i = 0$. Hence, the closed form solution corresponding to the global minimum for Eq. 1 is not possible. Thus, the above equation is represented in the following way as a *constrained optimization* function:

$$\min_{W} \|XW - Y\|_2^2,$$
$$s.t. \|W\|_1 \leq t, \tag{2}$$

where t is inversely proportional to λ. In the representation given in Eq. 2, both optimization function and the constraint are convex.

3.2 Network Architecture and Transfer Learning

We use the lung nodules dataset to fine-tune a 3D CNN trained on Sports-1M dataset [15]. The sports dataset comprises 1 million videos with 487 classes. In the absence of a large number of training examples from lung nodules, we use transfer learning strategy to obtain rich feature representation from a larger dataset (Sports-1M) for lung nodule characterization. The Sports-1M dataset is used to train a 3D CNN [5]. The network comprises 5 convolution, 5 max-pooling, 2 fully-connected and 1 soft-max classification layers. The input to the network is $3 \times 16 \times 128 \times 171$ where there are 16 non-overlapping slices in the input volume. The first 2 convolution layers have 64 and 128 filters respectively, whereas there are 256 filters in the last 3 layers. The outputs of the fully connected layers are of 4096 dimensions.

3.3 Multi-task Learning

Consider a problem with M tasks representing different attributes corresponding to a given dataset D. These tasks may be related and share some feature representation, both of which are unknown. The goal in Multi-task learning (MTL) is to perform joint learning of these tasks while exploiting dependencies in feature space so as to improve regressing one task using the others. In contrast to multi-label learning, tasks may have different features in MTL. Each task has model parameters denoted by W_m, used to regress the corresponding task m. Moreover, when $\mathbf{W} = [W_1, W_2 \dots W_M] \in \mathbb{R}^{M \times d}$ represents a rectangular matrix, rank is considered as an extension to the cardinality. In that case, trace norm, which is the sum of singular values is a replacement to the ℓ_1-norm. Trace norm, also known as nuclear norm is the convex envelope of the rank of a matrix (which is non-convex), where the matrices are considered on a unit ball. By replacing ℓ_1-norm with trace norm in Eq. 1, the trace norm regularized least square loss function is given by:

$$\min_{\mathbf{W}} \sum_{i=1}^{M} \|X_i W_i - Y_i\|_2^2 + \rho \|\mathbf{W}\|_*, \tag{3}$$

where ρ tunes the rank of the matrix $\mathbf{W}$, and trace-norm is defined as: $\|\mathbf{W}\|_* = \sum_{i=1} \sigma_i(\mathbf{W})$ with σ representing singular values.

Another regularizer, pertinent to MTL, is the regularization on the graph representing the relationship between the tasks [16,17]. Consider a complete graph $G = (V, \mathcal{E})$, such that nodes V represent the tasks and the edges $\mathcal{E}$ encode any relativity between the tasks. The complete graph can be represented as a structure matrix $S = [e^1, e^2 \ldots e^{\|\mathcal{E}\|}]$ and the difference between all the pairs connected in the graph is penalized by the following regularizer:

$$\|\mathbf{W}S\|_F^2 = \sum_{i=1}^{\|\mathcal{E}\|} \|\mathbf{W}e^i\|_2^2 = \sum_{i=1}^{\|\mathcal{E}\|} \left\|\mathbf{W}_{e_a^i} - \mathbf{W}_{e_b^i}\right\|_2^2. \tag{4}$$

Herein, e_a^i, e_b^i are the edges between the nodes a and b. The above regularizer can also be written as:

$$\|\mathbf{W}S\|_F^2 = \mathrm{tr}((\mathbf{W}S)^T(\mathbf{W}S)) = \mathrm{tr}(\mathbf{W}SS^T\mathbf{W}^T) = \mathrm{tr}(\mathbf{W}\mathcal{L}\mathbf{W}^T), \tag{5}$$

where 'tr' represents trace of a matrix and $\mathcal{L} = SS^T$ is the Laplacian matrix. Since there may exist disagreements between the scores from different experts (radiologists), we propose a scoring function to measure potential inconsistencies:

$$\Psi(j) = (e^{\frac{-\sum_i (x_i^j - \mu^j)^2}{2\sigma^j}})^{-1}. \tag{6}$$

The inconsistency measure corresponding to a particular example j is represented by $\Psi(j)$. x_i^j is the score given by the expert (radiologist) i and μ^j and σ^j denote mean and standard deviation of the scores, respectively. Here, for simplicity, we have dropped the index for the task; however, note that the inconsistency measure is computed for all the tasks. The final proposed graph regularized sparse least square optimization function with the inconsistency measure can then be written as:

$$\min_{\mathbf{W}} \sum_{i=1}^{M} \overbrace{\|(X_i + \Psi_i)W_i - Y_i\|_2^2}^{①} + \overbrace{\rho_1 \|\mathbf{W}S\|_F^2}^{②} + \overbrace{\rho_2 \|\mathbf{W}\|_1}^{③}, \tag{7}$$

where ρ_1 controls the level of penalty for graph structure and ρ_2 controls the sparsity. In the above optimization, the least square loss function ① considers tasks to be decoupled whereas ② and ③ consider the interdependencies between different tasks.

3.4   Optimization

The optimization function in Eq. 7 cannot be solved through standard gradient descent because the ℓ_1-norm is not differentiable at $\mathbf{W} = 0$. Since the optimization function in Eq. 7 has both smooth and non-smooth convex parts, estimating

---

Algorithm 1. Algorithm for the proposed MTL method

Input: Generated features from 3D CNN: X_M^N for M attributes and N examples
         Attributes scores: Y_M^N
Output: Coefficient matrix **W**
1: **Step 1** – **for** each task $i = 1$ to M and each example $j = 1$ to N **do**
            Solve equation (6) to find Ψ
         end for
2: **Step 2** – Formulate objective function as in equation (7)
3: **Step 3** – Use accelerated proximal gradient method to optimize equation (7)
4: **return W**

---

the non-smooth part can help solve the optimization function. Therefore, *accelerated proximal gradient method* [18,19] is employed to solve the Eq. 7. The accelerated proximal method is the first order gradient method with a complexity of $O(1/k^2)$, where k is the iteration counter. Note that in Eq. 7, the ℓ_1-norm comprises the non-smooth part and the proximal operator is used for its estimation. The steps in the proposed approach are summarized in Algorithm 1.

4   Experiments

4.1   Data

For evaluating our proposed approach, we used LIDC-IDRI dataset from Lung Image Database Consortium [3], which is one of the largest publicly available lung cancer screening datasets. There were 1018 CT scans in the dataset, where the slice thickness varied from 0.45 mm to 5.0 mm. The nodules having diameters larger than or equal to 3 mm were annotated by at most four radiologists.

The nodules which were annotated by at least three radiologists were used for the evaluations. There were 1340 nodules satisfying this criterion. We used the mean malignancy and attribute scores of different radiologists for experiments. The nodules have ratings corresponding to malignancy and the other six attributes which are (i) calcification, (ii) lobulation, (iii) spiculation, (iv) sphericity, (v) margin and (vi) texture. The malignancy ratings varied from 1 to 5 where 1 indicated benign and 5 represented highly malignant nodules. We excluded nodules with an average score equal to 3 to account for the indecision among the radiologists. Our final dataset consisted of 635 benign and 509 malignant nodules for classification. The images were resampled to have 0.5 mm spacing in each dimension.

4.2   Results

We used the 3D CNN trained on Sports-1M dataset [15] which had 487 classes. We fine-tuned the network using samples from lung nodule dataset. In order to generate the binary labels for the six attributes and the malignancy, we used the center point and gave positive (or negative) labels to samples having scores greater (or lesser) than the center point. In the context of our work, tasks represented six attributes and malignancy. We fine-tuned the network with these 7 tasks and performed 10 fold cross validation. By fine-tuning the network, we circumvented the need to have a large amount of training data. Since the 3D network was trained on image sequences with 3 channels and with at least 16 frames, we replicated the same gray level axial channel for the other two. Moreover, we also ensured that all input volumes have 16 slices by interpolation when necessary. We used the 4096-dimensional output from the first fully connected layer of the 3D CNN as a feature representation.

Table 1. Classification accuracy and mean absolute score difference of the proposed multi-task learning method in comparison with the other methods.

Methods	Accuracy	Mean score diff.
GIST features with LASSO	76.83%	0.6753
3D CNN MTL with trace norm	80.08%	0.6259
Proposed method (Eq. 7)	**91.26%**	**0.4593**

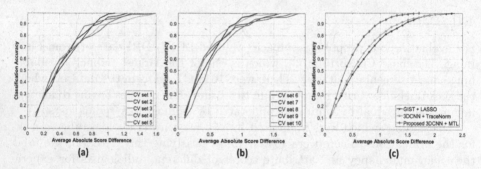

Fig. 3. Plots to show classification accuracy against various threshold values for average absolute score difference. The graphs in (a) and (b) represent results from 10 different cross validation (CV) sets. It can be seen that the classification accuracy increases, as we increase the threshold value for absolute score difference. The graph (c) shows the improved performance of the proposed method in comparison with GIST+LASSO and 3DCNN with Trace Norm.

To find the structure matrix S, we computed the correlation between tasks by finding an initial normalized coefficient matrix **W** using lasso with least square loss function and followed by computing the correlation coefficient matrix [17]. We then apply a threshold on the correlation coefficient matrix to obtain a binary graph structure matrix. For testing, we multiply the features from network trained on malignancy with the corresponding coefficient vector W to obtain the score.

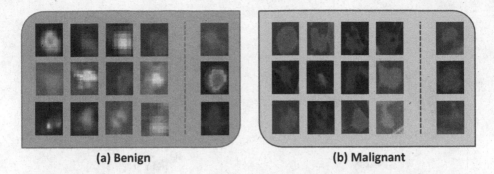

(a) Benign   (b) Malignant

Fig. 4. Qualitative results using our proposed approach. (a) and (b) show axial views of benign and malignant nodules respectively, where first three columns consist of successful cases (where prediction was within ±1 of the expert score) and the last column (after dotted line) shows failure cases.

For evaluation, we used metrics for both classification and regression. We calculated classification accuracy by considering classification to be successful if the predicted score lies in ±1 of the true score. We also reported average absolute score difference between the predicted score and the true score. Table 1 shows the comparison of our proposed Multi-task learning method with GIST features [20] +LASSO and 3D CNN Multi-task learning with trace norm. Our proposed graph regularized MTL outperforms the other methods with a significant margin. Our approach improves the classification accuracy over GIST features by about 15% and over trace norm regularization by 11%. Moreover, the average absolute score difference reduces by 32% and 27% when compared with GIST and trace norm respectively.

We also plotted classification accuracy against different thresholds for average absolute score difference. Figure 3(a) and (b) show the plot on different cross-validation sets. It can be noticed that across different validation sets, the predicted malignancy scores of around 70% of the nodules lie within a margin of ±0.6 which increases to around 90% when ±1 margin is used. Figure 3(c) shows the comparison with the other methods, where the proposed approach outperforms them over all values of average absolute score difference. Figure 4 shows the qualitative results from our proposed approach.

In order to evaluate the significance of transfer learning via fine-tuning, we project the features onto a low dimensional space. This is done by computing the proximity, between boundary points using t-distributed stochastic neighborhood embedding (t-SNE) [21]. As our feature space is high dimensional (4096-dimension), t-SNE is useful in revealing the structure of data at different scales. It can be seen in Fig. 5 that fine-tuning the network on the lung nodule dataset distinctively improves the separation between benign and malignant classes.

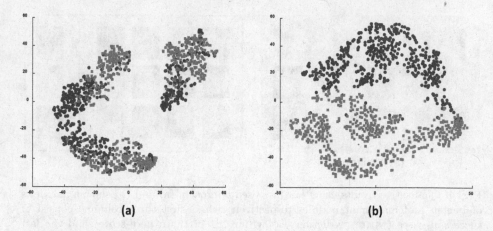

Fig. 5. Effect of fine-tuning on 3D CNN features. t-SNE visualization for features obtained from (a) pre-trained network and (b) network after fine-tuning. Separation between features belonging to two classes, i.e. benign nodules (represented in blue) and malignant nodules (shown in red) can be readily observed in (b). (Color figure online)

5   Discussion and Conclusion

In this work, we proposed a framework to stratify the malignancy of lung nodules using 3D CNN and graph regularized sparse multi-task learning. To the best of our knowledge, this is for the first time, transfer learning is employed over 3D CNN to improve lung nodule characterization. The task of data collection, especially in medical imaging fields, is highly regulated and the availability of experts for annotating these images is restricted. In this scenario, leveraging on the availability of crowdsourced and annotated data such as user captured videos can be instrumental in training discriminative models. However, given the diversity in data from these two domains (i.e. medical and non-medical user collected videos), it is vital to perform transfer learning from source domain (user collected videos) to the target domain (medical imaging data). To establish this observation and to visualize features, we used t-SNE to project high dimensional features onto a low dimensional space (2D space), where the separation between classes was evident in the case of transfer learning.

Moreover, in this work, we also empirically explored the importance of high-level nodule attributes such as calcification, sphericity, lobulation and others to improve malignancy determination. Rather than manually determining these attributes we used 3D CNN to learn discriminative features corresponding to these attributes. The 3D CNN based features from these attributes are fused in a graph regularized sparse multi-task learning.

Another important imaging modality for lung nodule diagnosis is Positron Emission Tomography (PET). It has been found that the combination of PET and CT can improve the diagnostic accuracy of solitary lung nodules [22]. With the increase in the availability of PET/CT scanners, our future work will involve their utilization for simultaneous detection and characterization of pulmonary nodules.

References

1. Stewart, B., Wild, C.P., et al.: World Cancer Report 2014. World, Mountain View (2016)
2. van Beek, E.J., Mirsadraee, S., Murchison, J.T.: Lung cancer screening: computed tomography or chest radiographs? World J. Radiol. **7**(8), 189 (2015)
3. Armato III, S., McLennan, G., Bidaut, L., McNitt-Gray, M.F., Meyer, C.R., Reeves, A.P., Zhao, B., Aberle, D.R., Henschke, C.I., Hoffman, E.A., et al.: The lung image database consortium (LIDC) and image database resource initiative (IDRI): a completed reference database of lung nodules on CT scans. Med. Phys. **38**(2), 915–931 (2011)
4. Shin, H., Roth, H.R., Gao, M., Lu, L., Xu, Z., Nogues, I., Yao, J., Mollura, D., Summers, R.M.: Deep convolutional neural networks for computer-aided detection: CNN architectures, dataset characteristics and transfer learning. IEEE Trans. Med. Imaging **35**(5), 1285–1298 (2016)
5. Tran, D., Bourdev, L., Fergus, R., Torresani, L., Paluri, M.: Learning spatiotemporal features with 3D convolutional networks. In: 2015 IEEE International Conference on Computer Vision (ICCV), pp. 4489–4497. IEEE (2015)
6. Uchiyama, Y., Katsuragawa, S., Abe, H., Shiraishi, J., Li, F., Li, Q., Zhang, C.T., Suzuki, K., Doi, K.: Quantitative computerized analysis of diffuse lung disease in high-resolution computed tomography. Med. Phys. **30**(9), 2440–2454 (2003)
7. El-Baz, A., Nitzken, M., Khalifa, F., Elnakib, A., Gimel'farb, G., Falk, R., El-Ghar, M.A.: 3D shape analysis for early diagnosis of malignant lung nodules. In: Székely, G., Hahn, H.K. (eds.) IPMI 2011. LNCS, vol. 6801, pp. 772–783. Springer, Heidelberg (2011). doi:10.1007/978-3-642-22092-0_63
8. Han, F., Wang, H., Zhang, G., Han, H., Song, B., Li, L., Moore, W., Lu, H., Zhao, H., Liang, Z.: Texture feature analysis for computer-aided diagnosis on pulmonary nodules. J. Digit. Imaging **28**(1), 99–115 (2015)
9. Way, T.W., Hadjiiski, L.M., Sahiner, B., Chan, H.P., Cascade, P.N., Kazerooni, E.A., Bogot, N., Zhou, C.: Computer-aided diagnosis of pulmonary nodules on CT scans: segmentation and classification using 3D active contours. Med. Phys. **33**(7), 2323–2337 (2006)
10. Lee, M., Boroczky, L., Sungur-Stasik, K., Cann, A., Borczuk, A., Kawut, S., Powell, C.: Computer-aided diagnosis of pulmonary nodules using a two-step approach for feature selection and classifier ensemble construction. Artif. Intell. Med. **50**(1), 43–53 (2010)
11. Kumar, D., Wong, A., Clausi, D.A.: Lung nodule classification using deep features in CT images. In: 2015 12th Conference on Computer and Robot Vision (CRV), pp. 133–138. IEEE (2015)
12. Buty, M., Xu, Z., Gao, M., Bagci, U., Wu, A., Mollura, D.J.: Characterization of lung nodule malignancy using hybrid shape and appearance features. In: Ourselin, S., Joskowicz, L., Sabuncu, M.R., Unal, G., Wells, W. (eds.) MICCAI 2016. LNCS, vol. 9900, pp. 662–670. Springer, Cham (2016). doi:10.1007/978-3-319-46720-7_77
13. Chen, S., Ni, D., Qin, J., Lei, B., Wang, T., Cheng, J.-Z.: Bridging computational features toward multiple semantic features with multi-task regression: a study of CT pulmonary nodules. In: Ourselin, S., Joskowicz, L., Sabuncu, M.R., Unal, G., Wells, W. (eds.) MICCAI 2016. LNCS, vol. 9901, pp. 53–60. Springer, Cham (2016). doi:10.1007/978-3-319-46723-8_7
14. Furuya, K., Murayama, S., Soeda, H., Murakami, J., Ichinose, Y., Yauuchi, H., Katsuda, Y., Koga, M., Masuda, K.: New classification of small pulmonary nodules by margin characteristics on highresolution CT. Acta Radiol. **40**(5), 496–504 (1999)

15. Karpathy, A., Toderici, G., Shetty, S., Leung, T., Sukthankar, R., Fei-Fei, L.: Large-scale video classification with convolutional neural networks. In: Proceedings of the IEEE Conference on Computer Vision and Pattern Recognition, pp. 1725–1732 (2014)

16. Evgeniou, T., Pontil, M.: Regularized multi-task learning. In: Proceedings of the Tenth ACM SIGKDD International Conference on Knowledge Discovery and Data Mining, pp. 109–117. ACM (2004)

17. Zhou, J., Chen, J., Ye, J.: MALSAR: multi-task learning via structural regularization (2012)

18. Nesterov, Y.: Introductory Lectures on Convex Optimization: A Basic Course, vol. 87. Springer Science & Business Media, Berlin (2013)

19. Parikh, N., Boyd, S., et al.: Proximal algorithms. Found. Trends® Optim. **1**(3), 127–239 (2014)

20. Oliva, A., Torralba, A.: Modeling the shape of the scene: a holistic representation of the spatial envelope. Int. J. Comput. Vis. **42**(3), 145–175 (2001)

21. van der Maaten, L., Hinton, G.: Visualizing data using t-SNE. J. Mach. Learn. Res. **9**(Nov), 2579–2605 (2008)

22. Wang, Y.X.J., Gong, J.S., Suzuki, K., Morcos, S.K.: Evidence based imaging strategies for solitary pulmonary nodule. J. Thorac. Dis. **6**(7), 872–887 (2014)

Brain Networks and Connectivity

Topographic Regularity for Tract Filtering in Brain Connectivity

Junyan Wang[1], Dogu Baran Aydogan[1], Rohit Varma[2], Arthur W. Toga[1], and Yonggang Shi[1(✉)]

[1] Laboratory of Neuro Imaging (LONI),
USC Stevens Neuroimaging and Informatics Institute,
Keck School of Medicine of University of Southern California,
Los Angeles, CA 90033, USA
yshi@loni.usc.edu
[2] Department of Ophthalmology, USC Roski Eye Institute,
Keck School of Medicine of University of Southern California,
Los Angeles, CA 90033, USA

Abstract. The preservation of the spatial relationships among axonal pathways has long been studied and known to be critical for many functions of the brain. Being a fundamental property of the brain connections, there is an intuitive understanding of topographic regularity in neuroscience but yet to be systematically explored in connectome imaging research. In this work, we propose a general mathematical model for topographic regularity of fiber bundles that is consistent with its neuroanatomical understanding. Our model is based on a novel group spectral graph analysis (GSGA) framework motivated by spectral graph theory and tensor decomposition. GSGA provides a common set of eigenvectors for the graphs formed by topographic proximity measures whose preservation along individual tracts in return is modeled as topographic regularity. To demonstrate the application of this novel measure of topographic regularity, we apply it to filter fiber tracts from connectome imaging. Using large-scale data from the Human Connectome Project (HCP), we show that our novel algorithm can achieve better performance than existing methods on the filtering of both individual bundles and whole brain tractograms.

1 Introduction

Tractography is an essential tool in studying human brain connectomes using diffusion MRI (dMRI). It has been successfully applied to reconstruct important anatomical bundles and connectivity matrices for graph-based assessment of brain connectivity [1]. On the other hand, it is also well-known that tractography tends to generate a large number of false positives and false negatives [2]. While various tract filtering and clustering methods have been proposed, they

Y. Shi—This work was in part supported by NIH grants R01EB022744, U01EY025864, K01EB013633, P41EB015922, U54EB020406, R01MH094343, and Research to Prevent Blindness.

© Springer International Publishing AG 2017
M. Niethammer et al. (Eds.): IPMI 2017, LNCS 10265, pp. 263–274, 2017.
DOI: 10.1007/978-3-319-59050-9_21

are usually driven by the geometry of fiber tracts rather than their biological relevance [3,4]. In addition, these methods rely heavily on the fine tuning of distance measures between tracts and heuristic selection of multiple parameters to achieve desired performance. Motivated by the wide presence of the topography-preserving property of anatomical connections in mammalian brains [5], we propose in this work a novel computational framework for tract filtering by measuring the topographic regularity of fiber tracts. Our method only involves the local analysis of topographic regularity and is generally applicable to both the reconstruction of individual fiber bundles and whole brain processing.

Topographic regularity is a common property in many brain networks [5]. The retinotopic organization of axons in the visual system, which involves almost half of the human brain, is an excellent demonstration of this property [6]. The retinotopy in the optic radiation is well-known from post-mortem studies [7]. Recent functional MRI studies showed that retinotopy is also followed in various pathways related to visual functions [5]. The somatotopic organization of the motor and sensory pathways [8], and the tonotopic organization of the auditory pathways [9] are also well-known examples where the fiber pathways follow a topography-preserving trajectory when they transmit sensory inputs to the cortical regions. Using data from tracer injection studies on macaque brains, the topographic organization of cortical connections to the striatum were also shown recently [10]. These regularities in brain pathways have great synergy to the recent proposition about the grid structure of fiber pathways [11].

While the topographic organization of brain pathways is a general principle, it has yet to be thoroughly investigated in tractography-based connectivity studies. A novel tractography-algorithm based on this principle was developed recently to model the topography-preserving connectomes in human brains [12]. In this work, we tackle the problem from a different perspective. We assume the fiber tracts have been generated from an arbitrary tractography algorithm and then filter the tracts based on their topographic regularity. Using tools from tensor decomposition, we quantify how topography is preserved as we traverse along each fiber tract. In contrast to the clustering approach that parcellate tracts into bundles, our method evaluates each tract separately by studying its topographic relation to a small set of neighboring tracts. In our experiments, we compare with spectral clustering methods, and demonstrate that our method can better improve the retinotopy of visual pathways and remove outlier tracts in whole brain tractography results.

2   Methods

2.1   Mathematical Definitions and Topographic Regularity

In neuroscience, topographic mapping is generally defined as: *point-to-point or region to region axonal connections that preserve spatial relationship between neurons* [5,13]. This definition implies that while nearby neurons are connecting to

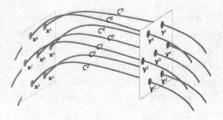

Fig. 1. An example of a topographically regular bundle with the mathematical notation used in this work.

other nearby neurons, the spatial relationships among their projection trajectories do not vary. In this paper, we mathematically model this neuroanatomical property and apply it to filter tracts obtained using dMRI based tractography (Fig. 1). Below we describe our framework and definitions needed to mathematically study topographic regularity within this context.

Definition 1 (Fiber tract). *A **fiber tract**, or streamline, denoted as $C = \{\mathbf{x}_i \in \mathbb{R}^3 | 0 \le i \le L\}$ is a finite set of evenly spaced points along a curve.*

Definition 2 (Tractogram). *A **tractogram**, $\mathcal{T}$, is a set of fiber tracts, $\mathcal{T} = \{C^0, C^1, C^2, \cdots \}$.*

Definition 3 (n-tract neighborhood). *Given a fiber tract in a tractogram, $C^0 \in \mathcal{T}$, the n-**tract neighborhood of** C^0, is the set of n spatially closest fiber tracts to C^0, including itself, and denoted by $\mathcal{N}_{C^0} = \{C^0, C^1, C^2, \cdots, C^{n-1}\}$.*

In this work, we define the distance from tract C^k to tract C^l as the 1-sided Hausdorff distance, that is:

$$d_{\mathcal{H}}(C^k, C^l) = \max_{\mathbf{x}_i^k \in C^k} \inf_{x_j^l \in C^l} \|\mathbf{x}_i^k - \mathbf{x}_j^l\| \tag{1}$$

where $\|\mathbf{x}_i^k - \mathbf{x}_j^l\|$ is the Euclidean distance between $\mathbf{x}_i^k$ and $\mathbf{x}_j^l$. $\mathbf{x}_i^k \in C^k$, is the ith point on the kth fiber tract.

Definition 4 (n-point neighborhood). *Given a fiber tract, C^0, its n-tract neighborhood $\mathcal{N}_{C^0} = \{C^0, C^1, C^2, \cdots, C^{n-1}\}$, and a point $\mathbf{x}_i^0 \in C^0$, the n-**point neighborhood of** $\mathbf{x}_i^0$ is defined as the set $\mathcal{N}_{\mathbf{x}_i^0} = \{\mathbf{x}_i^0, \mathbf{x}_i^1, \mathbf{x}_i^2, \cdots, \mathbf{x}_i^{n-1}\}$ such that $\mathbf{x}_i^k$, $k \in [1, 2, \ldots, n-1]$ is the spatially closest points to $\mathbf{x}_i^0$ on tract C^k.*

Based on the n-point neighborhood, we can define the proximity measure between every pair of points within an n-point neighborhood as follows.

Definition 5 (Topographic proximity measure). *Given an n-point neighborhood of C^0 around a point $\mathbf{x}_i^0 \in C^0$, we propose a measure of proximity between any pairs of $\{\mathbf{x}_i^k, \mathbf{x}_i^l\} \in \mathcal{N}_{\mathbf{x}_i^0}$ as follows:*

$$\rho(\mathbf{x}_i^k, \mathbf{x}_i^l) = e^{-d(\mathbf{x}_i^k, \mathbf{x}_j^k)/\sigma^2} \tag{2}$$

where σ is a model parameter and d is the normalized Euclidean distance computed as:

$$d(\mathbf{x}_i^k, \mathbf{x}_j^k) = \frac{\|\mathbf{x}_i^k - \mathbf{x}_i^l\|}{\max_{\{\mathbf{x}_i^k - \mathbf{x}_i^l\} \in \mathcal{N}_{\mathbf{x}_i^0}} \|\mathbf{x}_i^k - \mathbf{x}_i^l\|}. \tag{3}$$

*We call ρ the **topographic proximity measure**. In addition, we can define an $n \times n$ matrix $E_{\mathbf{x}_i^0}$ with elements $E_{\mathbf{x}_i^0}(k, l) = \rho(\mathbf{x}_i^k, \mathbf{x}_i^l)$, and $E_{\mathbf{x}_i^0}$ is called the **topographic proximity matrix** for the n-point neighborhood of $\mathbf{x}_i^0$.*

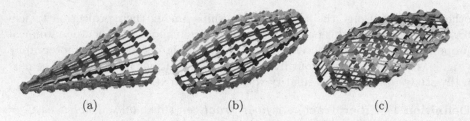

(a)   (b)   (c)

Fig. 2. Topographically regular bundles with invariant affinity graphs.

Note that the distance measure Eq. (3) and the topographic proximity measure Eq. (2) are rotation and translation-invariant. Besides, because of the normalization, they are scale-invariant as well. For example, for the fibers in Figs. 2(a) and (b) their topographic proximity matrices along the bundle are all identical despite the linear and nonlinear scaling. The twisting fiber bundle shown in Fig. 2(b) will also yield identical topographic proximity measures along the bundle due to the rotation invariance property. These properties agree with the topographic regularity concept in neuroanatomy. Finally we can define topographic regularity as follows:

Definition 6 (Topographic regularity). *A fiber tract C is **topographically regular** if $\Delta(E_\mathbf{x}) = 0 \quad \forall \mathbf{x} \in C$ or equivalently $\mathcal{E}_{TGR} = 1 - mean(\Delta(E_\mathbf{x})) = 1 \quad \forall \mathbf{x} \in C$. Here $0 \leq \Delta() \leq 1$ is called **topographic variation measure** and $\mathcal{E}_{TGR}$ is called **topographic regularity measure**.*

Our definition above interprets the neuroanatomical definition by quantifying the "spatial relationship between neuronal fibers" and the "preservation" of such relationship. We will clarify the mathematic definition of topographic variation and topographic regularity in the following section.

2.2   Spectral Graph Analysis for Modeling Topographic Regularity

To define the variation of the topographic proximity matrices along any fiber, we should first quantify the distance between any two of such matrices. A topographic proximity matrix can be viewed as an affinity matrix of a graph formed by points within an n-point neighborhood of certain point on a fiber tract. In the literature of graph matching [14], it is often argued that the distance between the graph affinity matrices can be captured by the distance between the eigenvalues of their affinity matrices. In the following, we will exploit this idea.

Suppose we have two topographic proximity matrices, E_X and E_Y. The distance between them can be written as:

$$\Delta_S(E_X, E_Y) = \|E_X - E_Y\|_F = \|S_X - S_Y\|_F, \tag{4}$$

where S_X and S_Y are eigenvalue matrices of E_X and E_Y, $\|\cdot\|_F$ is the Frobenius norm. The last equality holds true if and only if the two matrices share the same set of eigenvectors. Eigenvalues for graphs are also known as the graph spectrum,

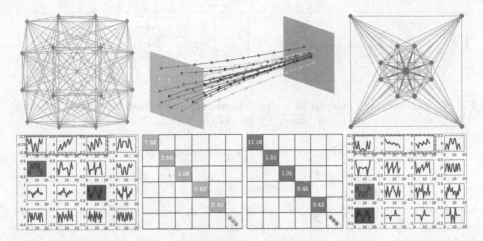

Fig. 3. Spectral graph analysis for nonrigidly deformed topographically regular bundle. The eigenvectors are arranged according to the magnitude of eigenvalues. The most dominant eigenvectors are shown at top left and the sequence goes from left to right and then top to bottom. (Color figure online)

and the associated analysis resides in the area of spectral graph theory [15]. However, graphs with identical spectra, namely isospectral/cospectral graphs, can be structurally distinct from each other. We refer the interested readers to [15] for details on this topic. Accordingly, we turn to look at the eigenvectors for graph modeling.

Eigenvectors have been proven critical in modeling graph structures in graph visualization [16] and graph partitioning [17]. We further demonstrate the characteristics of eigenvectors in modeling topographical regularity via an example illustrated in Fig. 3. In this example, we first generate a non-rigidly distorted yet topographically regular fiber bundle, as shown in the top middle of Fig. 3. For the point cloud at the two ends of the bundle we can define the topographic proximity matrices, which form two graphs as shown at the top left and top right of Fig. 3. The sorted eigenvalues and their associated eigenvectors to each graph are shown underneath the respective graphs. We can observe that the eigenvalues are different and difficult to compare, while there is some obvious analogy in the top eigenvectors (highlighted by the dashed boxes). In addition, we also found two pairs of identical eigenvectors from their eigenvector sets. We have highlighted the identical eigenvector pairs in red and blue.

In Fig. 4, we show another example of spectral analysis for a simple topographically irregular bundle. We only present the ends points due to limitted space. Because of the presence of a noisy fiber, we can observe a slight structural difference in the two graphs. After spectral analysis of the corresponding topographic proximity matrices, we observe certain minor differences in the eigenvalues of the two graphs. In addition, we observe that the top eigenvectors are identical while the last few eigenvectors are drastically different (magnitudes of their peaks and valleys do not match). These observations motivate us to model the topographical regularity using eigenvectors.

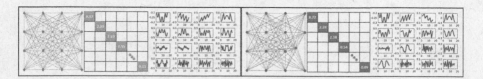

Fig. 4. Spectral graph analysis for a simple topographically irregular bundle. Left and right panels correspond to the two end points of the bundle. (Color figure online)

Intuitively, we consider the following matrix distance based on eigenvectors:

$$\Delta_{U_Y}(E_X, E_Y) = \inf_{\mathbf{off}(S_X)=0} \|E_X - U_Y S_X U_Y^T\|_F \tag{5}$$

where $\mathbf{off}(A)$ is the off diagonal part of A, U_Y is the matrix formed by eigenvectors of E_Y, and $\Delta_{U_Y}(E_X, E_Y)$ measures how well the eigenvectors of E_Y can be used to decompose E_X. This distance measure is not symmetric, i.e., $\Delta_{U_Y}(E_X, E_Y) \neq \Delta_{U_X}(E_X, E_Y)$, and, hence, it is biased. One way to symmetrize the measure is to use the $\Delta_{U_Y}(E_X, E_Y) + \Delta_{U_X}(E_X, E_Y)$. This method requires computing Eq. (5) $(L-1)$ times for any point along a tract consisting of L points. Therefore, it does not scale well for measuring topographic regularity of fiber tracts in massive tractograms. Alternatively, we adopt the following model:

$$\Delta_U(E_X, E_Y) \doteq \inf_{\mathbf{off}(S_X)=0} \|E_X - U S_X U^T\|_F + \inf_{\mathbf{off}(S_Y)=0} \|E_X - U S_Y U^T\|_F \tag{6}$$

where U is a matrix formed by a set of *common eigenvectors* for E_X and E_Y. This method requires computing Eq. (5) only once for a point. It will be $(L-1)$ times faster than the aforementioned exhaustive approach.

This formulation is closely related to simultaneous diagonalization [18] which is a special case of Tucker tensor decomposition [19]. These methods try to find the optimal eigenvectors and eigenvalues at the same time, while our idea is slightly different in that we are more interested in the common eigenvectors and we consider the projected eigenvalues from the common eigenvectors as a byproduct, which greatly simplifies the computation.

Given a tract $C = \{\mathbf{x}_1, \cdots, \mathbf{x}_L\}$, we can collect the topographic proximity matrices for all $\mathbf{x}_i \in C$ as a 3rd-order tensor $\mathbf{E} = \{E_{\mathbf{x}_i} | 1 \leq i \leq L\}$. To extract the common eigenvectors for the tensor $\mathbf{E}$, we adopt the following model:

$$\mathbf{u}^* = \operatorname*{argmax}_{\mathbf{u}} = \sum_i \|E_i \mathbf{u}\|_F^2, \quad \text{s.t. } \mathbf{u}^T \mathbf{u} = 1 \tag{7}$$

where we used E_i as a simplified notation for $E_{\mathbf{x}_i}$.

The intuition behind the above model is that we try to find the unit vector which is most similar to all the column vectors in the tensor. Since the column vectors are the topographic proximity measures, the optimal unit vector shall capture the dominant topographic proximity representation.

By differentiating the model and applying Lagrange multiplier, the optimal solution of the above is defined by:

$$\Sigma \mathbf{u}^* = \lambda \mathbf{u}^*, \ \Sigma = \begin{bmatrix} E_1^T E_1 \ E_2^T E_2 \ \cdots \ E_L^T E_L \end{bmatrix}. \tag{8}$$

Input : Tractogram $\mathcal{T} = \{C^1, C^2, C^3 ..., C^M\}$, Neighborhood size K, Threshold ratio η, parameter of topographic proximity measure σ

Output: Fiber Selection Label $\Phi = \{\phi_1, \phi_2, \phi_3 ..., \phi_M\}$

1 **foreach** $C^m \in \mathbf{X}$ **do**
2       $\mathbf{E}^m \leftarrow$ NeighborGraphConstruction$(C^m, \mathcal{T}, K, \sigma)$;
3       $\Sigma^m \leftarrow$ Eq. (9);
4   Λ, $U \leftarrow$ SVD (Σ^m); % By Eq. (9);
5       $k_{min} \leftarrow \mathrm{argmin}_k \{\Lambda(k) | k = 1, 2, ..., K\}$;
6       $\mathbf{u}^* \leftarrow U[:, k_{min}]$;
7       $S_i^{m*} \leftarrow \mathbf{diag}(\mathbf{u}^{*T} E_i^m \mathbf{u}^*)$; % By Eq. (11);
8       $\mathcal{E}_{TGR}^m \leftarrow \frac{1}{L_m} \sum_{i=1}^{L_m} \|S_i^{m*}\|_F / \|E_i^m\|_F$;% By Eq. (14);
9 **end**
10 $P \leftarrow$ CumulativeDensityEstimation$(\{\mathcal{E}_{TGR}^1, \mathcal{E}_{TGR}^2, \cdots, \mathcal{E}_{TGR}^M\})$;
11 **foreach** $C^m \in \mathcal{T}$ **do**
12       $\phi_m \leftarrow \mathbf{bool}(P(\mathcal{E}_{TGR}^m) < \eta)$;
13 **end**

Algorithm 1. Topographic regularity modeling of tractogram.

We shall call Eq. (7) *group spectral graph model* (GSGM). The above formulation also generalizes to multiple orthogonal vectors, and the optimal solution U^* is defined by:

$$\Sigma U^* = \Lambda^* U^*, \quad U^{*T} U^* = I \tag{9}$$

where I is identity matrix, Λ^* is the diagonal matrix from Lagrange multipliers and it becomes the eigenvalue matrix when the equality holds true. We shall call the optimal solution U^* the common eigenvectors of the tensor $\mathbf{E}$. And we shall call Eq. (9) group spectral graph analysis (GSGA).

With the common eigenvectors, we can solve the back-projected eigenvalues:

$$S_i^* = \underset{S_i}{\mathrm{argmin}} \|E_i - U^* S_i U^{*T}\|_F^2, \quad \text{s.t. } \mathbf{off}(S_i) = 0 \tag{10}$$

where $\mathbf{off}(S_i)$ is the off diagonal part of S_i. Note that $\|E_i - U^* S_i U^{*T}\|_F^2 = \|U^{*T} E_i U^* - S_i\|_F^2 = \|\mathbf{diag}(U^{*T} E_i U^* - S_i) + \mathbf{off}(U^{*T} E_i U^*)\|_F^2$, where $\mathbf{diag}(\cdot)$ extracts the diagonal elements from the matrix that it operates on. The last equality is a basic property of Frobenius norm, i.e. $\|A\|_F^2 = \sum_{ij} |a_{ij}|^2 = \sum_i |a_{ii}|^2 + \sum_{i \neq j} |a_{ij}|^2$. Resultantly,

$$S_i^* = \mathbf{diag}(U^{*T} E_i U^*) \tag{11}$$

Based on Eq. (6) and the above derivations, the topographic variation measure for the fiber tract C can be formulated as:

$$\Delta(E_i) = \frac{\|E_i - U^* S_i^* U^{*T}\|_F}{\|E_i\|_F}, \quad i = 1, \cdots, L \tag{12}$$

where the matrix distance is normalized for scale invariance. The topographic regularity measure can then be computed as:

$$\mathcal{E}_{TGR} = 1 - \frac{1}{L} \sum_i^L \Delta(E_i). \tag{13}$$

The more regular the fiber bundle is, the higher $\mathcal{E}_{TRG}$ shall be. However, an issue with this formulation is that this form uses the norm of the residual and the residual may contain noise. We alternatively use the following conceptually equivalent yet cleaner formulation.

$$\mathcal{E}_{TGR} = \frac{1}{L}\sum_i \frac{\|U^* S_i^* U^{*T}\|_F}{\|E_i\|_F} = \frac{1}{L}\sum_i \frac{\|S_i^*\|_F}{\|E_i\|_F} \tag{14}$$

The last equality holds because $\|U^* S_i^* U^{*T}\|_F^2 = \mathbf{Tr}(S_i^{*2})$ by definition. Note that $\|E_i\|_F = \|S_i\|_F$ and S_i is the true eigenvalue matrix of E_i. The above measure is essentially the ratio of back-projected eigenvalues against the true eigenvalues.

Regarding eigenvector selection we have the following observation. In Fig. 5, we find that the dominant eigenvectors for each graph in Fig. 3 are also the common eigenvectors from GSGA, while the eigenvectors associated to small eigenvalues in the three cases differ from each other. This means only the common eigenvectors associated to the small eigenvalues can capture the irregularity occurred in the fiber tracts. Therefore, we only use the common eigenvector corresponding to the smallest eigenvalue in the GSGA for the entire fiber. Our algorithm is summarized in Algorithm 1. The first part of the algorithm is GSGA and the second half is regularity ranking and thresholding. The regularity measure we defined in Eq. (14) can be used to rank all the fibers and we shall remove the lowest $\eta \times 100\%$ fibers according to the ranking.

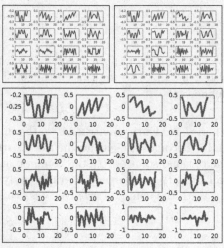

Fig. 5. GSGA for Fig. 4. The top left and top right are the eigenvectors for the orange and green graphs in Fig. 4. Common eigenvectors from GSGA for both of the graphs are shown at the bottom.

3   Experimental Results

We conducted both qualitative and quantitative evaluations to test our technique. In all the experiments we used data from the Q1–Q3 release of the Human Connectome Project (HCP) [20]. For all the experiments we computed fiber orientation distributions (FODs) using the algorithm in [21] and we used the iFOD1 algorithm of MRtrix3 [22] for tractography.

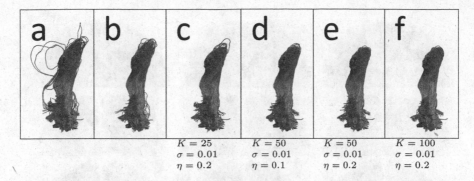

		$K = 25$	$K = 50$	$K = 50$	$K = 100$
		$\sigma = 0.01$	$\sigma = 0.01$	$\sigma = 0.01$	$\sigma = 0.01$
		$\eta = 0.2$	$\eta = 0.1$	$\eta = 0.2$	$\eta = 0.2$

Fig. 6. Example results for filtering visual pathway of subject 100307. (a) is the original optical radiation between V1 and LGN. (b) is the result from spectral clustering. (c)–(f) are results of our method with different parameter settings. K is the neighborhood size, σ is the weight in affinity measure and ρ is the ranking threshold value.

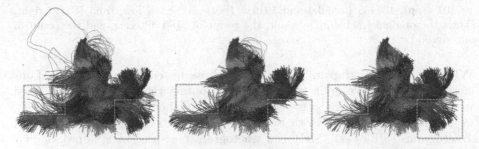

Fig. 7. Example results for optical radiation bundles for subject 106319 viewed near V1. The image on the left is the original bundle, the middle is the result of the conventional spectral clustering based filtering, and the right one is our result. The dashed yellow boxes highlight the differences in the results. (Color figure online)

3.1   Qualitative Evaluation

Visual Pathway Filtering: We reconstructed the optic radiation using the lateral geniculate nucleus (LGN) as *seed* and the primary visual cortex (V1) as the *include* regions. We used step size = 0.1 mm, angle = 6°, cutoff = 0.025, number = 25K as tractography parameters. Spurious fiber tracts were removed according to fiber pairwise distance. Results were obtained using our method and spectral clustering based tract filtering [23] are shown in Fig. 6. We can observe drastic improvements of our method compared to the conventional spectral clustering. We find that the parameter combination of $K = 100$, $\sigma = 0.01$ and $\eta = 0.2$ gives overall the most satisfactory results which we will use in our quantitative evaluations on large-scale HCP datasets.

In addition to outlier tract removal, our method also preserves topographically regular fiber tracts. Representative results are shown in Fig. 7. Our method does not only effectively remove outlier tracts but more importantly it also preserves topographically regular tracts.

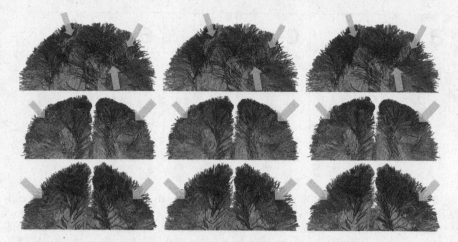

Fig. 8. Tract filtering for whole brain tractography (viewed near frontal lobe) of subject 100307 (top), 100408 (middle) and 101915 (bottom). Each row, from left to right, shows the original tractography result, the result of SIFT filtering, and the result of our method.

Whole Brain Tractogram Filtering: We also tested the applicability of our method on the whole brain tractograms. To obtain the tractograms, we used step size = 0.1 mm, angle = 6°, cutoff = 0.05, number = 100K. In these tests, we compared our method with Spherical-deconvolution Informed Filtering of Tractograms (SIFT) [24]. SIFT is a tractogram post-processing approach that aims to find the best tractogram subset that matches the underlying FOD field. We obtained the SIFT output using the `tcksift` command of MRtrix3. The results are shown in Fig. 8. From areas highlighted by the arrows, we can see that our method is more effective in removing spurious tracts running orthogonal to fibers immersing the cortex, thus significantly improving the topographical regularity in the filtered tracts than the SIFT filtered tractograms.

3.2 Quantitative Evaluation

The retinotopic organization of the visual cortex refers to a point-to-point mapping of the retinal space onto the visual cortex [6]. In [25], an automated technique was developed that assigns each vertex in the visual cortex two coordinates: angle and eccentricity. These coordinates have one-to-one correspondences on the retinal space. By leveraging this anatomical information, Aydogan and Shi recently proposed a validation

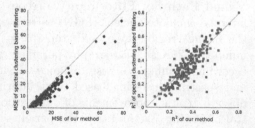

Fig. 9. Quantitative comparison of our method against spectral clustering based filtering for retinotopic organization. The MSE from our method is uniformly smaller and the R^2 values are comparable.

measure of retinotopic organization for visual pathway fiber bundles based on the eccentricity component [12]. They observed that the eccentricity values form a "U" shape function of the cross-section of the optical radiation projecting onto V1. Thus, the goodness-of-fit measures for the quadratic eccentricity regression, such as mean-squared-error (MSE) and coefficient of determination (R^2), are natural measures of topographic regularity for visual pathway fiber bundles. In this experiment, we also adopt these two measures for comparison. For quantitative evaluation we used 215 subjects from the Q1–Q3 release of HCP. The results are shown in Fig. 9. It is observed that our method consistently yields better fits that is measured with MSE. There is no significant difference in fit quality in terms of R^2.

4 Conclusion

In this work, we proposed a mathematical model of topographical regularity for tractograms. Our idea is to establish topographic representation for each point on the fiber and then use its variation to quantify the whole fiber's topographic regularity. Using spectral graph theory and tensor decomposition, we proposed a mathematical topographic regularity definition that is well consistent with its neuroscientific understanding. We applied our model to filter visual pathway and whole brain tractograms obtained using data from HCP subjects. Both qualitative and quantitative evaluations show promising results compared to other filtering approaches. We believe our contribution with this work is significant. We not only translated the well-known neuroanatomical information of topographic regularity to mathematical formulation but also provided a novel tool for filtering tractograms using this definition; which makes our filtering technique fundamentally different compared to other approaches in the literature.

References

1. Bullmore, E.T., Bassett, D.S.: Brain graphs: graphical models of the human brain connectome. Annu. Rev. Clin. Psychol. **7**(1), 113–140 (2011)
2. Thomas, C., Ye, F.Q., Irfanoglu, M.O., Modi, P., Saleem, K.S., Leopold, D.A., Picrpaoli, C.: Anatomical accuracy of brain connections derived from diffusion MRI tractography is inherently limited. Proc. Nat. Acad. Sci. **111**(46), 16574–16579 (2014)
3. O'Donnell, L.J., Westin, C.F.: Automatic tractography segmentation using a high-dimensional white matter atlas. IEEE Trans. Med. Imaging **26**(11), 1562–1575 (2007)
4. Aydogan, D.B., Shi, Y.: Track filtering via iterative correction of TDI topology. In: Navab, N., Hornegger, J., Wells, W.M., Frangi, A.F. (eds.) MICCAI 2015. LNCS, vol. 9349, pp. 20–27. Springer, Cham (2015). doi:10.1007/978-3-319-24553-9_3
5. Patel, G.H., Kaplan, D.M., Snyder, L.H.: Topographic organization in the brain: searching for general principles. Trends Cogn. Sci. **18**(7), 351–363 (2014)
6. Engel, S.A., Glover, G.H., Wandell, B.A.: Retinotopic organization in human visual cortex and the spatial precision of functional MRI. Cereb. Cortex **7**(2), 181–192 (1997)

7. Ebeling, U., Reulen, H.J.: Neurosurgical topography of the optic radiation in the temporal lobe. Acta Neurochir. **92**(1), 29–36 (1988)
8. Ruben, J., Schwiemann, J., Deuchert, M., Meyer, R., Krause, T., Curio, G., Villringer, K., Kurth, R., Villringer, A.: Somatotopic organization of human secondary somatosensory cortex. Cereb. Cortex **11**(5), 463–473 (2001)
9. Morosan, P., Rademacher, J., Schleicher, A., Amunts, K., Schormann, T., Zilles, K.: Human primary auditory cortex: cytoarchitectonic subdivisions and mapping into a spatial reference system. NeuroImage **13**(4), 684–701 (2001)
10. Lehman, J.F., Greenberg, B.D., McIntyre, C.C., Rasmussen, S.A., Haber, S.N.: Rules ventral prefrontal cortical axons use to reach their targets: implications for diffusion tensor imaging tractography and deep brain stimulation for psychiatric illness. J. Neurosci. **31**(28), 10392–10402 (2011)
11. Wedeen, V.J., Rosene, D.L., Wang, R., Dai, G., Mortazavi, F., Hagmann, P., Kaas, J.H., Tseng, W.Y.I.: The geometric structure of the brain fiber pathways. Science **335**(6076), 1628–1634 (2012)
12. Aydogan, D.B., Shi, Y.: Probabilistic tractography for topographically organized connectomes. In: Ourselin, S., Joskowicz, L., Sabuncu, M.R., Unal, G., Wells, W. (eds.) MICCAI 2016. LNCS, vol. 9900, pp. 201–209. Springer, Cham (2016). doi:10.1007/978-3-319-46720-7_24
13. Thivierge, J.P., Marcus, G.F.: The topographic brain: from neural connectivity to cognition. Trends Neurosci. **30**(6), 251–259 (2007)
14. Umeyama, S.: An eigendecomposition approach to weighted graph matching problems. IEEE Trans. Pattern Anal. Mach. Intell. **10**(5), 695–703 (1988)
15. Brouwer, A.E., Haemers, W.H.: Spectra of Graphs. Springer Science & Business Media, Heidelberg (2011)
16. Kruskal, J.B.: Multidimensional scaling by optimizing goodness of fit to a nonmetric hypothesis. Psychometrika **29**(1), 1–27 (1964)
17. Shi, J., Malik, J.: Normalized cuts and image segmentation. IEEE Trans. Pattern Anal. Mach. Intell. **22**(8), 888–905 (2000)
18. Bunse-Gerstner, A., Byers, R., Mehrmann, V.: Numerical methods for simultaneous diagonalization. SIAM J. Matrix Anal. Appl. **14**(4), 927–949 (1993)
19. Tucker, L.R.: Some mathematical notes on three-mode factor analysis. Psychometrika **31**(3), 279–311 (1966)
20. Essen, D.V., Ugurbil, K., et al.: The Human Connectome Project: a data acquisition perspective. NeuroImage **62**(4), 2222–2231 (2012)
21. Tran, G., Shi, Y.: Fiber orientation and compartment parameter estimation from multi-shell diffusion imaging. IEEE Trans. Med. Imaging **34**(11), 2320–2332 (2015)
22. Tournier, J.D., Calamante, F., Connelly, A.: MRtrix: diffusion tractography in crossing fiber regions. Int. J. Imaging Syst. Technol. **22**(1), 53–66 (2012)
23. Kammen, A., Law, M., Tjan, B.S., Toga, A.W., Shi, Y.: Automated retinofugal visual pathway reconstruction with multi-shell HARDI and FOD-based analysis. NeuroImage **125**, 767–779 (2016)
24. Smith, R.E., Tournier, J.D., Calamante, F., Connelly, A.: SIFT: spherical-deconvolution informed filtering of tractograms. NeuroImage **67**, 298–312 (2013)
25. Benson, N.C., Butt, O.H., Datta, R., Radoeva, P.D., Brainard, D.H., Aguirre, G.K.: The retinotopic organization of striate cortex is well predicted by surface topology. Curr. Biol.: CB **22**(21), 2081–2085 (2012)

Riccati-Regularized Precision Matrices
for Neuroimaging

Nicolas Honnorat[(✉)] and Christos Davatzikos

Department of Radiology, University of Pennsylvania, 3700 Hamilton Walk,
Richards Building, 7th Floor, Philadelphia, PA 19104, USA
nicolas.honnorat@uphs.upenn.edu

Abstract. The introduction of graph theory in neuroimaging has provided invaluable tools for the study of brain connectivity. These methods
require the definition of a graph, which is typically derived by estimating
the effective connectivity between brain regions through the optimization
of an ill-posed inverse problem. Considerable efforts have been devoted
to the development of methods extracting sparse connectivity graphs.

The present paper aims at highlighting the benefits of an alternative
approach. We investigate low-rank L2 regularized matrices recently introduced under the denomination of Riccati regularized precision matrices. We demonstrate their benefits for the analysis of cortical thickness
map and the extraction of functional biomarkers from resting state fMRI
scans. In addition, we explain how speed and result quality can be further improved with random projections. The promising results obtained
using the Human Connectome Project dataset, as well as, the numerous possible extensions and applications suggest that Riccati precision
matrices might usefully complement current sparse approaches.

Keywords: rs-fMRI · Precision · Sparse inverse covariance

1 Introduction

Resting-state functional MRI (rs-fMRI) studies of brain connectivity have
received a considerable amount of interest. Thanks to the continuous improvement of imaging techniques and the development of big data infrastructures,
large datasets are now available for conducting these investigations [17]. An
increasing effort has been devoted to the development of mathematical frameworks able to summarize these humongous datasets into robust and concise
causal models and biomarkers, with the hope of better describing cognition,
teasing out the mechanisms underlying brain diseases and defining novel clinical
dimensions [12]. Different measures of connectivity were proposed [18] and graph
theoretical approaches have been widely spread. [2]. The most straightforward
approaches assume that the time series observed during a rs-fMRI scan are generated by a multivariate Gaussian process and attempt to analyze its structure.
These studies typically start with the definition of locations in the gray matter

© Springer International Publishing AG 2017
M. Niethammer et al. (Eds.): IPMI 2017, LNCS 10265, pp. 275–286, 2017.
DOI: 10.1007/978-3-319-59050-9_22

once rs-fMRI have been registered, motion corrected, denoised and normalized. The connectivity between these nodes is measured by computing the covariance of their time series and a sparse graph built from the inverse of the covariance matrix, also known as precision matrix. These last two steps can be performed jointly, by directly estimating sparse precision matrices [6,18,19]. However, and despite very impressive recent development, the estimation of sparse precision matrices is still time-consuming for large matrices [6,11].

In this paper, we propose an alternative approach based on low-rank Riccati regularized precision matrices, introduced first by Witten and Tibshirani [20] and formalized by Honorio and Jaakkola [10]. As for sparse matrices, we measure network characteristics directly from these matrices [16,19]. Our approach offers several benefits such as a very competitive computational efficiency, which deteriorates only linearly with data dimension, straightforward practical and theoretical extensions. We demonstrate that reducing the dimension of the input neuroimaging signals via random projections [9] can simultaneously improve test-retest performances and reduce computational burden, and we present two extensions: the estimation of precision matrices at a population level, and the adaptation of Riccati penalties to regions of interests. These results were established using the data available for the hundred unrelated subjects of the HCP dataset [17]. An in-depth test-retest validation was carried out by reducing the spatial dimension of the resting state fMRI (rs-fMRI) scans with Glasser et al. parcellation [8]. In addition, we demonstrate that our approach can handle full resolution data and other modalities by analyzing cortical thickness maps.

The remainder of the paper is organized as follows. The methods combined in this work are presented in Sect. 2. Section 3 presents several variants of our approach addressing related neuroscience applications. The experimental results are presented in Sect. 4 and discussion concludes the paper.

2 Methods

The random projection method, described in Sect. 2.1, was used as a preprocessing step for reducing the dimensionality of our imaging data and filtering noise. We present, in Sect. 2.2, a generalization of Honorio and Jaakkola Riccati regularized precision matrices [10]. The Gaussian entropy introduced by Tononi, Sporns and Edelman [16] for measuring functional network integration is presented in Sect. 2.3. We used this measure for extracting biomarkers from Riccati regularized precision matrices.

2.1 Random Projection

Random projections were proposed for compressing high-dimensional measurement while preserving their Euclidean distance. The random projections proposed by Halko, Martinsson and Tropp in [9] achieve performances close to a truncated singular value decomposition (TSVD): when a data matrix X of size $N \times T$, $T < N$ is projected for creating a thinner matrix Y of size $N \times t$, $t < T$, the t non-zero singular values of Y are close to the t largest singular values of X. These random projections were proposed to accelerate the computation of singular value decompositions (SVD) [9].

[9] is straightforward to implement. Figure 1 provides the pseudo code of the random projection algorithm used for this work. This algorithm generates an orthogonal projection matrix by randomly combining matrix rows and orthonormalizing the basis obtained through the Gram-Schmidt process. As explained in [9] and reported in Sect. 4.1 for the HCP data, the quality of the projection basis can be significantly improved by running a few power iterations, but the cost of computation grows rapidly with the number of matrix rows.

---

input: data X of size $N \times T$, parameter t and number of power iteration q
1. form the $N \times t$ matrix Ω by sampling from Gaussian distribution $\mathcal{N}(0,1)$
2. $U \leftarrow \left(X^T X\right)^q X^T \Omega$
3. get W by orthonormalizing the columns of U with Gram-Schmidt process
4. $Y \leftarrow XW$
output: projected data Y, of size $N \times t$

Fig. 1. Random projection for dimensionality reduction [9].

2.2 Riccati Regularized Precision Matrices

Let X denote a matrix of size $N \times T$ containing N time series of T time points, normalized to zero mean and unit variance. The associated covariance matrix will be referred as $C = \frac{1}{T} X X^T$. Sparse, Tikhonov and Riccati regularized precision matrices are obtained by solving the following optimization problem:

$$\text{argmax}_{Q \succ 0} \left[\log \ \det Q - \langle C, Q \rangle - \rho R(Q)\right] \tag{1}$$

where an L1 norm is chosen for R for generating sparse precision matrices [19], the trace of Q in the case of Tikhonov regularization [10], and R is the square of the Frobenius norm for Riccati regularized precision matrices [10]. As explained in [10,20], Riccati regularization is a ridge penalty on the components of the precision matrix whereas, when precision matrices are computed for solving a linear regression, Tikhonov regularization corresponds to a ridge penalty on the coefficients of a linear regression. In this work, we generalize the Riccati regularization described in [20] and [10] by introducing an invertible matrix V and working with the penalty:

$$R(Q) = \frac{1}{2} ||VQV^T||_2^2 \tag{2}$$

When V is a diagonal matrix, $V = diag(v)$, the penalty R becomes a squared weighted Frobenius norm, which can be expressed as follows:

$$R(Q) = \frac{1}{2} ||B \odot Q||_2^2 \tag{3}$$

$$B = vv^T \tag{4}$$

where $\odot$ denotes the Hadamard product. This specific case, which is easy to interpret and interesting for applications, will be referred as Hadamard-Riccati regularization.

An analytical solution of (1) is obtained by following the Honorio and Jaakkola derivation [10], which bears similarities with the derivation of the *Scout*(2,.) method of Witten and Tibshirani [20]. More precisely, the extrema of the objective (1) are found by solving:

$$Q^{-1} - C - \rho V^T V Q V^T V = 0 \tag{5}$$

Following [10], Q is obtained as a matrix geometric mean:

$$VQV^T = P = \left(\frac{1}{\rho}D\right) \# \left(D^{-1} + \frac{1}{4\rho}D\right) - \frac{1}{2\rho}D \tag{6}$$

$$\text{where } D = V^{-T}CV^{-1} = (\frac{1}{\sqrt{T}}V^{-T}X)(\frac{1}{\sqrt{T}}V^{-T}X)^T \tag{7}$$

According to the properties of geometric means of matrices $\#$, recalled in [13], the eigenvectors of D are also eigenvectors of P, and an eigenvalue p of P depends only on the eigenvalue d of D associated with the same eigenvector:

$$p(d) = \sqrt{\frac{d}{\rho}\left(\frac{1}{d} + \frac{d}{4\rho}\right)} - \frac{d}{2\rho}. \tag{8}$$

This property leads to the efficient computation of Q presented in Fig. 2. The computation of Hadamard-Riccati regularized precision matrices, for which matrices V are diagonal, is almost as fast as the original [10]. We found that random projections [9] are of prominent interest for the computation of Riccati regularized inverses. First, because they accelerate all the computations by reducing matrices dimensions. Second, because they provide a direct control of the rank of the rank-deficient part of the precision matrix Q. Lastly, because they reduce precision matrices noise by truncating the small singular values of the covariance matrices C. This protective effect is illustrated in Sect. 4.1.

---

input: time series X of size $N \times T$, parameter ρ and $N \times N$ invertible matrix V

1. $[U, S, Z] \leftarrow SVD\left(\frac{1}{\sqrt{T}}V^{-T}X\right)$; U left singular vectors, S contains singular values
2. form diagonal matrix $\Omega = diag(\omega_1, .., \omega_n)$ from singular values $s_1, .., s_m$:
   $$\omega_i = \sqrt{\frac{1}{\rho} + \frac{s_i^4}{4\rho^2}} - \frac{s_i^2}{2\rho} - \frac{1}{\sqrt{\rho}}$$
3. $W \leftarrow V^{-1}U$
4. $Q \leftarrow W\Omega W^T + \frac{1}{\sqrt{\rho}}V^{-1}V^{-T}$

output: Riccati-penalized precision matrix Q

Fig. 2. Computation of Riccati-penalized precision matrix Q, for input time series X, the penalization ρ and a $N \times N$ invertible matrix V.

2.3   Tononi-Sporns-Edelman Entropy

Tononi, Sporns and Edelman introduced a measure of functional integration derived from precision matrices [16]. This measure will be referred as Tononi-Sporns-Edelman entropy (TSEe) in the sequel. Under the standard assumption that functional time series are Gaussian, TSEe measures the Gaussian entropy of a functional networks $\mathcal{N}$ as follows:

$$TSEe(Q, \mathcal{N}) = \frac{1}{2} logdet \left([Q]_{\mathcal{N}} \right) \tag{9}$$

where $[Q]_{\mathcal{N}}$ denotes the restriction of the precision matrix Q to the nodes in the network $\mathcal{N}$. TSEe is a standard measure of functional integration and has already been used for measuring the integration of the networks derived from sparse precision matrices [19]. In this work, TSEe was measured for Riccati regularized precision matrices as well. When the penalty R is constant over the network $\mathcal{N}$, the structure of the Riccati precision matrix can be exploited for accelerating TSEe computation. A constant penalty R over $\mathcal{N}$ corresponds indeed to a matrix V proportional to the identity for the nodes in $\mathcal{N}$:

$$[V]_{\mathcal{N}} = \alpha I \tag{10}$$

Under this assumption and following the notations of Fig. 2:

$$[Q]_{\mathcal{N}} = [W]_{\mathcal{N},:} \, \Omega \, [W]_{\mathcal{N},:}^{T} + \frac{1}{\alpha^2 \sqrt{\rho}} I \tag{11}$$

where $[W]_{\mathcal{N},:}$ denotes the restriction of the rows of W to the nodes in the network $\mathcal{N}$. Because Ω is a diagonal matrix with strictly positive diagonal components the following matrix can be computed in a single pass over $[W]_{\mathcal{N},:}$:

$$\overline{W} = [W]_{\mathcal{N},:} \, \Omega^{1/2} \tag{12}$$

Let s_i denote one of the m singular values of $\overline{W}$ and n the number of nodes of the network $\mathcal{N}$. The left singular vector of $\overline{W}$ associated to s_i is an eigenvector of $[Q]_{\mathcal{N}}$ and the associated eigenvalue λ_i is equal to $s_i^2 + \frac{1}{\alpha^2 \sqrt{\rho}}$. The remaining eigenvectors of $[Q]_{\mathcal{N}}$ are associated with the same eigenvalue: $\frac{1}{\alpha^2 \sqrt{\rho}}$. As a result, TSEe can be computed at the cost of a single SVD, as shown in Fig. 3.

---

input: network $\mathcal{N}$ containing n nodes, Riccati precision matrix
$Q = W \Omega W^T + \frac{1}{\sqrt{\rho}} V^{-1} V^{-T}$ with $[V]_{\mathcal{N}} = \alpha I$, Riccati penalty ρ

1. $\overline{W} \leftarrow [W]_{\mathcal{N},:} \, \Omega^{1/2}$
2. $[U, S, V] \leftarrow SVD(\overline{W})$ where $S = diag(s_1, .., s_m)$ and $m \leq n$ necessarily
3. $TSEe(Q, \mathcal{N}) \leftarrow \frac{(m-n)log(\alpha^4 \rho)}{4} + \frac{1}{2} \sum_{i=1}^{m} log \left(s_i^2 + \frac{1}{\alpha^2 \sqrt{\rho}} \right)$

output: TSEe for the network $\mathcal{N}$

Fig. 3. Efficient computation of the TSEe for constant Riccati penalties.

3   Applications

3.1   Robust Structural Distances

Cortical thickness (CT) is a scalar measured from structural MRI describing local cortical gray matter geometry [1,4]. The structural covariance matrix is obtained by computing CT covariance across a population, for all pairs of brain locations. Large structural covariances indicate that brain regions develop, age or suffer from a disease in similar ways across a population [1]. The inverse of a structural covariance C_S, obtained for a healthy population, can be used for defining a Mahalanobis distance d_S teasing out abnormal CT maps:

$$d_S(a,b) = \sqrt{(a-b)^T C_S^{-1}(a-b)} \tag{13}$$

This distance is small when the difference between CT maps a and b is likely to be observed in the healthy population, whereas large distances correspond to unusual CT variations. In this work, we introduce Riccati regularized structural precision matrices. We show experimentally that regularization and random projections improve structural distance robustness, in Sect. 5.

3.2   Shared Functional Networks

An increasing effort has been dedicated to the extraction of biomarkers capturing the specificities of individual rs-fMRI scans, with the aim of developing rs-fMRI based diagnostic tools. Because these scans are strongly affected by noise and subject motion, several regularization strategies were proposed such as the introduction of population averages [19].

In this work, rather than introducing a group average precision matrix and penalizing the differences between individual scans and the group average [19], we propose to perform a joint SVD (JSVD) when computing Riccati regularized precision matrices. This JSVD forces Riccati regularized precision matrices to share their eigenvectors. As a result, scan specificities are encoded in a reduced set of values, the eigenvalues of the Riccati regularized precision matrices, which can be interpreted as scan-specific loadings. This modeling offers many advantages for investigating neurodevelopment, aging and brain diseases [5,19]. The shared eigenvectors will be referred as shared functional networks in the sequel.

3.3   Functional Network Biomarkers

TSEe is an interesting functional biomarker. However, when small brain networks are investigated TSEe might be corrupted by a noise induced by the random variation of the other components in the precision matrix. To address this issue, we suggest to penalize more the components of the precision matrix corresponding to nodes outside the network of interest. We design a simple penalty to achieve this goal by choosing for V a diagonal matrix equal to the identity when restricted to the nodes of the network and to α times the identity, $\alpha > 1$, when restricted to the other nodes. As explained in Sect. 2.2 such a penalty is an Hadamard-Riccati penalty. When α is increased, this penalty gradually isolates the network of interest from the rest of the brain. As illustrated in Sect. 4.4, this effect can improve test-retest performances for some functional networks.

4   Experimental Validation

4.1   HCP Dataset

All the experiments presented in this work were carried out with the hundred unrelated subjects of the HCP dataset [17]. For each subject, four 15 min long rs-fMRI scans of 1200 time points are available, and several maps describing the local geometry of the cortex such as cortical thickness [7]. We used the rs-fMRI scans processed with the ICA+FIX pipeline with MSMAll registration and the cortical thickness map registered in the 32k Conte69 atlas, also registered with MSMAll [7]. Rs-fMRI scans were bandpass-filtered between 0.05 and 0.1 Hz by an equiripple finite impulse response filter and the first two hundred timepoints impacted by the temporal filtering were discarded. Cortical thickness maps outliers were discarded by thresholding each map independently at ± 4.4478 median absolute deviation from the median. This thresholding can be interpreted as a counterpart of the standard thresholding of Gaussian variable to three standard deviations from the mean robust to the presence of outliers [15]. All the time series and concatenated cortical thickness maps were normalized to zero mean and unit variance. The spatial dimension of the data was reduced by averaging the neuroimaging signals over Glasser et al. multi-modal parcellation [8]. The hundred eighty time series obtained for each hemisphere were normalized again to zero mean and unit variance.

The quality of the random projections (RP) was estimated by (1) concatenating the four rs-fMRI scans of each subject, (2) measuring for each subject the proportion of the squared Frobenius norm of the signal kept by the random projections, and (3) comparing the singular values of the time series before and after random projections. The results presented in Fig. 4 demonstrate that RP behaves almost like a perfect truncated SVD (TSVD) after only three power iterations.

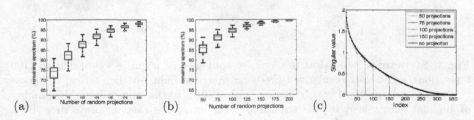

Fig. 4. RP for the functional data. Remaining spectrum for increasing number of random projections (a) without power iterations (b) three power iterations ($q = 3$) (c) For the first subject: singular values before and after random projections ($q = 3$).

The results also suggest that the 4000 timepoints time series can be randomly projected into a dimension 200 with negligible information loss, even without power iterations.

4.2 Robust Structural Distances

Riccati regularized structural precision matrices reliability was measured by the split sample negative log likelihood, a measure decreasing with reproducibility. More precisely, the dataset was randomly split a hundred times into two groups of fifty subjects. For each split, the CT maps of the two groups were concatenated and normalized to zero mean and unit variance separately. A precision matrix Q was computed for the first group and its negative log likelihood was measured by:

$$NLL(Q) = \langle C, Q \rangle - \log \ \det Q \tag{14}$$

where C is the structural covariance obtained from the second group. This test-retest procedure estimates the ability of the precision matrices learned for the first group to fit/generalize to the remaining HCP subjects. The results reported in Fig. 5(a) demonstrate that the reliability of structural precision matrices is improved by TSVD and RP and reaches an optimum at small dimension and for a moderate penalty $\rho = 0.5$. RP and TSVD results are very close, for large dimensions and large penalties. For the sake of simplicity, V was set to the identity for these experiments.

We measured the ability of our method to handle large data by computing structural precision matrices at full Conte69 32 k atlas resolution and both hemisphere simultaneously (59412 nodes total). On a standard office computer running an Intel Core i5-200 CPU 3.3 GHz and 8 Gb RAM, without random projections, the Riccati precisions were obtained in 12.47 s on average (over 100 runs). A random projection to dimension seven followed by the computation of

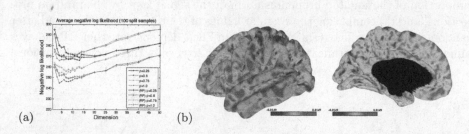

(a)   (b)

Fig. 5. Structural precision (a) Average split sample negative log-likelihood (100 repetitions) of Riccati regularized precision matrices built for the cortical thickness (CT) averaged over the 180 parcellation, with respect to the "dimension": the number of singular values kept by the truncated SVD or by the random projection (RP). Dimension 50 corresponds to the original data, without RP or TSVD. Four different Riccati penalties ρ were tested. (b) one of the seven modes of CT variation obtained at full brain resolution for the left hemisphere, $\rho = 100.0$ and RP into seven dimensions. This map corresponds to a column of the matrix W defined in Fig. 2.

the Riccati precision required 0.28 s on average (over 100 runs) and captured CT variation modes similar to the one presented in Fig. 5(b). By comparison, sparse precision matrices are typically obtained in two hours for 20000 nodes without GPU acceleration [11].

4.3 Shared Functional Networks

The joint SVD (JSVD) method [3] was used in this work for defining shared functional networks. We compared the ability of JSVD, TSVD, and RP to robustly capture individual function by computing first Riccati regularized precision matrices for all the rs-fMRI scans of the hundred unrelated HCP subjects, for different dimensions and penalties ρ. Because functional networks are usually described for correlations or partial correlations, we derived partial correlations from all these precision matrices. We compared the methods by measuring the average intraclass correlation coefficient (ICC) of the partial correlations. We measured if the repeated scans of a single subject were producing partial correlations more similar to each other than scans of different subjects. We measured an $ICC(C, 1)$ [14]. For the sake of simplicity, V was set to the identity for these experiments. The results of Fig. 6(a) clearly demonstrate that JSVD better captures the specificities of subjects brain function.

We checked the reliability/reproducibility of JSVD results by concatenating the first two and last two scans of each subject, computing JSVD, TSVD and RP Riccati regularized matrices for the first scans and measuring the negative log likelihood obtained with the last scans. As indicated in Fig. 6(b), we observed that JSVD matrices generalize slightly less than their TSVD and RP counterparts. These results suggest that a given population is much better described using JSVD, at the cost of a small decrease of generalizability to other populations.

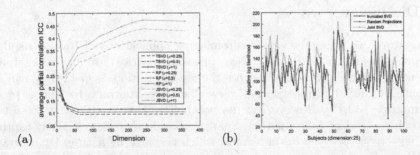

(a)   (b)

Fig. 6. Shared functional networks better capture subject specificities but generalize slightly less. (a) average ICC observed for the partial correlations derived from the Riccati precision matrices of the entire dataset, for different dimensions and penalties ρ. TSVD and RP results differ only at small dimension. (b) for each subject: negative log likelihood of the precision matrices obtained for the first two scans of the subject, evaluated with the last two scans. RP and TSVD results are close. JointSVD precisions, obtained for all the subjects simultaneously, generalize slightly less. The dimension was set to 25 and ρ to 0.25.

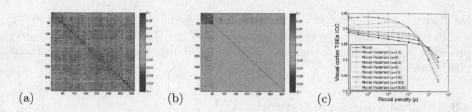

Fig. 7. Biomarkers extracted from Hadamard-Riccati precision matrices. (a) Riccati regularized precision matrix (b) Hadamard Riccati regularized precision matrix (c) Visual cortex TSEe ICC w.r.t Riccati penalties ρ and non ROI suppression α

4.4   Functional Network Biomarkers

TSEe measures the integration of a functional subnetwork, and can, therefore, be considered as a biomarker. We observed that when TSEe is computed for Riccati regularized precision matrices, the test-retest reproducibility of this biomarker can sometimes be improved by penalizing the precisions involving nodes not part of the subnetwork of interest. During our experiments, the visual cortex was considered as the network of interest and we compared the ICC measured for different Riccati Hadamard penalizations. As explained in Sect. 3.3, the vector v defining the Hadamard Riccati penalty was set to 1 for the nodes inside the visual cortex and α for the other nodes. The original Riccati penalty [10] corresponds to $\alpha = 1$. Figure 7(a) and (b) illustrates the effects of parameter α. For large α values, the precisions outside the visual cortex are almost discarded and the Hadamard-Riccati penalization has the same effect as a restriction of the entire analysis to the visual cortex. This effect was beneficial in terms of biomarker ICC for small penalties, and detrimental for large penalties.

5   Discussion

In this work, we present several neuroimaging applications of Riccati regularized precisions matrices. Because these precision matrices are low rank, stored efficiently, and the SVD required for their computation is fast, they can be computed at full brain resolution very efficiently, contrary to sparse precision matrices [10,19]. However, we do not believe that confronting these two approaches would be fully relevant. Sparse precision matrices elegantly capture the connectivity between brain regions, which is sparse by nature. By contrast, Riccati regularized matrices are designed for extracting the connectivity of large graphs where some homogeneity/redundancy is present, and hence suitable for a low-rank description. We could claim that the first approach captures the integration of brain regions, whereas the second exploits the segregation of brain function. For this reason, we think that a combined framework, generating precisions matrices sparse for long range connections and low-rank for small range connections, should ideally leverage the benefits of both approaches.

Because Riccati regularized and Tikhonov regularized precision matrices are computed in a similar fashion [10], their main differences reside in the larger flexibility offered by the Riccati regularized matrices. Contrary to the Tikhonov penalization which acts only on the diagonal of the precision, the Riccati regularization penalizes all the components of the matrix, which offers more freedom for designing penalties. A comparison of the eigenvalue transformation induced by the two penalties also suggest that the information corresponding to the large covariance eigenvalues is slightly better preserved into Riccati regularized precision matrices. The possibility of merging both penalties into a larger analytic framework is an interesting open question.

The experiments presented in this paper have the potential to stimulate novel applications. For instance, similarly to Sect. 3.1, robust structural distances could be derived from the other cortical measures provided by Freesurfer [4] such as areal distortion and cortical curvature, and for HCP myelin maps obtained by combining T1 and T2 weighted MRI scans [7,17]. In addition, we emphasize that, by considering symmetric Riccati penalties only, we have restricted our investigations to optimization problems that can be solved efficiently but we have missed large families of applications. Asymmetric penalties would involve more elaborate algebraic Riccati equations and hopefully stimulate novel neuroimaging applications of control theory.

6 Conclusion

In this paper, we propose an integrated approach for the extraction of neuroimaging biomarkers. We measure the entropy of brain networks defined by computing Riccati penalized precision matrices. We demonstrate how these biomarkers can be improved by reducing data dimension via random projection. We highlight several neuroscience applications for which Riccati regularized precision matrices offer novel perspectives. These applications were all validated by processing the hundred unrelated subjects of the HCP dataset. We hope that the promising results obtained, both in terms of speed and test-retest performances and the broad range of possible theoretical refinements, will encourage further developments and additional neuroimaging applications.

Acknowledgments. Data were provided by the Human Connectome Project, WU-Minn Consortium (PI: D. Van Essen and K. Ugurbil; 1U54MH091657) funded by the 16 NIH Institutes and Centers that support the NIH Blueprint for Neuroscience Research; and by the McDonnell Center for Systems Neuroscience at Washington University. This work was supported by NIH grant R01 EB022573.

References

1. Alexander-Bloch, A., Giedd, J., Bullmore, E.: Imaging structural co-variance between human brain regions. Nat. Rev. Neurosci. **14**(5), 322–336 (2013)
2. Bullmore, S.: Complex brain networks: graph theoretical analysis of structural and functional systems. Nat. Rev. Neurosci. **10**, 186–198 (2009)

3. Cardoso, J., Souloumiac, A.: Jacobi angles for simultaneous diagonalization. SIAM J. Matrix Anal. Appl. **17**, 161–164 (1996)
4. Dale, A., Fischl, B., Sereno, M.: Cortical surface-based analysis. I. segmentation and surface reconstruction. Neuroimage **9**, 179–194 (1999)
5. Eavani, H., Satterthwaite, T.D., Gur, R.E., Gur, R.C., Davatzikos, C.: Unsupervised learning of functional network dynamics in resting state fMRI. In: Gee, J.C., Joshi, S., Pohl, K.M., Wells, W.M., Zöllei, L. (eds.) IPMI 2013. LNCS, vol. 7917, pp. 426–437. Springer, Heidelberg (2013). doi:10.1007/978-3-642-38868-2_36
6. Fan, J., Liao, Y., Liu, H.: An overview of the estimation of large covariance and precision matrices. Econom. J. **19**(1), C1–C32 (2016)
7. Glasser, M.F., Sotiropoulos, S.N., Wilson, J.A., Coalson, T.S., Fischl, B., Andersson, J.L., Xu, J., Jbabdi, S., Webster, M., Polimeni, J.R., Van Essen, D.C., Jenkinson, M.: The minimal preprocessing pipelines for the human connectome project. Neuroimage **80**, 105–124 (2013)
8. Glasser, M., Coalson, T., Robinson, E., Hacker, C., Harwell, J., Yacoub, E., Ugurbil, K., Andersson, J., Beckmann, C., Jenkinson, M., Smith, S., Van Essen, D.: A multi-modal parcellation of human cerebral cortex. Nature **536**, 171–178 (2016)
9. Halko, N., Martinsson, P., Tropp, J.A.: Finding structure with randomness: probabilistic algorithms for constructing approximate matrix decompositions. SIAM Rev. **53**(2), 217–288 (2011)
10. Honorio, J., Jaakkola, T.: Inverse covariance estimation for high-dimensional data in linear time and space: spectral methods for riccati and sparse models. In: Proceedings of the 2013 Conference on Uncertainty in Artifical Intelligence (2013)
11. Hsieh, C.J., Sustik, M.A., Dhillon, I.S., Ravikumar, P.K., Poldrack, R.: Big and quic: sparse inverse covariance estimation for a million variables. In: Advances in Neural Information Processing Systems, pp. 3165–3173 (2013)
12. Insel, T., Cuthbert, B., Garvey, M., Heinssen, R., Pine, D.S., Quinn, K., Sanislow, C., Wang, P.: Research domain criteria (rdoc): toward a new classification framework for research on mental disorders. Am. J. Psychiatry **167**(7), 748–751 (2010)
13. Lim, Y.: The matrix golden mean and its applications to riccati matrix equations. SIAM J. Matrix Anal. Appl. **29**(1), 54–66 (2006)
14. McGraw, K., Wong, S.: Forming inferences about some intraclass correlation coefficients. Psychol. Methods **1**(1), 30–46 (1996)
15. Rousseeuw, P.J., Croux, C.: Alternatives to the median absolute deviation. J. Am. Stat. Assoc. **88**(424), 1273–1283 (1993)
16. Tononi, G., Sporns, O., Edelman, G.: A measure for brain complexity: relating functional segregation and integration in the nervous system. Proc. Nat. Acad. Sci. USA (PNAS) **91**, 5033–5037 (1994)
17. Van Essen, D., Smith, S., Barch, D., Behrens, T., Yacoub, E., Ugurbil, K., WU-Minn HCP Consortium: The WU-Minn human connectome project: an overview. NeuroImage **80**, 62–79 (2013)
18. Varoquaux, G., Craddock, R.C.: Learning and comparing functional connectomes. NeuroImage **80**, 405–415 (2013)
19. Varoquaux, G., Gramfort, A., Poline, J., Thirion, B.: Brain covariance selection: better individual functional connectivity models using population prior. In: Advances in Neural Information Processing Systems (2010)
20. Witten, D., Tibshirani, R.: Covariance-regularized regression and classification for highdimensional problems. J. R. Stat. Soc. **71**(3), 615–636 (2009)

Multimodal Brain Subnetwork Extraction Using Provincial Hub Guided Random Walks

Chendi Wang[1(✉)], Bernard Ng[2], and Rafeef Abugharbieh[1]

[1] Biomedical Signal and Image Computing Lab,
The University of British Columbia, Vancouver, Canada
chendi.wang.judy@gmail.com
[2] The Department of Statistics, The University of British Columbia,
Vancouver, Canada

Abstract. Community detection methods have been widely used for studying the modular structure of the brain. However, few of these methods exploit the intrinsic properties of brain networks other than modularity to tackle the pronounced noise in neuroimaging data. We propose a random walker (RW) based approach that reflects how regions of a brain subnetwork tend to be inter-linked by a provincial hub. By using provincial hubs to guide seed setting, RW provides the exact posterior probability of a brain region belonging to each given subnetwork, which mitigates forced hard assignments of brain regions to subnetworks as is the case in most existing methods. We further present an extension that enables multimodal integration for exploiting complementary information from functional Magnetic Resonance Imaging (fMRI) and diffusion MRI (dMRI) data. On synthetic data, our approach achieves higher accuracy in subnetwork extraction than unimodal and existing multimodal approaches. On real data from the Human Connectome Project (HCP), our estimated subnetworks match well with established brain systems and attain higher inter-subject reproducibility.

Keywords: Neuroimaging · Brain subnetwork extraction · Provincial hubs · Random walker · Posterior probability · Multimodal integration

1 Introduction

The human brain comprises functionally interacting regions that are physically connected by anatomical fiber pathways. The brain network can be abstracted as a graph $G = (V; E)$ where V is a collection of brain nodes and E the edges reflecting connections between the brain nodes. One can gain insights into the fundamental architectures and function of the brain from its modular structure [1], which can be extracted by clustering brain nodes into subnetworks (also referred to as communities) using community detection methods [2, 3]. Existing community detection methods that exploit network metrics typically use modularity to optimize a graph partitioning measure [2, 4]. However, such subnetwork extraction remains challenging due to the pronounced noise in neuroimaging data. Few methods exploited the intrinsic properties other than modularity of brain networks. Informative module-related network metrics

© Springer International Publishing AG 2017
M. Niethammer et al. (Eds.): IPMI 2017, LNCS 10265, pp. 287–298, 2017.
DOI: 10.1007/978-3-319-59050-9_23

like hubs, within-module degree score, participant coefficient and centrality can be estimated given a subnetwork assignment [4]. However, those network metrics have not been used to inform the subnetwork extraction process. Previous studies on anatomical [5, 6] and functional networks [7, 8] suggest the presence of "provincial hubs" [9], hubs that are highly connected to nodes within a subnetwork. These provincial hubs are thought to be responsible for the formation and stability of the subnetworks [9]. Given the critical role of provincial hubs, we argue that incorporating provincial hubs to guide the subnetwork extraction would be beneficial.

Currently, functional magnetic resonance imaging (fMRI) and diffusion MRI (dMRI) are the most widely used modalities to estimate functional connectivity (FC) and anatomical connectivity (AC) for brain subnetwork extraction purposes. Reliable subnetwork extraction remains challenging given the pronounced noise and acquisition limitations in both modalities. Specifically, FC estimates suffer from many false positive connections due to confounds such as scanner drifts, head movements and physiological noise [10]. AC estimates are prone to false negatives (missing connections) arising from related partial volume effects and crossing fiber problems during tractography [11]. We argue that combining the complementary information in FC and AC could help alleviate the problems linked to individual modalities. Benefits from integrating fMRI and dMRI modalities for connectivity estimation were demonstrated in [12–14]. As for multimodal subnetwork extraction, most existing integration methods aimed to fuse the connectivity matrices from different modalities to estimate common patterns, such as representative multiview spectral clustering (MVSC) [15], and related co-training methods [16–18]. Other models added in techniques such as regularization (COREG) [19] and overlapping subnetwork assumption (CSORD) [20]. Limitations of these existing multimodal methods include the lack of exploitation of intrinsic brain properties and the posterior probability of subnetwork assignments.

In this paper, we propose a Random Walker (RW) based approach which utilizes intrinsic brain properties to guide the brain subnetwork extraction. Through an iterative optimization process, we update RW model architecture based on feedback from provincial hub properties from the previous iteration. The feedback mechanism enables incorporation of the network information within iterations to efficiently identify improved subnetwork assignments. In the RW model [21] (Sect. 2.1), the manner in which nodes are clustered into groups based on probabilities of walking to seeds closely resembles the mechanism where brain regions within a subnetwork are inter-linked via provincial hubs. Compared to other seeded based methods like k-means [22], RW guarantees the global optimum with a convex energy function [21] and the model is more straightforward for incorporating provincial hub properties. The RW with prior model [23] is in fact well suited to incorporate a feedback from network properties via prior edges connecting nodes to augmented seeds. We thus deploy a feedback informed optimization model based on RW with prior model (Sect. 2.2), which also facilitates multimodal integration (Sect. 2.3). Further, most clustering methods produce hard subnetwork assignments, which forces all nodes to be assigned into subnetworks. By using RW, we can infer the probability of a node being assigned to a subnetwork, and further investigate non-significant nodes which do not belong to any subnetwork (Sect. 2.4).

2 Method

2.1 Notation Overview of Used RW Model

Given a weighted graph G, a set of weighted edges $w_{ij} \in E$, and a set of d nodes V, comprising labeled nodes (seeds) V_S, and unlabeled nodes, V_U, such that $V_S \cup V_U = V$, we wish to assign each node $v_i \in V_U$ with a label from set $\{1, 2, \ldots K\}$. We define set $M = \{m^1, m^2, \ldots, m^K\}$ as subnetwork structure, in which each subset m^k, $k \in 1 \sim K$ of M is a set of nodes within subnetwork k. The RW approach [21] assigns to each unlabeled node the probability, x_i^k, that a random walker starting from that node i first reaches a seed assigned to label k. Each unlabeled node is then assigned to the label for which it has the highest probability, i.e., $y_i = max_k x_i^k$. The minimization of $x^{kT} L x^k$ yields the probability x^k, where L ($d \times d$) is the Laplacian matrix of the graph defined as:

$$L_{v_i v_j} = \begin{cases} d^i & if\ i = j, \\ -w_{ij} & if\ v_i\ and\ v_j\ are\ adjacent\ nodes, \\ 0 & otherwise. \end{cases} \tag{1}$$

where $d^i = \sum_j w_{ij}$. By partitioning the Laplacian matrix into labeled L_S ($K \times K$) and unlabeled L_U ($d\text{-}K \times d\text{-}K$) blocks:

$$L = \begin{bmatrix} L_S & B \\ B^T & L_U \end{bmatrix}, \tag{2}$$

and denoting an $|V_S| \times 1$ indicator vector as $f_i^k = \begin{cases} 1 & if\ y_i = k \\ 0 & if\ y_i \neq k \end{cases}$, the minimization of $x^{kT} L x^k$ with respect to x_U^k is given by the linear equation as:

$$L_U x_U^k = -B f^k. \tag{3}$$

2.2 Feedback Informed Optimization Model

Given the important role of provincial hubs in forming and stabilizing the subnetwork [9], we propose an iterative optimization RW model by introducing an prior edge based on the RW posterior probability to reflect the affinity between a node and a seed. We deploy the RW with prior model [23] with an exact closed-form posterior probability update. Specifically, we use the posterior probability from the previous iteration as the prior in the RW with prior model [23] as below:

$$\left(L_U + \gamma \sum_{r=1}^{K} \Lambda_U^r\right) x_U^k = \lambda_U^k + B f^k, \tag{4}$$

where λ_i^k is a prior, that represents the probability of node i belonging to subnetwork k, and Λ^k is a diagonal matrix with the values of λ^k. According to [23], the incorporation of priors in (4) yields the same solution as would be obtained for the RW probabilities on an augmented graph in Fig. 1, which maintains the robustness of the RW algorithm. In this augmented graph, we denote the set $H = \{h^1, h^2, \ldots h^K\}$ as the augmented seeds (red "floating" seeds), which are generated by the subnetwork extraction result from the previous iteration. The blue edges in Fig. 1 are node-to-node edges w_{ij}, and we define the red edges, $\lambda_i^k, k \in 1 \sim K$ as the "prior edges" connecting nodes to floating augmented seeds. Here γ is used to modulate the degree of the incorporation of prior. The corresponding Laplacian matrix in our proposed model is:

$$L = \begin{bmatrix} L_S & B \\ B^T & L_U + \gamma I \end{bmatrix}, \tag{5}$$

where in B, $B_{i,k} = -\gamma \lambda_i^k$, I is an identity matrix, and the element in the right bottom unlabeled block is derived from the following:

$$d_{L_U}^i + \sum_{k=1}^{K} -B_{i,k} = d_{L_U}^i + \gamma \sum_{k=1}^{K} \lambda_i^k = d_{L_U}^i + \gamma, \tag{6}$$

where $\sum_{k=1}^{K} \lambda_i^k = 1$, as the probability of a node walking to all seeds sum to unity.

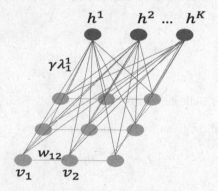

Fig. 1. Augmented graph model for our augmented RW with prior model. The use of prior is equivalent to using K labeled "floating" augmented nodes in red that correspond to each label and are connected to each node in blue. (Color figure online)

Based on the augmented graph model (one floating augmented seed per subnetwork), we extend our model to contain multiple augmented seeds per subnetwork. The reason for using multiple seeds could be the possible over-parcellation, which naturally splits a provincial hub into multiple seeds [24]. Further, using multiple seeds can increase robustness of the model by mitigating the problems caused by noisy connections between subnetworks, which we empirically observed the outperformance of using multiple seeds. We denote a new set of seeds, $HM = \{H^1, H^2, \ldots H^K\}$, where each subnet $H^k = \{h_1^k, h_2^k, \ldots, h_{n_k}^k\}$ represents the set of multiple seeds that belong to subnetwork k, $k \in \{1, 2, \ldots, K\}$. We define the prior edge from a node i to one of the augmented seeds h_j^k in the subnetwork k as the split version of the prior edge connecting to a single augmented seed in (7):

$$\mu_i^{h_j^k} = w_{i,h_j^k} \lambda_i^k, j = 1 \sim n_k, \tag{7}$$

accordingly, the corresponding B will be updated as $B_{i,h_j^k} = -\gamma \mu_i^{h_j^k}$.

We automatically set seeds based on network properties of provincial hubs, which have high within-module degree Z score and low participation coefficient P score [4], defined as:

$$Z_i \frac{d^i(m_i - \bar{d}(m_i))}{\sigma^{d(m_i)}}; P_i = 1 - \sum_{m \in M} \left(\frac{d^i(m)}{d^i} \right)^2, \tag{8}$$

where m_i is the subnetwork containing node i, $d^i(m_i)$ is the within-module degree of i, i.e., the number of links between i and all the other nodes in m_i, and $\bar{d}(m_i)$ and $\sigma^{d(m_i)}$ are the respective mean and standard deviation of the within-module m_i degree distribution.

Then we update the seeds and corresponding prior edges by applying the posterior probabilities from the previous iteration as the prior edges until the subnetwork extraction results converge. Convergence is measured by the normalized mutual information (NMI) [25] between subnetwork assignments from two successive iterations. The initial seeds are set from a pre-partitioned subnetwork structure obtained on FC connectivity using Normalized cut (Ncuts) [26]. We have chosen Ncuts for its global optimality guarantees so that our seed setting is not prone to problems such as instability to initialization in k-means [22] or local minimums in hierarchical clustering [32]. Hence, the results of the extracted networks would be consistent regarding different Ncuts initialization parameters. We derived the prior edges in the first iteration using the average weights between a node and all the other nodes within a particular subnetwork, followed by a normalization to guarantee $\sum_{k=1}^K \lambda_i^k = 1$. The average weights have been chosen considering to increase robustness to noise.

2.3 Multimodal fMRI-dMRI Integration

We extend the proposed feedback informed iterative optimization model to enable multimodal RW integration (henceforth referred to as mmRW) based on the assumption that subnetworks captured via multiple imaging modalities share common provincial hubs. By alternating the connectivity modalities for the node-to-node edges within the iterative model in Sect. 2.2 (where the graph weights in the current iteration is defined by FC, the weights in the next iteration will be defined by AC), provincial hubs can be used to guide the feedback information propagation across modalities until the subnetwork assignments from different modalities converge, as measured by NMI.

We base our connectivity estimation on a fingerprint formulation [27], where we derive the connectivity matrices $\mathbf{C}$ by estimating the cross-correlation between the fingerprint profiles of each brain node pair. The AC fingerprint profile for each brain node is defined as the fiber connection strength to the remaining brain nodes, namely the number of tracts connecting two nodes normalized by the node sizes. The FC fingerprint profile is defined as the cross-correlation between the time courses of a particular node and all the remaining nodes in the brain. We note that we set negative C_{ij} to zero given the currently unclear interpretation of negative connectivity [28]. Further, we map $\mathbf{C}$ to the graph weights w using a Gaussian kernel, where σ is the decaying parameter for the kernel estimation:

$$w_{ij} = \exp\left(-\frac{(1 - C_{ij})^2}{2\sigma^2}\right).$$ (9)

2.4 Posterior Probability

One major gain of using RW model is that it offers a confidence value that a given node belongs to a particular subnetwork (as represented by the probability). Thus the posterior probability derived from the RW model provides users with options to discard those non-significant nodes with low probability belonging to any subnetwork.

2.5 Parameter Selection

We estimate the free parameter γ to guide the feedback incorporation in our proposed model based on modularity, Q, a quantitative fitness function measure of the graph partitioning [4]. We stress the prior edges when relatively reasonable graph partitioning has been achieved from the previous iteration based on relatively higher Q value and vice versa. We set the other free parameter σ to be the typically used average non-zero values of connectivity distance which was computed as $1 - C_{ij}$.

For examining the subnetwork extraction on thresholded brain graphs, we examine a range of graph densities of [0.005, 0.5] at an interval of 0.005 to test the robustness of our approach, where the local thresholding [29] of the brain graph was used.

The number of seeds needed within each subnetwork is dependent on the graph density. Denser graphs require more seeds to tackle the noisy connection problem. Empirically, we set n_k to 15 for density [0.005, 0.1], 20 for density [0.105, 0.3], and 25 for density [0.305, 0.5].

For the stopping criteria for convergence, we empirically set the threshold for NMI (from successive iterations) between subnetwork assignments within the same modality to 0.99, and between inter-modality to 0.8. All the results in our experiments have reached convergence.

3 Materials

Synthetic Data. We generated 200 synthetic datasets that cover a wide variety of network configurations using the technique from [20]. Each dataset comprised $d = 500$ regions and 4 scans of 1200 time points as in the real data. We set the number of subnetworks, N, to a random value between 10 and 20 in each dataset. The number of

ROIs in each subnetwork was set to $\lceil d/N \rceil + c$ with c being a random number between -2 and 2, and ROIs were randomly assigned to subnetworks. We generated a $d \times d$ adjacency matrix, Σ, which was taken as the ground truth based on the network configurations. Next, we built an AC matrix, Σ_A, by randomly setting $p_1\%$ of the values in Σ to 0 to model how AC estimates contain false negatives, and built a FC matrix, Σ_F, by randomly setting $p_2\%$ of the values in Σ to 1 to model how FC estimates are prone to false positives. p_1 and p_2 were randomly chosen from $[0, 20]$. Two sets of time series were then generated by drawing random samples from $N(0, \Sigma_A)$ and $N(0, \Sigma_F)$. Then Gaussian noise was added to the time series with signal-to-noise ratio (SNR) randomly set between -6 and -3 dB. Finally, AC and FC matrices were simulated by computing the Pearson's correlation of these noisy time series.

Real Data. We used the resting state fMRI (RS-fMRI) and dMRI scans of 77 unrelated healthy subjects (36 males and 41 females, ages ranging from 22 to 35) from the HCP dataset [30]. Two sessions of RS-fMRI and one session dMRI data were available for multimodal integration. Details for acquisition can be found in [30]. In addition to preprocessing already applied [31], we regressed out motion artifacts, mean white matter and cerebrospinal fluid signals, and principal components of high variance voxels [32], followed by bandpass filtering with cutoff frequencies of 0.01 and 0.1 Hz. Given the preprocessed dMRI data [31], we applied global tractography based on constant solid angle orientation distribution function and Gibbs tracking by MITK package [33], which produces relatively more reliable AC estimates compared to conventional tractography strategy. We then used the Willard atlas [34] which has 499 ROIs to define regions of interest (ROIs). Voxel time courses within ROIs were averaged to generate region time courses. The region time courses were demeaned, normalized by the standard deviation, and concatenated across subjects. The Pearson's correlation values between the region time courses were taken as estimates of FC fingerprint profiles. To compute the fiber count between ROIs, which were taken as AC fingerprint profile estimates, we warped the Willard atlas onto the b = 0 volume of each subject. Subject-wise AC fingerprint profiles were concatenated for a group-level fingerprint profile.

4   Results and Discussion

4.1   Synthetic Data

We compared our mmRW against our unimodal RW using (4), unimodal Ncuts methods (NC), multimodal methods MVSC [15], COREG [19], and CSORD [20]. For unimodal techniques, we reported their performance using both FC and AC estimates. On 200 synthetic datasets, we assessed each method by computing the Dice coefficient (DC) between the ground truth and estimated subnetwork labels as: $DC = 2|L_{est} \cap L_{gnd}| / (L_{est} + L_{gnd})$, where L_{gnd} is the set of ROIs in the ground truth subnetwork, and L_{est} is the set of ROIs in the estimated subnetwork matched to L_{gnd} using Hungarian assignment [35]. mmRW achieved significantly higher DC than each contrasted method at $p = 10^{-5}$ based on Wilcoxon signed rank test (Fig. 2). We note that the numbers of subnetworks were set to the ground truth subnetwork numbers for all methods for simplification.

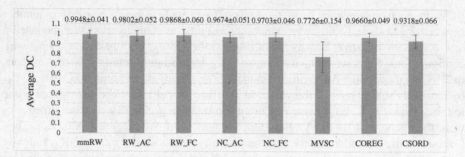

Fig. 2. Subnetwork extraction accuracy on synthetic data. Our mmRW approach achieved significantly higher DC than unimodal and existing multimodal methods.

4.2 Real Data

Due to the lack of the ground truth, we first evaluated our approach by examining the overlap between our extracted subnetworks and a well-established brain systems comprising 14 subnetworks presented in [36] which we took as the pseudo ground truth. We derived the connectivity matrix based on the Willard atlas [34]. Both the atlas and corresponding subnetwork assignment [36] were manually inspected and edited by neurologists, which included intensive user selection. 142 out of 499 ROIs in the Willard atlas were classified as significant brain nodes, we thus compared the DC on those significant nodes between the estimated and the established subnetwork assignments using our approach against unimodal and representative existing multimodal approaches. We set the number of subnetworks to 14 as the number of the established brain systems. As shown in Fig. 3, mmRW approach achieved significantly higher average DC over a range of graph densities compared to each contrasted method at $p = 10^{-7}$ based on Wilcoxon signed rank test. We observed that the results of using unimodal RW iterative model based on FC data can attain better results compared to AC based results. We conclude that FC would be a better modality for subnetwork extraction. But adding AC in always improved the accuracy, which confirms the benefit of multimodal integration. We note that the low DC from CSORD could be caused by

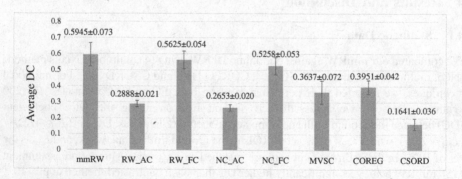

Fig. 3. Subnetwork extraction overlap to well-established brain system [36] on real data from HCP. Our mmRW approach achieved significantly higher DC than contrasted methods.

the implicit overlapping subnetwork assumption embedded in the approach while the pseudo ground truth has a non-overlapping subnetwork setting.

In order to utilize the posterior probability derived from our approach, we selected to show the subnetwork extraction results of an exemplar brain graph which achieved the highest DC = 0.7682 to the established brain systems [36] using mmRW. Amongst the 103 matched nodes out of the 142 significant nodes in the Willard atlas, the average posterior probabilities of a node belonging to the assigned subnetwork is 0.6473 with a minimum value at 0.3118. On the other hand, an average value at 0.4689 and a minimum value at 0.1156 of probabilities have been found in the remaining 357 non-significant Willard nodes, which further confirmed that the nodes with lower probabilities derived from our approach matched with those non-significant nodes excluded from 14 established brain systems. We further visualize the posterior probabilities by the size of nodes in Fig. 4(a and b). Here users have the option to discard non-significant nodes using desired thresholds of probability. Qualitatively, mmRW identified all commonly found subnetworks in the literature [36]. The extracted dorsal default mode subnetwork (dDMN), visuospatial subnetwork and left executive control subnetwork (LECN) are shown in Fig. 4(c–e) as exemplar results.

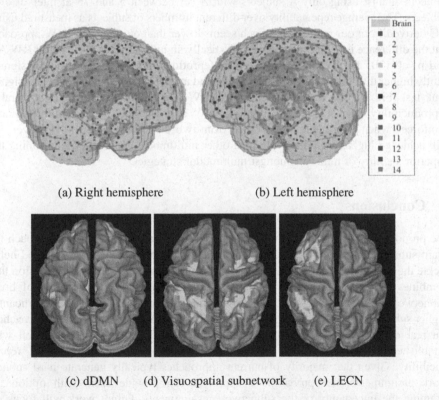

(a) Right hemisphere   (b) Left hemisphere

(c) dDMN   (d) Visuospatial subnetwork   (e) LECN

Fig. 4. Subnetwork extraction results on an exemplar brain graph. (a and b) Probabilities of a node being assigned to a given subnetwork (color-coded in 14 subnetworks), the larger size of a node indicates a higher probability. (c and e) Exemplar subnetworks identified by mmRW. (Color figure online)

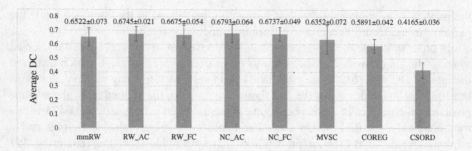

Fig. 5. Inter-subject reproducibility on real data from HCP. Multimodal RW approach achieved comparable DC to unimodal RW approach, but significantly higher DC than existing multimodal methods.

We next evaluated the inter-subject subnetwork reproducibility using the repeatability of the group subnetwork extraction results with respect to the numbers of subjects. Specifically, we compared the group subnetwork assignments generated from all 77 subjects against using only A subjects with A set between 5 and 75 at interval of 5 subjects. The average repeatability over different numbers of subjects as measured using DC derived from our mmRW approach seems lower than our unimodal RW approach, but the difference is negligible and not statistically significant at p = 0.5614 for RW AC and p = 0.1205 for RW FC. However, the reproducibility of our approach is significantly higher than contrasted multimodal method at p = 10^{-2} based on Wilcoxon signed rank test (Fig. 5). We note that multimodal RW approach only achieved comparable reproducibility compared to our unimodal RW approach since the stability was not reinforced when information was pooled from two different modalities. However, we still achieved higher reproducibility than other multimodal approaches, confirming the superior stability of mmRW amongst multimodal strategies.

5   Conclusions

We proposed a provincial hub guided random walker based optimization approach for brain subnetwork extraction that exploits intrinsic brain properties. Our method helps tackle the pronounced noise in neuroimaging data. We also presented an extension that combines information from fMRI and dMRI data for better identification of brain subnetworks. On synthetic data, we showed that our approach achieved significantly higher subnetwork identification accuracy than a number of state-of-the-art approaches. On real data, we demonstrated that our estimated subnetworks matched well with established brain systems and attained comparable or higher inter-subject reproducibility. Given that majority of current approaches typically generate hard subnetwork assignments, our probabilistic approach can provide users with options to examine the uncertainty of the subnetwork assignments. Future work will focus on studying the roles of low probability nodes and their possible biological meaning, e.g. them residing within overlapping subnetworks or simply being insignificant.

References

1. Bullmore, E., Sporns, O.: Complex brain networks: graph theoretical analysis of structural and functional systems. Nat. Rev. Neurosci. **10**, 186–198 (2009)
2. Nicolini, C., Bordier, C., Bifone, A.: Community detection in weighted brain connectivity networks beyond the resolution limit. Neuroimage **146**, 28–39 (2017)
3. Taya, F., de Souza, J., Thakor, N.V., Bezerianos, A.: Comparison method for community detection on brain networks from neuroimaging data. Appl. Netw. Sci. **1**, 8 (2016)
4. Rubinov, M., Sporns, O.: Complex network measures of brain connectivity: uses and interpretations. Neuroimage **52**, 1059–1069 (2010)
5. Hagmann, P., Cammoun, L., Gigandet, X., Meuli, R., Honey, C.J., Wedeen, V.J.: Mapping the structural core of human cerebral cortex. PLoS Biol. **6**(7), e159 (2008)
6. Sporns, O., Betzel, R.F.: Modular brain networks. Ann. Rev. Psychol. **67**, 613–640 (2016)
7. Meunier, D., Lambiotte, R., Fornito, A., Ersche, K.D., Bullmore, E.T.: Hierarchical modularity in human brain functional networks. Front. Neuroinform. **3**, 37 (2009)
8. Meunier, D., Lambiotte, R., Bullmore, E.T.: Modular and hierarchically modular organization of brain networks. Front. Neurosci. **4**, 200 (2010)
9. Guimerà, R., Nunes Amaral, L.A.: Functional cartography of complex metabolic networks. Nature **433**, 895–900 (2005)
10. Murphy, K., Birn, R.M., Bandettini, P.: Resting-state fMRI confounds and cleanup. Neuroimage **80**, 349–359 (2013)
11. Alexander, A.L., Hasan, K.M., Lazar, M., Tsuruda, J.S., Parker, D.L.: Analysis of partial volume effects in diffusion-tensor MRI. Magn. Reson. Med. **45**, 770–780 (2001)
12. Venkataraman, A., Rathi, Y., Kubicki, M., Westin, C.-F., Golland, P.: Joint modeling of anatomical and functional connectivity for population studies. IEEE Trans. Med. Imaging **31**, 164–182 (2012)
13. Ng, B., Varoquaux, G., Poline, J.-B., Thirion, B.: A novel sparse graphical approach for multimodal brain connectivity inference. In: Ayache, N., Delingette, H., Golland, P., Mori, K. (eds.) MICCAI 2012. LNCS, vol. 7510, pp. 707–714. Springer, Heidelberg (2012). doi:10.1007/978-3-642-33415-3_87
14. Abdelnour, F., Voss, H.U., Raj, A.: Network diffusion accurately models the relationship between structural and functional brain connectivity networks. Neuroimage **90**, 335–347 (2014)
15. Chen, H., Li, K., Zhu, D., Jiang, X., Yuan, Y., Lv, P., Zhang, T., Guo, L., Shen, D., Liu, T.: Inferring group-wise consistent multimodal brain networks via multi-view spectral clustering. IEEE Trans. Med. Imaging **32**, 1576–1586 (2013)
16. Dodero, L., Gozzi, A., Liska, A., Murino, V., Sona, D.: Group-wise functional community detection through joint laplacian diagonalization. In: Golland, P., Hata, N., Barillot, C., Hornegger, J., Howe, R. (eds.) MICCAI 2014. LNCS, vol. 8674, pp. 708–715. Springer, Cham (2014). doi:10.1007/978-3-319-10470-6_88
17. An, M., Ho, H.P., Staib, L., Pelphrey, K., Duncan, J.: Multimodal MRI analysis of brain subnetworks in autism using multi-view EM. In: 2010 Conference Record of the Forty Fourth Asilomar Conference on Signals, Systems and Computers, pp. 786–789 (2010)
18. Wang, B., Jiang, J., Wang, W., Zhou, Z., Tu, Z.: Unsupervised metric fusion by cross diffusion. In: IEEE Conference on Computer Vision and Patter Recognition (2012)
19. Kumar, A., Daum, H.: Co-regularized multi-view spectral clustering. In: Advances in Neural Information Processing Systems, pp. 1413–1421 (2011)

20. Yoldemir, B., Ng, B., Abugharbieh, R.: Coupled stable overlapping replicator dynamics for multimodal brain subnetwork identification. In: Ourselin, S., Alexander, D.C., Westin, C.-F., Cardoso, M.J. (eds.) Information Processing in Medical Imaging, pp. 770–781. Springer International Publishing, Cham (2015)

21. Grady, L.: Random walks for image segmentation. IEEE Trans. Pattern Anal. Mach. Intell. **28**, 1–17 (2006)

22. Jain, A.K.: Data clustering: 50 years beyond K-means. Pattern Recognit. Lett. **31**, 651–666 (2010)

23. Grady, L.: Multilabel random walker image segmentation using prior models. In: IEEE Computer Society Conference on Computer Vision and Pattern Recognition, pp. 763–770 (2005)

24. Nicolini, C., Bifone, A.: Modular structure of brain functional networks: breaking the resolution limit by surprise. Sci. Rep. **6**, 19250 (2016)

25. Witten, I.H., Frank, E.: Data Mining: Practical Machine Learning Tools and Techniques. Morgan Kaufmann, Burlington (2005)

26. van den Heuvel, M., Mandl, R., Hulshoff Pol, H.: Normalized cut group clustering of resting-state FMRI data. PLoS ONE **3**, e2001 (2008)

27. Johansen-Berg, H., Behrens, T.E.J., Robson, M.D., Drobnjak, I., Rushworth, M.F.S., Brady, J.M., Smith, S.M., Higham, D.J., Matthews, P.M.: Changes in connectivity profiles define functionally distinct regions in human medial frontal cortex. Proc. Natl. Acad. Sci. U. S. A. **101**, 13335–13340 (2004)

28. Skudlarski, P., Jagannathan, K., Calhoun, V.D., Hampson, M., Skudlarska, B.A., Pearlson, G.: Measuring brain connectivity: diffusion tensor imaging validates resting state temporal correlations. Neuroimage **43**, 554–561 (2008)

29. Wang, C., Ng, B., Abugharbieh, R.: Modularity reinforcement for improving brain subnetwork extraction. In: Ourselin, S., Joskowicz, L., Sabuncu, M.R., Unal, G., Wells, W. (eds.) MICCAI 2016. LNCS, vol. 9900, pp. 132–139. Springer, Cham (2016). doi:10.1007/978-3-319-46720-7_16

30. Van Essen, D.C., Smith, S.M., Barch, D.M., Behrens, T.E.J., Yacoub, E., Ugurbil, K.: The WU-Minn human connectome project: an overview. Neuroimage **80**, 62–79 (2013)

31. Glasser, M.F., Sotiropoulos, S.N., Wilson, J.A., Coalson, T.S., Fischl, B., Andersson, J.L., Xu, J., Jbabdi, S., Webster, M., Polimeni, J.R., Van Essen, D.C., Jenkinson, M.: The minimal preprocessing pipelines for the Human Connectome Project. Neuroimage **80**, 105–124 (2013)

32. Behzadi, Y., Restom, K., Liau, J., Liu, T.T.: A component based noise correction method (CompCor) for BOLD and perfusion based fMRI. Neuroimage **37**, 90–101 (2007)

33. Neher, P.F., Stieltjes, B., Reisert, M., Reicht, I., Meinzer, H.-P., Fritzsche, K.H.: MITK global tractography. In: Haynor, D.R., Ourselin, S. (eds.) SPIE Medical Imaging, p. 83144D. International Society for Optics and Photonics (2012)

34. Richiardi, J., Altmann, A., Milazzo, A.C., Chang, C., Chakravarty, M.M., Banaschewski, T., Barker, G.J., Bokde, A.L.W., Bromberg, U., Büchel, C., Conrod, P., Fauth-Bühler, M., Flor, H., Frouin, V., Gallinat, J., Garavan, H., Gowland, P., Heinz, A., Lemaître, H., Mann, K.F., Martinot, J.-L., Nees, F., Paus, T., Pausova, Z., Rietschel, M., Robbins, T.W., Smolka, M.N., Spanagel, R., Ströhle, A., Schumann, G., Hawrylycz, M., Poline, J.-B., Greicius, M.D., Consortium, I.: Correlated gene expression supports synchronous activity in brain networks. Science **348**, 1241–1244 (2015)

35. Kuhn, H.W.: The Hungarian method for the assignment problem. Nav. Res. Logist. Q. **2**, 83–97 (1955)

36. Shirer, W.R., Ryali, S., Rykhlevskaia, E., Menon, V., Greicius, M.D.: Decoding subject-driven cognitive states with whole-brain connectivity patterns. Cereb. Cortex **22**, 158–165 (2012)

Exact Topological Inference for Paired Brain Networks *via* Persistent Homology

Moo K. Chung[1(✉)], Victoria Villalta-Gil[2], Hyekyoung Lee[3], Paul J. Rathouz[1], Benjamin B. Lahey[4], and David H. Zald[2]

[1] University of Wisconsin-Madison, Madison, USA
mkchung@wisc.edu
[2] Vanderbilt University, Nashville, USA
[3] Seoul National University, Seoul, South Korea
[4] University of Chicago, Chicago, USA

Abstract. We present a novel framework for characterizing paired brain networks using techniques in hyper-networks, sparse learning and persistent homology. The framework is general enough for dealing with any type of paired images such as twins, multimodal and longitudinal images. The exact nonparametric statistical inference procedure is derived on testing monotonic graph theory features that do not rely on time consuming permutation tests. The proposed method computes the exact probability in quadratic time while the permutation tests require exponential time. As illustrations, we apply the method to simulated networks and a twin fMRI study. In case of the latter, we determine the statistical significance of the heritability index of the large-scale reward network where every voxel is a network node.

1 Introduction

There are many studies related to paired images: longitudinal studies with two repeat scans [7], multimodal imaging study involving PET and MRI [13] and twin imaging studies [15]. The paired images are usually analyzed by relating voxel measurements that match across two images in a mass univariate fashion at each voxel. Compared to the paired image setting, paired brain networks have not been often analyzed possibly due to the lack of problem awareness and analysis frameworks.

In this paper, we present a new unified statistical framework that can integrate paired networks in a holistic fashion by pairing every possible combination of voxels across two images. This is achieved using a hyper-network that connects multiple smaller networks into a larger network. Although hyper-networks are frequently used in machine learning [16], the concept has not been often used in medical imaging. Jie et al. used the hyper-network framework from the resting-state fMRI in classifying MCI from AD in a machine learning framework [9]. Bezerianos et al. constructed the hyper-network from the coupling of EEG activity of pilots and copilots operating an aircraft albeit using ad-hoc procedures without an explicit model specification [1]. Motivated particularly by

© Springer International Publishing AG 2017
M. Niethammer et al. (Eds.): IPMI 2017, LNCS 10265, pp. 299–310, 2017.
DOI: 10.1007/978-3-319-59050-9_24

the science of [1], we rigorously formulate the problem of characterizing paired networks as a single hyper-network with physically nonexistent hyper-edges connecting between two existing networks.

Graph theory is often used framework for analyzing brain networks mainly due to easier accessibility and interpretation. Since we do not know the exact statistical distribution of many graph theory features, resampling techniques such as the permutation tests have been mainly used in estimating the null distribution and computing p-values. The availability of inexpensive and fast computers made the permutation tests a natural choice for computing p-values when underlying distributions are unknown. However, even with fast computers, permutation test is still extremely slow even for small-scale problems. There is a strong need for fast inference procedures. We propose a new exact inference procedure for graphs and networks. The method speeds up the computation by counting the number of permutations combinatorially instead of empirically computing them by numerically generating large number of permutations.

Our main contributions are as follows.

1. The new formulation of the hyper-network approach for paired images. We show that hyper-networks can be effectively used as a baseline model for paired twin fMRI. The proposed holistic framework is applied to a twin fMRI study in determining the statistical significance of the brain network differences and the heritability of the reward network.
2. Showing that the topological structure of the sparse hyper-network has a monotonic nestedness. This is used to define monotonic graph features and subsequently in computing *topologically aware* distance between networks.
3. The derivation of the probability distribution of the combinatorial test procedure on graph theory feature vectors that do not rely on resampling techniques such as the permutation tests. While the permutation tests require exponential run time, our exact combinatorial approach requires quadratic run time.

2   Sparse Hyper-Network

Consider a collection of n paired images

$$(x_1, y_1), (x_2, y_2), \ldots, (x_n, y_n).$$

We assume x_k and y_k are related either genetically (twin or sibling images), scanwise (multimodal images of the same subject) or longitudinally. We further assume (x_k, y_k) are independently but identically distributed for different i. Let $\mathbf{x} = (x_1, \ldots, x_n)^\top$ and $\mathbf{y} = (y_1, \ldots, y_n)^\top$ be the vectors of images. We set up a hypernetwork by relating the paired vectors at different voxels v_i and v_j:

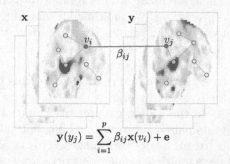

$$\mathbf{y}(y_j) = \sum_{i=1}^{p} \beta_{ij} \mathbf{x}(v_i) + \mathbf{e}$$

Fig. 1. The schematic of hyper-network construction on paired image vectors $\mathbf{x}$ and $\mathbf{y}$. The image vectors $\mathbf{y}$ at voxel v_j is modeled as a linear combination of the first image vector $\mathbf{x}$ at all other voxels. The estimated parameters β_{ij} give the hyper-edge weights.

$$\mathbf{y}(v_j) = \sum_{i=1}^{p} \beta_{ij}\, \mathbf{x}(v_i) + \mathbf{e} \tag{1}$$

for some zero-mean noise vector $\mathbf{e}$ (Fig. 1). The parameters $\beta = (\beta_{ij})$ are the weights of the hyper-edges between voxels v_i and v_j that have to be estimated. We are constructing a *physically nonexistent artificial network* across different images. For fMRI, (1) requires estimating over billions of connections, which is computationally challenging. In practice however, each application will likely to force β to have a specific structure that may reduce the computational burden. For this study, we will consider a reduced model relevant to our genetic imaging application:

$$\mathbf{y}(v_j) = \beta_{ij}\, \mathbf{x}(v_i) + \mathbf{e}. \tag{2}$$

The scientific motivation for using the reduced model will be explained in Sect. 6. Without loss of generality, we can center and scale $\mathbf{x}$ and $\mathbf{y}$ such that

$$\sum_{k=1}^{n} x_k(v_i) = \sum_{k=1}^{n} y_k(v_i) = 0,$$

$$\|\mathbf{x}(v_i)\|^2 = \mathbf{x}^\top(v_i)\mathbf{x}(v_i) = \|\mathbf{y}(v_i)\|^2 = \mathbf{y}^\top(v_i)\mathbf{y}(v_i) = 1 \tag{3}$$

for all voxels v_i.

In many applications, we have significantly more number of voxels (p) than the number of images (n), so model (2) is an under-determined system and belongs to the *small-n large-p problem* [5]. It is necessary to regularize the model using a sparse penalty:

$$\widehat{\beta}(\lambda) = \arg\min_{\beta} \frac{1}{2} \sum_{i,j=1}^{p} \| \mathbf{y}(v_j) - \beta_{ij}\, \mathbf{x}(v_i) \|^2 + \lambda \sum_{i,j=1}^{p} |\beta_{ij}|, \tag{4}$$

where sparse parameter $\lambda \geq 0$ modulates the sparsity of the hyper-edges. The estimation $\widehat{\beta}$ is a function of λ. When $\lambda = 0$, (4) is a least-squares problem and we obtain $\widehat{\beta}_{ij}(0) = \mathbf{x}^\top(v_i)\mathbf{y}(v_j)$, which is referred to as the *cross-correlation*. The cross-correlation is invariant under the centering and scaling.

3   Distance Between Networks

To study the topological characteristic of the hyper-network, the estimated edge weights $\widehat{\beta}_{ij}(\lambda)$ are binarized by assigning value 1 to any nonzero weight and 0 otherwise. Let G_λ be the resulting binary graph, i.e., unweighted graph, with adjacency matrix $A_\lambda = (a_{ij}(\lambda))$:

$$a_{ij}(\lambda) = \begin{cases} 1 & \text{if } \widehat{\beta}_{ij}(\lambda) \neq 0; \\ 0 & \text{otherwise.} \end{cases} \tag{5}$$

As λ increases, G_λ becomes smaller and nested in a sense that every edge weight gets smaller. This is *not* true for the binarization of other sparse network models. Our sparse hyper-network has this extra layer of additional structure that guarantees the nestedness.

Theorem 1. *The binary graph G_λ obtained from sparse model (4) satisfies*

$$G_{\lambda_1} \supset G_{\lambda_2} \supset \cdots \supset G_{\lambda_q} \qquad (6)$$

for any $0 \leq \lambda_1 \leq \lambda_2 \leq \ldots \leq \lambda_q \leq 1$.

Proof. By solving $d\widehat{\beta}(\lambda)/d\lambda = 0$ for $\lambda \neq 0$ and considering $\widehat{\beta}(0)$ separately, it can be algebraically shown that the solution of the optimization problem (2) is given by [5]

$$\widehat{\beta}_{ij}(\lambda) = \begin{cases} \mathbf{x}^\top(v_i)\mathbf{y}(v_j) - \lambda & \text{if } \mathbf{x}^\top(v_i)\mathbf{y}(v_j) > \lambda \\ 0 & \text{if } |\mathbf{x}^\top(v_i)\mathbf{y}(v_j)| \leq \lambda \\ \mathbf{x}^\top(v_i)\mathbf{y}(v_j) + \lambda & \text{if } \mathbf{x}^\top(v_i)\mathbf{y}(v_j) < -\lambda \end{cases} \qquad (7)$$

From (3) and the Cauchy-Schwarz inequality, we have $|\mathbf{x}^\top(v_i)\mathbf{y}(v_j)| \leq 1$. Thus, if $\lambda > 1$, $\widehat{\beta}(\lambda) = 0$. To avoid the trivial case of zero edge weights everywhere, we need $0 \leq \lambda \leq 1$. From (7), we have $|\widehat{\beta}_{ij}(\lambda_j)| \geq |\widehat{\beta}_{ij}(\lambda_{j+1})|$ for $0 \leq \lambda_j \leq \lambda_{j+1} \leq 1$. Subsequently, from (5), $a_{ij}(\lambda_j) \geq a_{ij}(\lambda_{j+1})$. Therefore, we have $G_{\lambda_j} \supset G_{\lambda_{j+1}}$. $\square$

The sequence of nested multi-scale graph structure (6) is called the *graph filtration* in persistent homology [11]. The graph filtration can be quantified using monotonic function B satisfying

$$B(G_{\lambda_1}) \leq B(G_{\lambda_2}) \leq B(G_{\lambda_3}) \leq \ldots \leq B(G_{\lambda_q}). \qquad (8)$$

The number of connected components, which is the zero-th Betti number β_0 and the most often used topological invariant in persistent homology, satisfies this condition. The size of the largest connected component satisfies a similar but opposite relation of monotonic decrease.

Given two different graph filtrations $\mathbf{G}^1 = \{G_\lambda^1 : 0 \leq \lambda \leq 1\}$ and $\mathbf{G}^2 = \{G_\lambda^2 : 0 \leq \lambda \leq 1\}$, define the distance between them as

$$D(\mathbf{G}^1, \mathbf{G}^2) = \sup_{\lambda \in [0,1]} \left| B(G_\lambda^1) - B(G_\lambda^2) \right|,$$

which can be discretely approximated as

$$D_q = \sup_{1 \leq j \leq q} \left| B(G_{\lambda_j}^1) - B(G_{\lambda_j}^2) \right|.$$

If we choose enough number of q such that λ_j are all the sorted edge weights, then $D(\mathbf{G}^1, \mathbf{G}^2) = D_q$. This is possible since there are only up to $p(p-1)/2$ number of unique edge weights in a graph with p nodes and $B(G_\lambda^1)$ and $B(G_\lambda^2)$

increase discretely. In practice, $\rho_j = j/q$ is chosen uniformly in $[0,1]$ or a divide-and-conquer strategy can be used to do adaptively grid the unit interval.

D satisfies all the axioms of a metric except identity. $D(\mathbf{G}^1, \mathbf{G}^2) = 0$ does not imply $\mathbf{G}^1 = \mathbf{G}^2$. Thus, D is *not* a metric. However, it will be shown in Sect. 4 that probability $P(D(\mathbf{G}^1, \mathbf{G}^2) = 0) = 0$ showing such event rarely happens in practice. Thus, D can be treated as a metric-like in applications without much harm.

4   Exact Topological Inference

We are interested in testing the null hypothesis H_0 of the equivalence of two monotonic graph feature functions:

$$H_0 : B(G_\lambda^1) = B(G_\lambda^2) \text{ for all } \lambda \in [0,1]$$

$$vs.$$

$$H_1 : B(G_\lambda^1) \neq B(G_\lambda^2) \text{ for some } \lambda \in [0,1].$$

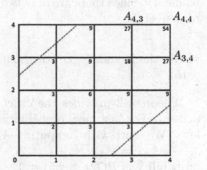

Fig. 2. $A_{u,v}$ are computed within the boundary (dotted red line). The red numbers are the number of paths from $(0,0)$. (Color figure online)

As a test statistic, we propose to use D_q. The test statistic takes care of the multiple comparisons by the use of supremum. Under the null hypothesis, we can derive the probability distribution of D_q combinatorially without numerically permuting images.

Theorem 2.

$$P(D_q \geq d) = 1 - \frac{A_{q,q}}{\binom{2q}{q}},$$

where $A_{u,v}$ satisfies $A_{u,v} = A_{u-1,v} + A_{u,v-1}$ with the boundary condition $A_{0,q} = A_{q,0} = 1$ within band $|u-v| < d$.

Proof. The proof is similar to the combinatorial construction of Kolmogorov-Smirnov (KS) test [2,5,8]. Combine two monotonically increasing vectors

$$(B(G_{\rho_1}^1), \ldots, B(G_{\rho_q}^1)), \quad (B(G_{\rho_1}^2), \ldots, B(G_{\rho_q}^2))$$

and arrange them in increasing order. Represent $B(G_{\rho_j}^1)$ and $B(G_{\rho_j}^2)$ as $\uparrow$ and $\rightarrow$ respectively. For example, $\uparrow\uparrow\rightarrow\uparrow\rightarrow\rightarrow\cdots$. There are exactly q number of $\uparrow$ and q number of $\rightarrow$ in the sequence. Treat the sequence as walks on a Cartesian grid. $\rightarrow$ indicates one step to the right and $\uparrow$ indicates one step up. Thus the walk starts at $(0,0)$ and ends at (q,q) (Fig. 2). There are total $\binom{2q}{q}$ possible number of paths, which forms the sample space. This is also the total number of possible permutations between the elements of the two vectors. The null assumption is that the two vectors are identical and there is no preference to one vector element to another. Thus, each walk is equally likely to happen in the sample space.

The values of $B(G^1{}_{\rho_j})$ and $B(G^2{}_{\rho_j})$ satisfying the condition $\sup_j |B(G^1{}_{\rho_j}) - B(G^2{}_{\rho_j})| < d$ are the integer coordinates of (u, v) on the path satisfying $|u - v| < d$. These are integer grid points within the boundary $v = u \pm d$ (dotted red lines in Fig. 2). Thus the probability can be written as

$$P(D_q \geq d) = 1 - P(D_q < d) = 1 - \frac{A_{q,q}}{\binom{2q}{q}}, \tag{9}$$

where $A_{u,v}$ be the total number of passible paths from $(0, 0)$ to (u, v) within the boundary. Since there are only two paths (either $\uparrow$ or $\rightarrow$), $A_{u,v}$ can be computed recursively as

$$A_{u,v} = A_{u-1,v} + A_{u,v-1}.$$

within the boundary. On the boundary, $A_{0,q} = A_{q,0} = 1$ since there is only one path. $\square$

Theorem 2 provides the exact probability computation for any number of nodes p. For instance, probability $P(D_4 \geq 2.5)$ is computed iteratively as follows. We start with computing $A_{1,1} = A_{0,1} + A_{1,0} = 2$, $A_{2,1} = A_{1,1} + A_{1,0} = 3, \cdots, A_{4,4} = A_{4,3} + A_{3,4} = 27 + 27 = 54$ (red numbers in Fig. 2). Thus the probability is $P(D_4 \geq 2.5) = 1 - 54/\binom{8}{4} = 0.23$. Few other examples that can be computed easily are

$$P(D_q = 0) = 0, \ P(D_q \geq 1) = 1, \ P(D_q \geq q) = 2/\binom{2q}{q}, \ P(D_q \geq q + 1) = 0.$$

Computing $A_{q,q}$ iteratively requires at most q^2 operations while permuting two samples consisting of q elements each requires $\binom{2q}{q}$ operations. Thus, our method can compute the p-value exactly substantially faster than the permutation test that is approximate and exponentially slow.

The asymptotic probability distribution of D_q can be also determined for sufficiently large q without computing iteratively as Theorem 2.

Theorem 3. $\lim_{q \to \infty} P\left(D_q/\sqrt{2q} \geq d\right) = 2 \sum_{i=1}^{\infty} (-1)^{i-1} e^{-2i^2 d^2}$.

The proof is not given here but the result follows from [8,14]. From Theorem 3, p-value under H_0 is computed as

$$p - \text{value} = 2e^{-d_o^2} - 2e^{-8d_o^2} + 2e^{-18d_o^2} \cdots,$$

where d_o is the *least integer greater than* $D_q/\sqrt{2q}$ in the data (Fig. 3-left). For any large observed value $d_0 \geq 2$, the second term is in the order of 10^{-14} and insignificant. Even for small observed d_0, the expansion converges quickly and 5 terms are sufficient.

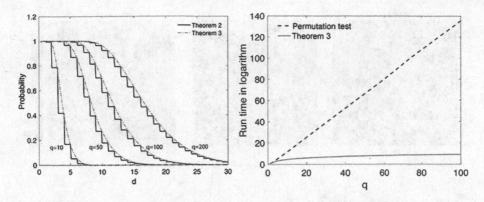

Fig. 3. Left: Convergence of Theorem 2 to 3 for $q = 10, 50, 100, 200$. Right: Run time of permutation test (dotted black line) *vs.* the combinational method in Theorem 2 (solid red line) in logarithmic scale. (Color figure online)

5 Validation and Comparison

The proposed method was validated and compared in two simulation studies against Gromov-Hausdorff (GH) distance. GH-distance was originally used to measure distance between two metric spaces. It was later adapted to measure distances in persistent homology, dendrograms [3] and brain networks [11]. Following [11], the computation of GH-distance is done done on graphs with1-correlation as edge weights. GH-distance is the difference in the L^∞-norm of corresponding single linkage matrices.

No Network Difference. The simulations were performed 1000 times and the average results were reported. There are three groups and the sample size is $n = 5$ in each group and the number of nodes are $p = 40$. In Groups I and II, data $x_k(v_i)$ at each node v_i was simulated as standard normal, i.e., $x_k(v_i) \sim N(0,1)$. The paired data was simulated as $y_k(v_i) = x_k(v_i) + N(0, 0.02^2)$ for all the nodes (Fig. 4). Using the proposed combinatorial method, we obtained the p-values of 0.6568 ± 0.3367 and 0.2830 ± 0.3636 for β_0 and the size of the largest connected component demonstrating that the method did not detect network differences as expected.

Using GH-distance, we obtained the p-value of 0.4938 ± 0.2919. The p-value was computed using the permutation test. Since there are 5 samples in each group, the total number of permutation is $\binom{10}{5} = 272$ making the permutation test exact and the comparison fair. Both methods seem to perform reasonably well. However, GH-distance method took about 950 s (16 min) while the combinatorial method took about 20 s in a computer.

Network Difference. Group III was generated identically and independently like Group I but additional dependency was added by letting $y_k(v_j) = x_k(v_1)/2$ for ten nodes indexed by $j = 1, 2, \ldots, 10$. This dependency gives high connectivity

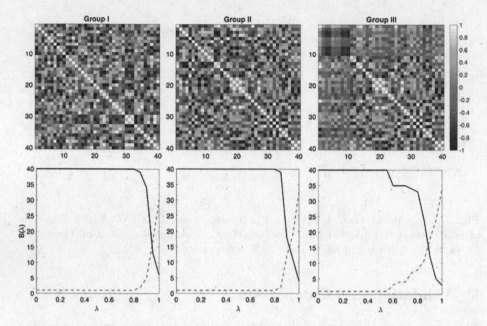

Fig. 4. Simulation studies. Group I and Group II are generated independently and identically. The resulting $B(\lambda)$ plots are similar. The dotted red line is β_0 and the solid black line is the size of the largest connected component. No statistically significant differences can be found between Groups I and II. Group III is generated independently but identically as Group I but additional dependency is added for the first 10 nodes (square on the top left corner). The resulting $B(\lambda)$ plots are statistically different between Groups I and II. (Color figure online)

differences between Groups I and III (Fig. 4). Using the proposed combinatorial method, we obtained the p-values of 0.0422 ± 0.0908 and 0.0375 ± 0.1056 for β_0 and the size of the largest connected component. On the other hand, we obtained 0.1145 ± 0.1376 for GH-distance. The proposed method seems to perform better in the presence of signal. The `MATLAB` code for performing these simulations is given in http://www.cs.wisc.edu/~mchung/twins.

6   Twin fMRI Study

The study consists of 11 monozygotic (MZ) and 9 same-sex dizygotic (DZ) twin pairs of 3 T functional magnetic resonance images (fMRI) acquired in Intera-Achiava Phillips MRI scanners with a 32 channel SENSE head coil. Subjects completed monetary incentive delay task of 3 runs of 40 trials [10]. A total 120 trials consisting of 40 \$0, 40 \$1 and 40 \$5 rewards were pseudo randomly split into 3 runs.

fMRI data went through spatial normalization to the template following the standard SPM pipeline. The fMRI dimensions after preprocessing are $53 \times 63 \times 46$ and the voxel size is 3 mm cube. There are a total of $p = 25972$ voxels in the template. After fitting a general linear model at each voxel, we obtained the

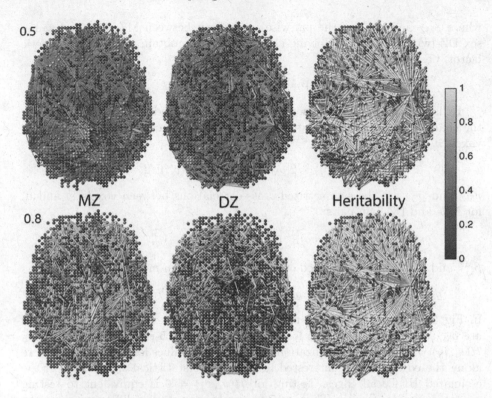

Fig. 5. Left, middle: Node colors are correlations of MZ- and DZ-twins. Edge colors are sparse cross-correlations at sparsity $\lambda = 0.5, 0.8$. Right: Heritability index (HI) at nodes and edges. MZ-twins show higher correlations compared to DZ-twins. Some low HI nodes show high HI edges. Using only the voxel-level HI feature, we may fail to detect such high-order genetic effects on the functional network.

contrast maps testing the significance of activity in the delay period for $5 trials relative to the control condition of $0 reward (Fig. 1). The paired contrast maps were then used as the initial images vectors $\mathbf{x}$ and $\mathbf{y}$ in the starting model (2).

We are interested in knowing *the extent of the genetic influence on the functional brain network* of these participants while anticipating the high reward as measured by activity during the delay that occurs between the reward cue and the target, and its statistical significance. The hyper-network approach is applied in extending the voxel-level univariate genetic feature called *heritability index* (HI) into a network-level multivariate feature. HI determines the amount of variation (in terms of percentage) due to genetic influence in a population. HI is often estimated using Falconer's formula [6] as a baseline. MZ-twins share 100% of genes while DZ-twins share 50% of genes. Thus, the additive genetic factor A, the common environmental factor C for each twin type are related as

$$\rho_{\text{MZ}}(v_i) = A + C, \tag{10}$$

$$\rho_{\text{DZ}}(v_i) = A/2 + C, \tag{11}$$

where ρ_{MZ} and ρ_{DZ} are the pairwise correlation between MZ- and and same-sex DZ-twins at voxel v_i. Solving (10) and (11), we obtain the additive genetic factor, i.e., HI given by

$$\mathcal{H}(v_i) = 2[\rho_{\mathrm{MZ}}(v_i) - \rho_{\mathrm{DZ}}(v_i)].$$

HI is a univariate feature measured at each voxel and does not quantify how the changes in one voxel is related to other voxels. We can determine HI across voxels v_i and v_j as

$$\mathcal{H}(v_i, v_j) = 2[\varrho_{\mathrm{MZ}}(v_i, v_j) - \varrho_{\mathrm{DZ}}(v_i, v_j)],$$

ϱ_{MZ} and ϱ_{DZ} are the symmetrized cross-correlations between voxels v_i and v_j for MZ- and DZ-twin pairs:

$$\varrho_{\mathrm{MZ}}(v_i, v_j) = (\widehat{\beta}_{ij}^{\mathrm{MZ}} + \widehat{\beta}_{ji}^{\mathrm{MZ}})/2, \quad \varrho_{\mathrm{DZ}}(v_i, v_j) = (\widehat{\beta}_{ij}^{\mathrm{DZ}} + \widehat{\beta}_{ji}^{\mathrm{DZ}})/2.$$

$\widehat{\beta}_{ij}^{\mathrm{MZ}}$ and $\widehat{\beta}_{ij}^{\mathrm{DZ}}$ are the estimated cross-correlations from model (4). Note that

$$\varrho_{\mathrm{MZ}}(v_i, v_i) = \rho_{\mathrm{MZ}}(v_i), \quad \varrho_{\mathrm{DZ}}(v_i, v_i) = \rho_{\mathrm{DZ}}(v_i), \quad \mathcal{H}(v_i, v_i) = \mathcal{H}(v_i).$$

In Fig. 5-left and -middle, the nodes are $\rho_{\mathrm{MZ}}(v_i)$ and $\rho_{\mathrm{DZ}}(v_i)$ while the edges are $\varrho_{\mathrm{MZ}}(v_i, v_j)$ and $\varrho_{\mathrm{DZ}}(v_i, v_j)$ for $\lambda = 0.5, 0.8$. In Fig. 5-right, we have $\mathcal{H}(v_i) = \mathcal{H}(v_i, v_i)$. The network visualization shows high HI values for almost everywhere along the edges. We are interested in testing the statistical significance of the estimated HI for all edges. Testing for $\mathcal{H}(v_i, v_j) = 0$ is equivalent to testing $\varrho_{\mathrm{MZ}}(v_i, v_j) = \varrho_{\mathrm{DZ}}(v_i, v_j)$. Thus, we test for hyper-network differences between twins using the test statistic D_q ($q = 100$ is used) (Fig. 6). For β_0 and the size of the largest connected component p-values are less than 0.00002 and 0.00001 respectively indicating very strong significance of MZ- and DZ- network difference and HI of the whole brain network.

7 Discussion

Hyper-Network. In this paper, we presented a unified statistical framework for for analyzing paired images using a hyper-network. Although we applied the framework in twin fMRI, the method can be easily applied to other paired image settings such as longitudinal and multimodal studies. The method can be further extended to triple images. Then we should start with the following hyper-network model

$$\mathbf{y}(v_j) = \sum_{i=1}^{p} \beta_{ij} \mathbf{x}(v_i) + \sum_{i=1}^{p} \gamma_{ij} \mathbf{z}(v_i) + \mathbf{e}. \tag{12}$$

Since we usually have more number of nodes p than the number of images n, it is necessary to introduce two separate sparse parameters in (12). Then, instead of building graph filtration over 1D, we need to build it over 2D sparse parameter space. This is related to multidimensional persistent homology [4, 12]. Extending the proposed method to triple image setting is left as a future study.

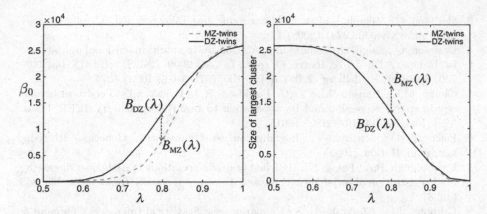

Fig. 6. The result of graph filtrations on twin fMRI data. The number of connected components (left) and the size of the largest connected component (right) are plotted over the sparse parameter λ. For each λ, MZ-twins tend to have smaller number of connected components but larger connected component. The dotted green arrow (D_q) where the maximum group separation occurs. (Color figure online)

Exact Topological Inference. We presented a combinatorial method for computing the probability that avoids time consuming permutation tests. Theorem 2 is the exact nonparametric procedure and does not assume any statistical distribution on graph features other than that they has to be monotonic. The technique is very general and applicable to any monotonic graph features such as node degree. Based on Stirling's formula, $q! \sim \sqrt{2\pi q}(\frac{q}{e})^q$, the total number of permutations in permuting two vectors of size q each is $\binom{2q}{q} \sim \frac{4^q}{\sqrt{2\pi q}}$. This is substantially larger than the quadratic run time q^2 needed in our method (Fig. 3). Even for small $q = 10$, more than tens of thousands permutations are needed for the accurate estimation the p-value. On the other hand, only up to 100 iterations are needed in our combinatorial method.

Acknowledgements. This work was supported by NIH grants 5 R01 MH098098 04 and EB022856 and NRF grant from Korea (NRF-2016R1D1A1B03935463). We thank Yoonsuck Choe of Texas A&M University and and Daniel Rowe of Marquette University for valuable discussions on permutation tests. We wish to thank anonymous reviewers for valuable comments that improved the revision.

References

1. Bezerianos, A., Sun, Y., Chen, Y., Woong, K.F., Taya, F., Arico, P., Borghini, G., Babiloni, F., Thakor, N.: Cooperation driven coherence: brains working hard together. In: 37th Annual International Conference of the IEEE Engineering in Medicine and Biology Society (EMBC), pp. 4696–4699 (2015)
2. Böhm, W., Hornik, K.: A Kolmogorov-Smirnov test for r samples. Institute for Statistics and Mathematics. Research report Series: Report, 105 (2010)

3. Carlsson, G., Memoli, F.: Persistent clustering and a theorem of J. Kleinberg. arXiv preprint arXiv:0808.2241 (2008)
4. Carlsson, G., Singh, G., Zomorodian, A.: Computing multidimensional persistence. In: Dong, Y., Du, D.-Z., Ibarra, O. (eds.) ISAAC 2009. LNCS, vol. 5878, pp. 730–739. Springer, Heidelberg (2009). doi:10.1007/978-3-642-10631-6_74
5. Chung, M.K., Hanson, J.L., Ye, J., Davidson, R.J., Pollak, S.D.: Persistent homology in sparse regression and its application to brain morphometry. IEEE Trans. Med. Imaging **34**, 1928–1939 (2015)
6. Falconer, D., Mackay, T.: Introduction to Quantitative Genetics, 4th edn. Longman, Harlow (1995)
7. Freeborough, P.A., Fox, N.C.: Modeling brain deformations in Alzheimer disease by fluid registration of serial 3D MR images. J. Comput. Assist. Tomogr. **22**, 838–843 (1998)
8. Gibbons, J.D., Chakraborti, S.: Nonparametric Statistical Inference. Chapman & Hall/CRC Press, Boca Raton (2011)
9. Jie, B., Shen, D., Zhang, D.: Brain connectivity hyper-network for MCI classification. In: Golland, P., Hata, N., Barillot, C., Hornegger, J., Howe, R. (eds.) MICCAI 2014. LNCS, vol. 8674, pp. 724–732. Springer, Cham (2014). doi:10.1007/978-3-319-10470-6_90
10. Knutson, B., Adams, C.M., Fong, G.W., Hommer, D.: Anticipation of increasing monetary reward selectively recruits nucleus accumbens. J. Neurosci. **21**, 159 (2001)
11. Lee, H., Chung, M.K., Kang, H., Kim, B.-N., Lee, D.S.: Computing the shape of brain networks using graph filtration and Gromov-Hausdorff metric. In: Fichtinger, G., Martel, A., Peters, T. (eds.) MICCAI 2011. LNCS, vol. 6892, pp. 302–309. Springer, Heidelberg (2011). doi:10.1007/978-3-642-23629-7_37
12. Lee, H., Kang, H., Chung, M.K., Lim, S., Kim, B.-N., Lee, D.S.: Integrated multimodal network approach to PET and MRI based on multidimensional persistent homology. Hum. Brain Mapp. **38**, 1387–1402 (2017)
13. Pichler, B.J., Kolb, A., Nägele, T., Schlemmer, H.-P.: PET/MRI: paving the way for the next generation of clinical multimodality imaging applications. J. Nuclear Med. **51**, 333–336 (2010)
14. Smirnov, N.V.: Estimate of deviation between empirical distribution functions in two independent samples. Bull. Moscow Univ. **2**, 3–16 (1939)
15. Thompson, P.M., Cannon, T.D., Narr, K.L., van Erp, T., Poutanen, V.P., Huttunen, M., Lonnqvist, J., Standertskjold-Nordenstam, C.G., Kaprio, J., Khaledy, M.: Genetic influences on brain structure. Nat. Neurosci. **4**, 1253–1258 (2001)
16. Zhang, B.-T.: Hypernetworks: a molecular evolutionary architecture for cognitive learning and memory. IEEE Comput. Intell. Mag. **3**, 49–63 (2008)

Multivariate Manifold Modelling of Functional Connectivity in Developing Language Networks

Ernst Schwartz[1,2][✉], Karl-Heinz Nenning[1], Gregor Kasprian[1],
Anna-Lisa Schuller[2], Lisa Bartha-Doering[2], and Georg Langs[1]

[1] Computational Imaging Research Lab and Division of Neuroradiology
and Musculoskeletal Radiology, Department of Biomedical Imaging
and Image-guided Therapy, Medical University Vienna, Vienna, Austria
ernst.schwartz@meduniwien.ac.at
[2] Department of Pediatrics and Adolescent Medicine, Medical University Vienna,
Vienna, Austria

Abstract. There is an increasing consensus in the scientific and medical communties that functional brain analysis should be conducted from a connectionist standpoint. Most connectivity studies to date rely on derived measures of graph properties. In this paper, we show that brain networks can be analyzed effectively by considering them as elements of the Riemannian manifold of symmetric positive definite matrices Sym^+. Using recently proposed methods for manifold multivariate linear modelling, we analyze the developing functional connectivity of a small cohort of children aged 6 to 13 of both genders with strongly varying handedness indices at both rest and task simultaneously. We show that even with small sample sizes we can obtain results that reflect findings on large cohorts, and that Sym^+ is a better framework for analyzing functional brain connectivity compared to Euclidean space.

1 Introduction

Functional connectivity (FC) of brains can be derived from covarying Blood-oxygen-level dependent (BOLD) signals in different parts of the brain using MRI. It is an established method for studying the human brain both at rest (rsFC) and while the subject is performing a specific task (tFC). Numerous studies have advocated the existence of intrinsic patterns in the layout of FC networks and their selective modulation during cognitive activation [1–3]. While there is a large body of work analyzing both rsFC and tFC using graph-theoretical methods [4,5], little work has been done to characterize FC as a whole from an intrinsic mathematical standpoint. Here, we show how using the Riemannian manifold of Symmetric Positive Definite (SPD) matrices improves the ability to model the global connectivity pattern and its relation to variables such as task condition, age, gender, or handedness.

G. Langs—This project was supported by FWF (KLI 544-B27, I 2714-B31) and OeNB (15356, 15929).

M. Niethammer et al. (Eds.): IPMI 2017, LNCS 10265, pp. 311–322, 2017.
DOI: 10.1007/978-3-319-59050-9_25

FC of two brain regions is determined from the covariance $\mathrm{Cov}(p_1, p_2)$ of the BOLD signal time courses p_1 and p_2 observed at distinct locations in the brain. Matrices $P, P_{ij}P_{ji} = \mathrm{Cov}(p_i, p_j), i, j \in 1 \ldots n$ representing networks of FC between n observed regions are elements of the space of Symmetric Positive Definite (SPD) matrices Sym_n^+. Positive-definiteness implies $\mathbf{v}^\top P \mathbf{v} > 0 \quad \forall \mathbf{v} \in \mathbb{R}^{+n}$, $P \in \mathrm{Sym}_n^+$, which renders elements of P interrelated. Euclidean operations do not accurately reflect this underlying geometry of the SPD manifold and can therefore lead to distorted results.

Related Work. SPD matrices are ubiquitous in their use in applied sciences in describing covariation. In computer vision, they have recently been used in the context of dictionary learning [6], dimensionality reduction [7] and image classification [8] to name a few. In neuroscience, the mathematical properties of SPD matrices have become of interest only recently. The geometric mean of a population of SPD matrices was used in [9] as prior for regularizing the estimation of FC. Parallel transport on Sym_n^+ has been used in [10] for decoding brain states from FC, while the authors in [11] performed classification of neurological diseases from FC matrices by applying kernel methods to intrinsic distances on Sym^+. Similarly, distances in Sym^+ have been applied for age regression in [12] by projecting them to the Euclidean space using locally linear embedding. Recently, Kim et al. [13], building upon the work of Fletcher [14] have adapted general linear modelling (GLM) for modelling diffusion tensor data.

Contribution. Using GLMs on the manifold of SPD matrices forms the basis of this paper. We demonstrate how it can by applied to analyzing the network architecture of the human brain directly using FC matrices. We show how it dramatically increases the capability to derive reliable results even from small datasets and that we obtain better contrasts between rest and task, a better representation of population means, and a more accurate capturing of correlates to outside variables when studying the full connectivity structure.

The remainder of this paper is organized as follows. We first give a brief introduction into the fundamental concepts of Riemannian geometry required for the intrinsic analysis of FC networks. We then demonstrate how manifold GLMs (MGLM) can be used to model a population of FC networks of children of different age, gender and handedness. We derive a robust core FC network and show how it is modulated by a language task. We compare our results to data collected on a large-scale cohort to demonstrate the validity of our results and the advantage of the proposed approach over standard Euclidean methods.

2   Methods

We first provide a brief background on Riemannian geometry of SPD matrices and the definition of MGLM which we will use for FC network modelling.

2.1   Brain Networks as Points on a Riemannian Manifold

A Riemannian manifold $\mathcal{M}$ is a manifold endowed with a smoothly varying inner product $\langle \cdot, \cdot \rangle_{T_P \mathcal{M}}$ defined in the tangent (vector) space $T_P \mathcal{M}$ of points

$P \in \mathcal{M}$. This smoothness property allows for length L of any path μ on $\mathcal{M}$ to be defined as the integral of the inner product $L(\mu) = \int \langle \mu'(t), \mu'(t) \rangle_{T_{\mu(t)}\mathcal{M}} dt$. A *geodesic* is the shortest path between any two points on $\mathcal{M}$ and therefore generalizes the notion of straight line to Riemannian manifolds. It is evident that this formulation induces a metric $d(P_1, P_2) = \inf L(\mu)$, $P_1, P_2 \in \mathcal{M}$ where μ is a curve joining P_1 and P_2 on $\mathcal{M}$.

All that is required to perform calculations on a Riemannian manifold are thus mappings between $\mathcal{M}$ and $T_P\mathcal{M}$ and back and a definition of an inner product in $T_P\mathcal{M}$. For $P, Q \in \mathcal{M} = \text{Sym}^+$, it can be shown that the operations

$$\text{Exp}_P(Q) : T_P\mathcal{M} \to \mathcal{M} = P^{\frac{1}{2}}\exp\left(P^{-\frac{1}{2}}QP^{-\frac{1}{2}}\right)P^{\frac{1}{2}} \tag{1}$$

$$\text{Log}_P(Q) : \mathcal{M} \to T_P\mathcal{M} = P^{\frac{1}{2}}\log\left(P^{-\frac{1}{2}}QP^{-\frac{1}{2}}\right)P^{\frac{1}{2}} \tag{2}$$

$$\left\langle Q_1, Q_2 \right\rangle_{T_P\mathcal{M}} = \text{Tr}\left(P^{-\frac{1}{2}}Q_1P^{-1}Q_2P^{-\frac{1}{2}}\right) \tag{3}$$

with exp and log the matrix exponential and logarithm satisfy all necessary conditions [15]. Due to the definition (2) of the logarithmic map, $\text{Log}_P(Q)$ can be viewed as a vector in $T_P\mathcal{M}$ joining P (the *root* of $T_P\mathcal{M}$) and $\text{Log}_P(Q)$ and thus forms the analogue of subtraction in Euclidean geometry. Respectively, $\text{Exp}_P(Q)$ effectively *adds* $\text{Exp}_P(Q)$ to P. It should be noted that while these mappings are defined in the whole tangent space $T_P\mathcal{M}$, they are one-to-one and onto only locally at its origin [15]. This makes the selection of an accurate root P paramount for further calculations.

2.2   General Linear Modelling of Functional Connectivity

Multiple linear regression between observations y_i and covariates x_{ij} is commonly performed by solving the minimization problem

$$\min_{\bar{M}\in\mathbb{R}^n, \mathbf{V}\in\mathbb{R}^{n\times K}} \sum_{i=1}^{N} \left\| \bar{M} + \sum_{j=1}^{K} \mathbf{V}_j x_{ij} - y_i \right\|_{\mathbb{R}^n}^2 \tag{4}$$

for which there exists a closed-form solution in the Euclidean setting. In the case where $y_i \in \text{Sym}_n^+$ and using the metric defined in Eqs. (3) and (4) corresponds to

$$\min_{\tilde{M}\in\mathcal{M}, \mathbf{V}_j\in T_P\mathcal{M}} \sum_{i=1}^{N} \left\| \text{Log}_{\tilde{y}_i}(y_i) \right\|_{T_{\tilde{y}_i}\mathcal{M}}^2$$
$$\text{where}$$
$$\tilde{y}_i = \text{Exp}_{\tilde{M}}\left(\sum_{j=1}^{K} \mathbf{V}_j x_{ij}\right) \text{ and } \left\| \text{Log}_{\tilde{y}_i}(\gamma) \right\|_{T_\gamma\mathcal{M}} = \left\langle \text{Log}_{\tilde{y}_i}(\gamma), \text{Log}_{\tilde{y}_i}(\gamma) \right\rangle_{T_\gamma\mathcal{M}} \tag{5}$$

which can be solved using gradient descent as proposed by Kim et al. [13]. In the case where the covariates x_{ij} are centered at the origin, $\bar{M}$ can be solved for separetely in (4) as $\bar{M} = \sum y_i / N$, $y_i \in \mathbb{R}^n$. In the case of $y_i \in \text{Sym}_n^+$, a similar approach can be taken by fixing the estimate $\tilde{M} \approx \bar{M}$ in (5) to correspond to the intrinsic mean of $y_{1...N}$ which can be found by minimizing

$$\min_{\tilde{M} \in \text{Sym}_n^+} \sum_{i=1}^{N} \left\langle \tilde{M}, y_i \right\rangle^2_{T_{\tilde{M}}\mathcal{M}}. \tag{6}$$

A recent comparison of approaches for solving (6) is given in [16]. Generally, the problem complexity is proportional to $n^3 N!$, which is prohibitive even in moderately sized populations. However, more efficient local solutions have recently been developed. We use the gradient descent method proposed in [17], which we initialize with the approximate geometric mean of [18] in order to reach an acceptable local minimizer of (6). We are thus able to solve the MGLM

$$\Gamma_{\text{Sym}^+} : \mathbb{R}^K \to \text{Sym}^+ = \text{Exp}_{\tilde{M}} \left(\sum_{j=1}^{K} \mathbf{V}_j x_j \right), \quad \mathbf{V}_j, \tilde{M} \in \text{Sym}^+, x_j \in \mathbb{R} \tag{7}$$

with population mean $\tilde{M}$, K model parameters $\mathbf{V}$ and covariates x.

3   Experiments

We conduct a series of experiments to demonstrate the advantage of performing analysis and modelling of FC networks in the Riemannian geometry of Sym^+. After briefly describing the dataset used, we show that its intrinsic Riemannian mean is better suited as its representative than the standard Euclidean mean. We then demonstrate how an MGLM can be used to model the modulation of rsFC under a task condition while accounting for covariate factors. Finally, we show how contrasts in Sym^+ derived from these factors relate to independent measures of brain function obtained on a seperate large dataset.

3.1   fMRI Acquisition and Processing

We aim at modelling the FC of 20 children aged 6 to 13 (mean 9.4 ± 2.14) of both genders (13 males) of varying handedness (determined using the Edinburgh Handedness Inventory to have mean 0.72 ± 0.49, range $[-0.77, 1]$). All children were scanned in a 3 Tesla Siemens TimTrio MRI scanner.

For each child, one *task* and one *rest* sequence were acquired during the same session (both gradient echo, single-shot echo planar imaging sequences with $\text{TE}/\text{TR} = 42/2000$ ms, slice thickness 4 mm). Under the *task* condition, the child had to complete an auditory semantic decision (ASD) task, age-matched in difficulty. The ASD task is presented as a block-design where the positive condition consists of the child listening to a sentence, at the end of which she has to indicate via button-press if the last word in the sentence semantically matches the sentence (for example "a long yellow fruit is a banana" (true) or "something you sit on is a spaghetti" (false), 70% true responses). The baseline condition is designed to control for both active listening and motor control and consists in reverse speech being presented to the child, after which in in 70% of the cases a tone occures, again prompting the child to press a button.

Both sequences are subjected to standard fMRI preprocessing steps. To reduce the dimensionality of our data, we use a recently proposed parcellation of the human cortex consisting of 180 anatomically and functionally defined regions on each hemisphere [19]. We average the signal in each parcel and estimate covariances using the shrinkage operator of [20]. This procedure results, for each case, in two FC matrices $M^{rest}, M^{task} \in \mathrm{Sym}_{360}^+$.

3.2 Comparing Euclidean and Riemannian Models of FC

We first evaluate the accuracy of (Eq. 6) in representing rsFC. We start by evaluating the representativeness of the intrinsic mean $\tilde{M}$ of $M_i^{rest}, i \in (1 \ldots 20)$. Because our dataset contains twice as many boys than girls, we work with the grand mean, defined as the unweighted average of all groups in the data (girls and boys in this case).

How well do individual entries in the intrinsic mean matrix $\tilde{M}$ represent the individual entries across the population? We compare the distribution of each entry in FC matrices M_i^{rest} to those of $\tilde{M}$ as well as those of the Euclidean grand mean $\hat{M}$ in Fig. 2a. We note that the distributions of both means deviate from that of the population, with the distribution of $\tilde{M}$ being much narrower. This shows that it is difficult to directly compare individual entries of $\hat{M}$ and $\tilde{M}$. However, the relative value and notably the sign of individual measures of average FC within $\hat{M}$ or $\tilde{M}$ should be representative of the population. We evelute the expected values $\mathbb{E}$ of the distributions using kernel density estimation (KDE), shown as vertical lines in Fig. 2a. This clearly indicates a bias towards anti-correlations for $\hat{M}$ ($\mathbb{E}[\hat{M}] = -0.0418$), whereas the $\mathbb{E}[\tilde{M}] = -0.0169$ allmost perfectly matches $\mathbb{E}[M] = -0.0173$.

Does the intrinsic mean better capture connectivity of the population? We compare mean FC of our relatively small dataset with published results obtained on a substantially larger population (n = 1000). Using the rsFC parcellations of Yeo et al. [2] and Power et al. [3] as references we evaluate the fraction of positive inter-parcel FC in both $\tilde{M}$ and $\hat{M}$ at varying thresholds (normalized with respect to the maximum in each $\tilde{M}$ and $\hat{M}$). As these parcellations represent functionally segregated cortical areas, these fractions should decrease rapidly. The results in Fig. 2b clearly indicate that $\tilde{M}$ more closely matches both parcellations as the fraction of inter-network edges declines more sharply at increasing thresholds than for $\hat{M}$. This shows that considering the geometry of Sym^+ allows the exploitation of smaller populations in FC analysis.

3.3 Multivariate Regression Between Brain States

It has been hypothesized that rsFC is modulated by specific cognitive tasks in a coherent manner [1]. Having determined the appropriateness of Sym^+ for the

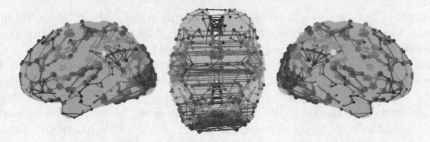

Fig. 1. $\tilde{M}^{0.5}$, the Karcher grand mean of 40 FC networks, 20 rsFC, 20 tFC, color coded for motor (green), auditory (red), vision (blue), task-positive (bright) and task-negative (dark) regions, thresholded at the 99th percentile of positive FC. (Color figure online)

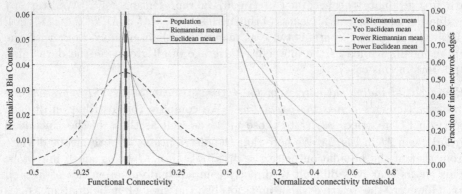

(a) FC histograms estimated using KDE   (b) Resting state networks integrities

Fig. 2. Evaluation of the accuarcy of the population means $\hat{M}$ and $\tilde{M}$ and their adherence to independent parcellations of rsFC.

analysis of rsFC data, we now show how the MGLM [13] can be used to model changes in the FC between *rest* and *task* conditions.

Does the joint intrinsic mean better reflect common characteristics of different brain states? The prerequisite for modelling changes in the FC induced by an ASD task is the definition of a common reference or intercept in the model (Eq. 7). We therefore again compute the grand mean of all 4 groups in $\{M^{\text{rest}}, M^{\text{task}}\}$, now containing both boys and girls in conditions *rest* and *task*. We use $\tilde{M}^{0.5}$ and $\hat{M}^{0.5}$ to denote the Riemannian and Euclidean grand means to indicate their expected position between *rest* and *task* conditions. In Fig. 3 we see that $\tilde{M}^{0.5}$ with Riemannian metric (Eq. 3) is most appropriate to describe both states, since the difference in distances to each individual case M_i between *task* and *rest* conditions is significantly reduced ($\rho < 1\text{e-}13$). More importantly it exhibits a balanced distance to the rest- and task-means as opposed to means and distances based in the Euclidean metric. Qualitative analysis of $\tilde{M}^{0.5}$ (Fig. 1) shows a highly structured bilateral network connecting densely interconnected primary cortical areas and sparsely connected association areas.

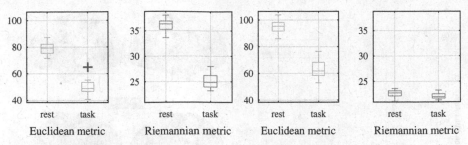

(a) Distances of individual cases to $\hat{M}^{0.5}$ (b) Distances of individual cases to $\tilde{M}^{0.5}$

Fig. 3. Distances between grand means $\tilde{M}^{0.5}$ and $\hat{M}^{0.5}$ and elements of $\{M_i^{\text{rest}}, M_i^{\text{task}}\}$

Does Riemannian multivariate effect modelling improve capturing the differences of task and rest? We use MGLM to describe the effects of age, gender, handedness and task state on the population of FC matrices $\{M^{\text{rest}}, M^{\text{task}}\}$. The model we use is

$$\Gamma_{\text{Sym+}} : M_i = \text{Exp}_{\tilde{M}^{0.5}}\left(\tilde{v}_1 \times \text{age} + \tilde{v}_2 \times \text{handedness} + \tilde{v}_3 \times \text{gender} + \tilde{v}_4 \times \text{state}\right)$$

$$\text{age} \in \mathbb{R}^+, \text{handedness} \in (-1, 1), \text{gender}, \text{state} \in \{-1, 1\}, \tilde{v}_i \in \text{Sym}_{360}^+$$

$$(8)$$

where state $= -1$ corresponds to the *rest* and state $= 1$ to the ASD *task* condition. Male gender is encoded as 1. The reference standard GLM is $\Gamma_\mathbb{R} = \hat{M}^{0.5} + \sum_{i=1}^{4} (\hat{v}_i \times \text{covariate}_i), \hat{v}_i \in \mathbb{R}^{360 \times 360}$ and the same encoding for the covariates. In order to evaluate the validity of $\Gamma_{\text{Sym+}}$ (8), we use it to simulate an average FC matrix $\tilde{M}^{\text{sim}}$ of a right-handed 9.3 year old boy at rest. We then vary the state in (8) and plot the correlation of the covariance profile (CP) of a parcel in the perisylvian language area (PSL, indicated by the dot in Fig. 4b) with publicly available data [21]. Figure 4b shows the comparison between $\tilde{M}^{\text{sim}}$ and the prediction $\hat{M}^{\text{sim}}$ of $\Gamma_\mathbb{R}$. $\tilde{M}^{\text{sim}}$ not only achieves overall higher maximum correlation with the ground truth ($R^2 = 0.61$, $\rho < 1\text{e-}37$ compared to $R^2 = 0.58$, $\rho < 1\text{e-}35$), but this maximum also lies closer to the expected value of state $= -1$ (vertical lines in Fig. 4b). In addition, the correlation shows a much clearer peak at the maximum, falls off more sharply towards the *task* state and turns less negative in the positive *task* limit. Notably, the correlation of both $\tilde{M}^{\text{sim}}$ and $\hat{M}^{\text{sim}}$ are greater than any correlation between the individual cases $\{M^{\text{rest}}, M^{\text{task}}\}$ and the reference (range $[-0.11, 0.48]$). Jointly, these results indicate that $\Gamma_{\text{Sym+}}$ yields a more comprehensive representation of the notion of rsFC and its modulation in tFC.

Motivated by these results, we performed a simple line search for the age exhibiting the highest correlation with the expected CP of PSL. Fixing all other model parameters, the maximum was found to be R2=0.64 at age 11.6 ($\rho < 1\text{e-}42$). The corresponding simulated rsFC CP for PSL is shown in Fig. 4b and accurately captures the bilateral covariance of PSL with language-associated ventro-lateral, temporal and pre-motor areas.

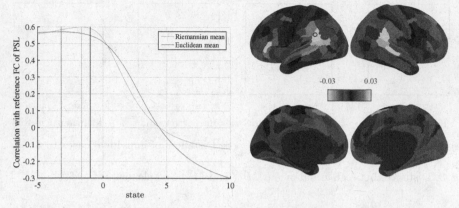

(a) Correlation of covariance profiles of PSL with varying rest/task effect.

(b) FC map of PSL in a simulated rsFC of a right-handed 11.6 year old boy at rest.

Fig. 4. Correlation of simulated connectivity profiles of PSL and ground truth with varying task effect and examplary CP showing increased FC in language-related areas.

Are constrasts between rsFC and tFC networks more meaningful when computed in Sym$_+$? Analoguously to standard GLMs, we define a network contrast β_v for an effect v as $\beta_v = \Gamma(v) - \Gamma(-v)$. Due to linearity of the Euclidean space, this reduces to $\hat{\beta}_v = \hat{v}$ for $\Gamma_\mathbb{R}$. In Sym$_+$ however, $\tilde{\beta}_v = \mathrm{Exp}_{\tilde{M}}(\tilde{v}) - \mathrm{Exp}_{\tilde{M}}(-\tilde{v})$. We show the pair-wise correlation between all contrasts $(\hat{v}_i, \hat{v}_j)\, i \neq j$ (Fig. 5a) and $(\tilde{v}_i, \tilde{v}_j)\, i \neq j$ (Fig. 5b). In $\Gamma_\mathbb{R}$, all correlations except those between age and handedness contrasts are significant ($\rho < 1e\text{-}48$). In $\Gamma_{\mathrm{Syn}+}$, all but the correlation between task and handedness contrast remain significant, albeit at a much

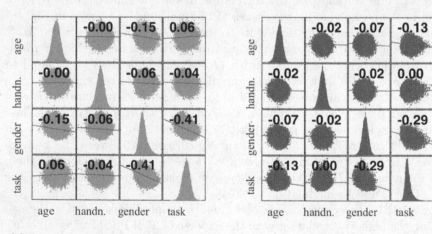

(a) Covariance between contrasts in $\Gamma_\mathbb{R}$ (b) Covariance between contrasts in $\Gamma_{\mathrm{Syn}+}$

Fig. 5. Correlation between contrasts in models $\Gamma_\mathbb{R}$ and $\Gamma_{\mathrm{Syn}+}$. Better seperability of model dimensions in $\Gamma_{\mathrm{Syn}+}$ is evident from a decrease in correlation.

lower level ($\rho < $ 1e-14). Importantly, $\Gamma_{\text{Syn}+}$ reduces the correlation between most dimensions of the model, while it shows increased correlation between age and handedness as well as age and task contrasts. This is intuitively appealing, since such as a negative correlation between the age and task contrasts indicate less modulation of rsFC under ASD task condition at an older age. Quantitatively, this signifies that MGLM enables a stronger separation of the effects of the different covariates. Additionally, these results help in elucidating the strong difference between the Euclidean means in Fig. 3, which might be due to a combination of the uneven distribution of the dataset between girls and boys, the definition of the grand mean and the strong correlation ($R^2 = 0.41$) between age and gender in $\Gamma_{\mathbb{R}}$.

Insights into the Nature of Rest/Task Contrasts. For a better understanding of the nature of the modulation of rsFC to tFC, we evaluate its correlation with publicly available task response maps. We use the degree weights, defined as the row-sums of the positive entries in $\hat{\beta}_{v_t}$ and $\tilde{\beta}_{v_t}$ as a proxy measure for the effect of performing an ASD task predicted by each model and correlate them with the collection of 86 task response maps published with [19]. We report the significant correlations, Bonferroni corrected for multiple comparisons in Table 1. We clearly observe that $\hat{\beta}_{v_t}$ strongly correlates with measures that can be associated to decrease in involuntary movement such as not tapping fingers or squeezing toes, while $\tilde{\beta}_{v_t}$ correlates strongly with higher-level contrasts related

Table 1. Table of significant correlation (Bonferroni corrected, $\rho < 0.01$) between node weight maps of FC task contrasts and HCP task contrast maps, more significant values in boldface. Note that the Riemannian model simulates significant contrasts for those tasks that are plausibly related to the task condition.

#	Task name	Task description	$R^2_{\text{Sym}+}$	$\rho_{\text{Sym}+}$	$R^2_{\mathbb{R}}$	$\rho_{\mathbb{R}}$
44	MOTOR	CUE vs avg. of other effectors	0.38	**6.63e-12**	0.06	1.91e+01
69	SOCIAL	View randomly moving geom. objects	0.31	**1.68e-07**	−0.03	4.94e+01
54	MOTOR	not tap right fingers	0.23	1.39e-03	0.31	**2.77e-07**
37	MOTOR	CUE visual instruction cue	0.30	**3.04e-07**	−0.05	3.05e+01
52	MOTOR	not tap left fingers	0.22	1.67e-03	0.30	**4.73e-07**
36	GAMBL	REWARD vs PUNISH	0.30	**6.95e-07**	0.15	2.76e-01
56	MOTOR	not avg. foot, hand and tongue motion	0.14	6.58e-01	0.30	**7.75e-07**
53	MOTOR	not squeeze right toes	0.14	8.27e-01	0.26	**4.63e-05**
51	MOTOR	not squeeze left toes	0.09	7.74	0.25	**2.17e-04**
65	LANG	MATH vs STORY	0.24	**3.79e-04**	0.08	1.12e+01
68	LANG	intercept of GLM vs listen to stories	0.24	**5.49e-04**	0.22	1.44e-03
70	SOCIAL	Theory of Mind ·	0.22	**1.41e-03**	−0.06	2.16e+01
55	MOTOR	not move tongue	0.03	5.28e+01	0.22	**1.81e-03**
6	WM	Zero-back task face images	−0.05	2.68e+01	−0.22	**2.16e-03**
7	WM	Zero-back task place images	0.01	7.68e+01	−0.21	**3.55e-03**
75	RELAT	Match objects based on verbal category	0.21	**7.30e-03**	−0.06	2.27e+01

to reward, language and relational processing tasks. These results show that the proposed modelling approach is significantly better at describing modulations affecting FC due to semantic processing than the classical approach.

Qualitative Analysis of Covariate Effects on FC. Having established the validity of performing multivariate regression in Sym^+ for the analysis of FC networks, we now give some qualitative results on their nature. We compute $\tilde{M}^{0.5} - \mathrm{Exp}_{\tilde{M}^{0.5}}(\sigma\tilde{v}_i), \sigma \in \{-1, 1\}$. The 0.01% connections most affected strongly positively and negatively by each model dimension $i = 1 \ldots 4$ are shown in Fig. 6, while $\hat{v}_{1\ldots4}$ are shown in Fig. 7, where we ommit the inverse due to the linearity

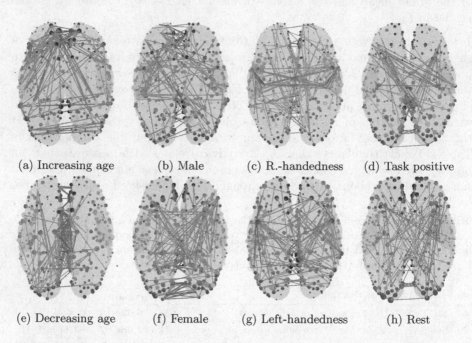

(a) Increasing age   (b) Male   (c) R.-handedness   (d) Task positive

(e) Decreasing age   (f) Female   (g) Left-handedness   (h) Rest

Fig. 6. Effect of varying individual covariates in $\Gamma_{\mathrm{Sym}+}$ (neurological right, strongest 0.01% increase and decrease shown, marker sizes indicative of positive node weights.)

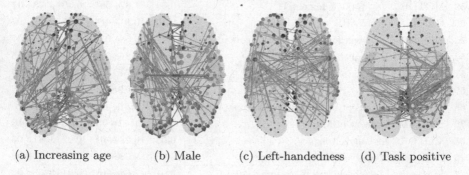

(a) Increasing age   (b) Male   (c) Left-handedness   (d) Task positive

Fig. 7. Effect of varying individual covariates in $\Gamma_{\mathbb{R}}$ (neurological right, strongest 0.01% increase and decrease shown, marker sizes indicative of positive node weights)

of each edge effect. While a detailed discussion of the neuroscientific interpretations of Fig. 6 is beyond the scope of this paper, the increased separation of covariate effects is clearly visible.

4   Conclusion

In this paper, we have shown that analysis of FC networks profits considerably when it is performed intrinsically on the manifold of SPD matrices. From a small dataset, we could derive numerous results elucidating the effects of covariates in structures where Euclidean methods would fail due to neglected interdependence between elements. This is particularly important if we study the relationship of FC to other variables such as age in smaller cohorts. While the neuroscientific implications of our results are the subject of future study, we have shown that results from the relatively small cohort are in line with results obtained from large scale studies.

References

1. Cole, M.W., Bassett, D.S., Power, J.D., Braver, T.S., Petersen, S.E.: Intrinsic and task-evoked network architectures of the human brain. Neuron **83**(1), 238–251 (2014)
2. Yeo, B.T., Krienen, F.M., Sepulcre, J., Sabuncu, M.R., Lashkari, D., Hollinshead, M., Roffman, J.L., Smoller, J.W., Zöllei, L., Polimeni, J.R., et al.: The organization of the human cerebral cortex estimated by intrinsic functional connectivity. J. Neurophysiol. **106**(3), 1125–1165 (2011)
3. Power, J.D., Cohen, A.L., Nelson, S.M., Wig, G.S., Barnes, K.A., Church, J.A., Vogel, A.C., Laumann, T.O., Miezin, F.M., Schlaggar, B.L., et al.: Functional network organization of the human brain. Neuron **72**(4), 665–678 (2011)
4. Ginestet, C.E., Fournel, A.P., Simmons, A.: Statistical network analysis for functional MRI: summary networks and group comparisons. Front. Comput. Neurosci. **8**, 51 (2014)
5. Betzel, R.F., Byrge, L., He, Y., Goñi, J., Zuo, X.N., Sporns, O.: Changes in structural and functional connectivity among resting-state networks across the human lifespan. Neuroimage **102**, 345–357 (2014)
6. Cherian, A., Sra, S.: Riemannian dictionary learning and sparse coding for positive definite matrices. arxiv preprint. arXiv:1507.02772 (2015)
7. Harandi, M., Salzmann, M., Hartley, R.: Dimensionality reduction on SPD manifolds: the emergence of geometry-aware methods. arxiv preprint. arXiv:1605.06182 (2016)
8. Huang, Z., Wang, R., Shan, S., Li, X., Chen, X.: Log-euclidean metric learning on symmetric positive definite manifold with application to image set classification. In: Proceedings of the 32nd International Conference on Machine Learning, ICML 2015, pp. 720–729 (2015)
9. Varoquaux, G., Gramfort, A., Poline, J.B., Thirion, B.: Brain covariance selection: better individual functional connectivity models using population prior. In: Advances in Neural Information Processing Systems, pp. 2334–2342 (2010)

10. Ng, B., Dressler, M., Varoquaux, G., Poline, J.B., Greicius, M., Thirion, B.: Transport on Riemannian manifold for functional connectivity-based classification. In: Golland, P., Hata, N., Barillot, C., Hornegger, J., Howe, R. (eds.) MICCAI 2014. LNCS, vol. 8674, pp. 405–412. Springer, Cham (2014). doi:10.1007/978-3-319-10470-6_51

11. Dodero, L., Minh, H.Q., San Biagio, M., Murino, V., Sona, D.: Kernel-based classification for brain connectivity graphs on the Riemannian manifold of positive definite matrices. In: IEEE 12th International Symposium on Biomedical Imaging (ISBI), pp. 42–45. IEEE (2015)

12. Qiu, A., Lee, A., Tan, M., Chung, M.K.: Manifold learning on brain functional networks in aging. Med. Image Anal. 20(1), 52–60 (2015)

13. Kim, H.J., Adluru, N., Collins, M.D., Chung, M.K., Bendlin, B.B., Johnson, S.C., Davidson, R.J., Singh, V.: Multivariate general linear models (MGLM) on Riemannian manifolds with applications to statistical analysis of diffusion weighted images. In: Proceedings of the IEEE Conference on Computer Vision and Pattern Recognition, pp. 2705–2712 (2014)

14. Fletcher, P.T.: Geodesic regression and the theory of least squares on Riemannian manifolds. Int. J. Comput. Vision 105(2), 171–185 (2013)

15. Pennec, X., Fillard, P., Ayache, N.: A Riemannian framework for tensor computing. Int. J. Comput. Vision 66(1), 41–66 (2006)

16. Jeuris, B., Vandebril, R., Vandereycken, B.: A survey and comparison of contemporary algorithms for computing the matrix geometric mean. Electr. Trans. Numer. Anal. 39(EPFL-ARTICLE-197637), 379–402 (2012)

17. Bini, D.A., Iannazzo, B.: Computing the Karcher mean of symmetric positive definite matrices. Linear Algebra Appl. 438(4), 1700–1710 (2013)

18. Bini, D.A., Iannazzo, B.: A note on computing matrix geometric means. Adv. Comput. Math. 35(2–4), 175–192 (2011)

19. Glasser, M., Coalson, T., Robinson, E., Hacker, C., Harwell, J., Yacoub, E., Ugurbil, K., Anderson, J., Beckmann, C., Jenkinson, M., et al.: A multi-modal parcellation of human cerebral cortex. Nature 536, 171–178 (2016)

20. Chen, Y., Wiesel, A., Eldar, Y.C., Hero, A.O.: Shrinkage algorithms for mmse covariance estimation. IEEE Trans. Sig. Process. 58(10), 5016–5029 (2010)

21. Van Essen, D.C., Smith, J., Glasser, M.F., Elam, J., Donahue, C.J., Dierker, D.L., Reid, E.K., Coalson, T., Harwell, J.: The brain analysis library of spatial maps and atlases (BALSA) database. NeuroImage 144, 270–274 (2017)

Hierarchical Region-Network Sparsity for High-Dimensional Inference in Brain Imaging

Danilo Bzdok[✉], Michael Eickenberg, Gaël Varoquaux,
and Bertrand Thirion

INRIA, Parietal Team, Saclay, France
danilo.bzdok@inria.fr

Abstract. Structured sparsity penalization has recently improved statistical models applied to high-dimensional data in various domains. As an extension to medical imaging, the present work incorporates priors on network hierarchies of brain regions into logistic-regression to distinguish neural activity effects. These priors bridge two separately studied levels of brain architecture: functional segregation into regions and functional integration by networks. Hierarchical region-network priors are shown to better classify and recover 18 psychological tasks than other sparse estimators. Varying the relative importance of region and network structure within the hierarchical tree penalty captured complementary aspects of the neural activity patterns. Local and global priors of neurobiological knowledge are thus demonstrated to offer advantages in generalization performance, sample complexity, and domain interpretability.

1 Introduction

Many quantitative scientific domains underwent a recent shift from the classical "long data" regime to the high-dimensional "wide data" regime. In the brain imaging domain, many contemporary technologies for acquiring brain signals yield many more variables per observation than total observations per data sample. This $n \ll p$ scenario challenges various statistical methods from classical statistics. For instance, estimating generalized linear models without additional assumptions yields an underdetermined system of equations. Many such ill-posed estimation problems have benefited from *sparsity* assumptions [3]. Those act as regularizer by encouraging zero coefficients in model selection. Sparse supervised and unsupervised learning algorithms have proven to yield statistical relationships that can be readily estimated, reproduced, and interpreted. Moreover, *structured sparsity* can impose domain knowledge on the statistical estimation, thus shrinking and selecting variables guided by expected data distributions [3]. These restrictions to model complexity are an attractive plan of attack for the >100,000 variables per brain map. Yet, what neurobiological structure best lends itself to exploitation using structured sparsity priors?

Neuroscientific concepts on brain organization were long torn between the two extremes *functional specialization* and *functional integration*. Functional specialization emphasizes that microscopically distinguishable brain regions are

M. Niethammer et al. (Eds.): IPMI 2017, LNCS 10265, pp. 323–335, 2017.
DOI: 10.1007/978-3-319-59050-9_26

solving distinct computational problems [14]. Conversely, functional integration emphasizes that neural computation is enabled by a complex interplay between these distinct brain regions [19]. However, local neuronal populations and global connectivity profiles are thought to go hand-in-hand to realize neural processes. Yet, probably no existing brain analysis method acknowledges that both functional design principles are inextricably involved in realizing mental operations.

Functional specialization has long been explored and interpreted. Single-cell recordings and microscopic tissue examination revealed the segregation of the occipital visual cortex into V1, V2, V3, V3A/B, and V4 regions [22]. Tissue lesion of the mid-fusiform gyrus of the visual system was frequently reported to impair recognition of others' identity from faces [11]. As a crucial common point, these and other methods yield neuroscientific findings naturally interpreted according to non-overlapping, discrete region compartments as the basic architecture of brain organization. More recently, the interpretational focus has shifted from circumscribed regions to network stratifications in neuroscience. Besides analyses of electrophysiological oscillations and graph-theoretical properties, studies of functional connectivity correlation and independent component analysis (ICA) became the workhorses of network discovery in neuroimaging [6]. As a common point of these other methods, neuroscientific findings are naturally interpreted as cross-regional integration by overlapping network compartments as the basic architecture of brain organization, in contrast to methods examining regional specialization.

Building on these two interpretational traditions in neuroscience, the present study incorporates neurobiological structure underlying functional segregation and integration into supervised estimators by hierarchical structured sparsity. Every variable carrying brain signals will be a-priori assigned to both region and network compartments to improve high-dimensional model fitting based on existing neurobiological knowledge. Learning algorithms exploiting structured sparsity have recently made much progress in various domains from processing auditory signals, natural images and videos to astrophysics, genetics, and conformational dynamics of protein complexes. The hierarchical tree penalties recently suggested for imaging neuroscience [12] will be extended to introduce neurobiologically plausible region and network priors to design neuroscience-specific classifiers. Based on the currently largest public neuroimaging repository (Human Connectome Project [HCP]) and widely used region [8] and network [18] atlases, we demonstrate that domain-informed supervised models gracefully tackle the curse of dimensionality, yield more human-interpretable results, and generalize better to new samples than domain-naive black-box estimators.

2 Methods

This paper contributes a neuroscience adaptation of hierarchical structured tree penalties to jointly incorporate region specialization and network integration priors into high-dimensional prediction. We capitalize on hierarchical group lasso to create a new class of convex sparse penalty terms. These conjointly acknowledge local specialization and global integration when discriminating defined psychological tasks from neural activity maps. Rather than inferring brain activity from psychological tasks by independent comparisons of task pairs, this approach simultaneously infers a set of psychological tasks from brain activity maps in a multivariate setting and allows for prediction in unseen neuroimaging data.

2.1 Rationale

3D brain maps acquired by neuroimaging scanners are high-dimensional but, luckily, the measured signal is also highly structured. Its *explicit dimensionality*, the number of brain voxels, typically exceeds 100,000 variables, while the number of samples rarely exceeds few hundreds. This $n \ll p$ scenario directly implies underdetermination of any linear model based on dot products with the voxel values. However, the *effective dimensionality* of functional brain scans has been shown to be much lower [7]. Two types of low-dimensional neighborhoods will be exploited by injecting accepted knowledge of regional specialization (i.e., region priors) and spatiotemporal interactions (i.e., network priors) into statistical estimation.

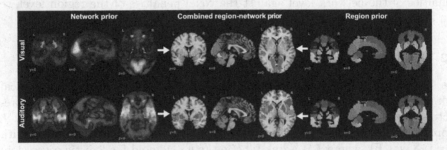

Fig. 1. Building blocks of the hierarchical region-network tree. Displays the a-priori neurobiological knowledge introduced into the classification problem by hierarchical structured sparsity. *Left:* Continuous, partially overlapping brain network priors (*hot-colored*, network atlas taken from [18]) accommodate the functional integration perspective of brain organization. *Right:* Discrete, non-overlapping brain region priors (*single-colored*, region atlas taken from [8]) accommodate the functional segregation perspective. *Middle:* These two types of predefined voxel groups are incorporated into a joint hierarchical prior of parent networks with their descending region child nodes. *Top to bottom:* Two exemplary region-network priors are shown, including the early cortices that process visual and sound information from the environment. (Color figure online)

Major brain networks emerge in human individuals before birth [9]. Their nodes have more similar functional profiles than nodes from different networks [2]. As a popular method for network extraction, ICA [6] yields continuous brain maps with voxel-level resolution. The region nodes of ICA network are spatially disjoint sets of voxel groups that

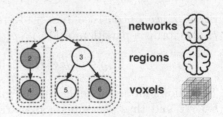

Fig. 2. Hierarchical tree prior.

agree with boundaries of brain atlases. Hence, each region from a brain atlas can be uniquely associated with one of the extracted ICA networks. Here, previously published network definitions obtained using ICA [18] and region definitions obtained from spatially constrained clustering [8] allowed constructing a hierarchy of global ICA networks with their assigned local cluster regions (Fig. 1). The ensuing network-region tree was used as a frequentist prior of expected weight distributions to advantageously bias supervised model fitting.

Specifically, this tree structure was plugged into hierarchical sparsity penalty terms [12]. It extends the group lasso [21] by permitting variable groups that contain each other in a nested tree structure. The first hierarchical level are the network groups with all the voxels of the brain regions associated with them. Each network node in turn descends into a second hierarchical level with brain regions of neighboring voxels (Fig. 2). Induced by the region-network sparsity tree, a child node enters the set of relevant voxel variables only if its parent node has been selected [3]. Conversely, if a parent node is deselected, also the voxel variables of all child nodes are deselected. Moreover, the coefficients of all region or all network groups can be weighed individually. Trading off the voxel penalties of the network level against the voxel penalties of the region level we can design distinct estimation regimes.

2.2   Problem Formulation

We formulate our estimation problem in the framework of regularized empirical risk minimization applied to linear models. The goal is to estimate a good predictor of psychological tasks given a single brain image. Let the set $\mathbf{X} \in \mathbb{R}^{n \times p}$ represent brain images of $p > 0$ voxels. We then minimize the risk $\mathcal{L}(\hat{y}, y)$ with $\hat{y} = f(\mathbf{X}\hat{\mathbf{w}} + \hat{\mathbf{b}})$, where f is a link function (e.g., sigmoid for logistic regression, identity for linear regression), and $\mathcal{L}$ usually represents an appropriate negative loglikelihood. We incorporate an informative prior through regularization:

$$\hat{\mathbf{w}}, \hat{\mathbf{b}} = \operatorname{argmin}_{w,b} \mathcal{L}(f(\mathbf{X}\mathbf{w} + \mathbf{b}), y) + \lambda \Omega(\mathbf{w}),$$

where $\lambda > 0$ and Ω is the regularizer. Brain *regions* are defined as disjoint groups of voxels. Let $\mathcal{G}$ be a partition of $\{1, \ldots, p\}$, i.e.

$$\bigcup_i g_i = \{1, \ldots, p\} \text{ and } g_i \cap g_j = \emptyset \quad \forall i \neq j$$

Brain *networks* consist of one or several brain regions. The set of brain networks $\mathcal{H}$ also forms a partition of $\{1, \ldots, p\}$ that is consistent with $\mathcal{G}$ in the sense that

$$\forall g \in \mathcal{G}, h \in \mathcal{H}, \quad \text{either } g \subset h \text{ or } g \cap h = \emptyset.$$

This allows for an unambiguous assignment of each region $g \in \mathcal{G}$ to one network $h \in \mathcal{H}$ and thus generates a tree structure. A root node is added to contain all voxels. For a brain image $\mathbf{w} \in \mathbb{R}^p$ and a group g, the vector $\mathbf{w}_g \in \mathbb{R}^{|g|}$ is defined as the restriction of $\mathbf{w}$ to the coordinates in g. The penalty structured by network and region information can then be written as

$$\Omega(\mathbf{w}) = \alpha \sum_{h \in \mathcal{H}} \eta_h \|\mathbf{w}_h\|_2 + \beta \sum_{g \in \mathcal{G}} \eta_g \|\mathbf{w}_g\|_2.$$

As originally recommended [21], we set $\eta_g = 1/\sqrt{|g|}$ to account for discrepancy in group sizes. The hierarchy-level-specific factors $\alpha > 0$ and $\beta > 0$ can tradeoff region-weighted and network-weighted models against each other. Decreasing α leads to less penalization of brain networks and thus the tendency for fully active groups and dense brain maps. If at the same time β is increased to induce group sparsity, then only the structure of brain regions encoded by $\mathcal{G}$ is acknowledged. Conversely, if β is chosen sufficiently small and α increased, the detected structure will derive from $\mathcal{H}$, leading to the selection of brain networks rather than regions.

Please note that the above tradeoff enables predominance attributed to either brain regions or networks, although the penalty structure remains hierarchical. If the network penalty layer sets a network group to zero, then all the contained region groups are forced to have activity zero. Conversely, if a brain region has non-zero coefficients, then necessarily the network containing it must be active. This relation is asymmetric, the roles of $\mathcal{G}$ and $\mathcal{H}$ cannot be swapped: A brain region can set all its coefficients to zero without forcing the corresponding network to zero. A brain network can be active without its subregions being active. When evaluating the tradeoff in (α, β), this needs to be taken into account.

The prediction problem at hand is a multiclass classification. We choose to attack this using one-versus-rest scheme on a binary logistic regression. The one-versus-rest classification strategy is chosen to obtain one weight map per class for display and model diagnostics. Its loss can be written as

$$\sum_{i=1}^{n} \log(1 + \exp(-y_i \langle x_i, \mathbf{w} \rangle)) + \lambda \Omega(\mathbf{w}),$$

if $y \in \{-1, 1\}$ and with $x_i \in \mathbb{R}^p$ the training sample brain images. We optimize parameters $\mathbf{w}$ using an iterative forward-backward scheme analogous to the FISTA solver for the lasso [5].

2.3 Hyperparameter Optimization

Stratified and shuffled training sets were repeatedly and randomly drawn from the whole dataset with preserved class balance and submitted to a nested cross-validation (CV) scheme for model selection and model assessment. In the inner CV layer, the logistic regression estimators have been trained in a one-versus-rest design that distinguishes each class from the respective 17 other classes (number of maximal iterations $= 100$, tolerance $= 0.001$). In the outer CV layer, grid search selected among candidates for the respective λ parameter by searching between 10^{-2} and 10^1 in 9 steps on a logarithmic scale. Importantly, the thus selected sparse logistic regression classifier was evaluated on an identical test set in all analysis settings.

2.4 Implementation

All experiments were performed in Python. We used *nilearn* to process and resphape the extensive neuroimaging data [1], *scikit-learn* to design machine-learning data processing pipelines [16], and *SPAMs* for numerically optimized implementations of the sparse learners (http://spams-devel.gforge.inria.fr/). All Python scripts that generated the results are accessible online for reproducibility and reuse (http://github.com/banilo/ipmi2017).

2.5 Data

As the currently biggest open-access dataset in brain imaging, we chose brain data from the HCP [4]. Neuroimaging data with labels of ongoing psychological processes were drawn from 500 healthy HCP participants. 18 HCP tasks (cf. [7], Table 1) were selected that are known to elicit reliable neural activity across participants. The HCP data incorporated $n = 8650$ first-level activity maps from 18 diverse paradigms in a common $60 \times 72 \times 60$ space of 3 mm isotropic gray-matter voxels. Hence, the present analyses were based on task-labeled HCP maps of neural activity with $p = 79{,}941$ z-scored voxels.

3 Experimental Results

3.1 Benchmarking Hierarchical Tree Sparsity Against Common Sparse Estimators

Hierarchical region-network priors have been systematically evaluated against other popular choices of sparse classification algorithms in an 18-class scenario (Fig. 3). Logistic regression with ℓ_1/ℓ_2-block-norm penalization incorporated a hierarchy of previously known region and network neighborhoods for a neurobio-logical bias of the statistical estimation ($\alpha = 1, \beta = 1$). Vanilla logistic regression with ℓ_1-penalization and ℓ_1-ℓ_2-elastic-net penalization do not assume any previously known special structure. These classification estimators embrace a vision of neural activity structure that expects a minimum of topographically and functionally independent brain voxels to be relevant. Logistic regression with (sparse) group sparsity imposes a structured ℓ_1/ℓ_2-block norm (with additional ℓ_1 term) with a known region atlas of voxel groups onto the statistical estimation process. These supervised estimators shrink and select the coefficients of topographically compact voxel groups expected to be relevant in unison. Logistic regression with trace-norm penalization imposed low-rank structure [10]. This supervised classification algorithm expected a minimum of unknown "network" patterns to be relevant.

Across experiments with stratified and shuffled cross-validation (90%/10% train/test set) across pooled participant data, hierarchial tree sparsity was most successful in distinguishing unseen neural activity maps from 18 psychological tasks (89.7% multi-class accuracy, mean AUC 0.948 [$\pm$0.091 standard deviation]

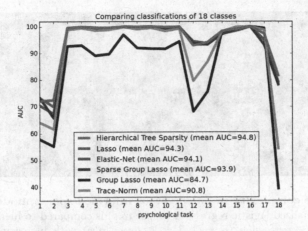

Fig. 3. Prediction performance across sparsity priors. Comparing the performance of logistic regression estimators with 6 different structured and unstructered sparse regularization penalties (*colors*) in classifying neural activity from 18 psychological tasks (cf. [7], Table 1). The area under the curve (AUC) is provided on an identical test set as class-wise measure (*y-axis*) and across-class mean (*legend*). Simultaneous knowledge of both region and network neighborhoods was hence most beneficial for predicting tasks from neural activity. (Color figure online)

mean precision 0.87, mean recall 0.92). It was closely followed by logistic regression structured by trace-norm regularization (89.4%, mean AUC 0.908 [±0.148], precision 0.86, recall 0.91). Lasso featured an average performance comparing to the other sparse estimators (88.6%, mean AUC 0.943 [±0.093], precision 0.86, recall 0.90). Elastic-Net, in turn, featured an average performance comparing to the other sparse estimators (88.1%, mean AUC 0.941 [±0.102], precision 0.85, recall 0.84). Introducing a-priori knowledge of brain region compartments by sparse group sparsity (87.9%, mean AUC 0.939 [±0.101], precision 0.85, recall 0.90) and by group sparsity (87.9%, mean AUC 0.847 [±0.173], precision 0.85, recall 0.90) performed worst.

In an important subanalysis, the advantage of the *combined* region-network prior was confirmed by selectively zeroing either the η_g coefficients of all *region* groups or the η_h coefficients of all *network* groups in the hierarchical prior. Removing region structure from the sparsity penalty achieved 88.8% accuracy, while removing network structure from the sparsity penalty achieved 87.1% accuracy. These results from priors with impoverished a-priori structure were indeed outperformed by the full region-network tree prior at 89.7% out-of-sample accuracy.

In sum, driving sparse model selection by domain knowledge of region-network hierarchies outcompeted all other frequently used sparse penalization techniques for high-dimensional data.

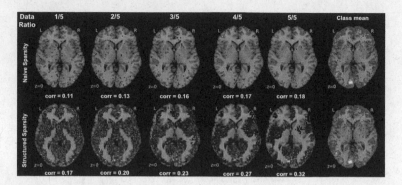

Fig. 4. Sample complexity in naive versus informed sparse model selection. Ordinary ℓ_1-penalized logistic regression (*upper row*) is compared to hierarchical-tree-penalized logistic regression ($\alpha = 1, \beta = 1$, *lower row*) with increasing fraction of the available training data to be fitted (*left to right columns*). For one example (i.e., "View tools") from 18 psychological tasks (cf. [7], Table 1), unthresholded axial maps of recovered model weights are quantitatively compared against the sample average of that class (*rightmost column*, thresholded at the 75th percentile). This notion of weight recovery was computed by Pearson correlation (*corr*). In the data-scarce scenario, ubiquitous in neuroimaging, hierarchical tree sparsity achieves much better support recovery. In the data-rich scenario, biologically informed logistic regression profits more from the available information quantities than biologically naive logistic regression.

3.2   Sample Complexity of Naive Versus Informed Sparse Model Selection

Subsequently, the sample complexity of ℓ_1-penalized and hierarchical-tree-penalized logistic regression ($\alpha = 1, \beta = 1$) was empirically evaluated and quantitatively compared (Fig. 4). Region-network priors should constrain model selection towards more neurobiologically plausible classification estimators. This should yield better out-of-sample generalization and support recovery than neurobiology-naive ℓ_1-constrained logistic regression in the data-scarce and data-rich scenarios. The HCP data with examples from 18 psychological tasks were first divided into 90% of training set (i.e., 7584 neural activity maps) and 10% of test set (i.e., 842 maps). Both learning algorithms were fitted based on the training set at different subsampling fractions: 20% (1516 neural activity maps), 40% (3033 maps), 60% (4550 maps), 80% (6067 maps), and 100% (7584 maps).

Regarding classification performance on the identical test set, ℓ_1-penalized versus hierarchical-tree-penalized logistic regression achieved 83.6% versus 88.7% (20% of training data), 85.0% versus 89.2% (40%), 86.8% versus 89.8% (60%), 88.9% versus 90.3% (80%), 88.6% versus 89.7% (100%) accuracy. Regarding model sparsity, the measure $s = \frac{||w||_1}{||w||_F}$ was computed from the model weights w of both penalized estimators for each of the 18 classes. The ℓ_1-penalized logistic regression yielded the mean sparsities 50.0, 45.4, 40.0, 30.9, and 24.0 after model fitting with 20% to 100% training data. The hierarchical-tree-penalized logistic regression yield the sparsities 163.2, 160.2, 132.1, 116.2, and 88.4 after fitting

20% to 100% of the training data. To quantitative a measure of support recovery, we computed Pearson correlation r between vectors of the z-scored model coefficients and the z-scored across-participant average maps for each class. ℓ_1-penalized versus hierarchical-tree-penalized logistic regression achieved a mean correlation r of 0.10 versus 0.13, 0.11 versus 0.13, 0.13 versus 0.17, 0.16 versus 0.22, and 0.19 versus 0.29 across classes based on 20% to 100% training data. Finally, regarding model variance, we quantified the agreement between ℓ_1-penalized versus hierarchical-tree-penalized model weights after fitting on 5 different 20%-subsamples of the training data. For each classifier, the absolute model weights were concatenated for all 18 classes, thresholded at 0.0001 to binarize variable selection, and mutual information was computed on all pairs of the 5 trained models. This agreement metric of model selection across fold pairs yielded the means 0.001 (ℓ_1) versus 0.506 (hierarchical tree).

Three observations have been made. First, in the data-scarce scenario (i.e., 1/5 of available training data), hierarchical tree sparsity achieved the biggest advantage in out-of-sample performance by 5.1% as well as better support recovery with weight maps already much closer to the respective class averages [20]. In the case of scarce training data, which is typical for the brain imaging domain, regularization by region-network priors thus allowed for more effective extraction of classification-relevant structure from the neural activity maps. Second, across training data fractions, the weight maps from ordinary logistic regression exhibited higher variance and more zero coefficients than hierarchical tree logistic regression. Given the usually high multicollinearity in neuroimaging data, this observation is likely to reflect instable selection of representative voxels among class-responsive groups due to the ℓ_1-norm penalization. Third, in the data-rich scenario (i.e., entire training data used for model fitting), neurobiologically informed logistic regression profited much more from the increased information quantities than neurobiologically naive logistic regression. That is, the region-network priors actually further enhanced the support recovery in abundant input data. This was the case although the maximal classification performance of $\approx$90% has already been reached with small training data fractions by the structured estimator. In contrast, the unstructured estimator approached this generalization performance only with bigger input data quantities.

3.3 Support Recovery as a Function of Region-Network Emphasis

Finally, the relative importance of the region and network group penalties within the hierarchical tree prior was quantified (Fig. 5). The group weight η_g of region priors was multiplied with a region-network ratio, while the group weight η_h of network priors was divided by that region-network ratio. For instance, a region-network ratio of 3 increased the relative importance of known region structure by multiplying $\beta = \frac{3}{1}$ to η_g of all region group penalties and multiplying $\alpha = \frac{1}{3}$ to η_h of all network group penalties (Table 1).

As the most important observation, a range between region-dominant and network-dominant structured penalties yielded quantitatively similar generalization to new data but qualitatively different decision functions manifested in the

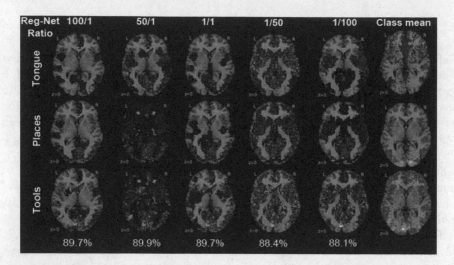

Fig. 5. Support recovery as a function of region and network emphasis. The relative strength of the region and network priors on the regularization is systematically varied against each other (i.e., α and β are changed reciprocally). Horizontal brain slices are shown with the voxel-wise weights for each class from the fitted predictive model. The region-network ratio (*columns*) weighted voxel groups to priviledge sparse models in function space that acknowledge known brain region neighborhoods (*left columns*) or known brain networks neighborhoods (*right columns*). Among the 18 classes (cf. [7], Table 1), the model weights are shown for 3 exemplary psychological tasks followed by participants lying in a brain imaging scanner (*from top to bottom*): tongue movement, viewing locations and tools. The 18-class out-of-sample accuracy *bottom* and the class-wise mean neural activity (*rightmost column*, thresholded at the 75th percentile) are indicated. Different emphasis on regions versus networks in hierarchical structured sparsity can yield very similar out-of-sample generalization. Favoring region versus network structure during model selection recovers complementary, non-identical aspects of the neural activity pattern underlying the psychological tasks.

Table 1. Out-of-sample performance by region-network emphasis

Reg-Net Ratio	100	50	10	5	2	1	$\frac{1}{2}$	$\frac{1}{5}$	$\frac{1}{10}$	$\frac{1}{50}$	$\frac{1}{100}$
Accuracy [%]	89.7	89.9	90.1	90.5	88.0	89.7	87.8	88.0	87.7	88.4	88.1

weight maps (Fig. 5, second and forth column). Classification models with many zero coefficients but high absolute coefficients in either region compartments or network compartments can similarly extrapolate to unseen neural activity maps. Second, these achieve classification performance comparable to equilibrated region-network priors that set less voxel coefficients to zero and spread the probability mass across the whole brain with lower absolute coefficients (Fig. 5, third column in the middle). Third, overly strong emphasis on either level of the hierarchical prior provides the neurobiologically informative results with maps of the most necessary region or network structure for statistically significant generalization (Fig. 5, leftmost and rightmost columns). In sum, stratifying the hierarchical tree penalty between region and network emphasis suggests that *class-specific region-network tradeoffs* enable more performant and more interpretable classification models for neuroimaging analyses [17].

4   Conclusion

Relevant structure in brain recordings has long been investigated according to two separate organizational principles: functional segregation into discrete brain regions [15] and functional integration by interregional brain networks [19]. Both organizational principles are however inextricable because a specialized brain region communicates input and output with other regions and a brain network subserves complex function by orchestrating its region nodes. Hierarchical statistical models hence suggest themselves as an underexploited opportunity for neuroimaging analysis. The present proof-of-concept study demonstrates the simultaneous exploitation of both neurobiological compartments for sparse variable selection and high-dimensional prediction in an extensive reference dataset. Introducing existing domain knowledge into model selection allowed privileging members of the function space that are most neurobiologically plausible. This statistically and neurobiologically desirable simplification is shown to enhance model interpretability and generalization performance.

Our approach has important advantages over previous analysis strategies that rely on dimensionality reduction of the neuroimaging data to tackle the curse of dimensionality. They often resort to preliminary pooling functions based on region atlases or regression against network templates for subsequent supervised learning on the ensuing aggregated features. Such lossy approaches of feature engineering and subsequent inference *(i)* can only satisfy either the specialization or the integration account of brain organization, *(ii)* depend on the ground truth being either a region or network effect, and *(iii)* cannot issue individual coefficients for every voxel of the brain. Hierarchical region-network sparsity addresses these shortcomings by estimating individual voxel contributions while benefitting from their biological multi-level stratification to restrict statistical complexity. Viewed from the bias-variance tradeoff, our modification to logistic regression entailed a large decrease in model variance but only a modest increase in model bias.

In the future, region-network sparsity priors could be incorporated into various pattern-learning methods applied in systems neuroscience. This includes supervised methods for whole-brain classification and regression in single- and multi-task learning settings. The principled regularization scheme could also inform unsupervised structure-discovery by matrix factorization and clustering algorithms [13]. Additionally, hierarchical regularization could be extended from the spatial activity domain to priors of coherent spatiotemporal activity structure. The deterministic choice of a region and network atlas could further be avoided by sparse selection of overcomplete region-network dictionaries. Ultimately, successful high-dimensional inference on brain scans is a prerequisite for predicting diagnosis, disease trajectories, and treatment response in personalized psychiatry and neurology.

Acknowledgement. The research leading to these results has received funding from the European Union Seventh Framework Programme (FP7/2007-2013) under grant agreement no. 604102 (Human Brain Project).

References

1. Abraham, A., Pedregosa, F., Eickenberg, M., Gervais, P., Mueller, A., Kossaifi, J., Gramfort, A., Thirion, B., Varoquaux, G.: Machine learning for neuroimaging with scikit-learn. Front. Neuroinform. **8**, 14 (2014)
2. Anderson, M.L., Kinnison, J., Pessoa, L.: Describing functional diversity of brain regions and brain networks. Neuroimage **73**, 50–58 (2013)
3. Bach, F., Jenatton, R., Mairal, J., Obozinski, G.: Optimization with sparsity-inducing penalties. Found. Trends Mach. Learn. **4**(1), 1–106 (2012)
4. Barch, D.M., Burgess, G.C., Harms, M.P., Petersen, S.E., Schlaggar, F.C.: Function in the human connectome: task-FMRI and individual differences in behavior. Neuroimage **80**, 169–189 (2013)
5. Beck, A., Teboulle, M.: A fast iterative shrinkage-thresholding algorithm for linear inverse problems. SIAM J. Imaging Sci. **2**(1), 183–202 (2009)
6. Beckmann, C.F., DeLuca, M., Devlin, J.T., Smith, S.M.: Investigations into resting-state connectivity using independent component analysis. Philos. Trans. R. Soc. Lond. B Biol. Sci. **360**(1457), 1001–1013 (2005)
7. Bzdok, D., Eickenberg, M., Grisel, O., Thirion, B., Varoquaux, G.: Semi-supervised factored logistic regression for high-dimensional neuroimaging data. In: Advances in Neural Information Processing Systems, pp. 3330–3338 (2015)
8. Craddock, R.C., James, G.A., Holtzheimer, P.E., Hu, X.P., Mayberg, H.S.: A whole brain FMRI atlas generated via spatially constrained spectral clustering. Hum. Brain Mapp. **33**(8), 1914–19289 (2012)
9. Doria, V., Beckmann, C.F., Arichia, T., Merchanta, N., Groppoa, M., Turkheimerb, F.E., Counsella, S.J., Murgasovad, M., Aljabard, P., Nunesa, R.G., Larkmana, D.J., Reese, G., Edwards, A.D.: Emergence of resting state networks in the preterm human brain. Proc. Natl. Acad. Sci. USA **107**(46), 20015–20020 (2010)
10. Harchaoui, Z., Douze, M., Paulin, M., Dudik, M., Malick, J.: Large-scale image classification with trace-norm regularization. In: 2012 IEEE Conference on Computer Vision and Pattern Recognition (CVPR), pp. 3386–3393. IEEE (2012)
11. Iaria, G., Fox, C.J., Waite, C.T., Aharon, I., Barton, J.J.: The contribution of the fusiform gyrus and superior temporal sulcus in processing facial attractiveness: neuropsychological and neuroimaging evidence. Neuroscience **155**(2), 409–422 (2008)
12. Jenatton, R., Gramfort, A., Michel, V., Obozinski, G., Bach, F., Thirion, B.: Multiscale mining of FMRI data with hierarchical structured sparsity. SIAM J. Imaging Sci. **5**(3), 835–856 (2012)
13. Jenatton, R., Obozinski, G., Bach, F.: Structured sparse principal component analysis. arXiv preprint arXiv:0909.1440 (2009)
14. Kanwisher, N.: Functional specificity in the human brain: a window into the functional architecture of the mind. Proc. Natl. Acad. Sci. USA **107**(25), 11163–11170 (2010)
15. Passingham, R.E., Stephan, K.E., Kotter, R.: The anatomical basis of functional localization in the cortex. Nat. Rev. Neurosci. **3**(8), 606–616 (2002)
16. Pedregosa, F., Varoquaux, G., Gramfort, A., et al.: Scikit-learn: machine learning in python. J. Mach. Learn. Res. **12**, 2825–2830 (2011)

17. Sepulcre, J., Liu, H., Talukdar, T., Martincorena, I., Yeo, B.T.T., Buckner, R.L.: The organization of local and distant functional connectivity in the human brain. PLoS Comput. Biol. **6**(6), e1000808 (2010)
18. Smith, S.M., Fox, P.T., Miller, K.L., Glahn, D.C., Fox, P.M., Mackay, C.E., Filippini, N., Beckmann, C.F.: Correspondence of the brain's functional architecture during activation and rest. Proc. Natl. Acad. Sci. USA **106**(31), 13040–13045 (2009)
19. Sporns, O.: Contributions and challenges for network models in cognitive neuroscience. Nat. Neurosci. **17**(5), 652–660 (2014)
20. Varoquaux, G., Gramfort, A., Thirion, B.: Small-sample brain mapping: sparse recovery on spatially correlated designs with randomization and clustering. arXiv preprint. arXiv:1206.6447 (2012)
21. Yuan, M., Lin, Y.: Model selection and estimation in regression with grouped variables. Philos. Trans. R. Soc. Lond. B Biol. Sci. **68**(1), 49–67 (2006)
22. Zeki, S.M.: Functional specialisation in the visual cortex of the rhesus monkey. Nature **274**(5670), 423–428 (1978)

A Restaurant Process Mixture Model for Connectivity Based Parcellation of the Cortex

Daniel Moyer[✉], Boris A. Gutman, Neda Jahanshad,
and Paul M. Thompson

Imaging Genetics Center,
University of Southern California, Los Angeles, USA
moyerd@usc.edu

Abstract. One of the primary objectives of human brain mapping is the division of the cortical surface into functionally distinct regions, i.e. parcellation. While it is generally agreed that at macro-scale different regions of the cortex have different functions, the exact number and configuration of these regions is not known. Methods for the discovery of these regions are thus important, particularly as the volume of available information grows. Towards this end, we present a parcellation method based on a Bayesian non-parametric mixture model of cortical connectivity.

Keywords: Human Connectome · Cortical parcellation · Bayesian non-parametrics

1 Introduction

Historically, researchers proposed and investigated regional brain parcellations through manual dissection and qualitative description [25]. The rise of non-invasive neuro-imaging coupled with advances in computing and computer vision allowed for the exploration of automated parcellation methods, both for fitting existing atlases to data and for data-driven discovery of functionally and structurally cohesive parcels [23]. The success of the former propelled the rise in interest and analyses of brain connectomics in the last decade [20]. Connectomics is a topic of interest within all scales of neuroscience; at the macro-scale, it is often defined by discrete networks of cortical gray matter regions as nodes with weighted or binary edges connecting them. In structural connectomics–the focus of this paper–the edge weights are usually based on counts of estimated structural connections recovered using diffusion MRI tractography, sometimes weighted by a microstructural measure.

A number of papers have focused on the converse, using the connection profile of either voxels or vertices, or in the case of functional MRI, the pairwise signal correlation for each vertex pair to define the parcellation of the cortex (see [4] and the references therein). For connectivity based parcellation (CBP) methods using structural connectivity, two modeling choices are required: (1) a spatial resolution of the grid on which connections are defined, and (2) the criteria on

© Springer International Publishing AG 2017
M. Niethammer et al. (Eds.): IPMI 2017, LNCS 10265, pp. 336–347, 2017.
DOI: 10.1007/978-3-319-59050-9_27

which clusters should be formed. In almost every existing method, connectivity measures are first estimated for a high resolution grid of atomic units (choice one), e.g. voxels or vertices, and the atomic units then combined under spatial constraints optimizing a desiderata (choice two).

The first decision is essentially a division of connectivity into two scales: the macro-region level and higher resolution voxel/vertex level, where our task is to learn from the former the regions of the latter. The second modeling choice is the criteria on which these atoms are clustered. Many popular choices come from more general clustering literature, e.g. within-group sum of squares (explained variance), within-group statistical distances, and mixture model likelihoods [4,15,24]. These criteria use the connectivity profiles of each meso-scale atom without regard to the network structure they induce at the macro-scale. In other words, they treat each vertex or voxel as a data point with an associated vector (its row in the meso-scale adjacency matrix), and then cluster based on this vector space. If one vertex is changed from one group to another, these methods generally do not re-evaluate the quality of all the groups, though on the macro-scale each of their connective profiles would have changed.

In the present work, we will address both these choices. We present a method framed in the context of generative models, specifically Bayesian non-parametric mixture models which place priors over all possible partitions of the higher resolution grid, and do not require the number of clusters to be predefined. One large classes of such priors are the so-called "restaurant processes", used here. We implement a continuum form of connectivity for our mixture components, and further leverage a conjugate likelihood-prior relationship to produce closed form marginal likelihoods for network interactions, allowing efficient sampling.

Our paper is organized as follows: we first define terminology, rigorously define the parcellation task, and describe the model as a whole. We then describe each of its components in closer detail. We then present results on two datasets, and discuss the model in relation to existing models and methods.

2   Model

Let Ω be the white matter/gray matter interface (the inner cortical surface), with the acknowledgment that Ω is in general composed of two disjoint sheets, each with a boundary at the medial wall. Fix a coordinate system over Ω, and define a parcellation P as any set of regions $\{E_i\}$ where $E_i \subset \Omega$, $\bigcup E_i = \Omega$, and $|\bigcap E_i| = 0$ (i.e. the regions E_i are almost disjoint). We assume there exists a latent parcellation P^* that accurately describes the cortical surface with respect to its underlying neuroanatomical structure. Our objective is the recovery of P^*, specifically using structural connectivity information, and without specifying the exact number of regions. In order to accomplish this, we construct a joint generative model of parcellations and connectivity.

We start by choosing a model of partitions. We use the distance dependent Chinese Restaurant Process (ddCRP) [2], a variant of the popular Chinese Restaurant Process (CRP) non-parametric Bayesian models. CRP models are most commonly used in mixture models, providing a prior over all possible label assignments for any number of label-parameter pairs. A main assumption of the CRP is the exchangeability of the data; the ddCRP removes this exchangeability assumption, allowing for non-trivial topologies of dependence between data points. This is discussed in Sect. 2.1 in detail. Briefly, ddCRP allows us to use non-parametric style mixture models on mesh grids, where we assume *a priori* that neighboring patches are dependent. For example, we assume there is spatial auto-correlation over the discrete manifold of the mesh. Practically speaking, the ddCRP is the component responsible for merging or splitting the parcels (clusters), and in general for their configuration.

We next choose a mixture component model; the distribution chosen here will generate the observed network between estimated regions from the ddCRP. We choose to follow the style of the Infinite Relational Model [1,12], where we model interactions between clusters instead of the profiles of the clusters themselves. Thus, we need a separate parameter for each *pair* of regions. Before diving into this however, it is important to consider the form of our connectivity data. Structural connectivity is estimated using streamlines (tractography), usually via identifying tracts which intersect the cortical surface at two locations. Thus, the evidence of connectivity is a set of endpoint pairs on Ω.

In traditional connectivity analysis, these endpoints are counted by region pair, and a graph is formed from the resulting count statistics. These representations abstract away both knowledge of region geometry such as surface area, curvature etc., as well as topological information, i.e. region adjacency; this is the information we will be using in the ddCRP model. While it is possible to ignore these conflicting motives and directly kluge a graph to a spatial patch model, we instead attempt to retain spatial intuition in our connectivity representation.

Consider $\Omega \times \Omega$, the set of all possible tract endpoints intersecting the cortical surface. We model the observation of these pairs of endpoints as a spatial point process on $\Omega \times \Omega$. Assuming that each tract is independently recovered[1], this process is the Poisson point process. That is, for any region pair $E_i \times E_j \subset \Omega \times \Omega$, the number of tract endpoint pairs observed in that region pair is Poisson distributed with parameter $\int_{E_i} \int_{E_j} \lambda(x,y) dy dx$. Here $\lambda : \Omega \times \Omega \to \mathbb{R}^+$ is a non-negative rate function assumed to be integrable over all $\Omega \times \Omega$. For Poisson processes, λ completely characterizes the process. While we discuss further the Poisson point process in Sect. 2.2, in the view of the overall model it is important to note one convenient property: disjoint regions have independent counts.

Moving back to the mixture components, we make the following simplifying assumption on the form of the tract endpoint process: each region pair interacts in a homogenous manner. That is, we assume λ is constant over any pair of parcels. Thus, for any finite configuration of K parcels we have on order K^2 non-negative scalar parameters to estimate, and these parameters are the rate parameters for Poisson spatial processes generating the evidence of connectivity. We choose to use the Gamma distribution to model these parameters (i.e.,

---

[1] It is important to make the distinction between physical fascicles and recovered tracts. Here, we define the latter to be the reconstructed tractography.

each pair of parcels (g_i, g_j) draws a rate λ_{ij} from a Gamma prior). As shown in Sect. 2.2, the conjugacy of the Gamma distribution with the homogenous Poisson process allows for closed form marginal distributions, and thus efficient collapsed sampling methods. We also choose to use the mesh faces $\{f_m\}_{m=1}^M$ as the elements of our ddCRP-mixture. This is because connectivity is usually defined over intersections of tracts with areal units, and both the ddCRP as well as the Poisson process naturally operate over such regions.

Putting this all together, and leaving the meaning of c_m for the next section, the model is as follows:

$$c_m, g_i \sim \text{ddCRP}(\alpha, Adj)$$
$$\lambda_{ij} \sim \text{Gamma}(a, b)$$
$$D_{ij} \sim \text{Poisson Point Process}(\lambda_{ij})$$

2.1   The Distance Dependent Chinese Restaurant Process (ddCRP)

As suggested by its name, distance directed Chinese Restaurant Process is a variant of the Chinese Restaurant Process (CRP), often used in non-parametric Bayesian mixture models as a prior over possible mixture components (i.e. a distribution over distributions). Let α be some positive constant concentration parameter, and let G_0 be a prior distribution over mixture component parameters (for us, a gamma distribution). The original CRP mixture model [17] describes an endless stream of customers (data) entering a restaurant with an infinite number of tables (clusters). Each customer either chooses (with prescribed probability dependent on α) to sit at an existing table (which has a particular component distribution) or sit an unoccupied table (draw a new component distribution from the prior). Up to the indexing of the tables, for any finite number of observations any number of clusters and configuration of cluster associations is possible.

In the original CRP, the data are assumed to be exchangeable; that is, the joint likelihood of any observations is invariant under permutations of observation indices. However, in our spatial context we have a topology of face adjacencies. Permutations of the face indexes are non-trivial, and thus the faces are not exchangeable. To model this, the ddCRP allows each customer to choose another customer (possibly itself) to sit with based on its dependencies. This forms a directed graph of seating choices; table assignments are then made to each group of customers who have chosen to sit with each other, i.e. each connected component of the seating choice graph. Mixture components are drawn for each table from G_0, and only then are the actual data drawn from each mixture component. Clearly this is a two stage procedure. In our context, this means each face will choose to be in a cluster with one of its neighbors or itself.

As above, let $\{f_m\}_{m=1}^M$ be the set of mesh faces, and let $\{c_m\}_{m=1}^M$ be the corresponding assignments, where each $c_m \in \{1, \ldots, M\}$. We draw c_m conditioned adjacency information Adj as follows:

$$p(c_m = j | Adj) \propto \begin{cases} 1 & \text{if } j \text{ is adjacent to } i \\ \alpha & \text{if } m = j \\ 0 & \text{otherwise} \end{cases}$$

We denote each cluster of faces as g_k for $k \in \{1, \ldots, K\}$, where K is the number of clusters. Due to our restriction of c_m to the indices of faces adjacent to f_m, each g_k is a contiguous region, and the set of groups forms a valid parcellation of Ω. We note that the original ddCRP is defined for more general distance functions.

2.2   Mixture Components: Poisson-Gamma

The evidence of pairwise interaction between regions in structural connectivity is the set of tract endpoints $D = \{(x_t, y_t)\}_{t=1}^T$. Since the regional clusters are defined over discrete grids of areal atoms (mesh faces), these are naturally aggregated to count measures over each pair of sub-regions. For any pair of regions $(g_i, g_j) \subset \Omega \times \Omega$, define $D_{ij} = \{(x_t, y_t) \in g_i \times g_j\}$. We model the counts $|D_{ij}|$ using the Poisson process with fixed intensity λ_{ij}, where the area $g_i \times g_j$ contains a random count $|D_{ij}|$ distributed

$$|D_{ij}| \sim Poisson\left(\int_{g_i \times g_j} \lambda \, dx dy\right)$$

Using the independence assumption of the tract endpoints, the likelihood of any configuration of tract endpoints can then be written

$$\mathcal{L}(D) = \prod_{g_i, g_j} \exp\left\{-\int_{g_i \times g_j} \lambda_{ij} dx dy\right\} \lambda_{ij}^{|D_{ij}|}$$

We use a Gamma prior for the λ_{ij} parameters, the conjugate prior of the Poisson distribution. Using the Gamma distribution allows us derive a simple closed form marginal distribution for D_{ij} that "integrates out" the λ_{ij}'s, leaving a likelihood in terms of prior parameters a, b. It is as follows:

$$P(D_{ij}|a,b) = \int P(D_{ij}, \mu | a, b) d\mu = \int P(D_{ij}|\mu) P(\mu|a,b) d\mu$$

$$= \int \underbrace{\exp\left\{-\int_{g_i} \int_{g_j} \lambda dA\right\} \prod_{t=1}^{|D_{ij}|} \lambda}_{\text{Homogeneous Point Process}} \times \underbrace{\frac{b^a}{\Gamma(a)} \exp(-b\lambda) \lambda^{a-1}}_{\text{Gamma Prior}} d\lambda$$

$$= Z(a,b) \int \underbrace{\exp\left\{-(|g_i \times g_j| + b)\lambda\right\} \lambda^{|D_{ij}|+a-1}}_{\text{Un-normalized Gamma Posterior}} d\lambda$$

$$= \frac{Z(a,b)}{Z(a',b')} = \left(\frac{\beta}{|g_i \times g_j| + b}\right)^a \left(\frac{1}{|g_i \times g_j| + b}\right)^{|D_{ij}|} \frac{\Gamma(a + |D_{ij}|)}{\Gamma(a)}$$

Here, $Z(a,b) = \frac{b^a}{\Gamma(a)}$

2.3 Combined Model and Collapsed Sampling Scheme

We will estimate the model via Collapsed Gibbs Sampling, specifically using the closed form integral over λ_{ij} to avoid sampling the interaction parameters. Starting at iteration $\ell = 0$, we update each c_m^ℓ by the following conditional likelihood:

$$P(c_m^{\ell+1} = k|D) \propto P(c_m = k) \prod_{i,j} P(D_{ij}|a, b, c_m^{\ell+1} = k, \{c_r^{\ell+1}\}_{r<m}, \{c_s^\ell\}_{s>m})$$

Since we assume c_m is restricted by our mesh topology, we have only a small number of options to evaluate. We denote the seating graph edge c_m^ℓ as a "critical edge" if for any other node $f_{m'}$ such that $c_{m'} = m$ there exists a path to the face with index c_m^ℓ. Let g_{old} be f_m's previous component, and g_{crit} be the component of f_m without its own edge (its critical component). Without loss of generality we may further order each neighbor of f_m as f_n for $n = 1, \ldots, N$, and their groups as $g(n)$. Using these definitions, for triangle meshes we can write out all possible scenarios:

1. If c_m is not critical, and all neighbors are of the same component before the update, then we can simply choose c_m via $P(c_m = k)$, as there is no difference with respect to the induced components.
2. If c_m is not critical, but not surrounded by the same component, then we are asking essentially "Should c_m's previously induced component join one of its as of yet independent neighbors". Thus,

$$P(c_m^{\ell+1} = n|D) \propto P(c_m = n) \prod_k^K P(D_{*,k}|g_{new} = g_{old} \cup g_n, g_k)$$

$$\times \prod_{\substack{g_{\hat{n}}:\hat{n}\neq n \\ \hat{n}\neq old}}^N \prod_k^K P(D_{g(n),k}|g_{\hat{n}}, g_k)$$

for each neighbor n. Here $D_{*,k} = \{(x_t, y_t) \in g_{old} \cup g_n \times g_k\}$
3. If c_m is critical, then for each neighboring component (including the component $g_{old} \backslash g_{crit}$ in the neighbors) we have

$$P(c_m^{\ell+1} = n|D) \propto P(c_m = n) \prod_k^K P(D_{*,k}|g_{new} = g_{crit} \cup g_n, g_k)$$

$$\times \prod_{\hat{n}\neq n} \prod_k^K P(D_{\hat{n},k}|g_{\hat{n}}, g_k).$$

We iteratively update the face associates using $P(c_m^{\ell+1} = k|D)$, collecting samples after every pass. While this generates a posterior distribution over c_m, we simply take the maximum a posteriori (MAP) estimate as our selected parcellation.

In general, updates made in Gibbs sampling algorithms are done sequentially; this is because strong dependencies between concurrent updates will destabilize some samplers. However, in cases of low dependence approximate asynchronous parallel updates have been used with empirically strong results (so called "Hog-wild" updates [11]). In our case, most updates are either within components, or between small components (with correspondingly small interdependencies), so a small degree of parallelism is possible. In practice we use a compromise between the serial algorithm and the parallel version: we use a shared memory parallel sampler for calculating the likelihoods of a small batch c_i, then make a serial updates based on these likelihoods. This allows a roughly linear speed-up in the number of threads used, though there is a slowly scaling cost of the serial update.

2.4 Implementation Notes

In fixing a coordinate system, it is common to split the white matter/gray matter interface into two spheres, each with a null region where the corpus callosum bridges the longitudinal fissure. Thus, an easy system can be constructed using spherical coordinates and a marker for hemisphere.

The symmetry of each tract's endpoints requires careful consideration to avoid double counting; while the intuition of the model can be understood without thinking about the symmetry of the data, when evaluating joint probabilities it is important to only include each data point once. This can be achieved by only evaluating $P(D_{ij}|a, b)$ for $i \leq j$. When computing the parallel updates, in our experience it is much more efficient to keep the threads active but idle, and simply have a single thread do the serial update. This avoids the overhead of repeated thread spawns, which for some implementations/architectures can be costly.

3 Procedure and Results

In order to test our proposed model, we use two open datasets, one composed of 20 subjects each scanned twice from the Institute of Psychology, Chinese Academy of Sciences (IPCAS) subset of the Consortium for Reliability and Reproducibility (CoRR) dataset [26], and the other composed of 30 subjects from the Human Connectome Project (HCP) S900 release [22]. The pre-processing differs slightly between the datasets, to account for the different imaging parameters. In general the HCP dataset has higher resolution (both in voxel size and angular resolution) leading to different tractographies. On each dataset we compare the performance of the proposed method against two recommended alternatives: Ward's method, a greedy hierarchical clustering method [4], and Spectral Clustering [15].

3.1 Preprocessing and Tractography

IPCAS: T1-weighted (T1w) and diffusion weighted (DWI) images were obtained on 3T Siemens TrioTim by the original investigators [26] using an 8-channel head coil and 60 directions. Each subject was scanned twice, roughly two weeks apart. T1w images were processed with Freesufer's [5] recon-all pipeline to obtain a triangle mesh of the grey-white matter boundary registered to a shared spherical space [6]. We resample this space to a geodesic grid (where each face has approximately equal area) with 10,000 total faces, doing so only after computing tract intersections with the surface. Probabilistic streamline tractography was conducted using the DWI in 2 mm isotropic MNI 152 space, using Dipy's [7] implementation of constrained spherical deconvolution (CSD) [21] with a harmonic order of 6. Tractography streamlines were seeded at 2 random locations in each white matter voxel labeled by FSL's FAST. Streamline tracking followed directions randomly in proportion to the orientation function at each sample point at 0.5 mm steps, starting bidirectionaly from each seed point with 8 restarts per seed. As per Dipy's Anatomically Constrained Tractography (ACT) [19], we retained only tracts longer than 5 mm with endpoints in likely gray matter.

HCP: We used the minimally preprocessed T1-weighted (T1w) and diffusion weighted (DWI) images rigidly aligned to MNI space. Briefly, the preprocessing of these images included motion correction and eddy current correction (DWI), and linear and nonlinear alignment (betweek T1w and DWI). We used the HCP Pipeline (version 3.13.1) FreeSurfer protocol to run an optimized version of the recon-all pipeline that computes surface meshes in a higher resolution (0.7 mm isotropic) space. We again resample this space to an geodesic grid after computing tract intersections with the surface. Tractography was conducted using the DWI in the native 1.25 mm isotropic voxel size in MNI space. Probabilistic streamline tractography was performed as in IPCAS above.

3.2 Fitting and Results

We fit the proposed method using our parallel sampling scheme, using 60 passes of the sampler with 8 parallel threads (approximately 600,000 updates per subject), using $a = 1$, $b = 1$, and $\alpha = 0.01$. We use the MAP estimate as our results. We fitted Ward clustering by maximizing Explained Variance over a naïve search of every possible merge. For the Spectral Clustering method we use an exponential kernel, using the normalized cosine distance as a metric. We use a number of eigenvectors equal to the number of clusters. For both baselines we take the vector of connections as our feature vector. In both clustering schemes, we specify the number of clusters to be equal to that of the proposed method.

We assess cluster quality using a KL-divergence based measure. We take the number of tracts from each face f_m to each region g_i as the objective distribution, and measure how well this is approximated by the average number of tracts from $g(f_m)$ to g_i. These form two matrices of dimension $M \times K$. We then normalize these matrices to sum to one and measure their KL divergence as in [15]. If a cluster is well represented by its average connectivity profile, then this divergence will be low. For the IPCAS dataset we have an additional measure of Test-Retest reproducibility. This is measured by Normalized Mutual Information (NMI)[1,4], which measures cluster similarity without requiring similar

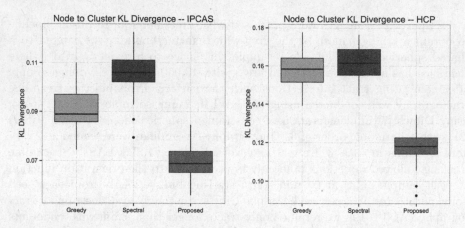

Fig. 1. Plots of the KL divergence based goodness of fit measure, for the three methods, on both datasets. Here, **lower** is better.

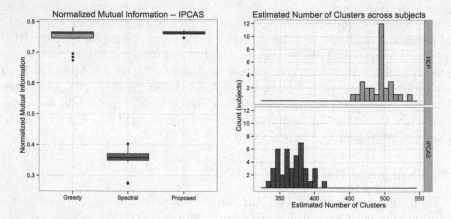

Fig. 2. Left: normalized mutual information between Test-Retest scans. Here, **higher** is better. Right: histograms of the number of clusters selected for each subject.

numbers of clusters. Let Z be a binary matrix of cluster assignments, where, for each row i, each entry Z_{ij} is 1 if f_i is in cluster j and zero otherwise. NMI is defined as $I(Z_1, Z_2)/\sqrt{(H(Z_1)H(Z_2)}$, where $I(\cdot, \cdot)$ is mutual information, $H(\cdot)$ is entropy, and Z_1 and Z_2 are the cluster assignments for the first and second scan respectively. (This uses the convention customary in information theory that $0 \log 0 = 0$). NMI is also invariant under permutations of labels. As can be seen in Figs. 1 and 2, the proposed method is performing well compared to the baseline methods. HCP dataset uses more clusters (around 250 per hemisphere) than the IPCAS dataset (around 175–200 per hemisphere). The difference here may be due in part to the higher resolution of the HCP dataset, leading to greater resolving power with respect to the regional connections. These averages are at the upper range of the number suggested by Van Essen et al. [23].

4   Discussion

This model draws on the wide range of previously proposed methods in connectivity based parcellation. Several non-parametric Bayesian methods have been proposed, in particular two excellent works Jbabdi et al. [10] and Baldassano et al. [1], both of whom use Normal-inverse-Wilshart conjugations as their mixture components (Baldassano et al. use a special case, the Normal-inverse-χ^2). These models also enjoy closed form marginal distributions, but do not have infinite divisibility (the distributions they model are not spatial processes). Jbabdi et al. whose work predates the ddCRP, use a Dirichlet Process with spatial priors as their partition prior. They then further define a hierarchical process on top of this that links multiple subjects. Baldassano et al. use the ddCRP directly, but model voxel connections, again without the aid of a spatial process. Instead, they model the aggregate connectivity as coming from a normal distribution.

The ddCRP is similar to a Markov Random Field model with a very strong spatial prior. These models have been successful in obtaining parcellations from functional connectivity [9, 18], though few if any have used Bayesian non-parametrics. This frame of reference leads us toward more traditional computer vision tasks such as pixel labeling, where as in many cases surface parcellation has been framed as vertex parcellation [3, 15, 24]. This is a small but relatively important conceptual difference; the pixel and mesh-face models have areal units, but vertex parcellations are graphs of infinitesimal points. The intuition of the former leads us toward the use of spatial processes.

A similar spatial process viewpoint of connectivity is proposed in Moyer et al. [14], but the discovery of new parcellations is not discussed. Poisson count processes for network interactions have also been explored in the literature [13], as have infinite relational variants [8] though usually in the context of network clustering via the stochastic blockmodel (i.e. clustering the regions themselves). These usually ignore spatial constraints.

Alternative methods to Bayesian models usually specify the number of clusters. Of note is Parisot et al. [15] and a subsequent work by the same authors [16], which propose spectral methods for the parcellation task, augmented with a pre-processing local agglomeration. These papers note the propensity for Spectral Clustering to form equi-areal clusters; as can be seen in Fig. 3, our method does not form equi-areal groups. Thus, it may be the case that a lower number of clusters for spectral clustering may perform better.

As there is a rich body of functional and anatomical knowledge regarding the cortex, parcellations based on connectivity information alone would need proper neuroanatomical, histological and functional validation, and more information from these sources would ideally be used to optimize parcellations. The model presented here uses only spatial constraints and connectivity to estimate feasible parcellations based on recoverable structural connections from imaging. However, we believe that the modeling techniques explored here can easily be imputed into larger, multi-modal models, and in general the improvements made may increase the accuracy and reproducibility of studies of connectivity patterns. These are critical to furthering our understanding of the living human brain.

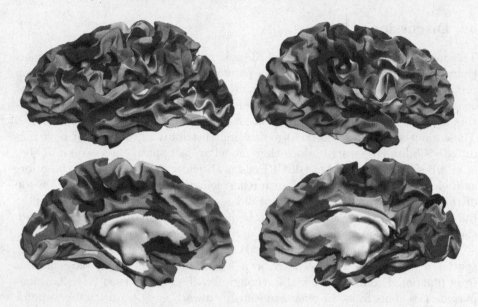

Fig. 3. An exemplar parcellation from an HCP subject. Region colors are random. (Color figure online)

Acknowledgements. This work was supported by NIH Grant U54 EB020403, as well as the NSF Graduate Research Fellowship Program. The authors would like to thank the reviewers as well as Greg Ver Steeg for multiple helpful conversations.

References

1. Baldassano, C., Beck, D.M., Fei-Fei, L.: Parcellating connectivity in spatial maps. PeerJ **3**, e784 (2015)
2. Blei, D.M., Frazier, P.I.: Distance dependent Chinese restaurant processes. J. Mach. Learn. Res. **12**(Aug), 2461–2488 (2011)
3. Clarkson, M.J., Malone, I.B., Modat, M., Leung, K.K., Ryan, N., Alexander, D.C., Fox, N.C., Ourselin, S.: A framework for using diffusion weighted imaging to improve cortical parcellation. In: Jiang, T., Navab, N., Pluim, J.P.W., Viergever, M.A. (eds.) MICCAI 2010. LNCS, vol. 6361, pp. 534–541. Springer, Heidelberg (2010). doi:10.1007/978-3-642-15705-9_65
4. Eickhoff, S.B., Thirion, B., Varoquaux, G., Bzdok, D.: Connectivity-based parcellation: critique and implications. Hum. Brain Mapp. **36**(12), 4771–4792 (2015)
5. Fischl, B.: Freesurfer. NeuroImage **2**(62), 774–781 (2012)
6. Fischl, B., et al.: High-resolution intersubject averaging and a coordinate system for the cortical surface. Hum. Brain Mapp. **8**(4), 272–284 (1999)
7. Garyfallidis, E., et al.: Dipy, a library for the analysis of diffusion MRI data. Front. Neuroinform. **8**(8) (2014)
8. Hinne, M., et al.: Probabilistic clustering of the human connectome identifies communities and hubs. PLoS ONE **10**(1), e0117179 (2015)
9. Honnorat, N., et al.: GraSP: geodesic graph-based segmentation with shape priors for the functional parcellation of the cortex. NeuroImage **106**, 207–221 (2015)

10. Jbabdi, S., Woolrich, M.W., Behrens, T.E.J.: Multiple-subjects connectivity-based parcellation using hierarchical Dirichlet process mixture models. NeuroImage **44**(2), 373–384 (2009)

11. Johnson, M., et al.: Analyzing hogwild parallel Gaussian Gibbs sampling. In: Advances in Neural Information Processing Systems, pp. 2715–2723 (2013)

12. Kemp, C., et al.: Learning systems of concepts with an infinite relational model (2006)

13. Moyer, D., et al.: Mixed membership stochastic blockmodels for the human connectome. MICCAI-Workshop on Bayesian and Graphical Models for Biomedical Imaging 5, 6

14. Moyer, D., Gutman, B.A., Faskowitz, J., Jahanshad, N., Thompson, P.M.: A continuous model of cortical connectivity. In: Ourselin, S., Joskowicz, L., Sabuncu, M.R., Unal, G., Wells, W. (eds.) MICCAI 2016. LNCS, vol. 9900, pp. 157–165. Springer, Cham (2016). doi:10.1007/978-3-319-46720-7_19

15. Parisot, S., Arslan, S., Passerat-Palmbach, J., Wells, W.M., Rueckert, D.: Tractography-driven groupwise multi-scale parcellation of the cortex. In: Ourselin, S., Alexander, D.C., Westin, C.-F., Cardoso, M.J. (eds.) IPMI 2015. LNCS, vol. 9123, pp. 600–612. Springer, Cham (2015). doi:10.1007/978-3-319-19992-4_47

16. Parisot, S., et al.: Group-wise parcellation of the cortex through multi-scale spectral clustering. NeuroImage **136**, 68–83 (2016)

17. Pitman, J., et al.: Combinatorial Stochastic Processes. Springer, Heidelberg (2002)

18. Ryali, S., et al.: A parcellation scheme based on von Mises-Fisher distributions and Markov random fields for segmenting brain regions using resting-state fMRI. NeuroImage **65**, 83–96 (2013)

19. Smith, R.E., et al.: Anatomically-constrained tractography: improved diffusion MRI streamlines tractography through effective use of anatomical information. NeuroImage **62**(3), 1924–1938 (2012)

20. Sporns, O., Tononi, G., Kötter, R.: The human connectome: a structural description of the human brain. PLoS Comput. Biol. **1**(4), e42 (2005)

21. Tournier, J.D., et al.: Resolving crossing fibres using constrained spherical deconvolution: validation using diffusion-weighted imaging phantom data. NeuroImage **42**(2), 617–625 (2008)

22. Van Essen, D.C, WU-Minn HCP Consortium et al.: The WU-Minn human connectome project: an overview. NeuroImage **80**, 62–79 (2013)

23. Van Essen, D.C., Glasser, M.F., Dierker, D.L., Harwell, J., Coalson, T.: Parcellations and hemispheric asymmetries of human cerebral cortex analyzed on surface-based atlases. Cereb. Cortex **22**(10), 2241–2262 (2012)

24. Yeo, B.T., et al.: The organization of the human cerebral cortex estimated by intrinsic functional connectivity. J. Neurophysiol. **106**(3), 1125–1165 (2011)

25. Zilles, K., Amunts, K.: Centenary of Brodmann's map–conception and fate. Nat. Rev. Neurosci. **11**(2), 139–145 (2010)

26. Zuo, X.N., et al.: An open science resource for establishing reliability and reproducibility in functional connectomics. Sci. Data 1 (2014)

On the Compactness, Efficiency, and Representation of 3D Convolutional Networks: Brain Parcellation as a Pretext Task

Wenqi Li[✉], Guotai Wang, Lucas Fidon, Sebastien Ourselin,
M. Jorge Cardoso, and Tom Vercauteren

Translational Imaging Group, Centre for Medical Image Computing (CMIC),
University College London, London, UK
wenqi.li@ucl.ac.uk

Abstract. Deep convolutional neural networks are powerful tools for learning visual representations from images. However, designing efficient deep architectures to analyse volumetric medical images remains challenging. This work investigates efficient and flexible elements of modern convolutional networks such as dilated convolution and residual connection. With these essential building blocks, we propose a high-resolution, compact convolutional network for volumetric image segmentation. To illustrate its efficiency of learning 3D representation from large-scale image data, the proposed network is validated with the challenging task of parcellating 155 neuroanatomical structures from brain MR images. Our experiments show that the proposed network architecture compares favourably with state-of-the-art volumetric segmentation networks while being an order of magnitude more compact. We consider the brain parcellation task as a pretext task for volumetric image segmentation; our trained network potentially provides a good starting point for transfer learning. Additionally, we show the feasibility of voxel-level uncertainty estimation using a sampling approximation through dropout.

1 Introduction

Convolutional neural networks (CNNs) have been shown to be powerful tools for learning visual representations from images. They often consist of multiple layers of non-linear functions with a large number of trainable parameters. Hierarchical features can be obtained by training the CNNs discriminatively.

In the medical image computing domain, recent years have seen a growing number of applications using CNNs. Although there have been recent advances in tailoring CNNs to analyse volumetric images, most of the work to date studies image representations in 2D. While volumetric representations are more informative, the number of voxels scales cubically with the size of the region of interest. This raises challenges of learning more complex visual patterns as well as higher computational burden compared to the 2D cases. While developing compact and effective 3D network architectures is of significant interest, designing 3D CNNs remains a challenging problem.

© Springer International Publishing AG 2017
M. Niethammer et al. (Eds.): IPMI 2017, LNCS 10265, pp. 348–360, 2017.
DOI: 10.1007/978-3-319-59050-9_28

The goal of this paper is to design a high-resolution and compact network architecture for the segmentation of fine structures in volumetric images. For this purpose, we study the simple and flexible elements of modern convolutional networks, such as dilated convolution and residual connection. Most of the existing network architectures follow a fully convolutional downsample-upsample pathway [3,4,11,13,15,16]. Low-level features with high spatial resolutions are first downsampled for higher-level feature abstraction; then the feature maps are upsampled to achieve high-resolution segmentation. In contrast to these, we propose a novel 3D architecture that incorporates high spatial resolution feature maps throughout the layers, and can be trained with a wide range of receptive fields. We validate our network with the challenging task of automated brain parcellation into 155 structures from T1-weighted MR images. We show that the proposed network, with twenty times fewer parameters, achieves competitive segmentation performance compared with state-of-the-art architectures.

A well-designed network could be trained with a large-scale dataset and enables transfer learning to other image recognition tasks [9]. In the field of computer vision, the well-known AlexNet and VGG net were trained on the ImageNet dataset. They provide general-purpose image representations that can be adapted for a wide range of computer vision problems. Given the large amount of data and the complex visual patterns of the brain parcellation problem, we consider it as a pretext task. Our trained network is the first step towards a general-purpose volumetric image representation. It potentially provides an initial model for transfer learning of other volumetric image segmentation tasks.

The uncertainty of the segmentation is also important for indicating the confidence and reliability of one algorithm [5,18]. The high uncertainty of labelling can be a sign of an unreliable classification. We demonstrate the feasibility of voxel-level uncertainty estimation using Monte Carlo samples of the proposed network with dropout at test time. Compared to the existing volumetric segmentation networks, our compact network has fewer parameter interactions and thus potentially achieves better uncertainty estimates with fewer samples.

2   On the Elements of 3D Convolutional Networks

Convolutions and Dilated Convolutions. To maintain a relatively low number of parameters, we choose to use small 3D convolutional kernels with only 3^3 parameters for all convolutions. This is about the smallest kernel that can represent 3D features in all directions with respect to the central voxel. Although a convolutional kernel with $5 \times 5 \times 5$ voxels gives the same receptive field as stacking two layers of $3 \times 3 \times 3$-voxel convolution, the latter has approximately 57% fewer parameters. Using smaller kernels implicitly imposes more regularisation on the network while achieving the same receptive field.

To further enlarge the receptive field to capture large image contexts, most of the existing volumetric segmentation networks downsample the intermediate feature maps. This significantly reduces the spatial resolution. For example, 3D U-net [3] heavily employs $2 \times 2 \times 2$-voxel max pooling with strides of two voxels in each dimension. Each max pooling reduces the feature responses of the previous layer to only 1/8 of its spatial resolution. Upsampling layers, such as deconvolutions, are often used subsequently to partially recover the high resolution of the input. However, adding deconvolution layers also introduces additional computational costs.

Recently, Chen et al. [2] used dilated convolutions with upsampled kernels for semantic image segmentation. The advantages of dilated convolutions are that the features can be computed with a high spatial resolution, and the size of the receptive field can be enlarged arbitrarily. Dilated convolutions can be used to produce accurate dense predictions and detailed segmentation maps along object boundaries.

In contrast to the downsample-upsample pathway, we propose to adopt dilated convolutions for volumetric image segmentation. More specifically, the convolutional kernels are upsampled with a dilation factor r. For M-channels of input feature maps $\mathbf{I}$, the output feature channel $\mathbf{O}$ generated with dilated convolutions are:

$$\mathbf{O}_{x,y,z} = \sum_{m=0}^{M-1} \sum_{i=0}^{2} \sum_{j=0}^{2} \sum_{k=0}^{2} \mathbf{w}_{i,j,k,m} \mathbf{I}_{(x+ir),(y+jr),(z+kr),m} ; \qquad (1)$$

where the index tuple (x, y, z) runs through every spatial location in the volumes; the kernels $\mathbf{w}$ consist of $3^3 \times M$ trainable parameters. The dilated convolution in Eq. (1) has the same number of parameters as the standard $3 \times 3 \times 3$ convolution. It preserves the spatial resolution and provides a $(2r + 1)^3$-voxel receptive field. Setting r to 1 reduces the dilated convolution to the standard $3 \times 3 \times 3$ convolution. In practice, we implement 3D dilated convolutions with a split-and-merge strategy [2] to benefit from the existing GPU convolution routines.

Residual Connections. Residual connections were first introduced and later refined by He et al. [7,8] for the effective training of deep networks. The key idea of residual connection is to create identity mapping connections to bypass the parameterised layers in a network. The input of a residual block is directly merged to the output by addition. The residual connections have been shown to make information propagation smooth and improve the training speed [7].

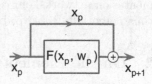

Fig. 1. A block with residual connections.

More specifically, let the input to the p-th layer of a residual block as $\mathbf{x}_p$, the output of the block $\mathbf{x}_{p+1}$ has the form: $\mathbf{x}_{p+1} = \mathbf{x}_p + F(\mathbf{x}_p, \mathbf{w}_p)$; where $F(\mathbf{x}_p, \mathbf{w}_p)$ denotes the path with non-linear functions in the block (shown in Fig. 1). If we stack the residual blocks, the last layer output $\mathbf{x}_l$ can be expressed as: $\mathbf{x}_l = \mathbf{x}_p + \sum_{i=p}^{l-1} F(\mathbf{x}_i, \mathbf{w}_i)$. The residual connections enables direct information propagation from any residual block to another in both forward pass and back-propagation.

Effective Receptive Field. One interpretation of the residual network is that they behave like ensembles of relatively shallow networks. The unravelled view of the residual connections proposed by Veit et al. [19] suggests that the networks with n residual blocks have a collection of 2^n unique paths.

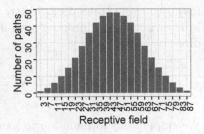

Without residual connections, the receptive field of a network is generally considered fixed. However, when training with n residual blocks, the networks utilise 2^n different paths

Fig. 2. Histogram of the receptive fields.

and therefore features can be learned with a large range of different receptive fields. For example, the proposed network with 9 residual blocks (see Sect. 3) has a maximum receptive field of $87 \times 87 \times 87$ voxels. Following the unravel view of the residual network, it consists of 2^9 unique paths. Figure 2 shows the distribution of the receptive field of these paths. The receptive fields range from $3 \times 3 \times 3$ to $87 \times 87 \times 87$, following a binomial distribution. This differs from the existing 3D networks. For example, Deepmedic [11] model operates at two paths, with a fixed receptive field $17 \times 17 \times 17$ and $42 \times 42 \times 42$ respectively. 3D U-net [3] has a relatively large receptive field of about $88 \times 88 \times 88$ voxels. However, there are only eight unique paths and receptive fields.

Intuitively, given that the receptive field of a deep convolutional network is relatively large, the segmentation maps will suffer from distortions due to the border effects of convolution. That is, the segmentation results near the border of the output volume are less accurate due to the lack of input supporting window. We conduct experiments and demonstrate that the proposed networks generate only a small distortion near the borders (See Sect. 4). This suggests training the network with residual connections reduces the effective receptive field. The width of the distorted border is much smaller than the maximum receptive field. This phenomenon was also recently analysed by Luo et al. [14]. In practice, at test time we pad each input volume with a border of zeros and discard the same amount of border in the segmentation output.

Loss Function. The last layer of the network is a softmax function that gives scores over all labels for each voxel. Typically, the end-to-end training procedure minimises the cross entropy loss function using an N-voxel image volume $\{x_n\}_{n=1}^N$ and the training data of C-class segmentation map $\{y_n\}_{n=1}^N$ where $y_n \in \{1, \ldots, C\}$ is:

$$\mathcal{L}(\{x_n\}, \{y_n\}) = -\frac{1}{N} \sum_{n=1}^N \sum_{c=1}^C \delta(y_n = c) \log F_c(x_n), \tag{2}$$

where δ corresponds to the Dirac delta function, $F_c(x_n)$ is the softmax classification score of x_n over the c-th class. However, when the training data are severely unbalanced (which is typical in medical image segmentation problems), this formulation leads to a strongly biased estimation towards the majority class. Instead of directly re-weighting each voxel by class frequencies, Milletari et al. [16] propose a solution by maximising the mean Dice coefficient directly, i.e.,

$$\mathcal{D}(\{x_n\}, \{y_n\}) = \frac{1}{C} \sum_{c=1}^{C} \frac{2 \sum_{n=1}^{N} \delta(y_n = c) F_c(x_n)}{\sum_{n=1}^{N} [\delta(y_n = c)]^2 + \sum_{n=1}^{N} [F_c(x_n)]^2}. \tag{3}$$

We employ this formulation to handle the issue of training data imbalance.

Uncertainty Estimation Using Dropout. Gal and Ghahramani demonstrated that the deep network trained with dropout can be cast as a Bayesian approximation of the Gaussian process [5]. Given a set of training data and their labels $\{\mathbf{X}, \mathbf{Y}\}$, training a network $F(\cdot, \mathbf{W})$ with dropout has the effect of approximating the posterior distribution $p(\mathbf{W}|\{\mathbf{X}, \mathbf{Y}\})$ by minimising the Kullback-Leibler divergence term, i.e. $\mathrm{KL}(q(\mathbf{W})\|p(\mathbf{W}|\{\mathbf{X}, \mathbf{Y}\}))$; where $q(\mathbf{W})$ is an approximating distribution over the weight matrices $\mathbf{W}$ with their elements randomly set to zero according to Bernoulli random variables. After training the network, the predictive distribution of test data $\hat{\mathbf{x}}$ can be expressed as $q(\hat{\mathbf{y}}|\hat{\mathbf{x}}) = \int F(\hat{\mathbf{x}}, \mathbf{W}) q(\mathbf{W}) d\mathbf{W}$. The prediction can be approximated using Monte Carlo samples of the trained network: $\hat{\mathbf{y}} = \frac{1}{M} \sum_{m=1}^{M} F(\hat{\mathbf{x}}, \mathbf{W}_m)$, where $\{\mathbf{W}_m\}_{m=1}^{M}$ is a set of M samples from $q(\mathbf{W})$. The uncertainty of the prediction can be estimated using the sample variance of the M samples.

With this theoretical insight, we are able to estimate the uncertainty of the segmentation map at the voxel level. We extend the segmentation network with a $1 \times 1 \times 1$ convolutional layer before the last convolutional layer. The extended network is trained with a dropout ratio of 0.5 applied to the newly inserted layer. At test time, we sample the network N times using dropout. The final segmentation is obtained by majority voting. The percentage of samples which disagrees with the voting results is computed at each voxel as the uncertainty estimate.

3 The Network Architecture and Its Implementation

3.1 The Proposed Architecture

Our network consists of 20 layers of convolutions. In the first seven convolutional layers, we adopt $3 \times 3 \times 3$-voxel convolutions. These layers are designed to capture low-level image features such as edges and corners. In the subsequent convolutional layers, the kernels are dilated by a factor of two or four. These deeper layers with dilated kernels encode mid- and high-level image features.

Residual connections are employed to group every two convolutional layers. Within each residual block, each convolutional layer is associated with an element-wise rectified linear unit (ReLU) layer and a batch normalisation layer [10]. The ReLU, batch normalisation, and convolutional layers are arranged in the pre-activation order [8].

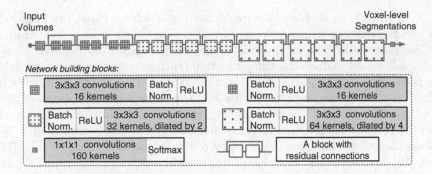

Fig. 3. The proposed network architecture for volumetric image segmentation. The network mainly utilises dilated convolutions and residual connections to make an end-to-end mapping from image volume to a voxel-level dense segmentation. To incorporate features at multiple scales, the dilation factor of the dilated convolutions is gradually increased when the layer goes deeper. The residual blocks with identity mapping enable the direct fusion of features from different scales. The spatial resolution of the input volume is maintained throughout the network.

The network can be trained end-to-end. In the training stage, the inputs to our network are $96 \times 96 \times 96$-voxel images. The final softmax layer gives classification scores over the class labels for each of the $96 \times 96 \times 96$ voxels. The architecture is illustrated in Fig. 3.

3.2   Implementation Details

In the training stage, the pre-processing step involved input data standardisation and augmentation at both image- and subvolume-level. At image-level, we adopted the histogram-based scale standardisation method [17] to normalised the intensity histograms. As a data augmentation at image-level, randomisation was introduced in the normalisation process by randomly choosing a threshold of foreground between the volume minimum and mean intensity (at test time, the mean intensity of the test volume was used as the threshold). Each image was further normalised to have zero mean and unit standard deviation. Augmentations on the randomly sampled $96 \times 96 \times 96$ subvolumes were employed on the fly. These included rotation with a random angle in the range of $[-10°, 10°]$ for each of the three orthogonal planes and spatial rescaling with a random scaling factor in the range of $[0.9, 1.1]$.

All the parameters in the convolutional layers were initialised according to He et al. [6]. The scaling and shifting parameters in the batch normalisation layers were initialised to 1 and 0 respectively. The networks were trained with two Nvidia K80 GPUs. At each training iteration, each GPU processed one input volume; the average gradients computed over these two training volumes were used as the gradients update. To make a fair comparison, we employed the Adam optimisation method [12] for all the methods with fixed hyper-parameters. The learning rate lr was set to 0.01, the step size hyper-parameter β_1 was 0.9

and β_2 was 0.999 in all cases, except V-Net for which we chose the largest lr that the training algorithm converges ($lr = 0.0001$). The models were trained until we observed a plateau in performance on the validation set. We do not employ additional spatial smoothing function (such as conditional random field) as a post-processing step. Instead of aiming for better segmentation results by adding post-processing steps, we focused on the dense segmentation maps generated by the networks. As we consider brain parcellation as a pretext task, networks without explicit spatial smoothing are potentially more reusable. We implemented all the methods (including a re-implementation of Deepmedic [11], V-net [16], and 3D U-net [3] architecture) with Tensorflow[1].

4   Experiments and Results

Data. To demonstrate the feasibility of learning complex 3D image representations from large-scale data, the proposed network is learning a highly granular segmentation of 543 T1-weighted MR images of healthy controls from the ADNI dataset. The average number of voxels of each volume is about $182 \times 244 \times 246$. The average voxel size is approximately $1.18\,mm \times 1.05\,mm \times 1.05\,mm$. All volumes are bias-corrected and reoriented to a standard Right-Anterior-Superior orientation. The bronze standard parcellation of 155 brain structures and 5 non-brain outer tissues are obtained using the GIF framework [1]. Figure 5 (left) shows the label distribution of the dataset. We randomly choose 443, 50, and 50 volumes for training, test, and validation respectively.

Overall Evaluation. In this section, we compare the proposed high-resolution compact network architecture (illustrated in Fig. 3; denoted as *HC-default*) with three variants: (1) the HC-default configuration without the residual connections, trained with cross-entropy loss function (*NoRes-entropy*); (2) the HC-default configuration without residual connections, trained with Dice loss function (*NoRes-dice*); and (3) the HC-default configuration trained with an additional dropout layer, and makes predictions with a majority voting of 10 Monte Carlo samples (*HC-dropout*). For the dropout variant, our dropout layer employed before the last convolutional layer consists of 80 kernels.

Additionally, three state-of-the-art volumetric segmentation networks are evaluated. These include 3D U-net [3], V-net [16], and Deepmedic [11]. The last layer of each network architecture is replaced with a 160-way softmax classifier.

We observe that training these networks with the cross entropy loss function (Eq. 2) leads to poor segmentation results. Since the cross-entropy loss function treats all training voxels equally, the network may have difficulties in learning representations related to the minority classes. Training with the Dice loss function alleviates this issue by implicitly re-weighting the voxels. Thus we train all networks using the Dice loss function for a fair comparison.

---

[1] The source code is available at https://github.com/gift-surg/HighRes3DNet.

Table 1. Comparison of different 3D convolutional network architectures.

Architecture	Multi-layer fusion	Num. param	Loss type	DCS (%)	STD (%)
HC-default	Residual	0.81M	Dice loss	82.05	2.96
HC-dropout	Residual	0.82M	Dice loss	**84.34**	**1.89**
NoRes-entropy	N/A	0.81M	Cross entr.	39.36	1.13
NoRes-dice	N/A	0.81M	Dice loss	75.47	2.97
Deepmedic [11]-dice	Two pathways	0.68M	Dice loss	78.74	1.72
3D U-net [3]-dice	Feature forwarding	19.08M	Dice loss	80.18	6.18
V-net [16]	Feature forwarding	62.63M	Dice loss	74.58	1.86

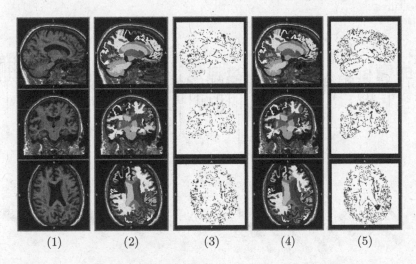

(1)   (2)   (3)   (4)   (5)

Fig. 4. Visualisations of segmentation results. (1) slices from a test image volume, segmentation maps and false prediction maps generated by HC-dropout (2, 3), and 3D U-net-dice (4, 5).

We use the mean Dice Coefficient Similarity (DCS) as the performance measure. Table 1 and Fig. 5 (right) compare the performance on the test set. In terms of our network variants, the results show that the use of Dice loss function largely improves the segmentation performance. This suggests that the Dice loss function can handle the severely unbalanced segmentation problem well. The results also suggest that introducing the residual connections improved the segmentation performance measured in mean DCS. This indicates that the residual connections are important elements of the proposed network. By adopting the dropout method, the DCS can be further improved by 2% in DCS.

With a relatively small number of parameters, our HC-default and HC-dropout outperform the competing methods in terms of mean DCS. This suggests that our network is more effective for the brain parcellation problem. Note that V-net has a similar architecture to 3D U-net and has more parameters, but

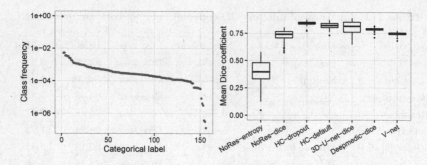

Fig. 5. Left: label distribution of the dataset; right: comparison of different network architectures.

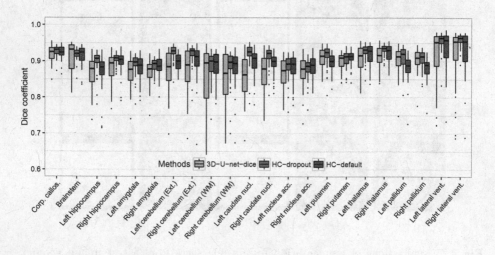

Fig. 6. Segmentation performance against a set of key structures.

does not employ the batch normalisation technique. The lower DCS produced by V-net suggests that batch normalisation is important for training the networks for brain parcellation.

In Fig. 6, we show that the dropout variant achieves better segmentation results for all the key structures. Figure 4 presents an example of the segmentation results of the proposed network and 3D U-net-Dice.

Receptive Field and Border Effects. We further compare the segmentation performance of a trained network by discarding the borders in each dimension of the segmentation map. That is, given a $d \times d \times d$-voxel input, at border size 1 we only preserve the $(d-2)^3$-voxel output volume centred within the predicted map. Figure 7 plots the DCS and standard errors of segmentation according to the size of the segmentation borders in each dimension. The results show that the distorted border is around 17 voxels in each dimension. The border effects do not severely decrease the segmentation performance. In practice, we pad the volume images with 16 zeros in each dimension, and remove the same amount of borders in the segmentation output.

The Effect of Number of Samples in Uncertainty Estimations. This section investigates the number of Monte Carlo samples and the segmentation performance of the proposed network. Figure 8 (left) suggests that using 10 samples is enough to achieve good segmentation. Further increasing the number of samples has relatively small effects on the DCS. Figure 8 (right) plots the voxel-wise segmentation accuracy computed using only the voxels with an uncertainty less than a threshold. The voxel-wise accuracy is high when the threshold is small. This indicates that the uncertainty estimation reflects the confidence of the network. Figure 9 shows an uncertainty map

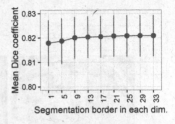

Fig. 7. Empirical analysis of the segmentation borders. Voxels near to the volume borders are classified less accurately.

generated by the proposed network. The uncertainties near the boundaries of different structures are relatively higher than the other regions.

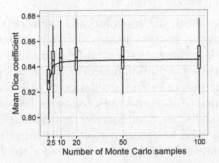 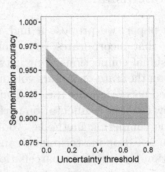

Fig. 8. Evaluation of dropout sampling. Left: the segmentation performance against the number of Monte Carlo samples. Right: voxel-level segmentation accuracy by thresholding the uncertainties. The shaded area represents the standard errors.

Currently, our method takes about 60 s to predict a typical volume with $192 \times 256 \times 256$ voxels. To achieve better segmentation results and measure uncertainty, 10 Monte Carlo samples of our dropout model are required. The entire process takes slightly more than 10 min in total. However, during the Monte Carlo sampling at test time, only the dropout layer and the final prediction layer are randomised. To further reduce the computational time, the future software could reuse the features from the layers before dropout, resulting in only a marginal increase in runtime when compared to a single prediction.

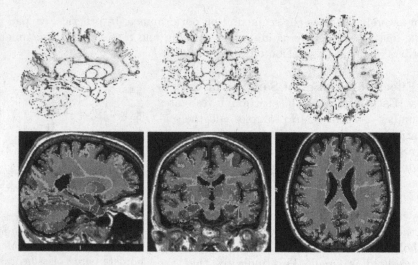

Fig. 9. Voxel-level segmentation uncertainty estimations. Top row: uncertainty map generated with 100 Monte Carlo samples using dropout. Bottom row: uncertainty map thresholded at 0.1.

5   Conclusion

In this paper, we propose a high-resolution, 3D convolutional network architecture that incorporates large volumetric context using dilated convolutions and residual connections. Our network is conceptually simpler and more compact than the state-of-the-art volumetric segmentation networks. We validate the proposed network using the challenging task of brain parcellation in MR images. We show that the segmentation performance of our network compares favourably with the competing methods. Additionally, we demonstrate that Monte Carlo sampling of dropout technique can be used to generate voxel-level uncertainty estimation for our brain parcellation network. Moreover, we consider the brain parcellation task as a pretext task for volumetric image segmentation. Our trained network potentially provides a good starting point for transfer learning of other segmentation tasks.

In the future, we will extensively test the generalisation ability of the network to brain MR scans obtained with various scanning protocols from different data centres. Furthermore, we note that the uncertainty estimations are not probabilities. We will investigate the calibration of the uncertainty scores to provide reliable probability estimations.

Acknowledgements. This work was supported through an Innovative Engineering for Health award by the Wellcome Trust and EPSRC [WT101957, NS/A000027/1], the National Institute for Health Research University College London Hospitals Biomedical Research Centre (NIHR BRC UCLH/UCL High Impact Initiative), UCL EPSRC CDT Scholarship Award [EP/L016478/1], a UCL Overseas Research Scholarship, a UCL Graduate Research Scholarship, and the Health Innovation Challenge Fund by the Department of Health and Wellcome Trust [HICF-T4-275, WT 97914]. The authors would like to acknowledge that the work presented here made use of Emerald, a GPU-accelerated High Performance Computer, made available by the Science & Engineering South Consortium operated in partnership with the STFC Rutherford-Appleton Laboratory.

References

1. Cardoso, M.J., Modat, M., Wolz, R., Melbourne, A., Cash, D., Rueckert, D., Ourselin, S.: Geodesic information flows: spatially-variant graphs and their application to segmentation and fusion. IEEE Trans. Med. Imaging **34**(9), 1976–1988 (2015)
2. Chen, L.C., Papandreou, G., Kokkinos, I., Murphy, K., Yuille, A.L.: DeepLab: Semantic image segmentation with deep convolutional nets, atrous convolution, and fully connected CRFs (2016). arXiv:1606.00915
3. Çiçek, Ö., Abdulkadir, A., Lienkamp, S.S., Brox, T., Ronneberger, O.: 3D U-Net: learning dense volumetric segmentation from sparse annotation. In: Ourselin, S., Joskowicz, L., Sabuncu, M.R., Unal, G., Wells, W. (eds.) MICCAI 2016. LNCS, vol. 9901, pp. 424–432. Springer, Cham (2016). doi:10.1007/978-3-319-46723-8_49
4. Dou, Q., Chen, H., Yu, L., Zhao, L., Qin, J., Wang, D., Mok, V.C., Shi, L., Heng, P.A.: Automatic detection of cerebral microbleeds from MR images via 3D convolutional neural networks. IEEE Trans. Med. Imaging **35**(5), 1182–1195 (2016)
5. Gal, Y., Ghahramani, Z.: Dropout as a Bayesian approximation: representing model uncertainty in deep learning. In: ICML (2016)
6. He, K., Zhang, X., Ren, S., Sun, J.: Delving deep into rectifiers: surpassing human-level performance on imagenet classification. In: ICCV (2015)
7. He, K., Zhang, X., Ren, S., Sun, J.: Deep residual learning for image recognition. In: CVPR (2016)
8. He, K., Zhang, X., Ren, S., Sun, J.: Identity mappings in deep residual networks. In: Leibe, B., Matas, J., Sebe, N., Welling, M. (eds.) ECCV 2016. LNCS, vol. 9908, pp. 630–645. Springer, Cham (2016). doi:10.1007/978-3-319-46493-0_38
9. Huh, M., Agrawal, P., Efros, A.A.: What makes ImageNet good for transfer learning? (2016). arXiv:1608.08614
10. Ioffe, S., Szegedy, C.: Batch normalization: accelerating deep network training by reducing internal covariate shift. In: ICML (2015)
11. Kamnitsas, K., Ledig, C., Newcombe, V.F., Simpson, J.P., Kane, A.D., Menon, D.K., Rueckert, D., Glocker, B.: Efficient multi-scale 3D CNN with fully connected CRF for accurate brain lesion segmentation. Med. Image Anal. **36**, 61–78 (2017)
12. Kingma, D., Ba, J.: Adam: A method for stochastic optimization (2014). arXiv:1412.6980
13. Kleesiek, J., Urban, G., Hubert, A., Schwarz, D., Maier-Hein, K., Bendszus, M., Biller, A.: Deep MRI brain extraction: a 3D convolutional neural network for skull stripping. NeuroImage 129 (2016)
14. Luo, W., Li, Y., Urtasun, R., Zemel, R.: Understanding the effective receptive field in deep convolutional neural networks. In: NIPS (2016)
15. Merkow, J., Marsden, A., Kriegman, D., Tu, Z.: Dense volume-to-volume vascular boundary detection. In: Ourselin, S., Joskowicz, L., Sabuncu, M.R., Unal, G., Wells, W. (eds.) MICCAI 2016. LNCS, vol. 9902, pp. 371–379. Springer, Cham (2016). doi:10.1007/978-3-319-46726-9_43

16. Milletari, F., Navab, N., Ahmadi, S.A.: V-Net: Fully convolutional neural networks for volumetric medical image segmentation. In: International Conference on 3D Vision (2016)
17. Nyúl, L.G., Udupa, J.K., Zhang, X.: New variants of a method of MRI scale standardization. IEEE Trans. Med. Imaging **19**(2), 143–150 (2000)
18. Shi, W., Zhuang, X., Wolz, R., Simon, D., Tung, K., Wang, H., Ourselin, S., Edwards, P., Razavi, R., Rueckert, D.: A multi-image graph cut approach for cardiac image segmentation and uncertainty estimation. In: International Workshop on Statistical Atlases and Computational Models of the Heart (2011)
19. Veit, A., Wilber, M., Belongie, S.: Residual networks are exponential ensembles of relatively shallow networks. In: NIPS (2016)

Discovering Change-Point Patterns in Dynamic Functional Brain Connectivity of a Population

Mengyu Dai[1]([✉]), Zhengwu Zhang[2,3], and Anuj Srivastava[1]

[1] Department of Statistics, Florida State University, Tallahassee, FL, USA
mengyu.dai@stat.fsu.edu
[2] Statistical and Applied Mathematical Sciences Institute,
Research Triangle Park, NC, USA
[3] Department of Statistical Science, Duke University, Durham, NC, USA

Abstract. This paper seeks to discover common change-point patterns, associated with functional connectivity (FC) in human brain, across multiple subjects. FC, represented as a covariance or a correlation matrix, relates to the similarity of fMRI responses across different brain regions, when a brain is simply resting or performing a task under an external stimulus. While the dynamical nature of FC is well accepted, this paper develops a formal statistical test for finding *change-points* in times series associated with FC observed over time. It represents instantaneous connectivity by a symmetric positive-definite matrix, and uses a Riemannian metric on this space to develop a graphical method for detecting change-points in a time series of such matrices. It also provides a graphical representation of estimated FC for stationary subintervals in between detected change-points. Furthermore, it uses a temporal alignment of the test statistic, viewed as a real-valued function over time, to remove temporal variability and to discover common change-point patterns across subjects, tasks, and regions. This method is illustrated using HCP database for multiple subjects and tasks.

Keywords: Functional connectivity · Change-point · Riemannian metric · Covariance estimation · Function alignment

1 Introduction

Learning about structural and functional connectivity in human brain is of great interest from multiple perspectives. The human connectome project (HCP) investigates these connectivities in order to understand brain functionality and to diagnose cognitive abilities of individual subjects. While structural connectivity is inferred using diffusion tensor - magnetic resonance imaging (DT-MRI) data, functional connectivity (FC) is estimated using functional MRI (fMRI) data. FC is usually defined as *statistical dependencies among remote neurophysiological events* [17]. These dependencies are expressed as quantifications of similarity, or *correlations*, between simultaneous functional measurements of neuronal activities across regions in human brain. Functional MRI measures the

© Springer International Publishing AG 2017
M. Niethammer et al. (Eds.): IPMI 2017, LNCS 10265, pp. 361–372, 2017.
DOI: 10.1007/978-3-319-59050-9_29

blood oxygen level dependent (BOLD) contrast signals of each brain voxel over a period of time. The short-term FC is often represented as a covariance or correlation matrix of fMRI data over a small time window, with the matrix size being the number of brain regions being considered. In the early days, FC associated with individual tasks or stimuli was treated as fixed or static over time. However, recent studies [13–15] have revealed strong evidence that FC is a dynamic process and evolves over time, even in the resting state. Our primary interest is to investigate and characterize the dynamic nature of FC between different anatomical brain regions during performances of certain tasks and resting states.

A dynamical FC model is bound to provide insight into fundamental working of brain networks [10]. (For a review on recent progress in analyzing FC, please refer to [14,17].) A critical part in modeling dynamical FC is to quantify changes that occur over time during observation intervals. For example, some recent studies have developed tests for temporal changes in coherence pattern of multiple regions of interest(ROI) [18]. [15] introduced Dynamic Connectivity Regression (DCR), which is a data-driven technique useful for detecting temporal change points in functional connectivity between brain regions. [5] presented a modified DCR on single-subject data that increases accuracy with a small number of observations and reduces the number of false positives. In case FC is represented by a covariance or a correlation matrix of fMRI signals, a sliding (time) window is used commonly to estimate the correlation matrix. Lindquist et al. [10] discuss some alternatives to moving window-based correlation estimation.

While these studies focused on testing whether FC is static or dynamic, or seek temporal change-points for *individual* subjects, we additionally analyze FC in a *group* of individuals and seek some common patterns in performances of specific tasks. We take different partitionings of human brain into functional units or regions and represent instantaneous FC as symmetric, positive definite matrices (SPDMs), with entries denoting covariances of localized functional signals under resting state or under external stimuli. We use a sliding window to segment multivariate time series into overlapping blocks, and compute covariance matrix for each block. The original time series data (BOLD signal) can thus be converted in to an indexed sequence of SPDMs and one of the goal is now to detect if these matrices denote a stationary process or if the underlying distribution changes at some time points. The actual test is performed using the graphical approach introduced in [1], where one constructs minimal spanning trees (MSTs) connecting the observed SPDMs. We utilize a Riemannian structure on the space of SPDMs to define and compute geodesic distances between correlation matrices, and to facilitate construction of MSTs. Computation of edge length distributions across temporal partitions of MSTs lead to a test statistic for change-point detection.

The change-point patterns for a group of people are expected to be similar especially when the fMRI is recorded in a well-designed experiment where different tasks are given at fixed intervals. However, different brains may react differently to external stimuli and the response times can be different. It might be hard to discern the commonality of change-point patterns across subjects from the raw change point data. Thus, temporal alignment naturally plays an important role in discovering underlying patterns and reducing the confounding variation in the time domain. We apply temporal alignment at the level of test statistics to detect and discover some common patterns FC dynamics for a group of individuals.

The rest of this paper as follows. In Sect. 2, we describe the mathematical components of the our proposed framework, including: representation of FC using covariance matrices, a Riemannian structure on the space of SPDMs, a graphical approach for detecting change-points, a method for reconstructing connectivity network in homogeneous sub-intervals and the temporal alignment method to discovery common change-point patterns. Section 3 presents several experimental results using HCP fMRI data.

2 Methodology

The proposed framework, for discovering dynamic patterns in FC over a population, is made up of several current and novel components. Figure 1 shows a systematic overview of the proposed framework. We describe it next.

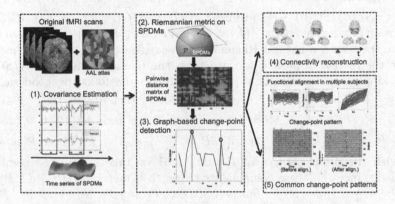

Fig. 1. A systematic overview of our proposed framework for FC change-point study.

2.1 Covariance Estimation

The first problem is to estimate a correlation or a covariance matrix that represents instantaneous (or short-term) functional connectivity between anatomical regions of interest. To specify this matrix, we segment the brain into d regions and then represent the functional connectivity at any time using a $d \times d$ covariance matrix of corresponding BOLD signals over small intervals. In this paper we take a simple approach and use the standard sample covariance matrix of signal over a temporal window. (There are more sophisticated ways of estimating covariance matrix, see for example [9], and those can easily be applied here.)

We segment multivariate time series into overlapping blocks with equal sizes. The block-size should be large enough to result in a positive definite covariance, but not too large to smooth over the subtle changes that are critical to assess temporal evolution of FC. Additionally, the step size for moving the window should be large enough to reduce dependency in successive covariance matrices. If the step is too small, then only few points differ in successive blocks, and the successive covariance will be highly correlated. In the experiments presented later, we use a step to window-size ratio of at least 0.2.

2.2 Riemannian Structure on SPDMs

In order to quantify differences in FC, represented by covariance matrices, we need a metric structure on the space of SPDMs. While there are several Riemannian structures used in the literature [16], we briefly summarize a convenient one taken from [7]; please refer to these papers for details.

Let $\mathcal{P}$ be the space of $n \times n$ SPDMs, and let $\tilde{\mathcal{P}}$ be its subset of matrices with determinant one. Recall that for any square matrix $G \in SL(n)$, one can decompose it uniquely as $G = PS$ where $P \in \tilde{\mathcal{P}}$ and $S \in SO(n)$. The quotient space $SL(n)/SO(n)$ is the set of all orbits of the type $[G] = \{GS | S \in SO(n)\}$, for $G \in SL(n)$. Thus, one can identify $\tilde{\mathcal{P}}$ with the quotient space $SL(n)/SO(n)$ via a map $\pi : SL(n)/SO(n) \to \tilde{\mathcal{P}}$, given by $\pi([G]) = \sqrt{\tilde{G}\tilde{G}^t}$, for any $\tilde{G} \in [G]$. The inverse map of π is given by: $\pi^{-1}(\tilde{P}) = [\tilde{P}] \equiv \{\tilde{P}S | S \in SO(n)\} \in SL(n)/SO(n)$. Now, we start with a natural Riemannian metric on $SL(n)$, the trace metric, and use the map π to push it forward from the quotient space $SL(n)/SO(n)$ to $\tilde{\mathcal{P}}$. Skipping the details, this process leads to the following geodesic distance in $\tilde{\mathcal{P}}$. For any $\tilde{P}_1, \tilde{P}_2 \in \tilde{\mathcal{P}}$, $d_{\tilde{\mathcal{P}}}(\tilde{P}_1, \tilde{P}_2) = \|A_{12}\|$ where $A_{12} = \log(P_{12})$ and $P_{12} = \sqrt{\tilde{P}_1^{-1} \tilde{P}_2^2 \tilde{P}_1^{-1}}$. Since for any $P \in \mathcal{P}$ we have $\det(P) > 0$, we can express $P = (\tilde{P}, \frac{1}{n} \log(det(P)))$ with $\tilde{P} = \frac{P}{\det(P)^{1/n}} \in \tilde{\mathcal{P}}$. Thus, $\mathcal{P}$ is identified with the product space of $\tilde{\mathcal{P}} \times \mathbb{R}_+$ and we take a weighted combinations of distances on these components to reach a metric on $\tilde{\mathcal{P}}$: $d_{\mathcal{P}}(I, P)^2 = d_{\tilde{\mathcal{P}}}(I, \tilde{P})^2 + \frac{1}{n} (log(det(P)))^2$. For two SPDMs P_1 and P_2, let $P_{12} = P_1^{-1} P_2 S_{12}$ for the optimal $S_{12} \in SO(n)$ (coming from Procrustes alignment) and $P_{12} \in \mathcal{P}$, we have $\det(P_{12}) = \det(P_2)/\det(P_1)$. Therefore, the resulting squared geodesic distance between P_1 and P_2 is $d_{\mathcal{P}}(P_1, P_2)^2 = d_{\tilde{\mathcal{P}}}(I, \tilde{P}_{12})^2 + \frac{1}{n} (log(det(P_2)) - log(det(P_1)))^2$. Once we have a metric on SPDMs, we can use that to define and compute sample means on $\mathcal{P}$ as follows. The sample Karcher mean of a given set of SPDMs is given by $\theta_P = \arg\min_{\theta_P \in \mathcal{P}} \sum_{i=1}^{n} d_{\mathcal{P}}(\theta_P, P_i)^2$, where $\{P_i \in \mathcal{P}\}$ is the given set. The algorithm for computing Karcher mean is a standard one and is not repeated here. We refer the reader to [7] for those details.

2.3 Change-Point Detection Using MST

The next issue is to detect change-points in a SPDM time series using a metric-based approach. We adapted a graph-theoretical method introduced by Chen and Zhang in [1] for solving this problem. There have been earlier works on graph-based methods for a two-sample test, but these authors extended the framework to arbitrary metric spaces.

Let $X_1, X_2, \ldots, X_T$ be random variables taking values on a manifold M, and let F_0 and F_1 denote two probability distribution functions on M. We are interested in testing the null hypothesis that all X_is are samples from the same distribution, against an alternative that all points after a certain time τ follow a different distribution. That is,

$$H_0 : X_t \sim F_0, \ t = 1, 2, \ldots, T, \qquad H_1 : \exists\, 1 \leq \tau < T, \ X_i \sim \begin{cases} F_1, & t > \tau \\ F_0, & \text{otherwise,} \end{cases}$$

This test is phrased for a single change-point, at time τ, but one can repeat this test for different τs to detect multiple change-points.

The test statistic $Z(\tau)$ for this test is defined as follows. First compute all the pairwise distances between all X_t under the chosen metric on M. Then, use these distances to form a minimal spanning tree (MST) connecting the set $\{X_t, t = 1, 2, \ldots, T\}$ in M. An MST is a connected graph such that: (1) each X_t is a node in the graph, (2) if any two points are connected by an edge then the weight of that edge is given by the pairwise distance between those points, and (3) the sum of weights of all connected edges is the smallest amongst all such graphs. Note that the MST is independent of the ordering of the given points, and can be computed/stored for the whole sequence in one shot. To test whether there is a change-point at a $\tau \in \{1, 2, \ldots, T-1\}$, we divide X_ts into two groups: $\{X_1, \ldots, X_\tau\}$, and $\{X_{\tau+1}, \ldots, X_T\}$. Let $R(\tau)$ represent the number of edges that connect points across two groups in MST. Intuitively, if τ is a change-point then the two groups represent an appropriate clustering of points and only a small number of edges connect across those clusters. In contrast, if the two groups are from the same distribution, then we expect a large number of edges in MST going across the two groups. Chen and Zhang [1] show that under H_0 $R(\tau)$ has a distribution with mean and variance given by: $E(R(\tau)) = p_1(\tau)|G|$, $Var(R(\tau)) = p_2(\tau)|G| + (\frac{1}{2}p_1(\tau) - p_2(\tau))\sum_i |G_i|^2 + (p_2(\tau) - p_1^2(\tau))|G|^2$, where $p_1(\tau) = \frac{2\tau(T-\tau)}{T(T-1)}$, $p_2(\tau) = \frac{4\tau(\tau-1)(T-\tau)(T-\tau-1)}{T(T-1)(T-2)(T-3)}$ and $|G_i|$ is defined as the number of edges in subgraph of G containing all edges that connect to node X_i. Now, standardize $R(\tau)$ using $Z(\tau) = -\frac{(R(\tau)-E(R(\tau)))}{\sqrt{Var(R(\tau))}}$ to reach the test statistic. This test statistic is then tested for a given confidence level for accepting or rejecting the null hypothesis. According to [1], a value of $Z(\tau) \geq 3$ implies a change-point detection at 0.95 confidence level, and $Z(\tau) \geq 4$ implies a change-point detection at 0.99 confidence level. The change-point detection algorithm is as follows:

Algorithm 1. *1. For a given **ordered** set of points $\{X_t \in M, t = 1, 2, \ldots, T\}$, compute D, the $T \times T$ pairwise geodesic distance matrix.*
2. Use D to form a minimal spanning tree (MST) connecting all the points.
3. For a fixed τ, count $R(\tau)$, the number of edges in this MST between first group: $\{X_1, \ldots, X_\tau\}$, and the second group $\{X_{\tau+1}, \ldots, X_T\}$.
4. Calculate $E(R(\tau))$ and $Var(R(\tau))$, and use them to standardize $R(\tau)$, resulting in $Z(\tau)$. If $Z(\tau) \geq 3$, a change-point is detected (at 0.95 confidence level).

To detect multiple change-points in a time sequence of SPDMs in our setting, we use a large moving window approach. Given a large window of fixed length, we detect whether midpoint in the window is a change-point, and we repeat after shifting the window to the right. Before we proceed further, we outline some limitations of the framework outlined so far. First, in the above algorithm, we divide SPDMs into two groups to detect whether the SPDMs before and after a certain time have different statistical distributions, but for multivariate time series with more than one change-point, the SPDMs in a divided group may not exactly follow one statistical distribution during the corresponding subintervals. In this situation, applying the above algorithm for the whole time series, with multiple change-points, will contradict with the original assumption that the time series only follow one specific distribution after a change-point. Second, the graph-based approach is not suitable for detecting change-points at the beginning and at the end of the time series.

2.4   Estimation of Connectivity Graphs for Displays

Given a specific covariance matrix, denoting stationary FC over a sub-interval between any two change-points, we are interested in estimating and visualizing a graph representing the connectivity of different brain regions. We accomplish this using graphical Lasso [6]. Let the observation period $[0, T]$ be subdivided into several sub-intervals by detected change-points at τ_1, τ_2, etc. For each sub-interval $[\tau_j, \tau_{j+1}]$ we compute the Karcher mean of all SPDMs over this sub-interval; call it $\bar{P}_j \in \mathcal{P}$. Then, we use this mean SPDM to estimate the associated precision matrix using: $\hat{\Theta}_j = \underset{\Theta \geq 0}{\operatorname{argmin}} \left(\operatorname{tr}(\bar{P}_j \Theta) - \log \det(\Theta) + \rho \sum_{i \neq k} |\Theta_{ik}| \right)$, where $\rho > 0$ is a parameter controls density of the generated graph (Fig. 2 illustrates the effect of ρ on the resulting graph). Given the estimated precision matrix $\hat{\Theta}_i$, the adjacency matrix is obtained by thresholding, i.e. $(A_j)_{ik} = 1_{|\hat{\Theta}_{ik}| > \epsilon = 0.001}$. This adjacency matrix is then used to represent the undirected graph formed by the corresponding brain regions.

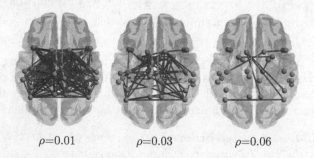

$\rho = 0.01$ $\rho = 0.03$ $\rho = 0.06$

Fig. 2. Estimated connectivity of 30 ROIs with different ρs.

We summarize the overall procedure for detecting change-point patterns in FC observations.

Algorithm 2. *1. Given fMRI time series data on a set of parcellated regions of interest, divide the fMRI data into T different time blocks using sliding windows of width W and step size S ($S < W$) and form a sequence of covariance matrices $\{P_1, P_2, \ldots, P_T\}$.*

2. Use Algorithm 1, to form a normalized test statistic $Z(\tau)$, for each $\tau \in \{2, \ldots, T-1\}$. And find those τ where $Z(\tau) > 3$; call them $\{\tau_j\}$. These denote the change-points of FC.

3. For each sub-interval $\{\tau_j, \tau_{j+1}\}$, find the Karcher mean of covariance matrices $\{P_{\tau_j}, \ldots, P_{\tau_{j+1}}\}$ to form $\bar{P}_j$. Use the mean SPDM to estimate the precision matrix and the adjacency matrix, which ultimately forms the graph.

2.5 Temporal Synchronization of Change-Point Statistics

Algorithm 2 enables us to detect change-points and estimate graphs associated with homogeneous sub-intervals, all for individual subjects. Additionally, it provides us with the test statistic $R(\tau)$ as a probabilistic measure of having a change-point at τ. Now we are interested in studying patterns of change-points associated with a population of individuals, while performing the same tasks. The question is: Are change-point patterns are similar of different for different individuals? Just visualizing $R(\tau)$ for different individual leads to no apparent structures. However, if we take into account the variable response times across individuals, and temporally align these functions, a pattern emerges.

To enable temporal registration, we fit a smooth function to each discrete $Z(\tau)$, obtained using Algorithm 1 for each subject, using cubic splines. Next, we use an elastic method based on the classical Fisher-Rao metric to obtain the best wrapping functions to perform the alignment [19]. Let $\{f_i\}$ be the set of fitted smooth functions on a normalized time interval, e.g. $[0, 1]$. Our goal is to find a set of warping functions $\{\gamma_i\}$, such that $\{f_i \circ \gamma_i\}$ are temporally aligned. Here $\gamma \in \Gamma$, and Γ is the set of all positive diffeomorphisms on $[0, 1]$ such that $\gamma(0) = 0$ and $\gamma(1) = 1$. For details, refer to [19]; we present final results here. Let q be the *square-root slope function* (SRSF) of the function f, defined as $q(t) = \text{sign}\{f(t)\}\sqrt{|f(t)|}$. To jointly register functions $\{f_1, \ldots, f_n\}$, one follows the following iterative procedure: initialize a template μ and iteratively solve for

$$\gamma_i = \arg \inf_{\gamma \in \Gamma} \|\mu - (q_i \circ \gamma)\sqrt{\dot{\gamma}}\|, i = 1, 2, \cdots, n, \text{ and } \mu = \frac{1}{n}\sum_{i=1}^{n}(q_i \circ \gamma_i)\sqrt{\dot{\gamma}_i} \quad . \quad (1)$$

Each optimization can be solved using the dynamic programming. Given the optimal γ_is, the aligned test score functions are $\{f_i \circ \gamma_i\}$, and enabling us to discover change-point patterns across population.

3   Experimental Results

In this section we demonstrate our framework using both simulated and real fMRI datasets taken from the HCP database.

3.1   Simulation Study

To illustrate the algorithm in situations with known ground truth, we simulate a d-dimensional time series data (with $T = 900$), with three sub-intervals coming three different multivariate normal distributions. Data points from $t = 1$ to $t = 300$ are simulated from $\mathcal{N}(0, \Sigma_1)$, from $t = 301$ to $t = 600$ are from $\mathcal{N}(0, \Sigma_2)$, and from $t = 601$ to $t = 900$ are from $\mathcal{N}(0, \Sigma_3)$, where Σ_1, Σ_2 and Σ_3 are randomly generated in such a way that $d_{\tilde{P}}(\Sigma_i, \Sigma_{i+1}) > 0.6$. To detect change-points we implemented Algorithm 2 using the parameter $W = 30$, $S = 20$, where W stands for the window size and S represents the step size for sliding windows. Figure 3 shows a plot of the test statistic, $Z(\tau)$ versus τ, for $d = 2$ in the left panel and $d = 10$ in the right panel. The detected change-points are marked using black circles, and one can clearly see the peak value of test statistic around the detected change-points, and this agrees with the ground truth.

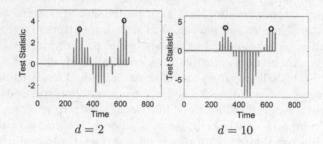

Fig. 3. Change-point detection on simulated data, with detections marked using circles.

3.2   Real Data Study

Next we consider task fMRI (tfMRI) data from Human Connectome Project (HCP) [2]. The majority of the HCP tfMRI data were acquired at 3T, which is considered to be the field strength currently most suitable for acquiring high quality data reliably from a large cohort of subjects. Acquisitions are based on blood oxygen level dependent (BOLD) contrast. A series of 4D imaging data were acquired for each subject while they were performing different tasks involving different neural systems, e.g. visual, motion and cognition systems. The acquired image is with an isometric spatial resolution of 2 mm and temporal resolution of 0.7 s. All fMRI data in HCP are preprocessed by removing spatial distortions, realigning volume to compensate for subject motion, registering the fMRI to the structural MRI, reducing the bias field, normalizing the 4D image to a global mean, masking the data with the final brain mask and aligning the brain to a standard space [8]. This preprocessed tfMRI is now ready for FC analysis.

To map the functional connectivity, we begin with the segmentation of brain into regions using an existing template, such as the AAL (Automated Anatomical Labeling) atlas [12]. Time series for each region in tfMRI are extracted using CONN functional connectivity toolbox [20] and AAL atlas (116 regions).

A [0.008, inf] (Hz) high-pass filter is used to de-noise the functional data. We evaluate the dynamic FC using the proposed method in two different tasks: (1) gambling and (2) social cognition.

Single Subject Dynamic FC for Gambling Task: The gambling task in HCP was adapted from the one developed in [11]. Participants play a card guessing game where they are asked to guess the number on a mystery card in order to win or loss money. Three different blocks are presented through out the task: reward blocks, neutral blocks and loss blocks. Brain regions that relate to this task include basal ganglia, ventral medial prefrontal and orbito-frontal. The basal ganglia contains multiple subcortical nuclei and is the part of brain that influences motivation and action selection. We selected four regions inside the basal ganglia: right Caudate, left Caudate, right Putamen and left Putamen, and studied FC using 4×4 SPDMs representing covariance of fMRI signal in these four regions. Algorithm 2 is applied and the results are shown in Fig. 4(a). It shows the evolution of the test statistic versus τ for two different choices of window size W. Despite different window sizes, the algorithm detects the same two change-points. This means that these four nodes formed three different connection patterns during the performance of the task. The three corresponding graphs are shown in Fig. 4(b).

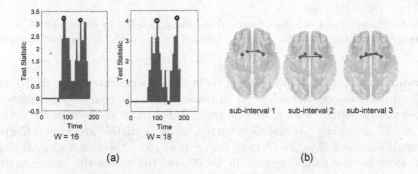

Fig. 4. FC change-point detection for four regions in basal ganglia in gambling task.

Single Subject Dynamic FC for Social Cognition Task: In this experiment, participants were presented with short video clips of objects (squares, circles, triangles) that either interaction in some way, or moved randomly on the screen [4]. After each video clip, participants judge whether the objects had (1) a mental interaction (an interaction that appears as if the shapes are affecting feelings and thoughts); (2) not sure or (3) no interaction. Each run of the task has 5 video blocks (2 Mental and 3 Random in the data used here). Possible brain regions that relate to this task are medial prefrontal cortex, temporal parietal junction, inferior and superior temporal sulcus [3]. Since this task has more time blocks (5 blocks) than the gambling data, we expect to detect more change-points. In this example, we use 14 regions in Occipital lobe, Parietal lobe and Temporal lobe, and the algorithm detects several change-points. Figure 5(a) shows the result using block size 16. Three major change-points are detected in these regions. We reconstruct the connectivity networks for the 14 ROIs using data in the four sub-intervals defined by the three detected change-points. Figure 5(b) shows the reconstructed networks. We can see that intermediate networks (during intervals 2 and 3) are more complex than the networks at the two ends.

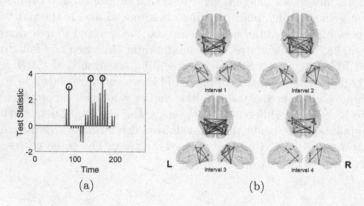

(a)   (b)

Fig. 5. FC change-point detection in social cognition task for 14 regions (ROI 50–63). (a) change-points with $W = 16$. (b) reconstructed FC networks for the four intervals.

Dynamical FC for Multiple Subjects: In this experiment, we use tfMRI data from multiple subjects (99 subjects) to demonstrate the change-point patterns in a population of individuals. We selected 8 ROIs (indexed 81–88 in the default atlas in [20], including Central Opercular Cortex, Parietal Operculum Cortex, Planum Polare and Heschl's Gyrus). Figure 6(a) plots the test scores $Z(\tau)$ for 99 subjects for the gambling task in HCP, and (d) shows the corresponding change-points for those subjects. Naturally FC changes occur at different times for different individuals, with barely any common pattern visible. However, the functional alignment allows us to get a better understanding of the shared patterns in these subjects. Figure 6(e) shows the aligned change-point pattern. After the alignment, one can clearly see that there are generally two or three change-points in all subjects. We also compared change-point patterns in task fMRI and resting fMRI using 20 subjects. For the same ROIs, we calculated the pairwise elastic distances (after pairwise alignments) between the test score functions in gambling task and resting state. Figure 6(f) shows these distances as a matrix. We can observe that change-point patterns are similar within the tasks but are significantly different from the resting state.

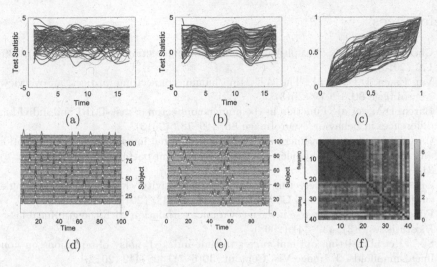

Fig. 6. Common FC change-point pattern of 8 ROIs in the gambling task for 99 subjects. (a) shows the fitted smooth test score functions. (b) shows the aligned test score functions. (c) shows the wrapping functions for alignment. (d) shows the change-point pattern before alignment. (e) shows the change-point pattern after alignment. (f) shows a comparison of the FC change-point pattern in gambling task with resting state.

4 Discussion

This paper develops a formal test for detecting change-points in FC using fMRI data, and seeks to discover common change-point patterns across subjects in a population. It represents instantaneous FCs as covariance matrices and studies changes in distributions of these SPDMs. The test statistic is based on minimal spanning trees between covariance matrices using Riemannian distances. The last step is to temporally align test statistics, treated as real-valued functions, to discover common patterns across subjects.

There is a potential for improvement in several parts of this proposed system. Firstly, the change-point test statistic assumes independent samples from the respective solutions, and a method tailored to the time-series data should perform better. Secondly, there is a possibility of trying correlation matrices, or precision matrices, and associated Riemannian metrics for representing instantaneous FC, and the performance can potentially improve. Finally, the temporal alignment can alternatively be performed at the raw data level, rather that at the test statistic level, followed by the rest of the pipeline.

Acknowledgments. This research was supported in part by NSF grants DMS 1621787 and CCF 1617397 to AS. ZZ was partially supported by NSF grant DMS-1127914 to SAMSI. Data were provided in part by the HCP, WU-Minn Consortium (Principal Investigators: David Van Essen and Kamil Ugurbil; 1U54MH091657).

References

1. Chen, H., Zhang, N.: Graph-based change-point detection. Ann. Stat. **43**(1), 139–176 (2015)
2. Van Essen, D.C., et al.: The WU-Minn human connectome project: an overview. NeuroImage **80**, 62–79 (2013)
3. Barch, D.M., et al.: Function in the human connectome: task-fMRI and individual differences in behavior. NeuroImage **80**, 169–189 (2013)
4. Castelli, F., et al.: Movement and mind: a functional imaging study of perception and interpretation of complex intentional movement patterns. NeuroImage **12**(3), 314–325 (2000)
5. Cribben, I., et al.: Detecting functional connectivity change points for single-subject fMRI data. Front. Comput. Neurosci. **7**(143) (2013)
6. Friedman, J., et al.: Sparse inverse covariance estimation with the graphical lasso. Biostatistics **9**(3), 432–441 (2008)
7. Su, J., et al.: Fitting optimal curves to time-indexed, noisy observations on non-linear manifolds. J. Image Vis. Comput. **30**(6–7), 428–442 (2012)
8. Glasser, M.F., et al.: The minimal preprocessing pipelines for the Human Connectome Project. NeuroImage **80**, 105–124 (2013)
9. Hinne, M., et al.: Bayesian estimation of conditional independence graphs improves functional connectivity estimates. PLoS Comput. Biol. **11**(11), e1004534 (2015)
10. Lindquist, M., et al.: Evaluating dynamic bivariate correlations in resting-state fMRI: a comparison study and a new approach. NeuroImage **101**, 531–546 (2014)
11. Delgado, M.R., et al.: Tracking the hemodynamic responses to reward and punishment in the striatum. J. Neurophysiol. **84**(6), 3072–3077 (2000)
12. Tzourio-Mazoyer, N., et al.: Automated anatomical labeling of activations in SPM using a macroscopic anatomical parcellation of the MNI MRI single-subject brain. NeuroImage **15**(1), 273–279 (2002)
13. Hindriks, R., et al.: Can sliding-window correlations reveal dynamic functional connectivity in resting-state fMRI? NeuroImage **127**, 242–256 (2016)
14. Hutchison, R.M., et al.: Dynamic functional connectivity: promise, issues, and interpretations. NeuroImage **80**, 360–378 (2013)
15. Monti, R.P., et al.: Estimating time-varying brain connectivity networks from functional MRI time series. NeuroImage **103**, 427–443 (2014)
16. Pennec, X., et al.: A Riemannian framework for tensor computing. Int. J. Comput. Vis. **66**(1), 41–66 (2006)
17. Friston, K.J.: Functional and effective connectivity: a review. Brain Connect. **1**(1), 13–36 (2011)
18. Poldrack, R.A.: Region of interest analysis for fMRI. Soc. Cogn. Affect. Neurosci. **2**(1), 67–70 (2007)
19. Srivastava, A., Klassen, E.: Functional and Shape Data Analysis. Springer, Heidelberg (2016)
20. Whitfield-Gabrieli, S., Nieto-Castanon, A.: Conn: a functional connectivity toolbox for correlated and anticorrelated brain networks. Brain Connect. **2**(3), 125–141 (2012)

Extracting the Groupwise Core Structural Connectivity Network: Bridging Statistical and Graph-Theoretical Approaches

Nahuel Lascano[1,2], Guillermo Gallardo-Diez[1], Rachid Deriche[1], Dorian Mazauric[3], and Demian Wassermann[1(✉)]

[1] Athena EPI, Université Côte d'Azur, Nice, Paris, France
{guillermo.gallardo-diez,rachid.deriche,demian.wassermann}@inria.fr
[2] Computer Science Department, FCEyN, Universidad de Buenos Aires,
Buenos Aires, Argentina
nlascano@dc.uba.ar
[3] ABS EPI, Université Côte d'Azur, Nice, Paris, France
dorian.mazauric@inria.fr

Abstract. Finding the common structural brain connectivity network for a given population is an open problem, crucial for current neuroscience. Recent evidence suggests there's a tightly connected network shared between humans. Obtaining this network will, among many advantages, allow us to focus cognitive and clinical analyses on common connections, thus increasing their statistical power. In turn, knowledge about the common network will facilitate novel analyses to understand the structure-function relationship in the brain.

In this work, we present a new algorithm for computing the core structural connectivity network of a subject sample combining graph theory and statistics. Our algorithm works in accordance with novel evidence on brain topology. We analyze the problem theoretically and prove its complexity. Using 309 subjects, we show its advantages when used as a feature selection for connectivity analysis on populations, outperforming the current approaches.

Keywords: Group-wise connectome · Core graph problem · Brain connectivity · Diffusion MRI

1 Introduction

Isolating the common brain connectivity network from a population is a main problem in current neuroscience [1–3]. Recent evidence suggests that there's a common and densely connected brain connectome across humans [4]. In this work we present a new approach for selecting these common connections, combining recent topological hypotheses [4] and current methods [2,3].

Finding the common brain connectome across subjects has the potential to increase our understanding of the relationship between function and structure in

© Springer International Publishing AG 2017
M. Niethammer et al. (Eds.): IPMI 2017, LNCS 10265, pp. 373–384, 2017.
DOI: 10.1007/978-3-319-59050-9_30

the brain. This relationship is one of the main open questions in neuroscience [1]. Moreover, knowledge about the most common connections in a population will facilitate clinical and cognitive Diffusion MRI analyses by reducing the number of surveyed connections, increasing the statistical power of those analyses. Finding the common connectome will also allow us to increase our knowledge about the brain structure by comparing core networks across different populations.

We formalize the problem of selecting the common connections combining graph theory and statistics. Then, we prove that the problem is NP-Hard and propose a polynomial-time algorithm to find approximate solutions. To do this, we develop an exact polynomial-time algorithm for a relaxed version of the problem and prove the algorithm's correctness and complexity.

Currently, the most used algorithm to extract a population's core structural connectivity network (CSNC) [2] uses an statistical approach: first, compute a connectivity matrix for each subject; then, analize each connection separately with a hypothesis test, using as null hypothesis that that edge is not present in the population; finally, construct a binary graph with the edges for which the null hypothesis was rejected. The main problem of Gong et al.'s [2] algorithm is that the resulting graph can be a set of disconnected subgraphs. Moreover, recent studies have shown that the brain has a *core* network tightly connected and a sparsely connected *outer* one [4]. In other words, this approach ignores the resulting network's topology. Also, performing statistical analyses in a feature set chosen by hypothesis testing incurs in the double dipping problem [5].

A newer approach to solve the CSCN problem, designed by Wassermann et al. [3], uses graph theory to get a connected CSCN: first, compute a binary connectivity graph for each subject using a threshold; for each possible connection compute the "cost" of including or excluding it from the common graph by evaluating in how many subjects that connection is present; finally, construct the binary graph with all the edges that is "cheaper" to include than to exclude and connect the resulting graph if it's disconnected, using the minimum possible cost. This algorithm guarantees that the resulting graph is connected, but the connection binarization discards significant information for the resulting common network. In other words, it discards information of the probability of each connection being in the brain. This is problematic because the resulting graph may include edges for which tractography assigned a very low existence probability across subjects. Also, the outer part of the brain, the connections which do not result in the core network, should also be sparsely connected [4], which this algorithm does not enforce.

In this work we propose, for the first time, a polynomial-time algorithm to obtain the CSCN of a population addressing the issues listed above. Our algorithm combines the recent graph-theoretical approach [3] with the statistical awareness of the most popular one [2]. We start by formalizing the problem, which allow us to prove that it's NP-Hard. We then propose a first algorithm that solves a relaxed version of the problem in an exact way. Finally, we adapt it to guarantee a connected result, agreeing with recent evidence on structural connectivity network topology [4]. We validate our approach using 300 subjects from the HCP database and comparing the performance of the networks obtained by our new approach, Wassermann et al.'s [3] and Gong et al.'s [2] predicting connectivity values from handedness in the core network.

2   Definitions, Problems and Contributions

We want to develop a new algorithm to extract the core structural connectivity network, a problem that implies working with different brains. Thus, we need to unify them into a common connectivity model. This allows us to model all brains with graphs in which each node represents a cortical or sub-cortical region, and each edge represents a white matter connection between two regions. We choose the Desikan parcellation [6] to uniformize the brain regions across subjects.

To compute the connectivity matrices we use a probabilistic tractography algorithm, which outputs one matrix per subject. The resulting matrices represent the existence probability of a connection across parcels in each subject [7]. As these are symmetric, we interpret the matrices as weighted undirected graphs.

Formally, we represent a sample of N brain structural networks by N complete weighted graphs $G_1 = (V, E, w_1), \ldots, G_N = (V, E, w_N)$ with a common node set V. We call $G_1, \ldots, G_N$ the *sample graphs*. Each graph G_i corresponds to a subject. Each vertex $v \in V$ represents a cortical or sub-cortical region. Each edge $e \in E = V \times V$ represents a white matter bundle connecting two regions. Finally, the weight $w_i(e) \in [0, 1]$ is the connection probability for the edge e in the subject i, obtained through tractography. Note that all graphs have the same ordered node set and all of them are complete: an edge weight, or connection probability, $w_i(e)$ of 0 represents an absent connection.

Using this formalization we express the general core structural connectivity network problem as follows: find a core graph $G^* = (V^*, E^*)$ densely connected such that G^* keeps the more *relevant* connections $E^* \subseteq E$ in the sample and discards the less *relevant* ones, for some definition of relevance and density.

We want a formalization of relevance that represents the probability that a connection is present across subjects. Thus, we choose to model the group-wise relevance $w^*(e)$ as the mean existence probability across subjects, factored by the standard deviation of these probabilities. Formally,

$$w^*(e) \triangleq \frac{\overline{w(e)}}{s(e)} \text{ where } \overline{w(e)} \triangleq \sum_{i=1}^{N} \frac{w_i(e)}{N}, \; s(e) \triangleq \sqrt{\sum_{i=1}^{N} \frac{\left(\overline{w(e)} - w_i(e)\right)^2}{N}}. \quad (1)$$

We use $w^*(e)$ as a statistical measure of edge presence across the population. Note that $w^*(e)$ is the statistic of a hypothesis z-test which assumes a media of 0 for the population weight of e. We choose the z-statistic because of the normal distribution's properties, e.g. linearity, even if other distributions, such as Beta distribution, may be more appropriate for modeling the probability. This statistic appropriate for within-group effects [8]. In any case, note that for the purpose of our contribution w^* can be any function $E \to \mathbb{R}$ which grows with the relevance of the edges in the sample.

We also want a formalization that represents the density of the core subgraph. We use the relationship between the number of edges of the core graph and the total statistical relevance w^* that those edges sum:

$$\alpha(w^*, E^*) \triangleq \frac{\sum_{e \in E^*} w^*(e)}{|E^*|}. \tag{2}$$

As we want also a sparse outer subgraph, we also define a representation of its density:

$$\beta(w^*, E^*) \triangleq \frac{\sum_{e \in E \setminus E^*} w^*(e)}{|E^*|}. \tag{3}$$

For simplicity, once we select E^* we can define V^* as

$$V^* = \{v \in V : \exists u \in V, (u, v) \in E^*\}, \tag{4}$$

the set of nodes that the edges in E^* cover. Then, we can reduce the problem of finding $G^* = (V^*, E^*)$ to find E^* alone. It should also be noted that once we obtain the edges in core graph E^* we also get the edges in the outer sparse subgraph, just by computing $E \setminus E^*$. Hence, the entire problem of finding the core and outer subgraphs can be reduced to find E^*. So we can express our objective informally as: choose $E^* \subseteq E$ such that $\alpha(w^*, E^*)$ (Eq. 2) is large and $\beta(w^*, E^*)$ (Eq. 3) small.

In accordance to recent evidence on the core network, we also want G^* to be connected. Let $\mathcal{E}^c$ be the family of sets of edges that induce a connected graph. We now formalize the problem of finding this common graph G^* in two different ways.

- The optimization version consists in computing:

$$\max_{E^* \in \mathcal{E}^c} f(w^*, E^*) = \lambda \alpha(w^*, E^*) - (1 - \lambda)\beta(w^*, E^*) \tag{5}$$

The parameter $\lambda \in [0, 1]$ can be adjusted to weight the relevance of the inner and the outer network. Note that if $\lambda = 1$, the solution to (5) only considers the density of the core network, and if $\lambda = 0$, it only considers the edges excluded of the core network.

- Given A and B, the decision version consists in finding $E^* \subseteq \mathcal{E}^c$ such that:

$$\begin{aligned} \alpha(w^*, E^*) \geq A \\ \beta(w^*, E^*) \leq B \end{aligned} \tag{6}$$

Having formalized the Core Structural Connectivity Network into an optimization and a decision problem, we proceed with one of our main theoretical contributions: proving that the problem is NP-Complete.

2.1 CSCN Problem's NP-Completeness

We have formalized the problem of the Core Structural Connectivity Network taking into account the density and connectedness of the core subgraph and the sparsity of the outer one. We will now prove that, with this formalization, the problem is NP-Complete.

Definition 1 (Core Structural Connectivity Network problem). *Given* $G_1 = (V, E, w_1), G_2 = (V, E, w_2), \ldots, G_N = (V, E, w_N)$ *weighted graphs (the sample graphs) with a common node set, a complete edges set $(E = V \times V)$ and* $w_1(e), w_2(e), \ldots, w_N(e) \in \mathbb{R}_{\geq 0} \; \forall e \in E$ *weights of their edges, and given A, B real numbers, find $G^* = (V^*, E^*)$ connected graph (the* core graph*) such that*

$$\alpha(w^*, E^*) \geq A$$

$$\beta(w^*, E^*) \leq B$$

for α and β as defined in Eqs. (2) and (3).

Here we prove that the *Core Structural Connectivity Network problem*, called CSCN, is NP-complete. In our reduction, we use the *Steiner Tree problem* [9], called ST in the following. Given an edge-weighted graph $G' = (V', E', w)$, a subset $S \subseteq V'$ of nodes, and a real $k \geq 0$, ST consists in determining if there exists a connected subgraph H such that $S \subseteq V(H)$ and $\sum_{e \in E(H)} w(e) \leq k$. The decision version of ST is NP-complete even if all weights are equal [9].

Instance of ST . Consider any edge-weighted graph $G' = (V', E', w)$ such that $w(e) = \frac{1}{2}$ for every $e \in E'$. Given $k \geq 0$, ST consists in determining if there exists a connected subgraph H such that $S \subseteq V(H)$ and $|E(S)| \leq 2k$. Without loss of generality, we assume that $|E'| \geq 2k$ and that G' is connected.

Reduction. We construct the instance of CSCN as follows. Let $s = |S|$ and let $t \geq 1$ be any positive integer. Let $G = (V, E, w^*)$ defined as follows. Let $V = V' \cup \{v_{i,j} \mid 1 \leq i \leq s, 1 \leq j \leq t\}$ and $E = V \times V$. Let $S = \{u_1, \ldots, u_s\}$. For every i, j, $1 \leq i \leq s$, $1 \leq j \leq t$, $w^*_{v_{i,j}, u_i} = 1$ and $w^*_{v_{i,j}, u} = 0$ for every $u \in V \setminus \{u_i\}$. Furthermore, for every $e \in E'$, set $w^*(e) = w(e) = \frac{1}{2}$, and for every $u, u' \in V'$ such that $\{u, u'\} \notin E'$, then set $w^*_e = 0$. Finally, we set $A = \frac{s.t+k}{s.t+2k}$ and $B = \frac{\frac{1}{2}(|E'|-2k)}{s.t+2k}$.

Lemma 1. *If $|E^*| < s.t + 2k$, then any solution for CSCN is not admissible because $\beta(w^*, E^*) > B$.*

Proof. Suppose that $|E^*| < s.t + 2k$. In order to minimize $\sum_{e \in E \setminus E^*} w^*(e)$, E^* must contain $\{\{v_{i,j}, u_i\} \mid 1 \leq i \leq s, 1 \leq j \leq t\}$ if $|E^*| \geq s.t$ (otherwise we select a subset of this set of edges). Indeed, by construction of G, we have $w^*_{v_{i,j}, u_i} = 1$ for every i, j, $1 \leq i \leq s$, $1 \leq j \leq t$. Then, if $|E^*| - s.t > 0$, E^* must contain $|E^*| - s.t$ edges of E', that is edges of E of weight $\frac{1}{2}$ each. Recall that there are exactly $s.t$ edges of weight 1, and the other edges have weight 0 or $\frac{1}{2}$.

There are two cases. First, suppose that $|E^*| \geq s.t$. We get that $\sum_{e \in E \setminus E^*} w^*(e) = \frac{1}{2}(|E'| - (|E^*| - s.t))$. Since $|E^*| - s.t < 2k$, then we get that $\sum_{e \in E \setminus E^*} w^*(e) = \frac{1}{2}(|E'| - (|E^*| - s.t)) > \frac{1}{2}(|E'| - 2k)$. Furthermore, since $|E^*| < s.t + 2k$, we get that $\frac{\frac{1}{2}(|E'| - (|E^*| - s.t))}{|E^*|} > \frac{\frac{1}{2}(|E'| - 2k)}{s.t + 2k}$. Thus, we proved that $\beta(w^*, E^*) = \frac{\sum_{e \in E \setminus E^*} w^*(e)}{|E^*|} > B$.

Second, suppose that $|E^*| < s.t$. We get that $\sum_{e \in E \setminus E^*} w^*(e) = s.t - |E^*| + \frac{|E'|}{2}$. Since $s.t - |E^*| + \frac{|E'|}{2} > \frac{1}{2}(|E'| - (|E^*| - s.t))$, we obtain the result by the arguments described for the first case.

Finally, if $|E^*| < s.t + 2k$, then there is no admissible solution for CSCN.   □

Lemma 2. *If $|E^*| > s.t + 2k$, then any solution for CSCN is not admissible because $\alpha(w^*, E^*) < A$.*

Proof. Suppose that $|E^*| > s.t + 2k$. In order to maximize $\sum_{e \in E^*} w^*(e)$, E^* must contain $\{\{v_{i,j}, u_i\} \mid 1 \leq i \leq s, 1 \leq j \leq t\}$ and $|E^*| - s.t$ edges of E'. Indeed, by construction of G, we have $w^*_{v_{i,j}, u_i} = 1$ for every i, j, $1 \leq i \leq s$, $1 \leq j \leq t$. Furthermore, $w^*(e) = \frac{1}{2}$ for every $e \in E'$. Recall that there are exactly $s.t$ edges of weight 1, and the other edges have weight 0 or $\frac{1}{2}$. We get that $\alpha(w^*, E^*) = \frac{s.t + \frac{1}{2}(|E^*| - s.t)}{|E^*|} < \frac{s.t + k}{s.t + 2k} = A$. Indeed, the average weight is lower when there are more edges of weight $\frac{1}{2}$ (the number of edges of weight 1 is the same in both ratios).

Finally, if $|E^*| > s.t + 2k$, then there is no admissible solution for CSCN.   □

By Lemmas 1 and 2, we get the following corollary.

Corollary 1. *Any solution for CSCN is such that $|E^*| = s.t + 2k$.*

We prove in Lemma 3 and in Lemma 4 that there is an admissible solution for CSCN if and only if there is an admissible solution for ST.

Lemma 3. *If there is an admissible solution for ST, then there is an admissible solution for CSCN.*

Proof. Suppose there is an admissible solution for ST. Let H be a connected subgraph such that $S \subseteq V(H)$ and $\sum_{e \in E(H)} w(e) = \frac{1}{2}|E(|H|) \leq k$. If $|E(H)| = 2k$, then set $E^* = E(H) \cup \{\{v_{i,j}, u_i\} \mid 1 \leq i \leq s, 1 \leq j \leq t\}$. If $|E(H)| < 2k$, then set $E^* = E(H) \cup \{\{v_{i,j}, u_i\} \mid 1 \leq i \leq s, 1 \leq j \leq t\} \cup F$, where $F \subseteq E'$ such that $F \neq E(H) = \emptyset$, $w^*(e) = \frac{1}{2}$ for every $e \in F$, and such that the graph induced by $E(H) \cup F$ is connected. The last condition comes from Corollary 1 in order to get the right number of edges in E^*. This condition is always possible to satisfy because G' is connected.

The graph induced by E^* is connected. Indeed, H is an admissible solution for ST, $E(H) \cup F$ is connected by construction, and $\{\{v_{i,j}, u_i\} \mid 1 \leq j \leq t\}$ is a set of edges all adjacent to $u_i \in S$ for every i, $1 \leq i \leq s$.

Furthermore, we get

$$\alpha(w^*, E^*) = \frac{\sum_{e \in E^*} w^*(e)}{|E^*|} = \frac{s.t + k}{s.t + 2k} = A$$

and

$$\beta(w^*, E^*) = \frac{\sum_{e \in E \setminus E^*} w^*(e)}{|E^*|} = \frac{\frac{1}{2}(|E'| - 2k)}{s.t + 2k} = B.$$

Finally, we proved that there is an admissible solution for CSCN.   □

Lemma 4. *If there is an admissible solution for* CSCN, *then there is an admissible solution for* ST.

Proof. Suppose there is an admissible solution for CSCN. Let $E^* \subseteq E$ be such that the graph induced by E^* is connected, and such that $\alpha(w^*, E^*) \geq \frac{s.t+k}{s.t+2k} = A$ and $\beta(w^*, E^*) \leq= \frac{\frac{1}{2}(|E'|-2k)}{s.t+2k} = B$.

We first prove that $\{\{v_{i,j}, u_i\} \mid 1 \leq i \leq s, 1 \leq j \leq t\} \subseteq E^*$. By Corollary 1, we know that $|E^*| = s.t + 2k$. Thus, it necessarily means that $\sum_{e \in E^*} w^*(e) \geq s.t + k$. By construction of G, the set of edges of weight 1 is $\{\{v_{i,j}, u_i\} \mid 1 \leq i \leq s, 1 \leq j \leq t\}$, that is $\{e \in E \mid w^*(e) > \frac{1}{2}\} = \{\{v_{i,j}, u_i\} \mid 1 \leq i \leq s, 1 \leq j \leq t\}$. We get that $\{\{v_{i,j}, u_i\} \mid 1 \leq i \leq s, 1 \leq j \leq t\} \subseteq E^*$ because, otherwise, we would have $\sum_{e \in E^*} w^*(e) < s.t + k$. Furthermore, every $e \in E^* \cap E'$ is such that $w^*(e) = \frac{1}{2}$. Indeed, otherwise, we would have $\sum_{e \in E^*} w^*(e) < s.t + k$.

Finally, since E^* is an admissible solution for CSCN, then it means that the graph induced by the set of edges $E^* \cap E'$ is connected and is such that for every u_i, $1 \leq i \leq s$, then there is an edge $e \in E^* \cap E'$ that is adjacent to u_i. By the previous remark, every edge in $E^* \cap E'$ has weight $\frac{1}{2}$. Thus, it means that there is $E^* \cap E'$ is an admissible solution for ST considering the graph G'. Indeed $|E^* \cap E'| = 2k$ and so $\sum_{e \in E^* \cap E'} w(e) = k$. □

We are now able to prove the NP-completeness of CSCN.

Theorem 1. CSCN *is NP-complete.*

Proof. The reduction is clearly polynomial. Furthermore, Lemma 3 and Lemma 4 prove the equivalence between CSĆN and ST. Since the decision version of ST is NP-complete even if all weights are equal [9], then we obtain the NP-completeness of the decision version of CSCN. □

We have proved that CSCN is NP-complete. Hence, to be able to solve it in reasonable time we need a relaxation to make it tractable or an approximate algorithm for the complete version. In this article we will propose both.

2.2 Relaxation of the CSCN Problem

The connectivity constraint is the main reason of the difficulty of the problem. In this section we solve a relaxed version of problem without that constraint. We then use this solution to approximate the full problem.

Theorem 2. *The decision version of* CSCN *without the connectivity constraint is in* P.

Proof. Assume that there exists an E^* that fulfills the constraints. Algorithm 1, in each step i, defines E^* as the i maximum weighted edges and tries to use that to fulfill the constraints. So if E^* has the $|E^*|$ maximum weighted edges

---

Algorithm 1. Maximum edges

Compute $w^*(e)$ for each $e \in E$
SORT(E)   ▷ sorts edges by w^* non-increasingly
for each $e \in E$ **do**
    $E^* \leftarrow E^* \cup e$
    if $\alpha(w^*, E^*) > A$ and $\beta(w^*, E^*) < B$ **then**
        return $True$
    end if
end for
return $False$

Algorithm 1 will find it. If not, then there are $e_j \in E^*$, $e_k \in E \setminus E^*$ such that $w^*(e_k) \geq w^*(e_j)$. Let $E' = (E^* \cup \{e_k\}) \setminus \{e_j\}$ another subset of E. Then

$$\alpha(w^*, E') = \frac{\sum_{e \in E'} w^*(e)}{|E'|} = \frac{\sum_{e \in E'} w^*(e)}{|E^*|} \geq \frac{\sum_{e \in E^*} w^*(e)}{|E^*|} = \alpha(w^*, E^*) \geq A$$

because the edges in E^* are the same as the ones in E' except from one that has a larger weight. For the same reason,

$$\beta(w^*, E') = \frac{\sum_{e \in E \setminus E'} w^*(e)}{|E'|} = \frac{\sum_{e \in E \setminus E'} w^*(e)}{|E^*|} \leq \frac{\sum_{e \in E \setminus E^*} w^*(e)}{|E^*|} = \beta(w^*, E^*) \leq B.$$

Thus, we found a new subset of E that still fulfills the constraints. We can repeat the process with E' (replace an edge with another one of larger weight) iteratively, always getting subsets that fulfills the constraints, until we cannot do this anymore. At that point we will have a subset that has only the maximum $|E^*|$ edges and fulfills the constraints. Thus, Algorithm 1 will find this subset.

We now need to prove Algorithm 1 runs in polynomial time in the size of $|E|$. The first operation, computing $w^*(e)$ for each e, implies computing the mean and standard deviation for each edge across the population, which can be done in $\mathcal{O}(N * |E|)$ (where N is the size of the population). The sorting can be done in $\mathcal{O}(|E| \log |E|)$. The main loop runs at most $|E|$ times, and in each loop it adds an edge to E^* (constant time if we use a linked list of edges), computes α and β and performs two float comparisons (constant time also). To compute α and β it is needed to iterate once again E (the part in E^* for α, the part in $E \setminus E^*$ for β) adding the weights together and then perform two divisions. This can be done in linear time in the size of E, and even quicker (constant time) if we keep the values of α and β across loops and update them with the weight of the edge that changed sets. Then, Algorithm 1 solves the CSCN in $\mathcal{O}(max(|E|^2, |E| * N))$ or in $\mathcal{O}(|E| * N)$ if a little optimization is used.   □

2.3   Heuristic Approach

As Algorithm 1 does not guarantee a connected result, we solve the original CSCN problem by first applying Algorithm 1 and then modifying the resulting core graph G^* to guarantee its connectedness, while decreasing the minimum possible the objective function f (defined in Eq. 5). For this, we use the same approach that Wassermann et al. [3]. Namely, we make a multigraph G_{cc} with the connected components of G^* as nodes, complete it with all the possible edges between those connected components, and run a Maximum Spanning Tree algorithm. This selects the edges needed to produce a connected subgraph with the maximum possible weight. For the full details, see Wassermann et al. [3]. This way we get a connected subgraph close to the best possible subgraph, which we obtained using Algorithm 1.

3   Experiments and Results

We formalized the CSCN problem in Sect. 2 and designed an algorithm to solve it in Sect. 2.3. Now we will asses the performance of our method. For this, we compare it with the most used [2] and with the recent one [3] in the task of connectivity prediction performance.

We use a subset of the HCP500 dataset [10]: all subjects aged 21–40 with complete dMRI protocol, totaling 309. We compute the weighted connectivity matrices between the cortical regions defined by the Desikan atlas [6] as done by Sotiropoulos et al. [10]. Examples of CSCN extracted with our algorithm at different λ levels are shown in Fig. 1, which was generated using Nilearn [11]. Some quantitative results are shown in Table 1.

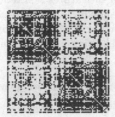 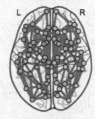 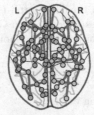

Fig. 1. Core structural connectivity network computed by our approach. On the left, we show the adjacency matrix for $\lambda = 0.5$. In the central and right panels, we show the resulting CSCN for $\lambda = 0.9$ and 0.99 respectively. The percentage of included connections in each figure are shown in Table 1.

3.1   Consistency of the Extracted Graph

To compare the stability across different algorithms for CSCN, we use an analysis based on Wassermann et al. [3]: we randomly take 500 subsets of 100 subjects each and computed the core graphs for all subsets. We then compute the number of *unstable connections*: connections that present in at least one core graph but not in all of them. Finally, in Table 2 we report each algorithm's *stability*:

$$\text{stability of the algorithm} \triangleq 1 - \frac{\#\{\text{unstable connections}\}}{\#\{\text{total connections}\}}. \tag{7}$$

Table 1. Characteristics of the resulting core and outer subgraphs for different values of λ. As stated above (in Eqs. 2 and 3) α and β represents the core's and outer's subgraph density respectively. The objective function is defined in Eq. 5. As it was expected, a bigger λ makes the algorithm prioritize a larger density in the core graph.

λ	% of connections	Objective	α	β
0.50	48.19%	0.4399	1.1466	0.2667
0.90	5.99%	2.0841	3.2208	8.1456
0.99	1.27%	3.9804	4.6925	66.5145

This measure quantifies the CSCN consistency across subsamples. Due to the homogeneity of our sample, we expect the CSCNs obtained by an algorithm to be similar across subsamples. Hence, a stabler algorithm is preferable.

3.2   Predicting Handedness-Specific Connectivity

We evaluate performance of the methods by using the generated core graphs as a feature selection for handedness specific connectivity. We use a nested Leave-$\frac{1}{3}$-Out procedure: the outer loop performs model selection on $\frac{1}{3}$ of the subjects using the core graph algorithm and the inner loop performs model fitting and prediction using the selected features.

Table 2. Stability (Eq. 7) of the algorithms and amount of features selected by linear regression in the core graph relating the weights with handedness. Our procedure gets more features selected than Gong et al. [2] and Wassermann et al. [3], showing better statistical power. It's also more stable than Gong et al., showing improved consistency.

Algorithm	Features (mean)	Features (std)	Stability
Gong et al. [2]	0.066	0.256	0.364
Wassermann et al. [3]	0.415	0.723	0.644
Our approach ($\lambda = 0.50$)	1.042	1.269	0.528

Specifically, we first take $\frac{1}{3}$ subjects randomly and compute the core graph for those subjects using the three different algorithms. Then we add the weights for the selected edges for each subject, and select the features F that are more determinant of handedness using a linear least-squares regression and the Bonferroni correction for multiple hypotheses. This experiment is repeated 500 times. We quantify the amount of features that are selected after each procedure, which indicates how useful is the core graph algorithm for selecting the edges related to handedness. We show the results in Table 2.

To evaluate the prediction, we randomly take $\frac{1}{2}$ of the remaining subjects and fit a linear model on the features F to predict connectivity weights using the handedness of each subject. Finally, we predict the values of the features F from the handedness in the subjects left out. We quantify the quality of the

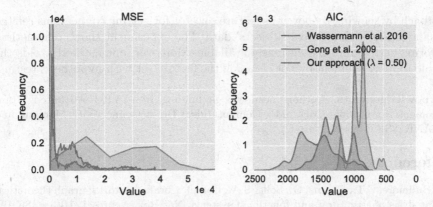

Fig. 2. Performance of core network as feature selection for a linear model for handedness specific connectivity. We evaluate model prediction (left) and fit (right) for Gong et al. [2] in green, Wassermann et al. [3] in blue and ours, in red. We show the histograms from our nested Leave-$\frac{1}{3}$-Out experiment. In both measures, our approach has more frequent lower values than Gong et al., showing a better performance. (Color figure online)

linear model fitting Akaike Information Criterion (AIC) and of the prediction performance with the mean squared error (MSE) of the prediction. For both measures a lower value indicates better performance. The outer loop is performed 500 times and the inner loop 100 times per outer loop, which totals 50,000 experiments. We show the results of this experiments in Fig. 2.

4   Discussion and Conclusion

We presented for the first time a polynomial algorithm to extract the core structural connectivity network of a population combining a graph-theoretical approach with statistic relevance of the connections, observing the recent evidence of the structural network topology.

Our results show that our algorithm outperforms, in the prediction experiment, the most used technique [2] as well as latest approaches [3]. In Table 2 we can see that our algorithm preserves, in average, more connections correlated with the handedness of the subjects. We can also see that despite being less stable than Wassermann et al.'s it is stabler than Gong et al.'s. Both results imply that our algorithm has better consistency and statistical power.

Figure 2 shows that, in the handedness prediction experiment, our method outperforms Gong et al.'s and Wassermann et al's: the number of cases with low AIC and MSE is larger in our case. This means the mean error of the prediction is usually smaller with our algorithm, which implies it selects features more closely related to the handedness of the subjects. Hence, in terms of model fitting and prediction, our CSCN heuristic works better as a linear model relating connectivity with a demographic aspect of the population.

In terms of theoretical contributions, we formalized the problem, proved its difficulty and gave a novel algorithm for dealing with it. We then validated our approach by showing its power as feature selector for getting connections related to handedness with 300 real subjects' data. The experiment shows our method performs better than the currently available. Moreover, our method avoids the double dipping problem by not choosing the feature set with hypothesis testing.

Acknowledgements. Authors acknowledge funding from ERC Advanced Grant agreement No. 694665: CoBCoM - Computational Brain Connectivity Mapping and the ANR-NSF grant NeuroRef.

References

1. Bullmore, E.T., Sporns, O., Solla, S.A.: Complex brain networks: graph theoretical analysis of structural and functional systems. Nat Rev. Neurosci. **10**(3), 186–198 (2009)
2. Gong, G., He, Y., Concha, L., Lebel, C., Gross, D.W., Evans, A.C., Beaulieu, C.: Mapping anatomical connectivity patterns of human cerebral cortex using in vivo diffusion tensor imaging tractography. Cereb. Cortex **19**(3), 524–536 (2009)
3. Wassermann, D., Mazauric, D., Gallardo-Diez, G., Deriche, R.: Extracting the core structural connectivity network: guaranteeing network connectedness through a graph-theoretical approach. In: Ourselin, S., Joskowicz, L., Sabuncu, M.R., Unal, G., Wells, W. (eds.) MICCAI 2016. LNCS, vol. 9900, pp. 89–96. Springer, Cham (2016). doi:10.1007/978-3-319-46720-7_11
4. Bassett, D.S., Porter, M.A., Wymbs, N.F., Grafton, S.T., Carlson, J.M., Mucha, P.J.: Robust detection of dynamic community structure in networks. Chaos **23**, 013142 (2013). doi:10.1063/1.4790830
5. Kriegeskorte, N., Simmons, W.K., Bellgowan, P.S.F., Baker, C.I.: Circular analysis in systems neuroscience: the dangers of double dipping. Nat. Neurosci. **12**, 535–540 (2009)
6. Desikan, R.S., Ségonne, F., Fischl, B., Quinn, B.T., Dickerson, B.C., Blacker, D., Buckner, R.L., Dale, A.M., Maguire, R.P., Hyman, B.T., Albert, M.S., Killiany, R.J.: An automated labeling system for subdividing the human cerebral cortex on MRI scans into gyral based regions of interest. NeuroImage **31**(3), 968–980 (2006)
7. Jbabdi, S., Sotiropoulos, S.N., Haber, S.N., Van Essen, D.C., Behrens, T.E.J.: Measuring macroscopic brain connections in vivo. Nat. Publ. Group **18**(11), 1546–1555 (2015)
8. Brown, C.J., Miller, S.P., Booth, B.G., Zwicker, J.G., Grunau, R.E., Synnes, A.R., Chau, V., Hamarneh, G.: Predictive subnetwork extraction with structural priors for infant connectomes. In: Ourselin, S., Joskowicz, L., Sabuncu, M.R., Unal, G., Wells, W. (eds.) MICCAI 2016. LNCS, vol. 9900, pp. 175–183. Springer, Cham (2016). doi:10.1007/978-3-319-46720-7_21
9. Garey, M.R., Johnson, D.S.: Computers and Intractability: A Guide to the Theory of NP-Completeness. W. H. Freeman & Co., New York (1979)
10. Sotiropoulos, S.N., Jbabdi, S., Xu, J., Andersson, J.L., Moeller, S., Auerbach, E.J., Glasser, M.F., Hernandez, M., Sapiro, G., Jenkinson, M., Feinberg, D.A., Yacoub, E., Lenglet, C., Van Essen, D.C., Ugurbil, K., Behrens, T.E.: Advances in diffusion MRI acquisition and processing in the Human Connectome Project. NeuroImage **80**(3), 125–143 (2013)
11. Abraham, A., Pedregosa, F., Eickenberg, M., Gervais, P., Mueller, A., Kossaifi, J., Gramfort, A., Thirion, B., Varoquaux, G.: Machine learning for neuroimaging with scikit-learn. Front. Neuroinform. **8**(February), 14 (2014)

Estimation of Brain Network Atlases Using Diffusive-Shrinking Graphs: Application to Developing Brains

Islem Rekik[1], Gang Li[2], Weili Lin[2], and Dinggang Shen[2(✉)]

[1] CVIP, Computing, School of Science and Engineering,
University of Dundee, Dundee, UK
irekik@dundee.ac.uk
[2] Department of Radiology and BRIC,
University of North Carolina at Chapel Hill, Chapel Hill, NC, USA
dgshen@med.unc.edu

Abstract. Many methods have been developed to spatially normalize a population of *brain images* for estimating a mean image as a population-average atlas. However, methods for deriving a network atlas from a set of *brain networks* sitting on a complex manifold are still absent. Learning how to average brain networks across subjects constitutes a key step in creating a reliable mean representation of a population of brain networks, which can be used to spot abnormal deviations from the healthy network atlas. In this work, we propose a novel network atlas estimation framework, which guarantees that the produced network atlas is *clean* (for tuning down noisy measurements) and *well-centered* (for being optimally close to all subjects and representing the individual traits of each subject in the population). Specifically, for a population of brain networks, we first build a tensor, where each of its frontal-views (i.e., frontal matrices) represents a connectivity network matrix of a single subject in the population. Then, we use tensor robust principal component analysis for jointly denoising all subjects' networks through cleaving a sparse noisy network population tensor from a clean low-rank network tensor. Second, we build a graph where each node represents a frontal-view of the unfolded clean tensor (network), to leverage the local manifold structure of these networks when fusing them. Specifically, we progressively shrink the graph of networks towards the centered mean network atlas through non-linear diffusion along the *local* neighbors of each of its nodes. Our evaluation on the developing functional and morphological brain networks at 1, 3, 6, 9 and 12 months of age has showed a better centeredness of our network atlases, in comparison with the baseline network fusion method. Further cleaning of the population of networks produces even more centered atlases, especially for the noisy functional connectivity networks.

1 Introduction

The study of brain connectivity propelled the development of the field of brain connectomics, where the connectivity between different brain regions is usually

© Springer International Publishing AG 2017
M. Niethammer et al. (Eds.): IPMI 2017, LNCS 10265, pp. 385–397, 2017.
DOI: 10.1007/978-3-319-59050-9_31

measured using functional (e.g., resting state fMRI) or structural brain imaging (e.g., diffusion MRI) [1]. A connectome is a brain network or a graph, where each node represents an anatomical/functional region of interest (ROI) in the brain and the weight between two nodes encodes biological information. This can also be represented as a symmetric matrix, where each of its values represents a connectivity measurement between a pair of ROIs. More importantly, big connectomic data are rapidly exploding with emerging international research initiatives aiming to massively collect large high-quality brain images with structural, diffusion and functional modalities such as UK Biobank [2], the Developing Human Connectome Project in Europe, and the Baby Connectome Project, which extends the Human Connectome Project from birth through early childhood [3]. Part of analyzing a large number of brain networks is to learn how to effectively average them, which indeed constitutes a key step in creating a reliable and meaningful mean representation of a population of brains. This can be used to spot deviations from the normal network atlas (e.g., cases with brain disorder/disease) as well as provide a principled understanding of the developing and aging trajectories of brain connectivities [1].

Broadly, connectomic data analysis methods targeted different neuroscientific and clinical applications such as population-based (or individual-based) brain parcellation using connectomes [4], extracting the connected core or backbone of connectivity networks of a population [5], and connectome-based feature extraction for brain disease/disorder diagnosis [1,6]. However, the problem of effectively fusing a population of brain networks nested in a complex manifold, which can shed new light on brain connectivity, was somewhat overlooked. On the other hand, a variety of methods have been developed to spatially normalize a population of brain images to estimate a 'mean image' (i.e., a population template or image atlas), which were further refined to estimate a sharp atlas that is well-centered and more representative of each individual image [7]. To fill in this gap, we aim to estimate a population-based *network atlas* that is *clean* and *centered*. Both these crucial traits are considered to define a good representative atlas of a corrupted or noisy population of networks.

Specifically, since fMRI has low signal-to-noise ratio possibly induced by non-neural noise, its derived functional connectivity strength between pairs of ROIs can be spurious or noisy. To address this issue, particularly when producing network atlas for functional networks, we first build a tensor where each of its frontal-views represents a connectivity network matrix of a single subject in the population. Since brain network is intrinsically sparse, we encourage sparsity in its noisy components (i.e., sparse noise). Hence, we propose to use tensor robust principal component analysis introduced in [8] to cleave a sparse noisy population network tensor from a clean low-rank network tensor. Next, we propose to estimate a well-centered atlas from the *unfolded clean tensor*. Since at a subject level, some brain regions wire similarly to one another, a low-rank representation is appropriate for brain network atlas representation. Furthermore, at a population level, since brain networks of different healthy subjects share similar connectivity patterns, then jointly decomposing and denoising them may better preserve their similarities.

Recently, Wang et al. introduced in [9] a robust method to non-linearly fuse different matrices, each matrix encoding a specific type of genomic similarities between a set of patients. Broadly, given N networks, each network is iteratively updated through diffusing the global structure of the averaged remaining $(N-1)$ networks across its local structure. Then the fused network is obtained through simply averaging the N diffused networks. A key limitation of such an approach is that it completely ignores the pairwise associations between different networks in the diffusion/fusion process. Particularly, it simply averages all remaining networks without considering their proximity or relationship to the current network. To address this issue, we propose to explore the underlying data distribution during the fusion process for network atlas estimation, through modeling of their relationships using a graph as introduced in [10] for image atlas estimation. This will better preserve the topology of the manifold, where the individual networks sit as they smoothly diffuse and fuse toward a *well-centered* network. This is an important characteristic of an atlas, where it occupies a position near to all the individuals of a population, which implies that it well captures the individual characteristics of each subject in the population while generating their mean. It is worth noting that our graph shrinkage strategy differs from [10] in two major aspects: (1) our graph is made of graphs (connectomes) instead of images (i.e., a graph of graphs), and (2) the graph shrinkage is performed through diffusion instead of diffeomorphic warping.

The main contributions of our work can be summarized as follows: (1) introducing the concept of a *clean and centered network atlas* to capture connectomic data characteristics of a population, (2) proposing a *joint* denoising of brain networks through modeling the network population as a tensor, (3) further improving network fusion strategy introduced in [9] by modeling each frontal-view of the unfolded clean tensor as a 'network node' in *a graph that shrinks through manifold-guided diffusion*, and (4) evaluating our approach on both functional and morphological brain networks of *developing* infants.

2   Estimation of Clean and Centered Network Atlas Using Diffusive-Shrinking Graphs

In this section, we briefly present the framework introduced in [9] for similarity network fusion (SNF), and extend it to our aim. We denote tensors by boldface Euler script letters, e.g., $\mathcal{X}$. Matrices are denoted by boldface capital letters, e.g., $\mathbf{X}$, and scalars are denoted by lowercase letters, e.g., x. For easy reference and enhancing the readability, we have summarized the major mathematical notations in Table 1.

2.1   Conventional Similarity Network Fusion Method

Suppose we have a population of N brain networks, where each brain network is subject-specific and can be represented as a graph (or connectome) $C = (V_C, E_C)$. The vertices V_C denote ROIs in the brain and the edges E_C

Table 1. Major mathematical notations used in this paper.

Mathematical notation	Definition
$\mathcal{X}$	Tensor in $\mathbb{R}^{n_1 \times n_2 \times n_3}$
$\mathbf{X}$	Connectivity matrix in $\mathbb{R}^{n_1 \times n_2}$ or frontal-view of tensor $\mathcal{X}$
$\mathbf{A}$	Population-based network atlas
$\mathbf{P}_k$	Global normalization of the connectivity matrix $\mathbf{X}_k$ of individual k
$\mathbf{S}_k$	Local normalization of the connectivity matrix $\mathbf{X}_k$ of individual k
N_i	Set of neighboring ROIs to the ith ROI in the brain network
N_k^g	Set of neighboring networks to a network $\mathbf{P}_k$ in a subgraph g
$\mathcal{L}$	Tubal low-rank tensor (clean tensor)
$\mathbf{L}_k$	Frontal-view of the clean tensor or brain network matrix
$\mathcal{E}$	Sparse tensor (noise)
$d(\mathbf{L}_k, \mathbf{L}_{k'})$	Distance between two brain networks $\mathbf{L}_k$ and $\mathbf{L}_{k'}$
$C = (V_C, E_C)$	Connectome or brain network graph of a single subject
V_C	Nodes or brain ROIs
E_C	Edges connecting pairs of brain ROIs in a single subject
$G = (V_M, E_M)$	Graph of brain networks representing the network population manifold
V_M	Set of network nodes or brain networks in the population
E_M	Edges connecting pairs of brain networks

are weighted by a connectivity strength. We represent edge weights by an $m \times m$ similarity matrix $\mathbf{X}$ with $\mathbf{X}(i,j)$ denoting the connectivity between ROI i and ROI j. Our goal is to estimate a *network atlas* $\mathbf{A}$, that captures both the local traits of each individual network $\mathbf{X}_k$ and the global traits of the population of networks $\{\mathbf{X}_1, \ldots, \mathbf{X}_k, \ldots, \mathbf{X}_N\}$. To this end, for each individual k in the population, we define a *global* matrix $\mathbf{P}_k$ that carries the connectivity strength of each ROI to *all* other ROIs and a *local* matrix $\mathcal{S}_k$ that encodes the similarity to *nearest* similar ROIs for each ROI in the brain network (or local affinity in the connectome graph C). These are defined as follows based on [9]:

$$\mathbf{P}_k(i,j) = \begin{cases} \frac{\mathbf{X}_k(i,j)}{2\sum_{l \neq i} \mathbf{X}_k(i,l)} & j \neq i \\ 1/2, & j = i \end{cases} \tag{1}$$

$$\mathbf{S}_k(i,j) = \begin{cases} \frac{\mathbf{X}_k(i,j)}{\sum_{l \in N_i} \mathbf{X}_k(i,l)} & j \in N_i \\ 0, & otherwise \end{cases} \tag{2}$$

We identify the set of ROIs N_i in an individual brain network that are neighbors to ROI i in the network graph C using KNN (K-nearest neighbors). $\mathbf{S}_k$ carries the sparse local traits of each individual network $\mathbf{X}_k$.

The basic idea of similarity network fusion proposed in [9] is to consider each individual network $\mathbf{P}_k$ of the population as a single view, then iteratively update it through diffusing the average global structure of other $(N-1)$ views from the population along the fixed local sparse structure $\mathbf{S}_k$ of the network. This is achieved through the following iterative equation:

$\mathbf{P}_k^t = \mathbf{S}_k \times \left(\frac{\sum_{k' \neq k} \mathbf{P}_{k'}^t}{N-1} \right) \times \mathbf{S}_k^T$, where $t \in \{0, \ldots, t^*\}$ denotes the diffusion iteration number and T denotes the matrix transpose operator. After each iteration t, $\mathbf{P}_k^t$ is normalized using Eq. 1. Finally, following t^* iterations, the fused network atlas is generated by averaging all updated diffused networks: $\mathbf{A} = \frac{1}{N} \sum_{k=1}^{N} \mathbf{P}_k^{t^*}$.

Whereas at a network-level SNF explores the local *inter-regional* relationships within each individual network through estimating the matrix $\mathbf{S}$, at a higher network manifold-level, it ignores the *inter-network* relationships during the diffusion process. In other words, when iteratively updating a single network, it weighs equally the contributions of other networks, as mathematically reflected by the diffusion kernel $\left(\frac{\sum_{k' \neq k} \mathbf{P}_{k'}^t}{N-1} \right)$. Additionally, although the diffusion of a global network along the local structure of a single network $\mathbf{S}_k$ may reduce some local noise in the original network $\mathbf{X}$, it may overlook noise that distributes randomly and sparsely in $\mathbf{X}$. To alleviate both shortcomings, we first propose to perform a *joint* denoising for all individual networks through modeling the network population as a tensor $\mathcal{X}$, then we devise a *diffusive-shrinking graph evolution strategy* through locally exploring the *clean* network manifold structure to estimate a well-centered network atlas.

2.2 Proposed Similarity Network Fusion Through Diffusive-Shrinking Graph

In this section we address the aforementioned limitations and detail the three steps for clean and centered network atlas estimation.

- **Step 1: Tensor-based network population denoising.** We first build a network tensor $\mathcal{X}$ by defining each of its frontal-views as a brain network from our population and then decompose this noisy network tensor into a tubal low- rank tensor (i.e., clean) and a sparse tensor (i.e., noise). The tensor denoising process is performed through mininizing the following equation using ADMM [8]:

$$\min_{\mathcal{L},\mathcal{E}} ||\mathcal{L}||_* + \lambda ||\mathcal{E}||_1, \ s.t. \ \mathcal{X} = \mathcal{L} + \mathcal{E} \in \mathbb{R}^{n_1 \times n_2 \times n_3} \tag{3}$$

$\mathcal{L}$ represents the low-rank clean tensor whereas $\mathcal{E}$ denotes the sparse noisy component of the tensor. In our case, $n_1 = n_2 = m$ (number of brain ROIs) and $n_3 = N$ (number of subjects in the population). The trade-off parameter λ is automatically set to $1/\sqrt{n_1 n_3}$ as detailed in [8].
- **Step 2: Tensor unfolding and graph building.** Motivated by the fact that a manifold representation can be effectively used to model the nonlinearity of samples in a population, we propose to model the manifold of brain networks using a graph for a more effective fusion of populations of networks with different distributions. Notably, graphs have demonstrated superb capability to model the nonlinearity of samples on a manifold [10]. To do so,

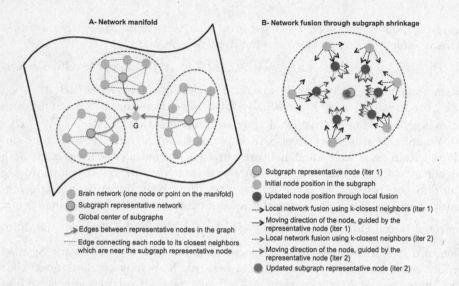

Fig. 1. Illustration of the proposed manifold-guided diffusive-shrinking graphs for network atlas estimation. (A) Modeling the manifold of brain networks as a graph partitioned into homogeneous subgraphs, where similar networks are clustered together. (B) Iterative sub-graph shrinking through locally diffusing and fusing each network node with its most similar neighboring nodes, in the direction of the global center of the manifold graph.

we first unfold the estimated clean tensor $\mathcal{L}$ into its frontal clean brain network views $\{\mathbf{L}_1, \ldots, \mathbf{L}_k, \ldots, \mathbf{L}_N\}$. Next, we build a graph $G = (E_M, V_M)$ to model the structure of the clean network population manifold. Each node in V_M represents a brain network $\mathbf{L}_k$ (or a graph). To compute a similarity between two networks $\mathbf{L}_k$ and $\mathbf{L}_{k'}$, we use the distance metric $d(\mathbf{L}_k, \mathbf{L}_{k'}) = 1 - (trace(\mathbf{L}_k \times \mathbf{L}_{k'}))/\|\mathbf{L}_k\|_F \times \|\mathbf{L}_{k'}\|_F)$ with $\|\cdot\|_F$ denoting Frobenius norm. Then, we define the symmetric $N \times N$ weighted graph edge matrix E_M, where two networks $\mathbf{L}_i$ and $\mathbf{L}_j$ are connected if $d(\mathbf{L}_i, \mathbf{L}_j) \neq 0$ and we set the weights on the diagonal to 0 to avoid self-connectedness. Our 'graph of graphs' is then built by implementing the following steps:

(1) Apply affinity propagation (AP) clustering method to V_M [11] to group similar network nodes (i.e., networks) using the network similarity distance d and define their representatives $\{\mathbf{P}_r\}$, so they can be fused in the same way.

(2) On a local level, each identified AP cluster defines a sub-graph, where similar nodes are connected with a weighted edge using distance d.

(3) To ensure that the local fusion of each node with nearby nodes is smooth, we average the representatives of all sub-graphs to generate a center global network $\mathbf{P}_C$ that will guide the fusion of sub-graphs.

(4) On a higher level, link all sub-graphs through connecting the representatives of all subgraphs to the global center.

Based on this graph, all brain networks in the manifold can be progressively diffused and fused in accordance to their connected networks, in the direction of the global center as illustrated in Fig. 1.

- **Step 3: Manifold-guided graph shrinkage through diffusion.** To ensure that the local fusion of each network node with nearby nodes is smooth, we average the representatives of all sub-graphs to generate a center global network. Then, we move each node (i.e., locally update each network) by fusing it with its closest neighboring nodes (i.e., networks) through an iterative process as in [10] in the direction of the global center. Since the representative nodes are moved, we subsequently update the global center. We then repeat these two steps while updating the global center until it becomes stable. Eventually, the as the original graph shrinks where all nodes will locate at the vicinity of the global center $\mathbf{P}_C$, where their averaging is more reliable and meaningful to produce the sought 'network atlas' (Fig. 1). The steps for diffusive-shrinking graph for network atlas estimation are detailed in Algorithm 1, where we denote by ⋄ the diffusion at a sub-graph level in G and by ⋄ the diffusion at a higher level in G.

3   Results

Evaluation Dataset. We evaluated the proposed framework on 35 typically developing infants, where each subject has 5 serial T1-w, T2-w MRI and resting-state fMRI (rsfMRI) scans acquired at 1, 3, 6, 9 and 12 months of age. We generated two types of brain networks for each subject.

Functional Brain Networks. After rsfMRI pre-processing (including motion correction), we performed infant brain image longitudinal registration from native space to MNI space using GLIRT where each rsfMRI was partitioned into 116 ROIs using AAL template, which includes both cerebral and cerebellar regions. For each subject, we computed the mean fMRI time-series signal in each ROI. Then, we created the 116×116 functional connectivity matrix where the connectivity strength between a pair of ROIs represents the correlation between their mean functional signals.

Morphological Brain Networks. After rigid alignment of longitudinal and cross-sectional infant structural MR images (i.e., T1-w and T2-w) and brain tissue segmentation, we reconstructed and parcellated the cortical surfaces into 35 cortical regions using in-house developed tools [12–14]. By computing the pairwise absolute difference in cortical thickness between pairs of regions of interest, we generate a 35×35 morphological connectivity matrix for each time point in each subject.

Evaluation. To evaluate the centeredness of the estimated brain network atlas, we compute the mean distance between the estimated network atlas and each individual network in the population using as metric d. Figure 2 shows the mean distance computed using the proposed network atlas estimation method and the conventional SNF method [9]. The smaller the evaluation distance the more centered is the atlas with respect to the individual networks on the network

---

Algorithm 1. Diffusive-shrinking graph strategy for network atlas estimation

1: **INPUTS:**
   Set of N brain networks: $\{\mathbf{L}_1, \ldots, \mathbf{L}_k, \ldots \mathbf{L}_N\}$
2: **for** each brain network $\mathbf{L}_k$ **do**
3:    **for** each pair of ROIs i and j in $\mathbf{L}_k$ **do**
      $\mathbf{S}_k(i,j) = \frac{\mathbf{L}_k(i,j)}{2\sum_{l \neq i} \mathbf{L}_k(i,l)}$ for $j \in N_i$, otherwise assign 0 (local network structure)

      $\mathbf{P}_k^0(i,j) = \frac{\mathbf{L}_k(i,j)}{2\sum_{l \neq i} \mathbf{L}_k(i,l)}$ if $j \neq i$, otherwise assign 1/2 (global network structure)
4:    **end for**
5: **end for**
6: Build graph $G = (E_M, V_M)$ to model the network manifold structure using the distance d as a network similarity metric
7: Partition G into a set of sub-graphs and define the representative network nodes for each cluster using affinity propagation
8: Compute the graph global center $\mathbf{P}_C$ by averaging all the representative brain networks
9: For $t = 0$, set $\mathbf{P}_C^0 = \mathbf{P}_C$
10: **for** each diffusion iteration $t \in \{1, \ldots, t^*\}$ **do**
11:    **while** global center $\mathbf{P}_C^t$ is not stable **do**
12:       **for** each subgraph g of G **do** ($\diamond$)
13:          **for** each network $\mathbf{P}_k^t$ in the subgraph g **do**
          Diffuse the network along its N_k^g nearest nodes in g, which are close to the sub-graph representative node and update its position in the graph using:

          $\mathbf{P}_k^{t+1} = \mathbf{S}_k \times (\frac{\sum_{k' \in N_k^g} \mathbf{P}_{k'}^t}{N_k^g}) \times \mathbf{S}_k^T$

          $\mathbf{P}_k^{t+1} = \frac{\mathbf{P}_k^{t+1} + (\mathbf{P}_k^{t+1})^T}{2}$ (network normalization after diffusion)
14:          **end for**
15:          **for** each subgraph representative $\mathbf{P}_r^{t+1}$ **do** ($\diamond$)
          $\mathbf{P}_r^{t+1} = \mathbf{S}_r \times \mathbf{P}_C^t \times \mathbf{S}_r^T$ (move representative towards the center $\mathbf{P}_C^t$)
          $\mathbf{P}_r^{t+1} = \frac{\mathbf{P}_r^{t+1} + (\mathbf{P}_r^{t+1})^T}{2}$ (representative normalization)
          Update global center $\mathbf{P}_C^t$ by averaging the updated representative networks
16:          **end for**
17:       **end for**
18:    **end while**
19: **end for**
20: **OUTPUT:** Fusion step to produce a clean and centered network atlas: $\mathbf{A} = \frac{1}{N} \sum_{k=1}^{N} \mathbf{P}_k^{t^*}$

---

manifold. We used paired t-test to evaluate the statistical significance of our method in comparison with [9]. Clearly, our method produced more centered network atlases than conventional SNF ($p \ll 0.001$) at all acquisition timepoints (Fig. 2). When using functional networks, the denoising step led to more centered network atlases for both our method and SNF (Fig. 2). On the other hand, denoising morphological networks did not further improve the centeredness of the estimated atlases at different timepoints, which can be explained by the fact that fMRI is much noisier than structural T1/T2-w MR imaging. Figures 3 and 4 show that at each diffusion iteration, our method generated rapidly a more centered network atlas than the conventional SNF method. Figure 3-B displays the estimated functional network atlases using our method at different timepoints. A dramatic functional connectivity change occurs between 1 and 3 months of age, followed by a few sparsely distributed changes between 3 and 12 months of age. We also notice that in Fig. 4-B many cortical thickness-based connectivities become weaker (i.e. smaller absolute difference) as we transition from 1 to 3 months of age, which implies that different brain regions develop more similar cortical thicknesses. On the other hand, brighter connectivities appear in morphological network atlases between 3 and 12 months of ages, which shows that the cortical thickness becomes more spatially heterogeneous with age.

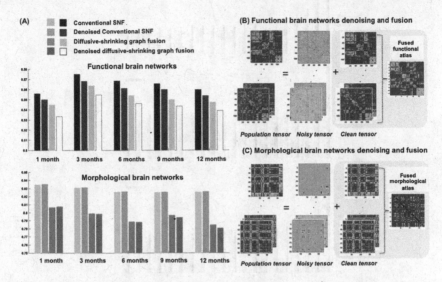

Fig. 2. Clean and centered network atlas evaluation. (A) Mean distance between the estimated network atlas and all individual networks in the population using conventional SNF method and our framework, with and without denoising. (B-C) Network denoising using tensor robust principal component analysis and fusion using the proposed diffusive-shriking graph strategy. We display both functional (B) and morphological (C) estimated network atlases at 9 months of age.

4. Discussion and Conclusion

We have proposed a diffusive-shrinking graph strategy that follows the local manifold structure of a set of brain networks to gradually fuse them through a diffusion process until reaching the final network atlas. Our results showed that our strategy significantly improves the atlas centeredness and pre-denoising (especially for functional networks) further centers the estimated clean atlases. Additionally, our method converges around 5–10 times faster than the conventional SNF method. While SNF converges when the number of iterations t exceeds 20 as noted in [9], the optimal number of iterations required for our method to converge is $t^* \sim 2$ for functional networks and $t^* \sim 4$ for morphological networks. Precisely, while the SNF mean distance slowly decreases with each diffusion iteration as the atlas becomes more centered (see red and white bars in Fig. 3 and dark blue and pink bars in Fig. 4), our mean distance dramatically drops during the first few iterations (black vs. yellow bars (without denoising) and red vs. white bars (with denoising) in Fig. 3) and then slightly increases and remains stable. This convergence behavior shows first that, following the manifold structure when diffusing, speeds up the convergence process

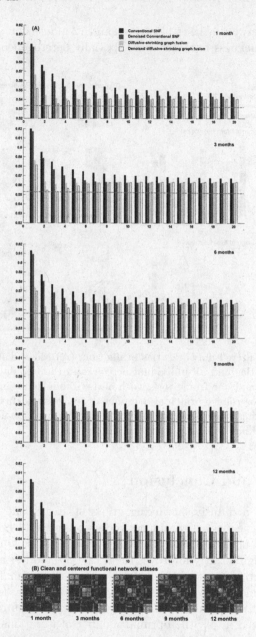

Fig. 3. (A) Evaluation of the estimated functional network atlases for developing infants (1, 3, 6, 9 and 12 months of age) using the conventional similarity network fusion method introduced in [9] and our proposed diffusive-shrinking graph method. We display the mean distance between estimated network atlas and all individuals in the population of networks at each diffusion iteration, with and without denoising. The dashed gray line shows that our method rapidly achieves the best accuracy within the first diffusion iterations ($t^* \sim 2$). (B) The estimated functional network atlases using our method. (Color figure online)

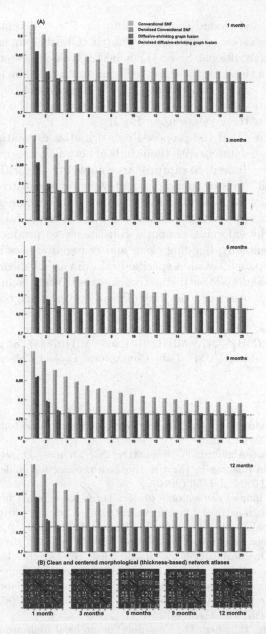

Fig. 4. (A) Evaluation of the estimated morphological network atlases for developing infants (1, 3, 6, 9 and 12 months of age) using the conventional similarity network fusion method introduced in [10] and our proposed diffusive-shrinking graph method. We display the mean distance between estimated network atlas and all individuals in the population of networks at each diffusion iteration, with and without denoising. The dashed gray line shows that our method rapidly achieves the best accuracy within the first diffusion iterations ($t^* \sim 4$). (B) The estimated morphological network atlases using our method. (Color figure online)

to the optimal t^*, and second that over-diffusion $t > t^*$ decenters the network atlas as it becomes closer to the identify matrix. Clearly, our method have two advantages over conventional SNF: (1) a better atlas centeredness (shown in Fig. 2-A), and (2) a significantly decreased computational time (shown in Figs. 3 and 4). We also notice that, when denoising, the diagonals of the denoised tensor may take non- zero values. This is not problematic since the diffusion process automatically resets these values using Eq. 1.

It is worth noting that the proposed network atlas estimation framework is appropriate for large datasets with thousands of networks where the network distribution is complex. Indeed, to capture this complexity, Algorithm 1 can include several hierarchical levels of subgraphs and their representatives that progressively diffuse as they approach the global center of the whole graph. Since our framework overlooks the network distribution in the temporal domain, we will further extend it by enforcing temporal consistency to produce a *longitudinal* network atlas. Eventually, building clean and centered atlases for healthy individuals as well as patients with a specific brain disease or disorder will help us better identify *population-based* distinctive changes in brain connectivity, thereby providing reliable features or biomarkers for an accurate diagnosis.

Acknowledgments. This work is also supported in part by National Institutes of Health grants (MH100217, MH108914 and MH107815) a grant from NIH (1U01MH110274) and UNC/UMN Baby Connectome Project Consortium.

References

1. Brown, C., Hamarneh, G.: Machine learning on human connectome data from MRI arXiv:1611.08699v1 (2016)
2. Miller, K., Alfaro-Almagro, F., Bangerter, N., Thomas, D., et al.: Multimodal population brain imaging in the UK Biobank prospective epidemiological study. Nat. Neurosci. **19**, 1523–1536 (2016)
3. Fallik, D.: The human connectome project turns to mapping brain development, from birth through early childhood. Neurol. Today **16**, 7–9 (2016)
4. Glasser, M., Coalson, T., Robinson, E., Hacker, C.D., et al.: A multi-modal parcellation of human cerebral cortex. Nature **536**, 171–178 (2016)
5. Wassermann, D., Mazauric, D., Gallardo-Diez, G., Deriche, R.: Extracting the core structural connectivity network: guaranteeing network connectedness through a graph-theoretical approach. In: Ourselin, S., Joskowicz, L., Sabuncu, M.R., Unal, G., Wells, W. (eds.) MICCAI 2016. LNCS, vol. 9900, pp. 89–96. Springer, Cham (2016). doi:10.1007/978-3-319-46720-7_11
6. Chen, X., Zhang, H., Shen, D.: Ensemble hierarchical high-order functional connectivity networks for MCI classification. In: Ourselin, S., Joskowicz, L., Sabuncu, M.R., Unal, G., Wells, W. (eds.) MICCAI 2016. LNCS, vol. 9901, pp. 18–25. Springer, Cham (2016). doi:10.1007/978-3-319-46723-8_3
7. Wu, G., Jia, H., Wang, Q., Shen, D.: SharpMean: groupwise registration guided by sharp mean image and tree-based registration. NeuroImage **56**, 1968–1981 (2011)
8. Lu, C., Feng, J., Chen, Y., Liu, W., et al.: Tensor robust principal component analysis: exact recovery of corrupted low-rank tensors via convex optimization. In: CVPR, pp. 5249–5257 (2016)

9. Wang, B., Mezlini, A., Demir, F., Fiume, M., et al.: Similarity network fusion for aggregating data types on a genomic scale. Nat. Methods **11**, 333–337 (2014)

10. Ying, S., Wu, G., Wang, Q., Shen, D.: Hierarchical unbiased graph shrinkage (HUGS): a novel groupwise registration for large data set. Neuroimage **1**, 626–638 (2014)

11. Frey, B., Dueck, D.: Clustering by passing messages between data points. Science **315**, 972–976 (2007)

12. Li, G., Wang, L., Shi, F., et al.: Simultaneous and consistent labeling of longitudinal dynamic developing cortical surfaces in infants. Med. Image Anal. **18**, 1274–1289 (2014)

13. Wang, L., Shi, F., Lin, W., Gilmore, J.H., Shen, D.: Automatic segmentation of neonatal images using convex optimization and coupled level sets. NeuroImage **58**(3), 805–817 (2011)

14. Li, G., Nie, J., Wang, L., Shi, F., Gilmore, J.H., Lin, W., Shen, D.: NeuroImage **90**, 266–279 (2014)

A Tensor Statistical Model for Quantifying Dynamic Functional Connectivity

Yingying Zhu[1]([⊠]), Xiaofeng Zhu[1], Minjeong Kim[1], Jin Yan[2], and Guorong Wu[1]

[1] Department of Radiology and BRIC, UNC at Chapel Hill, Chapel Hill, NC, USA
zhuyingying2@gmail.com
[2] Department of Pharmacology and Cancer Biology, Duke University, Durham, NC, USA

Abstract. Functional connectivity (FC) has been widely investigated in many imaging-based neuroscience and clinical studies. Since functional Magnetic Resonance Image (MRI) signal is just an indirect reflection of brain activity, it is difficult to accurately quantify the FC strength only based on signal correlation. To address this limitation, we propose a learning-based tensor model to derive high sensitivity and specificity connectome biomarkers at the individual level from resting-state fMRI images. First, we propose a learning-based approach to estimate the intrinsic functional connectivity. In addition to the low level region-to-region signal correlation, latent module-to-module connection is also estimated and used to provide high level heuristics for measuring connectivity strength. Furthermore, sparsity constraint is employed to automatically remove the spurious connections, thus alleviating the issue of searching for optimal threshold. Second, we integrate our learning-based approach with the sliding-window technique to further reveal the dynamics of functional connectivity. Specifically, we stack the functional connectivity matrix within each sliding window and form a 3D tensor where the third dimension denotes for time. Then we obtain dynamic functional connectivity (dFC) for each individual subject by simultaneously estimating the within-sliding-window functional connectivity and characterizing the across-sliding-window temporal dynamics. Third, in order to enhance the robustness of the connectome patterns extracted from dFC, we extend the individual-based 3D tensors to a population-based 4D tensor (with the fourth dimension stands for the training subjects) and learn the statistics of connectome patterns via 4D tensor analysis. Since our 4D tensor model jointly (1) optimizes dFC for each training subject and (2) captures the principle connectome patterns, our statistical model gains more statistical power of representing new subject than current state-of-the-art methods which in contrast perform above two steps separately. We have applied our tensor statistical model to identify ASD (Autism Spectrum Disorder) by using the learned dFC patterns. Promising classification results have been achieved demonstrating high discrimination power and great potentials in computer assisted diagnosis of neuro-disorders.

© Springer International Publishing AG 2017
M. Niethammer et al. (Eds.): IPMI 2017, LNCS 10265, pp. 398–410, 2017.
DOI: 10.1007/978-3-319-59050-9_32

1   Introduction

Functional Magnetic Resonance Imaging (fMRI) provides a non-invasive way to study how human brain works. This imaging technique assumes that the change of cerebral blood flow is closely related with brain activity. When an area of the brain is in use, blood flow to that region correspondingly increases [1]. There are various fMRI studies in neuroscience research to understand how the healthy brain works [2], and how that normal function is disrupted in disease [3]. Resting-state fMRI (rs-fMRI) is one of the functional brain imaging techniques that is widely used to measure occurrence of regional interactions that a subject is not performing an explicit task [4]. In resting state, fluctuations in spontaneous neural activity are pre-assumed to underlie the Blood-Oxygen-Level Dependent (BOLD) signal fluctuations, which form inter-regional functional connectivity in human brain network [5]. Since the spatial patterns of resting-state functional brain network are stable and often are overlapped with known anatomical pathways, rs-fMRI has been widely implemented to explore the brain's functional organization and examine the altered connectivity in neurological or psychiatric diseases [6].

In current functional brain network studies, Pearson's correlation on BOLD signals is used to measure the strength of FC between two brain regions [5]. It is worth noting that such correlation based connectivity measure is exclusively calculated based on the observed BOLD signals and fixed for the subsequent data analysis. However, the BOLD signal usually has very poor signal-to-noise ratio and is mixed with substantial non-neural noise and artifacts. Therefore, it is hard for current state-of-the-art methods to determine a good threshold of FC strength which can effectively distinguish real and spurious connections [7].

For simplicity, many FC characterization methods assume that connectivity patterns in the brain do not change over the course of a resting-state fMRI scan. However, there is a growing consensus in the neuroimaging field, that the spontaneous fluctuations and correlations of signals between two distinct brain regions change with correspondence to cognitive states, even in a task-free environment [8]. Thus, dynamic FC patterns have been investigated recently mainly by using sliding window techniques [8,9]. Due to the large dimension of sliding window numbers and large number of brain regions, it is very difficult to represent the dynamic brain network compactly directly. Therefore, many different machine learning techniques has been proposed to reduce the dimension of dynamic brain FC patterns. The common strategy of those works is to reduce the dimension on sliding windows using clustering [10] or Principle Component Analysis (PCA) [11] along time. And the clustering coefficients or PCA coefficients are used as the compact representation for dynamic FC. However, these methods reduce the dynamic FC dimension at the cost of losing the local temporal changes along time. Furthermore, in all existing dynamic FC methods, the procedures of estimating functional connectivity and extracting connectome features are completely independent. Although both steps are very challenging, we would like to argue that these two steps can help each other in a collaborative manner. Specifically, accurate functional connectivity of individual subjects can derive

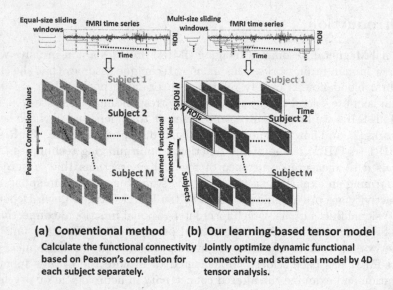

Fig. 1. The advantage of our 4D tensor method (b) over the conventional method (a).

more reasonable statistical model to better represent the whole population. On the other hand, the learned statistical model can provide additional population-based heuristics to address the uncertainty in measuring functional connectivity for individual subject. To that end, we propose a tensor-based statistical model which jointly optimizes the dynamic functional connectivity at the individual basis and learns the intrinsic connectome patterns for the whole population. Our proposed method is illustrated in Fig. 1, which consists of three parts:

First, we present a robust learning-based method to optimize FC from the BOLD signals in a fixed sliding window. In order to avoid the unreliable calculation of FC based on signal correlations, high level feature representation is of necessity to guide the optimization of FC. Specifically, our method seeks for module-wise network structure during the optimization of node-to-node functional connectivity, where the brain region within the same module should have similar connection patterns. Thus, we can optimize functional connections for each brain region based on not only the observed region-to-region signal correlations but also the similarity between high level module-to-module connection patterns. In turn, the refined FC can lead to more reasonable estimation of module-wise connections. Since brain network is intrinsically economic and sparse, sparsity constraint is used to control the number of connections during the joint estimation of principal connection patterns and the optimization of FC.

Second, we further extend the above FC optimization framework from one sliding window (capturing the static FC patterns) to a set of overlapped sliding windows (capturing the dynamic FC patterns). The leverage is that we arrange the FCs along time into a 3D tensor (cubic in Fig. 1) and we employ additional low rank constraint to penalize the oscillatory changes of FC in the temporal domain.

Third, in order to learn the statistical model of intrinsic feature representations derived from the dynamic functional connectivity (dFC) in the population, we arrange the estimated functional dynamics of all subjects into a 4D tensor (right of Fig. 1) with the subjects denoted by fourth dimension. Then we go one step further to alternatively (1) optimize the dFC within each subject-specific 3D tensor under the guidance of learned intrinsic feature representations, and (2) learn the statistical model which can represent majority variations of dynamic functional connectivity patterns in the population. In doing so, we can derive robust statistical model of dynamic functional connectivity and encode the characteristics of dFC for the new unseen subjects. It is worth noting that the output of our statistical model can be regarded as the imaging markers in identifying individuals having or at risk of neuro-disease.

2 Method

2.1 Optimize Functional Connectivity Within Sliding Window

To start our tensor-based statistical model of dFC, we first propose a robust FC optimization method given a sliding window. Let $\mathbf{x}_i \in \mathbb{R}^{W \times 1}$ denote the mean BOLD signal calculated in brain region $O_i, (i = 1, \cdots, N)$, where W is the length of time course within the sliding window and N is the total number of brain regions under consideration. Conventionally, a $N \times N$ connectivity matrix $\mathbf{S}$ is used to measure the FC in the whole brain, where each element s_{ij} quantitatively measures the strength of FC between region O_i and $O_j(i \neq j)$. Particularly, the strength of functional connectivity s_{ij} is assumed to be measurable based on Pearson's correlation $c(x_i, x_j)$ between observed BOLD signals $\mathbf{x}_i$ and $\mathbf{x}_j$, where big value of Pearson's correlation indicates strong functional connectivity. Thresholding on Pearson's correlation values is commonly used to remove the spurious connection. However, it is not easy to find a good threshold that works for all subjects.

Since fMRI is just an indirect reflection of brain activity, it is difficult to accurately quantify the FC strength only based on signal correlation. To alleviate this issue, we propose to optimize the reasonable functional connectivities, which should (1) be in consensus with the Pearson's correlation of low level signals between $\mathbf{x}_i$ and $\mathbf{x}_j$; (2) use the high level information such as module-to-module connection [12] to guide the measurement of low level region-to-region connectivity strength; and (3) represent sparsity since the brain network is intrinsically efficient to have sparse connections [13]. For convenience, we use $\mathbf{s}_i \in \mathbb{R}^{N \times 1}$ denote i-th column in connectivity matrix $\mathbf{S}$, which characters the connections of region O_i with respect to other brain regions. Also, we arrange all Pearson's correlation values into a $N \times N$ matrix $\mathbf{C} = \{c_{ij} | i, j = 1, \cdots, N\}$. Instead of calculating the connectivity s_{ij} just based on Pearson's correlation $c(\mathbf{x}_i, \mathbf{x}_j)$ between observed BOLD signals $\mathbf{x}_i$ and $\mathbf{x}_j$, we optimize the connectivity matrix $\mathbf{S}$ by integrating the above three criteria:

$$\arg \min_{\mathbf{S}} \|\mathbf{S} - \mathbf{C}\|_F^2 + \alpha \|\mathbf{S}\|_* + \gamma \|\mathbf{S}\|_1, \tag{1}$$

where α and γ are the scalars which balance the strength of the low rank constraint [14] on $\mathbf{S}$ (the second term) and the l_1 sparsity constraint [15] on $\mathbf{S}$ (the third term).

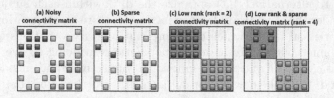

Fig. 2. The intuition behind low rank and sparsity constraint in optimizing functional connectivity.

Discussion. Specifically, the first term requires the optimized functional connectivity matrix $\mathbf{S}$ should be close to the observed Pearson's correlation matrix $\mathbf{C}$. Sparse representation technique has been used in [16] to establish the functional connection of one brain region to all other regions. As the toy examples shown in Fig. 2(a), there might be a lot of spurious connections (gray blocks) in the FC matrix calculated based on Pearson's correlation. After applying signal sparse representation at each brain regions independently, only a small number of connections remain such that the sparse constraint can make the estimation of FC more robust, as shown in Fig. 2(b).

It is clear that the l_1 norm is effective to remove redundant connections in functional connectivity [17]. However, one limitation of l_1 norm is that the modular relationship are not jointly considered [12]. Figure 2(b) shows the connection patterns obtained using l_1 norm, which shows no modular structure. Since brain network exhibit modular organization, we further introduce low rank constraint $\|\mathbf{S}\|_*$ to achieve strong modular organization. As shown in Fig. 2(c), the connection patterns are highly consistent within the same module but the intra modular regions are over connected. To achieve a reasonable sparse and modularized brain connections, we combine low rank and sparsity constraint on $\mathbf{S}$ to achieve connection patterns as shown in Fig. 2.

2.2 Characterize Dynamic Functional Connectivity by 3D Tensor Analysis

Here, we extend the learning-based FC optimization method to the temporal domain, in order to capture dynamics of functional connectivity. First, we follow the sliding window technique to obtain T overlapped multiple scale sliding windows which cover the whole time course for one subject. Let $\mathbf{S}^t$ denote for the FC matrix in sliding window t. Then we stack all $\mathbf{S}^t$ along time and form a tensor $\mathcal{S} = \{\mathbf{S}^t | t = 1, \cdots, T\} \in \mathbb{R}^{N \times N \times T}$ which represents the complete information of dynamic connectivity for each subject. Similarly, we can also construct another tensor $\mathcal{C} = \{\mathbf{C}^t | t = 1, \cdots, T\} \in \mathbb{R}^{N \times N \times T}$, where each

$\mathbf{C}^t = \{c_{i,j}^t | i, j = 1, \cdots, N\}$ is the $N \times N$ matrices in $t - th$ sliding window. Next, we propose a learning-based optimization method to characterize dFC using tensor analysis by:

$$\arg\min_{\mathcal{S}} \|\mathcal{S} - \mathcal{C}\|_F^2 + \alpha\|\mathcal{S}\|_* + \gamma\|\mathcal{S}\|_1, \tag{2}$$

Compared to the objective function in Eq. 1, the objective function here also encourages low rank on the brain connectivity patterns. Since brain in resting state generally transverses a small number of discrete stages during a short period of time [8], it is reasonable to apply low rank constraint on $\mathcal{S}$ (by minimizing nuclear norm $\|\mathcal{S}\|_*$) to penalize too rapid FC change in the temporal domain and also find the optimal connectivity patterns in each sliding window.

2.3 Conventional Linear PCA Statistical Model

The learned 3D tensor $\mathcal{S}_m$ for subject m is $N \times N \times T$ which can not be used as the dynamic FC feature representation due to the high dimension. Conventional work proposed to reshape $\mathcal{S}_m$ to a matrix $\mathbf{S}_m \in \mathbb{R}^{N^2 \times T}$, where each column stands for a connection pattern, then M subjects are stacked together to formulate a matrix $\mathbf{S}^\# \in \mathbb{R}^{N^2 \times MT}$ as shown in Fig. 3(a). A low dimensional principle connectome space $\mathbf{U}_{(c)} \in \mathbb{R}^{N^2 \times R}$ can be learned by decomposing $\mathbf{S}^\# \in \mathbb{R}^{N^2 \times MT}$ into a orthonormal space $\mathbf{U}_{(c)}$ and coefficients matrix using linear Principle Component Analysis (PCA),

$$\mathbf{S}^\# = \mathbf{U}_{(c)}\mathbf{F}^\#, \tag{3}$$

where $\mathbf{U}_{(c)}$ is the brain connectome space, $\mathbf{F}^\# = [\mathbf{F}_1, \cdots, \mathbf{F}_M] \in \mathbb{R}^{N^2 \times MT}$ is the projected coefficients for $\mathbf{S}^\#$ as shown in Fig. 3. The high dimensional dynamic FC $\mathbf{S}_m \in \mathbb{R}^{N^2 \times T}$ for subject m can be represented as a coefficients matrix $\mathbf{F}_m = \mathbf{U}_{(c)}^T \mathbf{S}_m \in \mathbb{R}^{R \times T}$. Since the sliding window number is large, this coefficients matrix is further normalized by the sliding window number T as the compact feature representation for dynamic FC patterns.

Conventional Method Issues. Conventional PCA based brain connectome space based method suffers from several issues: (1) How to set up optimal connection matrix threshold. (2) Temporal dynamics space is not modelled. Using

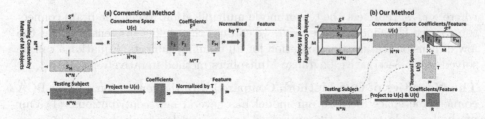

Fig. 3. The comparison of conventional linear principle component analysis brain connectome model and our proposed tensor analysis connectome model.

the matrix techniques, the conventional method can only model the connectome space on the population, but the temporal dynamics space are not modelled (shown in Fig. 3(a)).

2.4   Statistical Model of Dynamic Functional Connectivity by Tensor Analysis on Population

Motivated by those above issues in conventional method, we extend the linear PCA model to a non-linear tensor analysis model in order to learn the optimal connectivity matrices for each subject at different sliding windows from the data without setting thresholds and a better brain connectome representation space and temporal dynamic space based on population jointly. Suppose we have M training subjects in total. As demonstrated in the right of Fig. 1, we stack the individual-based 3D tensors to a population-based 4D tensor (with the fourth dimension stands for M training subjects). Specifically, let the subscript m denote for the subject index. We construct a 4D tensor $\mathbb{S} = \{\mathcal{S}_m | m = 1, \cdots, M\} \in \mathbb{R}^{N \times N \times T \times M}$ to include the dFC of all M training subjects. It is worth noting that different subject may have different number of sliding windows, here, $T = max(T_m), m = 1, \cdots, M$. We also construct another 4D tensor of Pearson's correlation values $\mathbb{C} = \{\mathcal{C}_m | m = 1, \cdots, M, t = 1, \cdots, T\} \in \mathbb{R}^{N \times N \times T \times M}$. Then, we learn the dynamic FC pattern using tensor analysis:

$$\arg \min_{\mathbb{S}} \|\mathbb{S} - \mathbb{C}\|_F^2 + \alpha \|\mathbb{S}\|_* + \gamma \|\mathbb{S}\|_1, \tag{4}$$

In order to learn the principle connectome space as conventional methods, we reshape the 4D tensor $\mathbb{S}$ to a 3D tensor $\mathcal{S}^\# \in \mathbb{R}^{N^2 \times T \times M}$, where 1st dimension stands for the vectorized connectivity matrix, 2nd dimension stands for the sliding windows and 3rd model stands for M subjects as shown in Fig. 3(b). We learn a low rank and sparse 4D tensor $\mathcal{S}$ and simultaneously decompose the reshaped tensor $\mathcal{S}^\#$ into a brain connetome space $\mathbf{U}_{(c)} \in \mathbb{R}^{R \times N^2}$, a temporal dynamic space $\mathbf{U}_{(t)} \in \mathbb{R}^{R \times T}$ and a coefficients tensor $\mathcal{F}^\# \in \mathbb{R}^{R \times R \times M}$ using the tensor high-order singular value decomposition as,

$$\arg \min_{\mathbf{U}_{(c)}, \mathbf{U}_{(t)}, \mathcal{F}^\#, \mathbb{S}} \|\mathbb{S} - \mathbb{C}\|_F^2 + \alpha \|\mathbb{S}\|_* + \gamma \|\mathbb{S}\|_1, \tag{5}$$

$$\mathcal{S}^\# = \mathcal{F}^\# \times_1 \mathbf{U}_{(c)} \times_2 \mathbf{U}_{(t)},$$

where $\times_1, \times_2$ represent the tensor mode multiplication. When the brain connectome space $\mathbf{U}_{(c)}$ and $\mathbf{U}_{(t)}$ are fixed, we can use the coefficients tensor $\mathcal{F}^\#$ as the low dimension feature representation for all training subjects. Equation 5 can be solved using Alternative Lagrange Multipliers method iteratively [14,15].

The Novelties of Our Method. Compared with the conventional linear PCA connectome space method, our model has several new contributions: (1) Our method is able to learn the optimized sparse and low rank dynamic FC patterns based on data without setting optimal thresholds for brain connectome matrices. (2) Tensor analysis enables our method to learn a low dimensional connectome space $\mathbf{U}_{(c)}$ along with a low dimensional temporal dynamic space $\mathbf{U}_{(t)}$ which models FC temporal changes. Therefore, our method is more suitable for modeling dynamic FC patterns as shown in Fig. 3(b).

Encode Dynamic FC Feature and Apply Classifier for New Subjects. In the testing stage, we assume that each testing subject is independent to others. Thus, we obtain the compact connectome representations for each testing subject separately. Specifically, We first construct the 3D tensor of Pearson's correlation $\mathcal{C}^* \in \mathbb{R}^{N \times N \times T}$. The goal here has two folds: (i) estimate the dynamic functional connectivity $\mathcal{S}^*$ (a 3D tensor with the same dimension as $\mathcal{C}^*$) for the underlying subject; and (ii) obtain the compact connectome feature representation $\mathbf{F}^* \in \mathbb{R}^{R \times R}$ by projecting to the subspace spanned by learned connectivity space $\mathbf{U}_{(c)}$, $\mathbf{U}_{(t)}$ on the training dataset. $\mathcal{S}^*$ can be learn using Eq. 2. After $\mathcal{S}^*$ is learned, we reshape it to a matrix $\mathbf{S}^{*\#} \in \mathbb{R}^{N^2 \times T}$ and compute the compact feature representations by projecting $\mathbf{S}$ onto the learned connectome space $\mathbf{U}_{(c)}$ and temporal dynamic space $\mathbf{U}_{(t)}$ from training data,

$$\mathbf{F}^* = \mathbf{U}_{(c)}^T \mathbf{S}^{*\#} \mathbf{U}_{(t)}, \tag{6}$$

where $\mathbf{F}^* \in \mathbb{R}^{R \times R}$ is the projected low dimensional feature representation on the trained connectome space and temporal dynamic space. We apply our trained classifier to the learned dynamic FC feature representation to determine the class label for each testing subject.

3 Experiment Results

In this section, we evaluate our proposed tensor connectome model of dynamic functional connectivity by comparing the discriminative power in identifying ASD subjects with conventional state-of-the-art methods.

Experiment Setup. We randomly partition all subjects into 10 non-overlapping approximately equal size sets. Then, we use one fold for testing and the remaining folds are used for training. The training subjects are further divided into 5 subsets for another 5-fold inner cross validation, where 4 folds are used as training subset and the last fold is used as the validation subset. We found that our method is able to achieve stable performance when $\alpha = 1, \gamma = 1$. The tensor connectome space $\mathbf{U}_{(c)}$ and temporal dynamic space $\mathbf{U}_{(t)}$ are learned from the subjects in the training subset. The low dimension connectome features representations of those training subjects, derived from the learned 4D tensor model, are further used to train the classic SVM (Support Vector Machine) for classification. Here, in order to show the power of our learned dynamic brain connectivity features, we only use a standard linear kernel SVM with l_2 norm penalty. The optimal parameters are determined based on validation subset. It is worth noting that any classification model can be applied to our learned dynamic FC feature representations. For each testing subject, we use the approach summarized in Sect. 2.4 to estimate the dynamic FC feature representations, which is considered as the connectome signature to identify the clinical label of the testing subject. For the competing methods, we apply our multiple scale sliding window strategy to calculate the dynamic functional connectivity feature representation (based on Pearson's correlation and optimal thresholding on validation dataset) for each subject. We first manually set up the sliding window size which ranges from 20 to 100 of the entire time course. It is worthy noting to mention that the brain connection patterns are unstable is the window size is smaller than 20. In optimizing the dynamic FC pattern, we set the shift of sliding window to 1 TR, in order to fully capture the dynamics of FC. In order to reduce feature dimension, we follow the work in to use classic PCA (Principle Component Analysis) model to encode the low dimensional connectome feature representation [11] for comparison.

Data Preprocessing. The subjects in our experiments were scanned for six and ten minutes during resting state, respectively, producing 180 time points and 300 time points at a repetition time (TR) of 2 s. We have corrected the head motion of the data first. It is worthy noting that this work focus on dynamic functional connectivity study and we assume that the dynamics caused by head motion are removed in motion correction. We further processed all these data using Data Processing Assistant for 0 the AAL template with 116 ROIs to the subject image domain and compute the mean BOLD signal in each ROI, where conventional method calculate the 116×116 connectivity matrix S based on the Pearson's correlation of mean BOLD signals between any pair of two distinct brain regions.

Evaluation Measurements. We use several quantitative measurements including Accuracy (ACC), Specificity (SPEC) and Sensitivity (SEN) to evaluate the classification performance using our learned tensor dynamic FC feature representation. In the following experiments, PCA represents Pearson's correlation based dynamic FC and feature coded using PCA. OURS represents the learned dynamic FC patterns by our 4D tensor method.

Subject Information. We conducted various experiments on resting-state fMRI images using two Autism data sets in order to demonstrate the generality of our method. We use the Autism Brain Imaging Data Exchange (ABIDE) database including both the data from NewYork University (NYU) and University of Minnesota (UM) site. Specifically, 45 NC and 45 ASD subjects are selected from the NYU site. 74 NC and 57 ASD subjects are selected from UM site.

Evaluation of Learned Dynamic FC Patterns in NC/ASD Classification Using the Same Dataset. We first evaluate the performance of our model using the same dataset for training and testing. 10-fold cross-validation strategy is employed here on UM and NYU dataset. The NC/ASD classification results using different sliding window setup on UM and NYU dataset are shown in Fig. 4(a) and (b) respectively. It is shown that, first, the optimal sliding window size is 40 for two datasets; secondly, multiple scale sliding window setup achieves the best performance for all methods on two datasets, which improves >1% in terms of Accuracy compared to best performance achieved by fixed sliding window size; our learned 4D tensor feature representation improves the performance at least 4.5% in terms of Accuracy compared with the conventional Pearson's correlation & PCA method using multiple scale sliding windows.

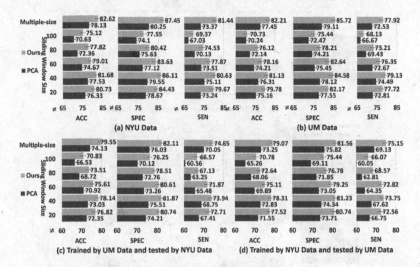

Fig. 4. Evaluation of learned dynamic FC patterns. (a) and (b) Use the same training and testing dataset. (c) and (d) Use different training and testing dataset.

Evaluation of Learned Dynamic FC Patterns in NC/ASD Classification Using Different Dataset. To evaluate the generalization of the learned dynamic FC pattern representations, we select the training data and testing data from different sites. Two experiments are conducted here: first, we split the NYU and UM data into ten non-overlapped folds and use 9 folds from NYU as the training data and one fold from UM as the testing data; then, we swicth the training and testing dataset. Figure 4(c) and (d) shows the performance of conventional Pearson's correlation patterns coded by PCA and our learned dynamic FC patterns with respect to different sliding window sizes. The performance is sensitive to different window size setting up. All competing methods achieve the best performance when the sliding window is 40 and multiple scale sliding window setting up improves the performance about >1% compared to sliding window size 40 for all competing methods. Compared with the conventional Pearson's correlation patterns coded by PCA [11], our learned dynamic FC pattern improves the ASD classification performance >4% on Accuracy using multiple scale sliding windows.

Validation of Learned Dynamic FC Patterns. To evaluate the learned dynamic FC patterns, we checked the learned dynamic connection patterns for vision function regions, such as Lingual gyrus, Cuneus, Parahippocampal gyrus, and for motion function such as Putamen, Globus Pallidus using the NYU ASD

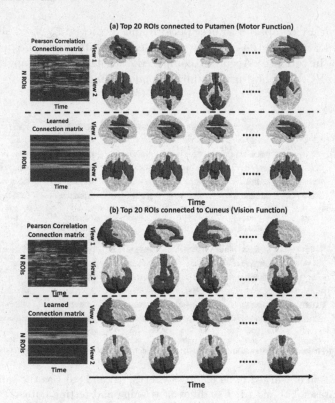

Fig. 5. Visualization of the top 20 connection along time of Putamen (motion function related) and Cuneus (relation to vision function) by the Pearson's correlation and our method.

dataset. We found that the connection patterns of those regions are inconsistent by the conventional Pearson's correlation and thresholding method. However, the connection pattern learned by our method is changing smoother along time for those regions, which is consistent with current neuroscience findings.

Figure 5(a) shows the visualization of the positive connected ROIs to the Putamen along time computed by conventional Pearson's correlation method and our method. Putamen is known to be related to motion function, since the fMRI time series are all collected during the resting and there is no motion task involved, the connection to putamen should be consistent and smooth along time. We found that the connection pattern by our method is stable along time. However, the connection pattern computed by the conventional Pearson's correlation method is changing randomly along time. We also show the connection pattern variations along time for the Cuneus in Fig. 5(b). Cuneus is known to be related to vision function. The connection patterns to Cuneus are supposed to be consistent along time since no vision tasks are involved in the resting state. Compared to the varying connection patterns along time calculated by conventional Pearson's correlation method, the connection patterns generated by our method resemble much better at different times.

4   Conclusion

In this work, we propose a novel learning-based method to discover both static and population based dynamic FC patterns from resting-state fMRI data using multiple linear tensor analysis. We evaluated the learned dynamic FC patterns by apply it as biomarkers for Autism identification and achieved promising results. Future work will explore the application of dynamic FC patterns on diagnosis of more neurological disorders such as, Alzheimer's diseases and Obesity.

References

1. Logothetis, N.K., Pauls, J., Augath, M., Trinath, T., Oeltermann, A.: Neurophysiological investigation of the basis of the fMRI signal. Nature **412**, 150–157 (2001)
2. Mousss, M.N., Steen, M.R., Laurienti, P.J., Hayasaka, S.: Consistency of network modules in resting-state fMRI connectome data. PLoS One **7**, 44428 (2012)
3. Bilello, M.: Correlating cognitive decline with white matter lesion and brain atrophy magnetic resonance imaging measurements in Alzheimer's disease. J. Alzheimers Dis. **48**(4), 987–994 (2015)
4. Biswal, B.B.: Resting state fMRI: a personal history. NeuroImage **62**, 938–944 (2012)
5. Heuvel, M., Pol, H.: Exploring the brain network: a review on resting-state fMRI functional connectivity. Eur. Neuropsychopharmacol. **20**, 519–534 (2010)
6. Miller, D.B., O'Callaghan, J.: Biomarkers of Parkinson's disease. Metabolism **64**, 40–46 (2015)
7. Power, J.D., Cohen, A.L., Nelson, S.M., Wig, G.S., Barnes, K.A., Church, J.A.: Functional network organization of the human brain. Neuron **72**, 665–678 (2011)
8. Hutchison, R.M., Womelsdorf, T., Allen, E.A., Bandettini, P.A., Calhoun, V.D., Corbetta, M.: Dynamic functional connectivity: promise, issues, and interpretations. Neuroimage **80**, 360–378 (2013)
9. Zhu, Y., Zhu, X., Zhang, H., Gao, W., Shen, D., Wu, G.: Reveal consistent spatial-temporal patterns from dynamic functional connectivity for autism spectrum disorder identification. In: Ourselin, S., Joskowicz, L., Sabuncu, M.R., Unal, G., Wells, W. (eds.) MICCAI 2016. LNCS, vol. 9900, pp. 106–114. Springer, Cham (2016). doi:10.1007/978-3-319-46720-7_13
10. Wee, C., Yap, P., Shen, D.: Diagnosis of autism spectrum disorders using temporally distinct resting-state functional connectivity networks. CNS Neurosci. Ther. **22**, 212–219 (2016)
11. Leonardi, N.: Principal components of functional connectivity: a new approach to study dynamic brain connectivity during rest. NeuroImage **83**, 937–950 (2013)
12. Heuvel, M.P., Sporns, O.: Rich-club organization of the human connectome. J. Neurosci. **31**, 75–86 (2011)
13. Bullmore, E., Sporns, O.: Complex brain networks: graph theoretical analysis of structural and functional systems. Nature **10**, 186–198 (2009)
14. Zhu, Y., Huang, D., De La Torre, F., Lucey, S.: Complex non-rigid motion 3D reconstruction by union of subspaces. In: CVPR (2014)

15. Zhu, Y., Lucey, S.: 3D motion reconstruction for real-world camera motion. In: CVPR (2011)
16. Wee, C., Yap, P., Zhang, D., Wang, L., Shen, D.: Group-constrained sparse fMRI connectivity modeling for mild cognitive impairment identification. Brain Struct. Funct. **219**, 641–656 (2014)
17. Zhu, Y., Lucey, S.: Convolutional sparse coding for trajectory reconstruction. IEEE Trans. Pattern Anal. Mach. Intell. **37**, 529–540 (2015)

Modeling Task fMRI Data via Deep Convolutional Autoencoder

Heng Huang[1(✉)], Xintao Hu[1], Milad Makkie[2], Qinglin Dong[2], Yu Zhao[2], Junwei Han[1], Lei Guo[1], and Tianming Liu[2]

[1] School of Automation, Northwestern Polytechnical University, Xi'an, China
huangheng2014@gmail.com
[2] Department of Computer Science and Bioimaging Research Center,
The University of Georgia, Athens, GA, USA

Abstract. Task-based fMRI (tfMRI) has been widely used to study functional brain networks. Modeling tfMRI data is challenging due to at least two problems: the lack of the ground truth of underlying neural activity and the intrinsic structure of tfMRI data is highly complex. To better understand brain networks based on fMRI data, data-driven approaches were proposed, for instance, Independent Component Analysis (ICA) and Sparse Dictionary Learning (SDL). However, both ICA and SDL only build shallow models, and they are under the strong assumption that original fMRI signal could be linearly decomposed into time series components with their corresponding spatial maps. As growing evidence shows that human brain function is hierarchically organized, new approaches that can infer and model the hierarchical structure of brain networks are widely called for. Recently, deep convolutional neural network (CNN) has drawn much attention, in that deep CNN has been proven to be a powerful method for learning high-level and mid-level abstractions from low-level raw data. Inspired by the power of deep CNN, in this study, we developed a new neural network structure based on CNN, called Deep Convolutional Auto-Encoder (DCAE), in order to take the advantages of both data-driven approach and CNN's hierarchical feature abstraction ability for the purpose of learning mid-level and high-level features from complex tfMRI time series in an unsupervised manner. The DCAE has been applied and tested on the publicly available human connectome project (HCP) tfMRI datasets, and promising results are achieved.

Keywords: Task-based fMRI · Deep learning · CNN · Autoencoder

1 Introduction

Task-based functional magnetic resonance imaging (tfMRI) has been a powerful noninvasive tool to study functional networks and cognitive behaviors of the human brain. It has significantly advanced our knowledge of brain regions/networks that are functionally involved in specific tasks. To model the very informative and complex tfMRI time series, a variety of methods have been proposed over the past decades, such as the general linear model (GLM) [1], as a model-driven approach, and independent component analysis (ICA) [2] and sparse dictionary learning [3], as data-driven

© Springer International Publishing AG 2017
M. Niethammer et al. (Eds.): IPMI 2017, LNCS 10265, pp. 411–424, 2017.
DOI: 10.1007/978-3-319-59050-9_33

approaches. However, these existing methods only build shallow models which can't meet the needs of modeling the hierarchical structures in tfMRI data [4, 5], and as a consequence, they might overlook other rich information contained in tfMRI data.

Recently, deep learning has attracted much attention in the field of machine learning and data mining [6], and it has been proven that deep learning approach is superb at learning high-level and mid-level features from low-level raw data [7]. A deep learning architecture usually consists of deep network layers by stacking multiple similar building blocks. The bottom layer receives an input and then passes the transformed versions of input to the next layer, all the way up from the bottom layer to the top layer. As a result, the architecture of a deep learning model acts as a hierarchical feature extractor as a whole. In the past several years, there have been growing bodies of literature that adopted deep learning models into fMRI data modeling applications, for instances, Plis et al. [8] used deep belief network (DBN) to learn physiologically important representations from fMRI data; Suk et al. [9] combined the Deep Auto-Encoder (DAE) with Hidden Markov Model (HMM) to investigate the functional connectivities in resting-state fMRI; and Huang et al. [10] use the restricted Boltzmann machines (RBM) to mine the latent sources in task fMRI data.

Among all available deep learning models, convolutional neural network (CNN) is one of the most popular methods. Basically, CNN is a variant of the feed-forward artificial neural network, and its connectivity between layers is inspired by cat's visual cortex. A recent study on neuroimaging data found similar structures in human brains [11], which suggested CNN might be naturally suitable for modeling fMRI data. In this study, we designed a new CNN structure for modeling tfMRI data, called deep convolutional auto-encoder (DCAE). The major advantages and novelties of our DCAE are that the whole training process is in an unsupervised manner and no single label is needed, and importantly, the DCAE structure inherits the powerful feature abstraction ability of traditional CNNs. To evaluate the effectiveness of our DCAE in modeling fMRI data, we proposed two novel validation approaches. First, we used theoretical models to verify that the hierarchical feature maps learned by DCAE are related to the underlying neural activities. Second, we performed a comparison study between high-level sparse dictionary learning (HL-SDL) with traditional shallow sparse dictionary learning (SL-SDL) to explore the induced influences when the model's depth increases. Experimental results on the human connectome project (HCP) tfMRI datasets demonstrated promising results.

2   Methods

Figure 1 summarizes the structure of the proposed deep convolutional autoencoder (DCAE), as well as the relations with the two validation studies. The DCAE model consists of two main components, the encoder, and the decoder, to model tfMRI data hierarchically. Specifically, after data preprocessing (Sect. 2.1), the whole-brain tfMRI signals in each subject are extracted and normalized (with zero mean and standard deviation). As shown in Fig. 1, for each voxel's signal, the encoder represents it as mid-level and high-level feature maps as the layer goes deeper, and then the decoder decodes these feature maps layer by layer and finally reconstructs the original signal at its top layer. The objective of the DCAE is to minimize the reconstruction errors of the entire training data sets (voxels' signals from all subjects) (Sects. 2.1, 2.2 and 2.3), and the whole training process is completely unsupervised. The two validation studies are performed in the feature maps and the hidden states of the top layer, respectively. The details of two validation studies will be presented in Sects. 2.4 and 2.5.

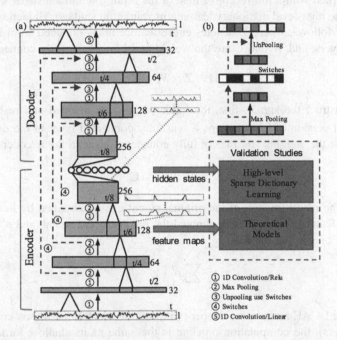

Fig. 1. Illustration of the DCAE structure with its two validation studies. (a) DCAE structure, the hidden states, and the feature maps, as well as their relationship with the validation studies. (b) The detailed processes of max pooling and unpooling.

2.1 Deep Convolutional Auto-Encoder (DCAE)

The DCAE model mainly consists of two components, the encoder and the decoder. The encoder is responsible for mapping the input signal into higher level feature maps, and the decoder does the opposite reconstruction work. To explain the basic ideas, we first ignore the max pooling operations and consider the situation when the model is shallow (both encoder and decoder only have 1 convolutional layer). For an input 1D fMRI signal x, the i-th feature map in the encoder is computed in a convolutional fashion:

$$z_i = f(p_i * x + b_i) \tag{1}$$

where $*$ denote 1D convolution, p_i and b_i are the filters and bias for i-th feature maps. f is the activation function. In this paper, except for the top convolutional layer in the decoder layer where we use linear activation function, we use the rectified nonlinearity unit (Relu) in all other convolutional layers. The benefits of using the Relu activation function have been broadly discussed in other prior literature studies [12].

Following the convolutional layer, we build a fully connected layer at the top of the encoder. The fully connected layer is used to keep the final hidden state in the encoder to have the same feature size as input, and at the same time to ensure that the hidden states are learned with a full receptive field of the input (the hidden states will be used to perform the high-level dictionary learning in validation studies). Hidden states H are computed as follows, where Z denotes entire feature maps obtained from lower convolutional layers, and W and C are the weight and bias of the fully connected layer.

$$H = Z \times W + C \tag{2}$$

To reconstruct the signal, first, the hidden states are mapped and reshaped to a reconstructed version of feature maps Z' via fully connected layer in the decoder. W' and C' denote the weights and bias of fully connected layer in the decoder.

$$Z' = H \times W' + C' \tag{3}$$

Finally, the reconstruction of the original signal can be obtained by linearly combining these feature maps, where $\hat{x}$ denoted the reconstructed signal, and p_i' and b_i' are the filter and bias in the decoder.

$$\hat{x} = \sum_i p_i' * z_i' + b_i' \tag{4}$$

When the DCAE model goes deeper (with more convolutional layers connected to previous layers), the computation pipeline is the same as its shallow form. The difference is that when there are more than 1 convolutional layers, the input will be transformed by different convolutional layers into different feature maps by a chain rule.

The parameters in the whole DCAE are optimized to minimize the mean square error between fMRI signals and their reconstructions. It should be noted that an additional l2 regularized term between feature maps in the top layer of the encoder and the bottom layer of the decoder is added to the cost function, which ensures that the fully connected layer does not randomly shuffle the timing order when reconstructing features maps in the decoder.

$$\min \frac{1}{2}||X - \hat{X}||_2^2 + \frac{1}{2}\lambda||Z - Z'||_2^2 \tag{5}$$

2.2 Max-Pooling and Unpooling in DCAE

In DCAE, the max pooling is applied on each layer after the convolutional layer. Max pooling is a down-sampling operation on features maps, and there are two major benefits by using max pooling. First, it substantially reduces the computational cost for the upper layer. Second, it gains translation-invariance. In the tfMRI field, the time shift phenomenon has been observed and reported in many studies [13, 14], given that an fMRI signal could be a shifted version of another signal. Some research studies have suggested that the phenomenon is caused by the hemodynamic response function (HRF) differences in different brain areas, while other researchers believe it is because of the dynamic causal effects in human brains. In traditional models, the phenomenon is often ignored. By introducing the translation-invariance property in DCAE, it becomes possible to learn a set of similar high-level features for shifted time series, which will be discussed in details later in the results sections.

In the decoder, we use the unpooling to inverse the max pooling. However, it should be noted that max pooling operation itself is not invertible, and we used two types of unpooling operations in this study. During training, we adopted the idea proposed by Zeiler and Fergus [15]. That is, we used the "switches" to record the location of the local max in each pooling regions, and these "switches" are then used to place corresponding local max value to its original position, as illustrated in Fig. 1(b). In validation studies (high-level sparse dictionary learning) when "switches" are not available, we simply use traditional up-sampling. A similar strategy has been used by [16] before, and similar to their conclusion, our results also suggested that using "switches" during training makes the structure learn a better representation of tfMRI data.

2.3   DCAE Parameter Settings and Model Training

Our parameter settings are summarized in Table 1. In this table, feature map numbers in each layer refer to how many representative feature forms for a signal we aim to obtain. The HCP motor task fMRI data we used in this study include six basic motor tasks. Therefore, we used relatively small feature map numbers, which ensures that the learned patterns are the most general patterns in HCP subjects' brains.

As far as we know, there has been no published studies that used the 1D CNN structure for tfMRI feature learning. Thus the most suitable length of the filter in each layer remains to be explored. Nonetheless, we conducted a variety of preliminary experiments, and have empirically chosen the filter length according to the recon-struction errors, as well as the performances in our validation studies. The results of our extensive experiments suggested that when the filters in the first layer have about twice the length than the filters in upper layers, it will obtain satisfactory results in both of reconstruction performance and our validation experiments. The parameters in this proposed model are optimized by minimizing the cost function in Eq. 5. Training was performed by utilizing GPU (NVidia Quadro M4000) for 20 epochs. It took approx-imately 40 min for training the DCAE model.

Table 1. Feature map number and filter length settings in this study.

Feature map/filter	Layer1	Layer2	Layer3	Layer4
Encoder	32/21	64/9	128/9	256/9
Decoder	128/9	64/9	32/9	1/21

2.4 Building Theoretical Models of Brain Responses

We use theoretical models of brain responses to validate the hierarchical feature maps learned by DCAE. Specifically, we aim to figure out whether the feature maps learned by DCAE model are associated with the real functional brain activities. In traditional studies, the theoretical brain responses (theoretical regressors) are generated by directly convoluting stimulus function (task stimulus design) with a hemodynamic response function (HRF) (Eq. 6), as shown in Fig. 2(a).

$$r_0(t) = h(t) * s(t) \tag{6}$$

where $r_0(t)$ is the basic task paradigm regressor which represents the dominant brain response pattern, $s(t)$ is the stimulus pattern, and $h(t)$ is the hemodynamic response function, respectively. Though useful, previous studies have limitations in interpreting neural activities due to that they assume a task stimulus only has one form of brain response. Meanwhile, in other studies, researchers have reported that the human brain processes information in a hierarchical way [4], and the responses of human brain are very rich and variable, even under the same stimulus condition. Inspired by these studies, we propose a novel method based on the idea that the variety of brain responses are the transformation forms of the basic theoretical response (Fig. 2b). Specifically, we extended the basic theoretical regressors into regressor groups via delay, derivative, integral, anti (inversed) operations, which are the most common transforms in signal processing. After extension, the regressor groups could contain a variety of possible functional human responses. We treat these theoretical models as the benchmarks of underlying neural activities and compare them with the feature maps learned by DCAE. The detailed comparisons will be discussed in the results section.

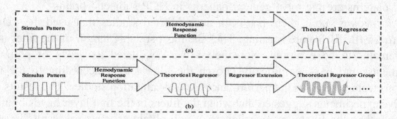

Fig. 2. Generating theoretical models of brain responses. (a) Traditional method and (b) our proposed method.

2.5 High-Level and Shallow Sparse Dictionary Learning

In addition to the validation study on feature maps, another validation study we conducted is the comparison between high-level sparse dictionary learning (HL-SDL) and shallow sparse dictionary learning (SL-SDL). Sparse Dictionary Learning (SDL) is an unsupervised learning algorithm which aims to find a basis set (dictionaries) in data along with its corresponding coefficients to sparsely represent the data. In fMRI, the coefficients are the spatial distribution of the corresponding functional networks [3]. Traditionally, the SDL is directly applied on fMRI data (denoted as SL-SDL in this study) and assumes that fMRI data could be linearly separated as dictionaries and their spatial distributions. Unlike traditional methods, we use the high-level representation obtained by DCAE (denoted as HL-SDL in this study) and do the same task as shallow SDL. Figure 3 illustrates the difference between SL-SDL and HL-SDL we proposed here. It should be noted here that during training, we set the final hidden state in the encoder has the same dimension size as the original fMRI time series, and we ensure that all the parameter settings of SL-SDL and HL-SDL are the same.

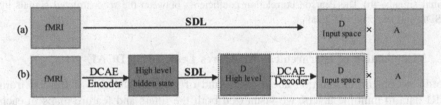

Fig. 3. (a) Shallow sparse dictionary learning, (b) high-level sparse dictionary learning. D is the learned basis set (dictionaries), and A is the corresponding matrix of coefficients.

3 Experimental Results

The DCAE model, HL-SDL and SL-SDL in this study are trained on six randomly selected HCP subjects tfMRI datasets, which contains 1,207,308 tfMRI time series. All of the results are evaluated on the separate validation datasets (the subject that were not used in training).

3.1 DCAE Reconstruction Error Analysis

First, to quantitatively examine the signal reconstruction ability of DCAE, the Pearson correlation coefficients between original tfMRI signals and reconstructed signals in the validation data were calculated. Figure 4a and b are the reconstruction results of DCAE and SL-SDL, respectively. Although both of the methods reconstructed the original signals quite well (most of the correlations are larger than 0.9), we can still see two main differences. First, DCAE has significantly better reconstruction performance (higher average correlations) compared to SL-SDL, as shown in Fig. 4. Second, when using DCAE to reconstruct the whole brain signals, there is a clear boundary between adjacent brain areas (highlighted with black arrows), while there is a less similar observation in SL-SDL.

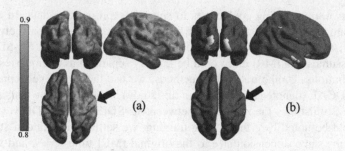

Fig. 4. Comparison of the performance in reconstructing the fMRI signals by different methods. (a) The Pearson correlation coefficients between the reconstructed signals by DCAE and the original signals. (b) The Pearson correlation coefficients between the reconstructed signals by SL-SDL and the original signals.

3.2   Visualization of Hierarchical Structures Learned by DCAE

In order to obtain an intuition about what kind of patterns DCAE has learned from tfMRI data in multiple layers, we visualized both the filters and feature maps in each layer. Figure 5(1) shows all 32 filters in the first layer and 16 randomly selected filters in other four layers. The filters in the first layer summarized the most common sub-shapes of tfMRI time series. For example, #B2 in Fig. 5(1) is a filter similar to bowl-shaped patterns in input data, #B3 is a single hemodynamic response shape, #B7 looks like a sin function pattern in tfMRI, and #D3 looks like a cos function models. Other filters such as #A1, #A8, #C8, #D7, and #D8 have reasonable, interpretable patterns. It is clear that DCAE has learned the low-frequency task-related filters in an unsupervised manner. Also, high-frequency filters can also be found, such as #A6, #B6, and #C1. For other layers visualized in Fig. 5(2)–(4), it is harder to tell, as their patterns are learned in higher levels. To further investigate the properties of higher layers, we focus on visualizing the feature maps. We utilized a technique called DeconvNet [15], which projected these mid-level and high-level feature maps back into

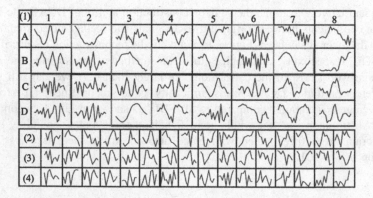

Fig. 5. (1)–(4) are the filters from layer 1 to layer 4. In (1), the filter rows are indexed with A–B and the columns are indexed with value 1–8.

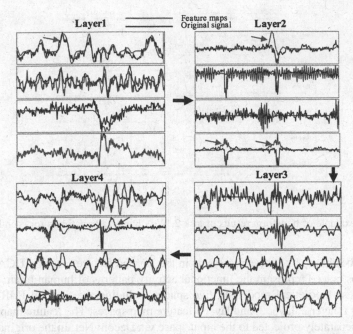

Fig. 6. Visualization of randomly selected 4 feature maps in each layer. The feature maps were projected (via the DeconvNet method) to the input space for visualization and comparison. Green arrows highlight some representative feature maps. (Color figure online)

the input space, to see what kinds of input will cause the activations. Figure 6 shows the 4 randomly selected feature maps with their original signals in each layer. A clear trend can be observed here. That is, in the first layer, all the feature maps have positive correlations with the original signals. We can postulate that the first layer focuses on modeling the shapes of tfMRI signals. While in the second layer, we observed the inverse correlation (highlighted with green arrows), which suggests that DCAE begins to have a logical abstraction of the input. When the depth increases, e.g., in the third layer and fourth layer, the feature maps become more complex. It is not just modeling the shapes and simple logics of the input, but we can also observe patterns with multiple frequencies in one feature map.

3.3   Interpreting Feature Maps via Theoretical Models of Brain Responses

In addition to the intuition about hierarchical structures in Sect. 3.2, we also aim to interpret the complex feature maps obtained by DCAE in a more rigorous, neuroscientifically meaningful way by utilizing the theoretical models in Sect. 2.5. As there are six basic stimulus patterns in the motor task, for each basic design, we obtained 42 types of transformations. Figure 7 shows the transform results of task 2. These theoretical models (regressors) are considered as benchmarks of the underlying brain activities.

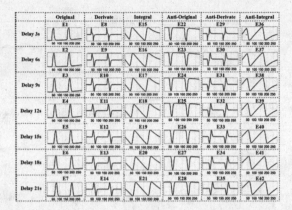

Fig. 7. An example of transform results of task 2. We obtain 42 transforms for each basic task

We should be able to find these regressors in the learned feature maps by DCAE, if the feature maps indeed represent the functional activity patterns of human brain. Thus we searched these theoretical models in five spaces including the original fMRI signals space, layer 1, layer 2, layer 3, and layer 4 feature map spaces. The feature maps in each layer were separately projected to the input space via DeconvNet. In the original signals space, the Pearson correlations between the theoretical models and all the voxel signals in the validation data were calculated, and the corresponding theoretical model is considered to be found once it has a voxel signal that has the correlation lager than 0.55 (empirically and experimentally determined). Figure 8 shows the correlation matrix in the original signal space. The correlation matrix is thresholded with 0.55, its x axis denotes the basic task design index, the y axis denotes the transform index of corresponding task (42 for each basic task), and the yellow block means the theoretical model is found. We can conclude from this result that the theoretical models widely exist in tfMRI signals. It is interesting that although the original signals are quite noisy, we still found 22 theoretical models.

Figure 8 shows the correlation matrices for layer 1 to layer 4 spaces. The correlations are calculated between the projected feature maps (in the validation data) and the

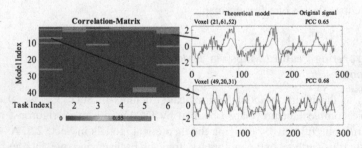

Fig. 8. Searching theoretical models in the original input space. The left subfigure shows the correlation matrix, where the deep color blue indicates the design patterns are not found in original signals space. (Color figure online)

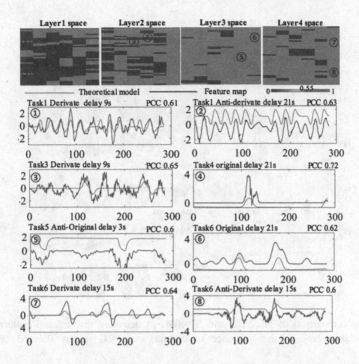

Fig. 9. Searching the theoretical models from layer 1 to layer 4, respectively. Corresponding feature maps and theoretical models were highlighted with red numbers. (Color figure online)

theoretical models. To ensure different layers are comparable, we limit our search space to the top 6000 feature maps with the highest activation values in each layer. A trend can be clearly observed: when the depth increases, more theoretical models are found in the feature maps. In summary, we found 35.7%, 48.4%, 53.6%, and 61.1% of theoretical models from layer 1 to layer 4, respectively. This experiment demonstrated that feature maps in DCAE are not randomly generated, but they are representations of underlying brain activities, and when the depth increases, its ability increase too (Fig. 9).

3.4 Comparison of HL-SDL and SL-SDL

In addition to analyzing feature maps in each layer, we also performed a validation study on the hidden state on the top layer of the encoder, called HL-SDL. Figure 3 already summarized the computational framework of HL-SDL and SL-SDL. Briefly, except that the input is different, the parameter settings for HL-SDL and SL-SDL are the same. Both models learned 400 dictionaries with 0.7 sparsity regularizer. As the original fMRI signal length is 284, to keep the dimensions, we set the output of the encoder in DCAE as 284. After training, the high-level features are decomposed as high-level dictionaries and corresponding spatial distributions. Then we use the decoder to project these high-level dictionaries (time series patterns) back to signal space. Figure 10 shows the results of task-related patterns. Although SL-SDL has

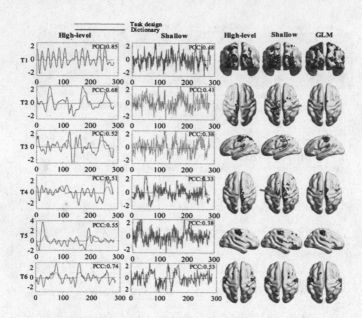

Fig. 10. The comparison of HL-SDL and SL-SDL in detecting task related patterns. GLM results are shown here as the reference of comparison. PCC means Pearson correlation coefficient.

learned all the six task patterns, these patterns are mixed with a large number of random noises, and their correlation values with task design are quite small (see PCCs in Fig. 10). On the other hand, the HL-SDL contained much less noises in both of the time series patterns and spatial maps. Combining this with the results in Sect. 3.3, we can conclude that the DCAE model filters noises in each layer, and at the same time, it keeps the relevant information of brain activities. In addition to these basic task-related patterns, we also observed more meaningful patterns in HL-SDL compared to SL-SDL. For example, some theoretical models we proposed in Sect. 2.4 can also be found, as shown in Fig. 11 with examples.

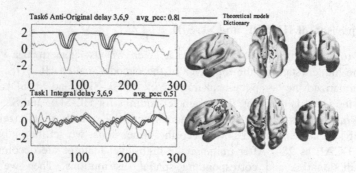

Fig. 11. Patterns that are only found in HL-SDL. avg_pc in this figure denotes the average correlation between the group of theoretical models and dictionary patterns.

4   Discussion and Conclusion

In this work, we proposed a novel variant of the convolutional neural network (CNN) - the deep convolutional autoencoder (DCAE). Our DCAE hierarchically models tfMRI data in an unsupervised manner. We used the HCP motor task as a testing bed in this study, and our experiments showed promising results. We summarize our results as three interesting observations. (1) By visualizing DCAE model, we found the feature maps gain a higher level abstraction of the fMRI signal along with the model depth increasing. (2) By using theoretical models of brain responses, we confirmed that the feature maps are not randomly generated, and the depth greatly influences the chance to find these theoretical models. (3) The comparison study of shallow sparse dictionary learning and the high-level dictionary learning showed that the high-level features are superior in task-related regions detection. At the same time, more intrinsic networks could be detected compared to traditional shallow sparse dictionary learning. In our future works, we will conduct more investigations into the feature maps learned by DCAE, and develop novel methods to examine spatial distributions of these feature maps on the entire brain, to provide more neuroscientific insights of the DCAE. We will also apply DCAE on clinical fMRI datasets to potentially reveal the altered brain network architectures in brain disorders.

References

1. Frston, K.J., et al.: Statistical parametric maps in functional imaging: a general linear approach. Hum. Brain Mapp. **2**, 189–210 (1995)
2. McKeown, M.J., Sejnowski, T.J.: Independent component analysis of fMRI data: examining the assumptions. Hum. Brain Mapp. **6**, 368–372 (1998)
3. Lv, J., et al.: Holistic atlases of functional networks and interactions reveal reciprocal organizational architecture of cortical function. IEEE TBME. **62**, 1120–1131 (2015)
4. Meunier, D., et al.: Hierarchical modularity in human brain functional networks. Front. Hum. Neurosci. **3**, 1–12 (2009)
5. Ferrarini, L., et al.: Hierarchical functional modularity in the resting-state human brain. Hum. Brain Mapp. **30**, 2220–2231 (2009)
6. Schmidhuber, J.J.: Deep learning in neural networks: an overview. Neural Netw. **61**, 85–117 (2014)
7. Bengio, Y., Courville, A., Vincent, P.: Representation learning: a review and new perspectives. IEEE Trans. Pattern Anal. Mach. Intell. **35**, 1798–1828 (2012)
8. Plis, S.M., et al.: Deep learning for neuroimaging: a validation study. Front. Neurosci. **8**, 1–11 (2014)
9. Suk, H.-I., et al.: State-space model with deep learning for functional dynamics estimation in resting-state fMRI. Neuroimage **129**, 292–307 (2016)
10. Huang, H., Hu, X., Han, J., Lv, J., Liu, N., Guo, L., Liu, T.: Latent source mining in FMRI data via deep neural network (2016)
11. De Valois, R.L., William Yund, E., Hepler, N.: The orientation and direction selectivity of cells in macaque visual cortex. Vis. Res. **22**, 531–544 (1982)
12. Nair, V., Hinton, G.E.: Rectified linear units improve restricted Boltzmann machines. In: Proceedings of the 27th ICML, pp. 807–814 (2010)

13. Aguirre, G.K., Zarahn, E., D'esposito, M.: The variability of human BOLD hemodynamic responses. Neuroimage **8**, 360–369 (1998)
14. Friston, K.J., Harrison, L., Penny, W.: Dynamic causal modelling. Neuroimage **19**, 1273–1302 (2003)
15. Zeiler, M.D., Fergus, R.: Visualizing and understanding convolutional networks. In: Fleet, D., Pajdla, T., Schiele, B., Tuytelaars, T. (eds.) ECCV 2014. LNCS, vol. 8689, pp. 818–833. Springer, Cham (2014). doi:10.1007/978-3-319-10590-1_53
16. Zhao, J., Mathieu, M., Goroshin, R., Lecun, Y.: Stacked what-where auto-encoders. arXiv Prepr. arXiv:1506.02351 (2015)

Diffusion Imaging

Director Field Analysis to Explore Local White Matter Geometric Structure in Diffusion MRI

Jian Cheng$^{(\boxtimes)}$ and Peter J. Basser$^{(\boxtimes)}$

SQITS, NIBIB, NICHD, National Institutes of Health, Bethesda, USA
jian.cheng@nih.gov, pjbasser@helix.nih.gov

Abstract. In diffusion MRI, a tensor field or a spherical function field, e.g., an Orientation Distribution Function (ODF) field, are estimated from measured diffusion weighted images. In this paper, inspired by microscopic theoretical treatment of phases in liquid crystals, we introduce a novel mathematical framework, called Director Field Analysis (DFA), to study local geometric structural information of white matter from the estimated tensor field or spherical function field. (1) We propose Orientational Order (OO) and Orientational Dispersion (OD) indices to describe the degree of alignment and dispersion of a spherical function in each voxel; (2) We estimate a local orthogonal coordinate frame in each voxel with anisotropic diffusion; (3) Finally, we define three indices to describe three types of orientational distortion (splay, bend, and twist) in a local spatial neighborhood, and a total distortion index to describe distortions of all three types. To our knowledge, this is the first work to *quantitatively* describe orientational distortion (splay, bend, and twist) in diffusion MRI. The proposed scalar indices are useful to detect local geometric changes of white matter for voxel-based or tract-based analysis in both DTI and HARDI acquisitions.

1 Introduction

Diffusion MRI is a unique non-invasive imaging technique to explore white matter in human brain. Diffusion Tensor Imaging (DTI) [3] is used to reconstruct a tensor field from diffusion weighted images (DWIs). High Angular Resolution Diffusion Imaging [13], without the assumption of Gaussian diffusion, is used to reconstruct a general function field from DWIs, e.g., an Orientation Distribution Function (ODF) or Ensemble Average Propagator (EAP) field. Exploring meaningful information from the reconstructed tensor field or spherical function field is of interest in many application areas, which makes diffusion MRI a powerful means to study white matter.

Some scalar indices have been proposed to be estimated voxel-wise from tensors/ODFs/EAPs. For DTI, the mean diffusivity and Fractional Anisotropy (FA) are widely used biologically meaningful descriptors [8]. For HARDI, the generalized FA [13], Orientation Dispersion (OD) [14], etc., were proposed for ODFs and EAPs. Some existing works have extracted local geometric information by considering spatial gradients of tensor field. [7] demonstrated that the norm of

© Springer International Publishing AG 2017
M. Niethammer et al. (Eds.): IPMI 2017, LNCS 10265, pp. 427–439, 2017.
DOI: 10.1007/978-3-319-59050-9_34

the spatial gradient of the tensor field can be useful for detecting boundaries between white matter, CSF and grey matter. [5] proposed tangents of scalar invariants and rotation tangents which are 2nd order tensors, and also proposed projecting the 3rd order spatial gradient tensor onto these 2nd order tangents to obtain the spatial direction with the largest change of scalar indices or rotation of tensors. Based on the rotation tangents of tensors, [10] proposed fiber curving and fiber dispersion indices. These studies are all based on spatial gradients of tensor fields from DTI. However, to our knowledge, there is no work making connections between general spherical function fields from HARDI data and local geometric structure (splay, bend and twist) of white matter.

Torsion and curvature of a fiber tract [2] were proposed based on the Frenet frame along the tract. [12] used Frenet frame as a prior to regularize the data and estimate ODFs in voxels. These works on the Frenet frame studied geometric information along a single tract. However, tractography is known to be sensitive to a large number of parameters, and any flaws in the reconstructed tracts due to noise or parameter selection will inevitably be reflected in the subsequently extracted geometric information. [9] proposed moving frames determined by the geometry of cardiac data, and calculated Maurer-Cartan connections. However this method cannot work for general diffusion MRI data, and did not consider the sign ambiguity in the frame.

Orientational order parameter is well-established to describe the degree of alignment in liquid crystals [1]. [11] calculated the order parameter map by estimating variance of microscopic diffusion parameters from the contrast between signals measured by directional and isotropic diffusion encoding. However, it cannot be used for general DTI and HARDI data.

In this paper, inspired by theoretical analysis of orientation and distortion for liquid crystals, we propose a unified framework, called Director Field Analysis (DFA), to study local geometric information of white matter. DFA works for both tensor field from DTI and spherical function field from HARDI. At the voxel level, (1) the Orientational Order index (OO) is defined for the spherical function in voxel with a given axis, e.g., the ODF with the principal direction, and the Orientational Dispersion index (OD) is defined as $1 - OO$. (2) The principal direction is extracted from the spherical function in a anisotropic voxel. In a local neighborhood level, (1) a local orthogonal frame is defined for each anisotropic voxel with the first axis as the extracted principal direction; (2) three distortion indices (splay, bend, twist) and a total distortion index are defined based on spatial directional derivatives of the principal direction.

2   Method: Director Field Analysis

2.1   Orientational Order and Dispersion

The NODDI model is increasingly used to study neurite orientation dispersion [14]. NODDI uses the Watson distribution in Eq. (1) to model the orientation distribution function with a single orientation,

$$f(\mathbf{u} \mid \boldsymbol{n}) = \frac{1}{4\pi \, M(1/2, 3/2, \kappa)} \exp(\kappa(\mathbf{u}^T \boldsymbol{n})^2), \qquad \mathbf{u} \in \mathbb{S}^2 \tag{1}$$

where M is the confluent hypergeometric function, $\boldsymbol{n} \in \mathbb{S}^2$ is a given axis. Note that the original formula in [14], which has no unit integral in $\mathbb{S}^2$, missed 4π. An orientation dispersion index (OD) was defined as $\mathrm{OD}_w = \frac{2}{\pi} \arctan(\frac{1}{\kappa})$, where we denote it as OD_w because it can not be used for ODFs with general shapes, with more than one peak.

For a general spherical function $f(\mathbf{u}), \mathbf{u} \in \mathbb{S}^2$, we propose the *orientational order index (OO)* from the theory of liquid crystals [1][1] to describe the orientation or dispersion of a general spherical function along a given axis $\boldsymbol{n}$:

$$\mathrm{OO}(\boldsymbol{n}) = \int_{\mathbf{u} \in \mathbb{S}^2} P_2(\mathbf{u}^T \boldsymbol{n}) f(\mathbf{u}) \mathrm{d}S = \int_{\mathbb{S}^2} \frac{3(\mathbf{u}^T \boldsymbol{n})^2 - 1}{2} f(\mathbf{u}) \mathrm{d}S \tag{2}$$

where P_2 is the second-order Legendre polynomial. By definition Eq. (2) is an *integral transform* in $\mathbb{S}^2$ which converts $f(\mathbf{u})$ to another spherical function $\mathrm{OO}(\boldsymbol{n})$, and the kernel is $P_2(\mathbf{u}^T \boldsymbol{n})$, similar to the Funk-Radon transform used in Q-Ball imaging [13], where the kernel is $\delta(\mathbf{u}^T \boldsymbol{n})$. We call Eq. (2) the *Orientational Order Transform (OOT)*. Although $\mathrm{OO}(\boldsymbol{n})$ is a spherical function, it is a scalar index when $\boldsymbol{n}$ is chosen as a physically meaningful axis, e.g., $f(\mathbf{u})$ takes its maximal value at $\boldsymbol{n}$. Let θ be the angle between $\mathbf{u}$ and axis $\boldsymbol{n}$, then $P_2(\mathbf{u}^T \boldsymbol{n}) = \frac{3\cos^2 \theta - 1}{2}$. Thus if $f(\mathbf{u})$ is a Probability Density Function (PDF) in sphere, then OO is $\langle \frac{3\cos^2 \theta - 1}{2} \rangle$, where $\langle \cdot \rangle$ signifies the expectation operation. $\langle \cos^2 \theta \rangle$ is the expectation of squared projected length of $\mathbf{u}$ onto the axis $\boldsymbol{n}$. By definition, when $f(\mathbf{u})$ is a PDF, then we have $\mathrm{OO} \in [-0.5, 1]$. If $f(\mathbf{u}) = \delta(\mathbf{u}^T \boldsymbol{n} - 1)$, i.e. the delta function along $\boldsymbol{n}$ axis, then $\mathrm{OO} = 1$. If $f(\mathbf{u}) = 0$, $\forall \mathbf{u} \in \mathbb{S}^2$ such that $\mathbf{u}^T \boldsymbol{n} \neq 0$, then $\mathrm{OO} = -0.5$. If $f(\mathbf{u})$ is the isotropic PDF, i.e. $f(\mathbf{u}) = \frac{1}{4\pi}$, then $\mathrm{OO} = 0$. In practice, if we choose the axis $\boldsymbol{n}$ such that $f(\mathbf{u})$ takes its global maximal value, then OO is normally non-negative. We define the *orientational dispersion*, $\mathrm{OD} = 1 - \mathrm{OO}$. Then $\mathrm{OD} \in [0, 1.5]$.

Axisymmetric Spherical Functions. When $f(\mathbf{u})$ is axisymmetric, and its axis is given by $\boldsymbol{n}_0$, i.e., $f(\mathbf{u}) = f'(\mathbf{u}^T \boldsymbol{n}_0)$, where $f'(x)$ is the corresponding scalar function defined in $[-1, 1]$, then OOT has a closed form:

$$\mathrm{OO}(\boldsymbol{n}) = \int_0^\pi \left(\int_0^{2\pi} P_2(\cos\theta \cos t + \sin\theta \cos t \sin\phi) \mathrm{d}t \right) f'(\cos\theta) \mathrm{d}\theta$$
$$= \frac{(1 + 3\cos(2\phi))\pi}{2} a_2 = \frac{1 + 3\cos(2\phi)}{4} \mathrm{OO}(\boldsymbol{n}_0) \tag{3}$$

where $\phi = \arccos(|\boldsymbol{n}^T \boldsymbol{n}_0|)$ is the angle between $\boldsymbol{n}$ and the axis $\boldsymbol{n}_0$, and $a_2 = \int_{-1}^1 P_2(x) f'(x) \mathrm{d}x$ is the second-order Legendre coefficient of $f'(x)$. Note that if $a_2 > 0$, when $\boldsymbol{n} = \boldsymbol{n}_0$, $\phi = 0$, then $\mathrm{OO} = 2\pi a_2$ is the global maximum of $\mathrm{OO}(\boldsymbol{n})$.

---

[1] https://en.wikipedia.org/wiki/Liquid_crystal.

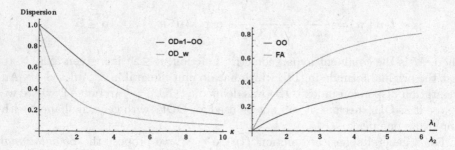

Fig. 1. Left: dispersion indices of a Watson distribution as functions of κ. Right: OO and FA of prolate tensors ($\lambda_2 = \lambda_3$) as functions of $\frac{\lambda_1}{\lambda_2}$.

In the following paper, without any ambiguity, we will use OO to denote $OO(n_0)$ for axisymmetric spherical functions.

Watson Distributions. The Watson distribution defined in Eq. (1) is axisymmetric with the axis n_0. Thus, based on the above analysis of axisymmetric spherical functions, we have $OO(n) = \frac{1+3\cos(2\phi)}{4}OO$, and

$$OO = \frac{3e^{\kappa}}{2\sqrt{\kappa\pi}\,\mathrm{Erfi}(\sqrt{\kappa})} - \frac{3+2\kappa}{4\kappa} \tag{4}$$

where $\mathrm{Erfi}(x) = \frac{2}{\sqrt{\pi}}\int_0^x \exp(t^2)\mathrm{d}t$ is the imaginary error function. Then $OD = 1 - OO$. The left part of Fig. 1 shows the above OD and OD_w as functions of κ, where the axis n is set as the Watson distribution's axis. Both dispersion indices decrease as κ increases. Based on the derivation of κ, OD_w is more sensitive for changes of κ when κ is small (<2), while it is less sensitive when κ is large (>2). Compared with OD_w, the change of OD is smoother for the change of κ over the entire range of κ.

Tensors. For a tensor $\mathbf{D}$ in DTI, OOT is defined for its ODF, i.e.,

$$\Phi(\mathbf{u} \mid \mathbf{D}) = \frac{1}{4\pi|\mathbf{D}|^{\frac{1}{2}}} \frac{1}{(\mathbf{u}^T \mathbf{D}^{-1} \mathbf{u})^{\frac{3}{2}}}. \tag{5}$$

which is a PDF on the unit sphere. When the three eigenvalues of $\mathbf{D}$ satisfies $\lambda_1 > \lambda_2 = \lambda_3 > 0$, $\Phi(\mathbf{u} \mid \mathbf{D})$ is axisymmetric with the axis v_1 that is the principal eigenvector of $\mathbf{D}$. OOT has a closed-form expression in Eq. (3), and

$$OO = \frac{\sqrt{\lambda_1 - \lambda_2}(2\lambda_1 + \lambda_2) - 3\lambda_1\sqrt{\lambda_2}\arctan\left(\sqrt{\frac{\lambda_1-\lambda_2}{\lambda_2}}\right)}{2(\lambda_1 - \lambda_2)^{\frac{3}{2}}}. \tag{6}$$

The right panel of Fig. 1 shows OO and FA as functions of λ_1/λ_2, where we set $n = v_1$. Both OO and FA increases as λ_1/λ_2 increases. Thus OO can be seen as a type of anisotropy index for tensors. For general tensors with $\lambda_1 > \lambda_2 > \lambda_3$, no such closed form solution like Eqs. (6) and (3) exist, but we can calculate OO using the spherical harmonic representation of the ODF.

Spherical Harmonic Representation. For a general spherical function $f(\mathbf{u})$, OO and OD can be analytically calculated from its rotated spherical harmonic coefficients. Considering $f(\mathbf{u})$ is a real function in sphere, it can always be linearly represented by the real Spherical Harmonic (SH) basis $\{Y_l^m(\mathbf{u})\}$, i.e., $f(\mathbf{u}) = \sum_{l,m} c_l^m Y_l^m(\mathbf{u})$, where $Y_l^m(\mathbf{u})$ is the real Spherical Harmonic (SH) basis. For any rotation matrix, the SH coefficients of the rotated function can be calculated with very high accuracy based on Wigner D-matrix[2], or based on fitting rotated function samples [6]. Let $\mathbf{R}$ be the rotation matrix which rotates the axis $\mathbf{n}$ to z-axis, and $\{a_l^m\}$ be the real SH coefficients of the rotated function $(Rf)(\mathbf{u}) = f(\mathbf{R}^{-1}\mathbf{u})$, considering the orthogonality of real SH basis and $Y_2^0(\theta, \phi) = \sqrt{\frac{5}{4\pi}} P_2(\cos\theta)$, we have

$$OO(\mathbf{n}) = \int_{\mathbf{u}\in\mathbb{S}^2} P_2(\mathbf{u}^T \mathbf{n}) f(\mathbf{u}) dS = \int_{\mathbf{u}\in\mathbb{S}^2} P_2(\cos\theta) \sum_{l,m} a_l^m Y_l^m(\theta,\phi) dS = \sqrt{\frac{4\pi}{5}} a_2^0 \quad (7)$$

Note that $OO(\mathbf{n})$ is only determined by the rotated SH coefficient a_2^0 which is only related to $\{c_2^m\}_{-2\leq m\leq 2}$ and the axis $\mathbf{n}$, based on the property of the SH basis. Thus $OO(\mathbf{n})$ is only related to the SH coefficients of $f(\mathbf{u})$ with $l = 2$.

Mixture Model. OOT in Eq. (2) is a linear transform. Thus if $f(\mathbf{u}) = \sum_i w_i f_i(\mathbf{u})$ is the ODF of a mixture of models, where $f_i(\mathbf{u})$ is the ODF for the i-th model, and w_i is the weight, then $OO(\mathbf{n}) = \sum_i w_i OO_i(\mathbf{n})$ is a mixture of OO functions. Figure 2 illustrates OO for a two-tensor model with a crossing angle ϕ, where two tensors share the same eigenvalues $[1.7, 0.2, 0.2] \times 10^{-3}\,\mathrm{mm}^2/\mathrm{s}$, the weights are 0.5 and 0.5, and one tensor component is along y-axis and the other one rotates from y-axis to x-axis. Based on Eqs. (3) and (6), OO for the mixture model can be analytically calculated.

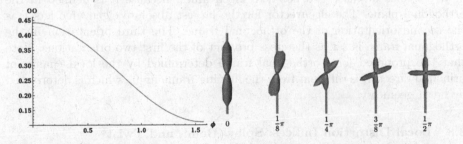

Fig. 2. OO for mixture tensor model. Left: OO as a function of the angle between two tensor components. Right: ODF glyphs for different crossing angles, where the yellow tube shows the y-axis to calculate OO. (Color figure online)

---

[2] https://en.wikipedia.org/wiki/Spherical_harmonics.

2.2   Director and Local Orthogonal Frame

In a voxel with anisotropic diffusion, the orientations where the anisotropic ODF takes its local peak (i.e., local maximal values) are normally considered as local fiber directions in that voxel. A normal peak detection algorithm for ODFs performs a grid search in a spherical mesh, then refines the solution using a gradient ascent on the continuous sphere. In order to avoid including small peaks produced by noise, only peaks whose value larger than a threshold percentage (e.g., 0.5) of the largest ODF value are counted.

We define a *director* as a vector v which is equivalent to its negative $-v$. Normally ODFs are antipodally symmetric, thus a peak is a director. After peak detection, for each voxel x, we obtain a discrete spherical function $g(\mathbf{u}, x) = \sum_i f(\mathbf{u}_i, x)\delta(\mathbf{u} - \mathbf{u}_i)$ from the continuous spherical function $f(\mathbf{u}, x)$, where $\{\mathbf{u}_i\}$ are local peaks. This discrete spherical function field is called a *director field*, or *peak field*. We propose extracting a local orthogonal frame in each anisotropic voxel from the detected peak field. The orthogonal frame has three orthogonal orientations. The first orientation is the principal direction where the ODF takes its global maximum $\mathbf{u}_1$, i.e. $f(\mathbf{u}_1, x) > f(\mathbf{u}_i, x), \forall i \neq 1$. We call it the *principal director* of the anisotropic voxel. The other two orientations are in the orthogonal plane of the principal direction. Considering $f(\mathbf{u})$ is normally antipodally symmetric in diffusion MRI, all these orientations are equivalent with their antipodal ones. Thus, we define a weighted sum of dyadic tensors in voxel x:

$$T_x = \sum_{y \in \Omega_x} \sum_i w(y, x) f(\mathbf{u}_i, y)(\mathbf{u}_i - (\mathbf{u}_i^T \mathbf{u}_1)\mathbf{u}_1)(\mathbf{u}_i - (\mathbf{u}_i^T \mathbf{u}_1)\mathbf{u}_1)^T \quad (8)$$

where Ω_x is a local neighborhood of voxel x, $w(y, x)$ is the spatial weight which is normally set to be proportional to $\exp(-\frac{\|y-x\|^2}{2\sigma^2})$, δ which is normally set as 1 voxel controls spatial weight concentration, $(\mathbf{u}_i - (\mathbf{u}_i^T \mathbf{u}_1)\mathbf{u}_1)(\mathbf{u}_i - (\mathbf{u}_i^T \mathbf{u}_1)\mathbf{u}_1)^T$ is the outer product of the projected orientation $\mathbf{u}_i$ onto the orthogonal plane of $\mathbf{u}_1$. T_x has at most two non-zero eigenvalues, because it is defined in the orthogonal plane. The eigenvector for the largest absolute eigenvalue is set as the second orientation of the orthogonal frame. The third orientation in the orthogonal frame is set as the cross product of the first two orientations. Note that the proposed local orthogonal frame determined by the local change of principal director, is different from the moving frame in [9], which is determined by heart geometry.

2.3   Local Distortion Indices: Splay, Bend, and Twist

There are three types of distortions (see footnote 1) for the director field as demonstrated in Fig. 3. (1) *splay*: bending occurs perpendicular to the director. (2) *bend*: the distortion is parallel to the director and molecular axis. (3) *twist*: neighboring directors are rotated with respect to one another, rather than aligned. These three fundamental distortions can describe complex geometric patterns.

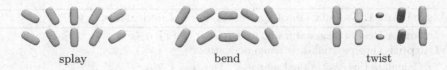

splay   bend   twist

Fig. 3. Demonstration of three types of distortions.

With the local orthogonal frame $\{\mathbf{u}_1(\boldsymbol{x}), \mathbf{u}_2(\boldsymbol{x}), \mathbf{u}_3(\boldsymbol{x})\}$ obtained at each anisotropic voxel $\boldsymbol{x}$, we propose three scalar indices to describe the three types of local orientational distortions of white matter, and a total distortion index as:

$$\text{Splay index:} \quad s = \sqrt{(\mathbf{u}_2^T \frac{\partial \mathbf{u}_1}{\partial \mathbf{u}_2})^2 + (\mathbf{u}_3^T \frac{\partial \mathbf{u}_1}{\partial \mathbf{u}_3})^2} \tag{9}$$

$$\text{Bend index:} \quad b = \sqrt{(\mathbf{u}_2^T \frac{\partial \mathbf{u}_1}{\partial \mathbf{u}_1})^2 + (\mathbf{u}_3^T \frac{\partial \mathbf{u}_1}{\partial \mathbf{u}_1})^2} \tag{10}$$

$$\text{Twist index:} \quad t = \sqrt{(\mathbf{u}_2^T \frac{\partial \mathbf{u}_1}{\partial \mathbf{u}_3})^2 + (\mathbf{u}_3^T \frac{\partial \mathbf{u}_1}{\partial \mathbf{u}_2})^2} \tag{11}$$

$$\text{Total distortion index:} \quad d = \sqrt{s^2 + b^2 + t^2} \tag{12}$$

where $\frac{\partial \mathbf{u}_1}{\partial \mathbf{u}_i}$, $i = 1, 2, 3$, is the spatial directional derivative of director field $\mathbf{u}_1(\boldsymbol{x})$ respectively along $\mathbf{u}_i$, i.e.,

$$\frac{\partial \mathbf{u}_1}{\partial \mathbf{u}_i} = \lim_{k \to 0} \frac{\mathbf{u}_1(\boldsymbol{x} + k\mathbf{u}_i) - \mathbf{u}_1(\boldsymbol{x} - k\mathbf{u}_i)}{2k} \tag{13}$$

We define these indices using squared value of $\mathbf{u}_j^T \frac{\partial \mathbf{u}_1}{\partial \mathbf{u}_i}$ to avoid the sign ambiguity of $\{\mathbf{u}_i\}$ and $\{\frac{\partial \mathbf{u}_1}{\partial \mathbf{u}_i}\}$.

It is challenging to numerically calculate the three spatial directional derivatives $\{\frac{\partial \mathbf{u}_1}{\partial \mathbf{u}_i}\}$, because the extracted local coordinate frame $\{\mathbf{u}_i(\boldsymbol{x})\}$ is ambiguous with respect to its sign. In other words, $\mathbf{u}_i$ is equivalent to $-\mathbf{u}_i$. We propose calculating the above spatial directional derivatives using rotation matrices. See Algorithm 1. The algorithm first calculates three rotation matrices respectively along x, y, z axes, which is analogous to the spatial gradient of a vector field. Then $\frac{\partial \mathbf{u}_1}{\partial \mathbf{u}_i}$ is numerically approximated by $\mathbf{u}_1(\boldsymbol{x} + \mathbf{u}_i) - \mathbf{u}_1(\boldsymbol{x} - \mathbf{u}_i)$, where $\mathbf{u}_1(\boldsymbol{x} + \mathbf{u}_i)$ and $\mathbf{u}_1(\boldsymbol{x} - \mathbf{u}_i)$ are approximated by the weighted mean of three rotated vectors along three axes. After $\{\frac{\partial \mathbf{u}_1}{\partial \mathbf{u}_i}\}$ are obtained, we can calculate the above four indices in Eqs. (9), (10), (11), and (12), from the directional derivatives.

3   Experiments

Synthetic Data Experiments. Figure 4 demonstrated these four distortion indices calculated from idealized tensor fields. The tensors were visualized using

---

Algorithm 1. Calculation of spatial directional derivatives.

Input: A local orthogonal frame field $\{\mathbf{u}_1(\boldsymbol{x}), \mathbf{u}_2(\boldsymbol{x}), \mathbf{u}_3(\boldsymbol{x})\}$
Output: Three spatial directional derivatives $\frac{\partial \mathbf{u}_1}{\partial \mathbf{u}_i}$, $i = 1, 2, 3$.
// Calculate three rotational matrices $\{M_i\}$, $i = 1, 2, 3$;
$\boldsymbol{o}_1 = [1, 0, 0]^T$, $\boldsymbol{o}_2 = [0, 1, 0]^T$, $\boldsymbol{o}_3 = [0, 0, 1]^T$;
for $i = 1, 2, 3$ **do**
$\quad$ | $\boldsymbol{v}_1 = \mathbf{u}_1(\boldsymbol{x} + \boldsymbol{o}_i)$, $\boldsymbol{v}_0 = \mathbf{u}_1(\boldsymbol{x} - \boldsymbol{o}_i)$;
$\quad$ | $\boldsymbol{v}_2 = (\boldsymbol{v}_1 + \boldsymbol{v}_0)/2$, $\boldsymbol{v}_2 = \frac{\boldsymbol{v}_2}{\|\boldsymbol{v}_2\|}$;
$\quad$ | Calculate rotation matrix $\mathbf{M}_i$ which rotates $\boldsymbol{v}_2$ to $\boldsymbol{v}_1$;
end
// Calculate spatial directional derivatives from rotation matrices ;
for $i = 1, 2, 3$ **do**
$\quad$ | **for** $j = 1, 2, 3$ **do**
$\quad\quad$ | $u_{i,j} = \mathbf{u}_i^T \boldsymbol{o}_j$;
$\quad\quad$ | **if** $u_{i,j} \geq 0$ **then**
$\quad\quad\quad$ | $\boldsymbol{p}_j = u_{i,j} \mathbf{M}_j \mathbf{u}_1$, $\boldsymbol{n}_j = u_{i,j} \mathbf{M}_j^T \mathbf{u}_1$;
$\quad\quad$ | **else**
$\quad\quad\quad$ | $\boldsymbol{p}_j = -u_{i,j} \mathbf{M}_j^T \mathbf{u}_1$, $\boldsymbol{n}_j = -u_{i,j} \mathbf{M}_j \mathbf{u}_1$;
$\quad\quad$ | **end**
$\quad$ | **end**
$\quad$ | $\boldsymbol{p}_0 = \boldsymbol{p}_1 + \boldsymbol{p}_2 + \boldsymbol{p}_3$, $\boldsymbol{p}_0 = \frac{\boldsymbol{p}_0}{\|\boldsymbol{p}_0\|}$;
$\quad$ | $\boldsymbol{n}_0 = \boldsymbol{n}_1 + \boldsymbol{n}_2 + \boldsymbol{n}_3$, $\boldsymbol{n}_0 = \frac{\boldsymbol{n}_0}{\|\boldsymbol{n}_0\|}$;
$\quad$ | **if** $\|\boldsymbol{p}_0 - \boldsymbol{n}_0\| \leq \|\boldsymbol{p}_0 + \boldsymbol{n}_0\|$ **then**
$\quad\quad$ | $\frac{\partial \mathbf{u}_1}{\partial \mathbf{u}_i} = \boldsymbol{p}_0 - \boldsymbol{n}_0$
$\quad$ | **else**
$\quad\quad$ | $\frac{\partial \mathbf{u}_1}{\partial \mathbf{u}_i} = \boldsymbol{p}_0 + \boldsymbol{n}_0$
$\quad$ | **end**
end

---

superquadric tensor glyphs. Figure 4 showed that (1) the four indices only depend on the orientations, not on the tensor or ODF shape; (2) splay, bend, twist indices provide complementary information about the orientational change, which demonstrate different types of orientational distortions. Note that the twist index for the third tensor field is actually a constant, the index value around the boundary is different due to the Neumann boundary condition used in the calculation. Although the results in Fig. 4 are for tensor fields, the distortion indices are actually determined by the local orthogonal frame field that can be calculated from a general spherical function field.

We compared the four distortion indices with the curving and dispersion indices proposed for tensor fields in [10]. The tensor field in Fig. 5 was used in [10]. It has three areas where the tensors rotate about its three eigenvectors respectively. Figure 5 shows that (1) splay index is similar with dispersion index, and bend index is similar with curving index; (2) the four distortion indices are

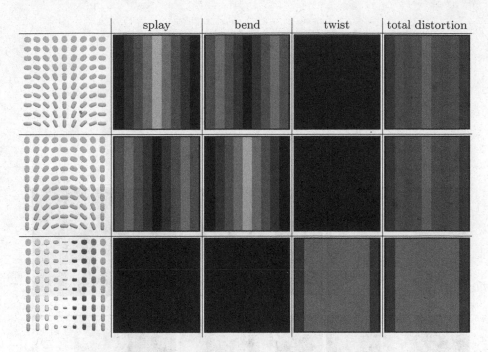

Fig. 4. Distortion indices calculated from different tensor fields.

independent of tensor shapes, while curving and dispersion indices are dependent on tensor shape; (3) when the principal directions are well aligned, all distortion indices are close to zero, because they are calculated based on the spatial difference of principal directions. Note that dispersion and curving indices in [10] are only for tensor fields, while the proposed distortion indices work for both tensor field and ODF field.

Real Data Experiments. The real data is from Human Connectome Project (HCP). It has three shells at $b = 1000, 2000, 3000 \, \text{s/mm}^2$, with 90 staggered directions per shell. Non-negative spherical deconvolution (NNSD) [4] was performed to estimate fiber ODFs from three shell DWI data. Peaks were detected from the estimated fODFs with GFA larger than 0.3. OO and OD were calculated from the spherical harmonic representation of fODFs along their principal peaks. Figure 6 demonstrated OO and OD maps from fODFs, and the total distortion map estimated from the local orthogonal frames of fODFs. The close-up views of fODFs, local orthogonal frames, the six proposed indices for the red region, which is the crossing area of Corpus Callosum and Fornix, were also visualized. The three orientations in the local orthogonal frame in each voxel were visualized using three tubes in red, blue and green color respectively. We performed whole brain streamline tractography on the fODF field using mrtrix[3]. The voxels with

---

[3] http://www.mrtrix.org.

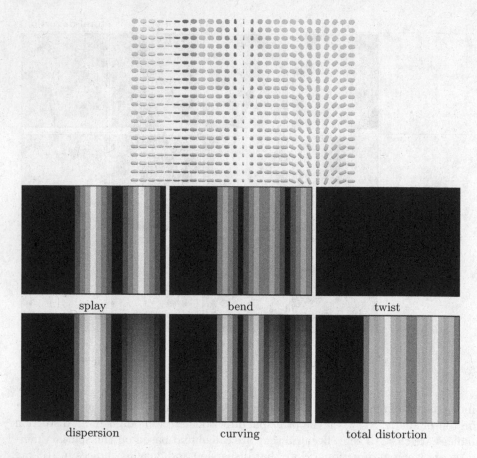

Fig. 5. Dispersion, curving [10], and the proposed four distortion indices calculated from a tensor field.

GFA larger than 0.3 were used as seed voxels to generate 10000 tracts by using tckgen in mrtrix. The obtained fiber tracts cross the red region were colored by the proposed six scalar indices and visualized using trackvis[4]. Figure 6 showed that (1) OO is high in anisotropic areas with well-aligned directions, while OD is high in isotropic or crossing areas. (2) the four distortion indices are low in areas with well aligned principal directions, and zero in isotropic voxels without peaks. (3) total distortion index is high in areas with highly curved fibers or crossing fibers. (4) Although splay, bend, twist indices may be separable (e.g., one is large while another one is close to zero) in synthetic data, in real data, these three types of distortions normally occur together, especially for bending and splaying.

---

[4] http://trackvis.org.

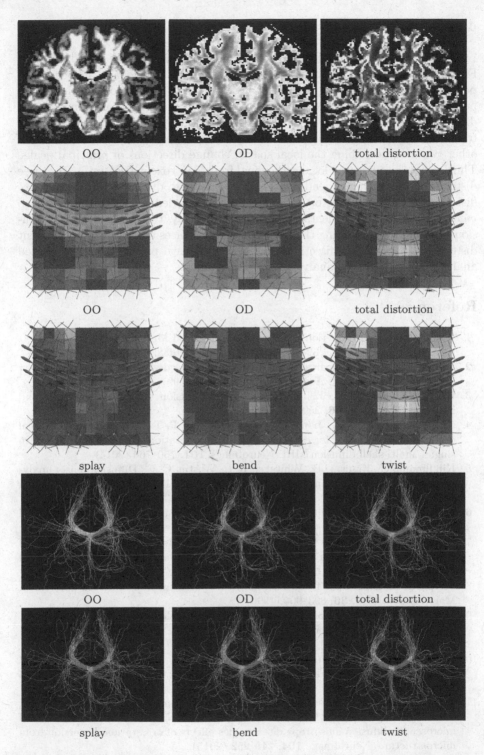

Fig. 6. First row: OO, OD and total distortion maps calculated from fODFs in multi-shell HCP data. 2–3 rows: the close-up views of fODFs, local orthogonal frames, the six proposed indices in the red region. 4–5 rows: fiber tracts cross the red region were colored by six indices. (Color figure online)

4 Conclusion

In this paper, we proposed a unified mathematical framework called Director Field Analysis (DFA) to analyze a spherical function field and its extracted peaks. First, we define the orientational order (OD) and the orientational dispersion (OD) indices in voxels. OD is more general and natural than previous dispersion index proposed in NODDI [14]. Second, we define a local orthogonal frame in each anisotropic voxel with the principal peak as its first axis, and the other two axes describing the local spatial change directions of principal peaks. Third, from the extracted local orthogonal frames in voxels, DFA estimates three distortion indices (splay, bend, twist) which is able to distinguish three types of distortions, and a total distortion index. To our knowledge, it is the first work to *quantitatively* describe orientational distortion (splay, twist, and bend) in diffusion MRI data. Considering the proposed scalar indices are sensitive to different distortions of principal directions, these indices have potential in voxel-based analysis and tract-based analysis for group studies.

References

1. Andrienko, D.: Introduction to Liquid Crystals, Bad Marienberg (2006). https://pdfs.semanticscholar.org/b241/d553a810d86fc6640cbf88b09d58ce54c57a.pdf
2. Basser, P.J.: New histological and physiological stains derived from diffusion-tensor MR images. Ann. N. Y. Acad. Sci. **820**, 123–138 (1997)
3. Basser, P.J., Mattiello, J., LeBihan, D.: MR diffusion tensor spectroscropy and imaging. Biophys. J. **66**, 259–267 (1994)
4. Cheng, J., Deriche, R., Jiang, T., Shen, D., Yap, P.-T.: Non-negative spherical deconvolution (NNSD) for estimation of fiber orientation distribution function in single-/multi-shell diffusion MRI. NeuroImage **101**, 750–764 (2014)
5. Kindlmann, G., Ennis, D.B., Whitaker, R.T., Westin, C.-F.: Diffusion tensor analysis with invariant gradients and rotation tangents. IEEE Trans. Med. Imaging **26**(11), 1483–1499 (2007)
6. Lessig, C., de Witt, T., Fiume, E.: Efficient and accurate rotation of finite spherical harmonics expansions. J. Comput. Phys. **231**(2), 243–250 (2012)
7. Pajevic, S., Aldroubi, A., Basser, P.J.: A continuous tensor field approximation of discrete DT-MRI data for extracting microstructural and architectural features of tissue. J. Magn. Reson. **154**(1), 85–100 (2002)
8. Pierpaoli, C., Basser, P.: Toward a quantitative assessment of diffusion anisotropy. Magn. Reson. Med. **36**, 893–906 (1996)
9. Piuze, E., Sporring, J., Siddiqi, K.: Maurer-Cartan forms for fields on surfaces: application to heart fiber geometry. IEEE Trans. Pattern Anal. Mach. Intell. **37**(12), 2492–2504 (2015)
10. Savadjiev, P., Kindlmann, G.L., Bouix, S., Shenton, M.E., Westin, C.-F.: Local white matter geometry from diffusion tensor gradients. NeuroImage **49**, 3175–3186 (2010)
11. Szczepankiewicz, F., Lasi, S., van Westen, D., Sundgren, P.C., Englund, E., Westin, C.-F., Ståhlberg, F., Lätt, J., Topgaard, D., Nilsson, M.: Quantification of microscopic diffusion anisotropy disentangles effects of orientation dispersion from microstructure. NeuroImage **104**, 241–252 (2015)

12. Savadjiev, P., Zucker, S.W., Siddiqi, K.: On the differential geometry of 3D flow patterns: generalized helicoids and diffusion MRI analysis. In: ICCV, pp. 1–8 (2007)
13. Tuch, D.S.: Q-ball imaging. Magn. Reson. Med. **52**, 1358–1372 (2004)
14. Zhang, H., Schneider, T., Wheeler-Kingshott, C.A., Alexander, D.C.: NODDI: practical in vivo neurite orientation dispersion and density imaging of the human brain. Neuroimage **61**(4), 1000–1016 (2012)

Decoupling Axial and Radial Tissue Heterogeneity in Diffusion Compartment Imaging

Benoit Scherrer[1(✉)], Maxime Taquet[1,2], Armin Schwartzman[3],
Etienne St-Onge[1], Gaetan Rensonnet[2], Sanjay P. Prabhu[1],
and Simon K. Warfield[1]

[1] Department of Radiology, Boston Children's Hospital, Boston, MA 02115, USA
`benoit.scherrer@childrens.harvard.edu`
[2] ICTEAM, Université catholique de Louvain, Louvain-la-neuve, Belgium
[3] University of California, San Diego, La Jolla, CA 92093, USA

Abstract. Diffusion compartment imaging (DCI) characterizes tissues
in vivo by separately modeling the diffusion signal arising from a finite
number of large scale microstructural environments in each voxel, also
referred to as compartments. The DIAMOND model has recently been
proposed to characterize the 3-D diffusivity of each compartment using
a statistical distribution of diffusion tensors. It enabled the evaluation of
compartment-specific diffusion characteristics while also accounting for
the intra-compartment heterogeneity. In its original formulation, however, DIAMOND could only describe symmetric heterogeneity, while tissue heterogeneity likely differs along and perpendicular to the orientation
of the fascicles. In this work we propose a new statistical distribution
model able to decouple axial and radial heterogeneity of each compartment in each voxel. We derive the corresponding analytical expression of
the diffusion attenuated signal and evaluate this new approach with both
numerical simulations and in vivo data. We show that the heterogeneity
arising from white matter fascicles is anisotropic and that the shape of
the distribution is sensitive to changes in axonal dispersion and axonal
radius heterogeneity. We demonstrate that decoupling the modeling of
axial and radial heterogeneity has a substantial impact of the estimated
heterogeneity, enables improved estimation of other model parameters
and enables improved signal prediction. Our distribution model characterizes not only the orientation of each white matter fascicle but also
their diffusivities; it may enable unprecedented characterization of the
brain development and of brain disease and injury.

Keywords: Diffusion-weighted imaging · Diffusion compartment
imaging · Tissue microstructure heterogeneity · Statistical modeling

1 Introduction

Diffusion-weighted magnetic resonance imaging (DW-MRI) measures the bulk
motion of water molecules diffusing during a short period of time in tissues

© Springer International Publishing AG 2017
M. Niethammer et al. (Eds.): IPMI 2017, LNCS 10265, pp. 440–452, 2017.
DOI: 10.1007/978-3-319-59050-9_35

and has emerged as a powerful imaging modality to non-invasively evaluate microstructural tissue features. Diffusion tensor imaging (DTI) [2] is often used to assess quantitative descriptors of the tissue microstructure such as the fractional anisotropy and the mean diffusivity. DTI, however, summarizes the diffusion in each entire voxel with a single diffusion tensor and has poor specificity to describe the nature of microstructural changes. Instead, an increasingly popular approach is diffusion compartment imaging (DCI). DCI considers that the signal in each voxel arises from a finite number of large scale microstructural environments in slow exchange (also referred to as compartments) such as distinct white matter fascicles with heterogeneous orientations or spaces filled with cerebrospinal fluid (CSF) due to partial voluming. The signal arising from each compartment is modeled with a biophysical model that describes our understanding of the signal generation based on some parameters that describe the compartment (e.g., axonal radius [1], axonal dispersion [15], etc.). Computation of the inverse problem enables, in turn, extraction of microstructural descriptors that best explain the measured signal. Most models focus on point estimates of microstructural parameters and have largely ignored the heterogeneous nature of in vivo tissues.

More recently, Scherrer *et al.* [12] proposed the DIAMOND model, a phenomenological biophysical and statistical hybrid model in which each compartment is modeled using a peak-shaped continuous statistical distribution of diffusion tensors. It enables the assessment of compartment-specific diffusion characteristics (compartment-specific values for fractional anisotropy, mean, axial and radial diffusivity, i.e. cFA, cMD, cAD and cRD, respectively) while also capturing the heterogeneity of each compartment, based upon the concentration of the distribution of tensors. The concentration of each distribution, however, is described using a single scalar parameter in the space of positive-definite symmetric matrices, and only isotropic heterogeneity can be modeled. In actual neural tissues, the axial and radial heterogeneity likely differ, *e.g.* due to axonal radius heterogeneity, axonal undulation or axonal dispersion.

In this work we propose a novel biophysical and statistical hybrid approach that decouples the modeling of axial and radial heterogeneity and allows the modeling of anisotropic heterogeneity in each compartment. Specifically, we propose to describe each compartment using a *non-central* matrix-variate Gamma distribution of diffusion tensors. We demonstrate that this choice enables the computation of a new analytical solution of the diffusion attenuated signal and propose the new asymmetric DIAMOND model. We evaluate asymmetric DIAMOND using both numerical simulations and in vivo data and demonstrate the impact of decoupling axial and radial heterogeneity.

The paper is organized as follows. Section 2 provides the theoretical derivation of the diffusion attenuation for compartments modeled by a non-central matrix-variate Gamma distribution of diffusion tensors. Section 3 describes the numerical simulations and in vivo experiments carried out to evaluate this approach, the results of which are reported in Sect. 4. Finally, we discuss the impact of our novel DCI model in Sect. 5.

2 Theory

The DIAMOND DCI model [12] extended the 1-dimensional apparent diffusion coefficient (ADC) statistical distribution model of Yablonskiy *et al.* [14] to model the 3-dimensional diffusivity of heterogeneous anisotropic compartments in tissues. The diffusion-weighted signal is considered to arise from a finite number N_c of large scale compartments in slow exchange. Furthermore, the signal arising from each compartment is considered to arise from the infinite number of spin packets composing the compartment such that spin packets interacting with a homogeneous portion of the microstructure undergoes 3-D Gaussian diffusion. The signal $S(\mathbf{g}, b)$ for a unit-norm gradient vector $\mathbf{g}$ and b-value b is obtained by summing the contribution of all the spin packets of all the compartments, with:

$$S(\mathbf{g}, b) = \sum_{j=1}^{N_c} S_j(\mathbf{g}, b), \quad S_j(\mathbf{g}, b) = S_0 \int_{\mathbf{D} \in \mathrm{Sym}^+(3)} P_j(\mathbf{D}) \exp\left(-b\mathbf{g}^T \mathbf{D} \mathbf{g}\right) d\mathbf{D}, \quad (1)$$

where S_0 is the non-DW signal, $S_0 \exp\left(-b\mathbf{g}^T \mathbf{D} \mathbf{g}\right)$ is the contribution of the spin packet described by $\mathbf{D}$ and $P_j(\mathbf{D})$ is a continuous distribution of diffusion tensors that describes the spin packet composition of the jth compartment. In [12], $P_j(\mathbf{D})$ was choosen to be a matrix-variate Gamma distribution which is a peak-shaped distribution defined over the space of positive-definite symmetric matrices $(\mathrm{Sym}^+(3))$ and allows computation of an analytical solution of the integral in (1). In this work we propose instead to model $P_j(\mathbf{D})$ using a *non-central* matrix-variate Gamma distribution which provides additional flexibility. Omitting the compartment index j to simplify the notations (but without loss of generality), $\mathbf{D} \in \mathrm{Sym}^+(3)$ has a non-central matrix-variate Gamma distribution with parameter $\kappa > 1$, $\mathbf{\Psi} \in \mathrm{Sym}^+(3)$ and $\mathbf{\Theta} \in \mathrm{Sym}(3)$ if it has density [4,9]:

$$P(\mathbf{D}; \kappa, \mathbf{\Psi}, \mathbf{\Theta}) = \frac{[\det(\mathbf{D})]^{\kappa-2}}{[\det(\mathbf{\Psi})]^{\kappa} \Gamma_3(\kappa)} \exp[-\mathrm{tr}(-\mathbf{\Theta} - \mathbf{\Psi}^{-1}\mathbf{D})] F_{0,1}(\kappa; \mathbf{\Theta}\mathbf{\Psi}^{-1}\mathbf{D}) \quad (2)$$

where $F_{0,1}$ is the hypergeometric (Bessel) function of matrix argument of order $(0,1)$ and $\mathbf{\Theta}$ is the noncentrality parameter that enables description of a non-symmetric peak-shaped distribution. Note that when $\mathbf{\Theta} = 0$, (2) reduces to the matrix-variate Gamma distribution used in DIAMOND [12].

Proposition 1. *Suppose* $\mathbf{D} \in \mathrm{Sym}^+(3)$ *has a non-central matrix-variate Gamma distribution with density (2). Then:*

$$S = S_0 \int_{\mathbf{D} \in \mathrm{Sym}^+(3)} P(\mathbf{D}) \exp\left(-b\mathbf{g}^T \mathbf{D} \mathbf{g}\right) d\mathbf{D} = S_0 \left(1 + b\mathbf{g}^T \mathbf{\Psi} \mathbf{g}\right)^{-\kappa} \exp\left(-\frac{b\mathbf{g}^T \mathbf{\Psi} \mathbf{\Theta} \mathbf{g}}{1 + b\mathbf{g}^T \mathbf{\Psi} \mathbf{g}}\right)$$

Proof. According to the parameterization (2), the moment generating function of $\mathbf{D}$ is given by [4]:

$$M_{\mathbf{D}}[\mathbf{Z}] = \mathbb{E}[\exp(\mathrm{tr}(\mathbf{Z}\mathbf{D}))] = [\det(I_3 - \mathbf{Z}\mathbf{\Psi})]^{-\kappa} \exp\left(\mathrm{tr}\left\{\left[(I_3 - \mathbf{Z}\mathbf{\Psi})^{-1} - I_3\right]\mathbf{\Theta}\right\}\right), \quad (3)$$

for $\mathbf{Z} \in \mathrm{Sym}(3)$ satisfying $I_3 - \mathbf{Z}\mathbf{\Psi} \in \mathrm{Sym}^+(3)$. Replacing $\mathbf{Z} = -b\mathbf{g}\mathbf{g}^T$ gives:

$$S = S_0 \, \mathbb{E}\left[\exp(-b\mathbf{g}^T\mathbf{D}\mathbf{g})\right] \tag{4}$$

$$= S_0\left[\det\left(I_3 + b\mathbf{g}\mathbf{g}^T\mathbf{\Psi}\right)\right]^{-\kappa} \exp\left(\mathrm{tr}\left\{\left[\left(I_3 + b\mathbf{g}\mathbf{g}^T\mathbf{\Psi}\right)^{-1} - I_3\right]\mathbf{\Theta}\right\}\right) \tag{5}$$

which is valid because $I_3 - \mathbf{Z}\mathbf{\Psi} = I_3 + b\mathbf{g}\mathbf{g}^T \in \mathrm{Sym}^+(3)$ for all $b > 0$ and $\mathbf{g} \in \mathbb{R}^3$. Using the Sherman-Morrison formula, the matrix inverse above can be simplified to $\left(I_3 + b\mathbf{g}\mathbf{g}^T\mathbf{\Psi}\right)^{-1} = I_3 - \frac{b\mathbf{g}\mathbf{g}^T\mathbf{\Psi}}{1 + b\mathbf{g}^T\mathbf{\Psi}\mathbf{g}}$. Because $\mathbf{g}$ is a column vector and $\mathbf{g}^T\mathbf{\Psi}$ is a row vector, the above expression (5) for S can be simplified using $\mathrm{tr}(\mathbf{g}\mathbf{g}^T\mathbf{\Psi}) = \mathbf{g}^T\mathbf{\Psi}\mathbf{g}$ and using the Sylvester's determinant theorem to:

$$S = S_0\left(1 + b\mathbf{g}^T\mathbf{\Psi}\mathbf{g}\right)^{-\kappa} \exp\left(-\frac{b\mathbf{g}^T\mathbf{\Psi}\mathbf{\Theta}\mathbf{g}}{1 + b\mathbf{g}^T\mathbf{\Psi}\mathbf{g}}\right). \tag{6}$$

$\square$

Equation (6) describes the signal arising from a compartment that can have anisotropic heterogeneity described by κ and $\mathbf{\Theta}$. The expectation of $\mathbf{D}$ for model (2) is $\mathbf{D}_0 = \mathbb{E}[\mathbf{D}] = \mathbf{\Psi}(\kappa I_3 + \mathbf{\Theta})$ [4], *i.e.* $\mathbf{D}_0$ is the *average tensor* describing the compartment from which compartment-specific parameters (cFA, cMD, cAD, cRD) can be extracted. We reparameterize (6) by setting $\mathbf{\Psi} = \mathbf{D}_0(\kappa I_3 + \mathbf{\Theta})^{-1}$:

$$S = S_0\left(1 + b\mathbf{g}^T\mathbf{D}_0(\kappa I_3 + \mathbf{\Theta})^{-1}\mathbf{g}\right)^{-\kappa} \exp\left(-\frac{b\mathbf{g}^T\mathbf{D}_0(\kappa I_3 + \mathbf{\Theta})^{-1}\mathbf{\Theta}\mathbf{g}}{1 + b\mathbf{g}^T\mathbf{D}_0(\kappa I_3 + \mathbf{\Theta})^{-1}\mathbf{g}}\right). \tag{7}$$

We verify that when $\mathbf{\Theta} = 0$, then $S = S_0\left(1 + \frac{b\mathbf{g}^T\mathbf{D}_0\mathbf{g}}{\kappa}\right)^{-\kappa}$ which is the signal modeled by the original DIAMOND [12]. Our aim is to define $\mathbf{\Theta}$ so that the axial and radial heterogeneity with respect to the major diffusion orientation can be modeled, and therefore so that the axial and radial heterogeneity along fascicles can be described. For this purpose we set $\mathbf{\Theta} = \mathbf{V}\,\mathrm{diag}\left(\kappa', 0, 0\right)\mathbf{V}^T$, $\kappa' > 0$ with $\mathbf{V}$ coming from the eigenvalue decomposition of $\mathbf{D}_0$ ($\mathbf{D}_0 = \mathbf{V}\,\mathrm{diag}\left(\lambda^{\|}, \lambda^{\perp}, \lambda^{\perp}\right)\mathbf{V}^T$), *i.e.* $\mathbf{V}$ describing the 3-D orientation of the diffusion in the compartment. With this choice, (7) simplifies to:

$$S = S_0\left(1 + b\mathbf{g}^T\mathbf{V}\left[\mathrm{diag}(\tfrac{\lambda^{\|}}{\kappa + \kappa'}, \tfrac{\lambda^{\perp}}{\kappa}, \tfrac{\lambda^{\perp}}{\kappa})\right]\mathbf{V}^T\mathbf{g}\right)^{-\kappa} \exp\left(-\frac{b\mathbf{g}^T\mathbf{V}\left[\mathrm{diag}(\tfrac{\lambda^{\|}\kappa'}{\kappa + \kappa'}, 0, 0)\right]\mathbf{V}^T\mathbf{g}}{1 + b\mathbf{g}^T\mathbf{V}\left[\mathrm{diag}(\tfrac{\lambda^{\|}}{\kappa + \kappa'}, \tfrac{\lambda^{\perp}}{\kappa}, \tfrac{\lambda^{\perp}}{\kappa})\right]\mathbf{V}^T\mathbf{g}}\right),$$
$$\tag{8}$$

which explicitly shows how the axial and radial tensor components are affected by the axial ($\kappa^{\|} = \kappa + \kappa'$) and radial ($\kappa^{\perp} = \kappa$) heterogeneities. Compared to the original DIAMOND approach, this only adds one free parameter to be estimated per compartment (κ'). We name this new approach asymmetric DIAMOND.

3   Methods

We considered a multi-compartment DCI model with up to $N_c = 3$ anisotropic compartments to represent up to 3 fascicles and one purely homogeneous isotropic compartment to represent freely diffusing water. Using Eq. (7) (because of its increased compactness compared to that of (8)), this leads to modeling the DW signal with:

$$S(\mathbf{g}, b) = S_0 \left[f_{\mathrm{iso}} \exp(-bD_{\mathrm{iso}}) + \right. \tag{9}$$

$$\left. \sum_{j=1}^{N_c} f_j \left(1 + b\mathbf{g}^T \mathbf{D}_{0,j} \left(\kappa_j I_3 + \mathbf{\Theta}_j \right)^{-1} \mathbf{g} \right)^{-\kappa_j} \exp\left(-\frac{b\mathbf{g}^T \mathbf{D}_{0,j} \left(\kappa_j I_3 + \mathbf{\Theta}_j \right)^{-1} \mathbf{\Theta}_j \mathbf{g}}{1 + b\mathbf{g}^T \mathbf{D}_{0,j} \left(\kappa_j I_3 + \mathbf{\Theta}_j \right)^{-1} \mathbf{g}} \right) \right],$$

where D_{iso} is the diffusivity of free water and $\{f_{\mathrm{iso}}, f_1, \ldots, f_{N_c}\}$ are the *apparent* volumic fractions of occupancy of each compartment. The parameters were estimated by considering a chi-squared objective function with offset noise level, also known as the corrected least squares method [10], to account for Rician noise. This was achieved by minimizing at each voxel $\mathcal{L} = \sum_{(\mathbf{g}, b)} \left(\tilde{S}(\mathbf{g}, b) - \sqrt{S(\mathbf{g}, b)^2 + \sigma^2} \right)^2$, where $\tilde{S}(\mathbf{g}, b)$ is the measured signal for the diffusion gradient $(\mathbf{g}, b)$ and σ is a noise parameter to be estimated. The numerical optimization was achieved with BOBYQA [11], a derivative-free bound-constrained optimization technique using an estimation procedure similar to that of [12] except that the apparent volumic fractions were not constrained to sum to 1 and that σ was added as an additional free parameter to be estimated in BOBYQA. Model order selection was achieved by comparing the Akaike information criterion of ball-and-sticks models with 1, 2 and 3 anisotropic compartments. Models of increasing complexity were then gradually estimated, from the ball-and-sticks to the multi-tensor to the full asymmetric DIAMOND model, similarly to [12].

Simulations. We generated synthetic phantoms with varying axonal orientation dispersions by simulating voxels with 10000 cylinders with orientations drawn from a Watson distribution [15] with increasing dispersion indices ($\rho \in [0, 0.1]$) and with $f_{\mathrm{iso}} = 0.3$. The signal was simulated 100 independent times with three Rician noise levels (noise free, 40 dB, and 30 dB) with the CUSP90 scheme [12] that images multiple non-zero b-values up to 3000 s/mm^2 with short echo time and therefore high SNR. We used gradient pulses with duration $\delta = 30$ ms and separation $\Delta = 40$ ms, as typically used on clinical scanners. We compared compartment-specific parameters obtained with DIAMOND to those obtained with asymmetric DIAMOND. The concentration parameters were converted to compartment heterogeneity indexes (cHI) valued in [0,1] with a transform similar to that of Zhang *et al.* [15]: $\mathrm{cHI}_j^{\bullet} = \frac{2}{\pi} \arctan(1/(\kappa_j^{\bullet} - 1))$ (0 = low heterogeneity; 1 = high heterogeneity).

We also generated synthetic phantoms with a varying axonal radius heterogeneity (see Fig. 2i, ii). The signal was simulated using Monte-Carlo simulations (Camino toolkit [5], 200000 walkers, 5000 time points, *i.e.* dt = 14 μs). We considered phantoms composed of cylinders whose radii were drawn from a Gamma distribution with different shape and scale parameters (r_α and r_β, respectively) We used the parameters: {substrate lattice size, number of cylinders, r_α, r_β} = $\{20\,\mu\mathrm{m}, 300, 50, 1.0 \times 10^{-8}\}$ (low radius heterogeneity) and $\{20\,\mu\mathrm{m}, 240, 3, 1.667 \times 10^{-7}\}$ (high radius heterogeneity) so that both the mean axonal radius r_{mean} and the intra-axonal volume fraction ρ were constant ($r_{mean} = 0.5\,\mu m$ and $\rho = 0.6$) between the experiments. The signal was simulated with the same CUSP90 ($\delta = 30\,ms, \Delta = 40\,ms, b \leq 3000\,s/mm^2$) and three Rician noise corruption levels (noise free, 40 dB, and 30 dB). We assessed the cHI of DIAMOND and the cHI$^{\parallel}$ and cHI$^{\perp}$ of asymmetric DIAMOND over 100 independent repetitions of each experiment. The latter experiments were reproduced using a multiple shell gradient scheme with 6 shells of 36 gradients each at b-values: $300, 700, 1500, 2800, 4500, 6000\,s/mm^2$ which achieved higher b-values, increasing the sensitivity to small axonal radii.

In Vivo Data. We acquired a CUSP90 scan of a healthy volunteer (FOV = 220 mm; matrix = 128×128; 71 slices; resolution = $1.7 \times 1.7 \times 2\,mm^3$; TR = 10704 ms; TE = 78 ms; <16 min) and compared the symmetric distribution parameter of DIAMOND to the decoupled distribution parameters of asymmetric DIAMOND. We quantitatively compared the impact of decoupling axial and radial heterogeneity by comparing the generalization error [3,13] of asymmetric DIAMOND and DIAMOND. The generalization error quantifies the capability of the models to accurately predict the signal for unobserved DW gradients and therefore provides a measure of how well the mechanisms underlying the signal formation are captured by different models. Significance testing between the distributions of generalization error of DIAMOND and of asymmetric DIAMOND was achieved using the non-parametric Kruskal-Wallis test ($p < 0.01$).

4   Results

Figure 1a, c shows that increasing axonal dispersion was captured by a modest increase in cHI with DIAMOND. In contrast, asymmetric DIAMOND identified substantially different contributions of the axial and radial heterogeneities (Fig. 1b, d): cHI$^{\parallel}$ was very mildly affected by axonal dispersion while cHI$^{\perp}$ reached values an order of magnitude larger than the heterogeneity of DIAMOND. The two models also captured increased dispersion by a decreased cAD and increased cRD. This is consistent with the expected behavior of water molecules enduring more restriction along the fascicle orientation and less restriction perpendicularly when dispersion increases. Interestingly, the cRD slope was more pronounced with asymmetric DIAMOND (+90%) than with DIAMOND (+41%). Finally, while f_{iso} was over-estimated with the two models, accounting for anisotropic heterogeneity with asymmetric DIAMOND provided an estimate of f_{iso} closer to the ground truth and less dependent on the amount of dispersion.

Figure 2 shows that axonal radius heterogeneity was captured by an increased cHI with DIAMOND, and by an increased cHI$^{\perp}$ but mostly unchanged cHI$^{\parallel}$ with asymmetric DIAMOND, as we could expect. The effect was milder than axonal dispersion (Fig. 1) but clearly present nonetheless. Moreover, we found that using higher b-values led to a higher contrast between low and high heterogeneity (Fig. 2d–f), *i.e.* provided higher sensitivity to axonal radius heterogeneity. Figure 2 also shows that when using realistic Monte-Carlo simulations of the diffusion in the intra- and extra-axonal space, and when representing both

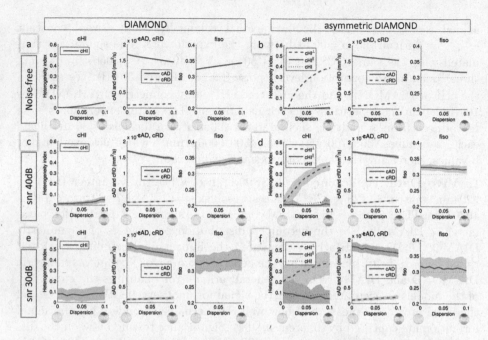

Fig. 1. Evaluation of DIAMOND and asymmetric DIAMOND parameters for a simulated increasing axonal dispersion and various noise levels. Shown are the symmetric and asymmetric compartment heterogeneity indexes (cHI, cHI$^\parallel$, cHI$^\perp$); the compartment axial diffusivity (cAD) and compartment radial diffusivity (cRD); and the fraction of isotropic diffusion (fiso). We superimposed in (b, d, f) the cHI from DIAMOND (dotted line) to facilitate the comparison with cHI$^\parallel$ and cHI$^\perp$.

intra- and extra-axonal diffusion with a single non-central matrix-variate Gamma distribution, the estimated heterogeneity in the homogeneous phantom was not null and anisotropic (cHI$^\perp$ > cHI$^\parallel$). This is expected as water molecules bounce on the cylinders surface, leading to local heterogeneities near the cylinders surface and to non-Gaussian diffusion, especially in the radial direction. We also verified that the baseline estimated heterogeneity was larger when using higher b-values (Fig. 2d–f.i), which is consistent with the known larger deviation from mono-exponential decay when using higher b-values.

Figure 3 reports the results from in vivo human data. Figure 3a shows that the local orientations of white matter fascicles captured by the orientations of the distribution expectations D_{0j} match the expected anatomy. Figure 3c–d shows that, overall, radial heterogeneity was found to be higher than axial heterogeneity throughout the brain. Quantitatively, we found that ≈80% of compartments verified cHI$^\perp$ > cHI$^\parallel$ in the WM, and ≈65% verified cHI$^\perp$ > 1.2 × cHI$^\parallel$ (*i.e.* values of cHI$^\perp$ at least 20% larger than cHI$^\parallel$). In addition, a number of regions of higher FA (first column) were found to be homogeneous with DIAMOND (Fig. 3b) but heterogeneous when decoupling axial and radial heterogeneity (low cHI$^\parallel$ and high cHI$^\perp$) with asymmetric DIAMOND (see Fig. 3b–d.i, ii).

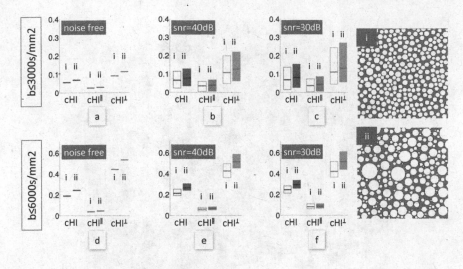

Fig. 2. Heterogeneity indexes estimated by DIAMOND and asymmetric DIAMOND in configurations with different axonal radius heterogeneity. (a–c) cHI (DIAMOND) and cHI$^\parallel$ and cHI$^\perp$ (asymmetric DIAMOND) for varying noise levels using the CUSP90 gradient scheme ($b \leq 3000\,\text{s/mm}^2$) (d–f) cHI and cHI$^\parallel$ and cHI$^\perp$ for varying noise levels using higher b-values ($b \leq 6000\,\text{s/mm}^2$). It shows that cHI$^\perp$ of asymmetric DIAMOND is more sensitive to detecting axonal radii heterogeneity. Moreover, increasing the maximum b-value provides additional sensitivity, especially when the SNR decreases.

Other regions were found to be heterogeneous with both DIAMOND and asymmetric DIAMOND (see iii). Finally, the body of the corpus callosum was found to have high heterogeneity (Fig. 3.iv). This heterogeneity was mostly isotropic (cHI$^\parallel$ ≈ cHI$^\perp$) in the coronal slice shown in Fig. 3, except near the inter-hemispheric plane (see Fig. 3.v) where the low cHI$^\parallel$ and high cHI$^\perp$ could be explained by change in axonal orientation, consistently with our simulations of axonal dispersion (Fig. 1).

Figure 4 shows a zoom of the heterogeneity in the single-fascicle voxels of the corpus callosum. First it shows that both DIAMOND and asymmetric DIAMOND found a substantial heterogeneity in this structure (see also Fig. 3.iv). Moreover, while the heterogeneity was mostly isotropic in the splenium (see Fig. 4.iii), it was anisotropic closer to the genu (cHI$^\parallel$ << cHI$^\perp$). The hypothesis of dispersion in this region (as suggested by Fig. 1 when cHI$^\parallel$ << cHI$^\perp$) is consistent with the detection of two fascicles in Fig. 4.ii by the model selection and by recent microscopic observations of dispersion in the corpus callosum using polarized light imaging [8].

Finally, Fig. 5 shows that accounting for the anisotropic nature of heterogeneity significantly reduces the generalization error ($p < 0.01$), *i.e.* it better captures the mechanisms underlying the signal formation and enables better prediction of the signal for DW gradients not used during the model estimation.

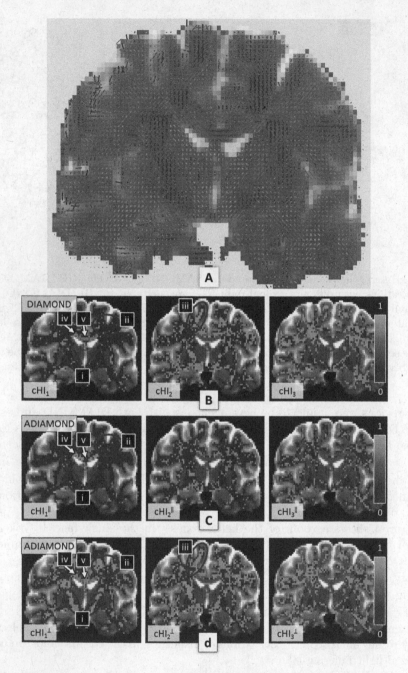

Fig. 3. Results from in vivo data (coronal views). (a) Fascicle orientations in each voxel estimated by asymmetric DIAMOND. (b) Symmetric compartment heterogeneity index cHI (DIAMOND) in the WM for each anisotropic compartment (c–d) Asymmetric cHI$^{\parallel}$ and cHI$^{\perp}$ (asymmetric DIAMOND) in the WM for each anisotropic compartment. In (b–d), the compartments were ordered by decreasing cFA (left to right columns).

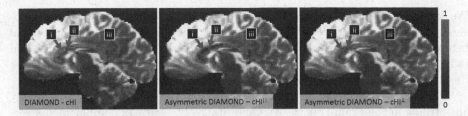

Fig. 4. Zoom of the heterogeneity in the CC (sagittal view). Only single fascicle voxels in the CC are shown. It shows that the heterogeneity is anisotropic ($cHI^{\perp} > cHI^{\|}$) near the genu (i) but isotropic ($cHI^{\|} \approx cHI^{\perp}$) in the splenium (iii). Region ii corresponds to a region where two fascicles were detected by our model order selection procedure.

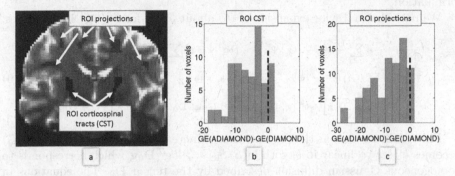

Fig. 5. (a) ROIs in which the generalization error was assessed, based on the highly anisotropic heterogeneity in these regions. (b–c) Histograms showing the reduction of the generalization error when using asymmetric DIAMOND instead of DIAMOND (negative result means a lower generalization error with asymmetric DIAMOND).

5   Discussion

Modeling the signal arising from compartments using a statistical distribution of diffusion tensors enables the description of compartment-specific tissue parameters (cAD, cRD) while accounting for the compartment microstructural heterogeneity and for the non-monoexponential decay in tissues. We proposed, for the first time, to use an asymmetric distribution to enable the separate modeling of axial and radial heterogeneities. We showed that, by using the non-central matrix-variate Gamma distribution, the integral in (1) had an analytic solution, the expression of which we provided in (7) and (8).

We found that using a symmetric distribution such as used in DIAMOND prevents the model from capturing a substantial part of the heterogeneity. This was verified with both simulations (Fig. 1) and with in vivo data (Fig. 3.i, ii). In contrast, using an asymmetric distribution provided an additional degree of freedom to separately capture axial and radial heterogeneity in white matter fascicles. We found that axial and radial heterogeneities were distinctly affected in presence of axonal dispersion and axonal radius heterogeneity ($cHI^{\perp} > cHI^{\|}$).

We also found that $cHI^{\parallel} \leq cHI \leq cHI^{\perp}$, *i.e.* that the estimated isotropic heterogeneity cHI with DIAMOND was always a compromise between axial and radial heterogeneity contributions. Importantly, we showed that decoupling axial and radial heterogeneities improved the estimation of other model parameters (see Fig. 1, more stable estimate of f_{iso} in presence of increased dispersion).

Our analysis using in vivo data showed that the heterogeneity was highly anisotropic in the brain (Fig. 3c–d). Quantitatively, $\approx 80\%$ of compartments verified $cHI^{\perp} > cHI^{\parallel}$ in the white matter. Moreover, we found that decoupling axial and radial heterogeneities enabled substantially better prediction of the signal for new diffusion gradients not used during the model estimation (Fig. 5). This shows both the importance and the impact of the new asymmetric DIAMOND formulation.

We note that a Taylor expansion of (6) about $b = 0$ for $0 \leq b\mathbf{g}^T \mathbf{\Psi}\mathbf{g} < 1$ gives:

$$
\begin{aligned}
\ln\left(\frac{S}{S_0}\right) &= -\kappa \sum_{q=1}^{\infty} \frac{(-1)^{q-1}}{q} \left(b\mathbf{g}^T \mathbf{\Psi}\mathbf{g}\right)^q - \left(b\mathbf{g}^T \mathbf{\Psi}\mathbf{\Theta}\mathbf{g}\right) \sum_{q=0}^{\infty} (-1)^q \left(b\mathbf{g}^T \mathbf{\Psi}\mathbf{g}\right)^q \\
&= \sum_{q=1}^{\infty} (-1)^q b^q \left(\mathbf{g}^T \mathbf{\Psi}\mathbf{g}\right)^{q-1} \mathbf{g}^T \mathbf{\Psi} \left(\frac{\kappa}{q}\mathbf{I}_3 + \mathbf{\Theta}\right) \mathbf{g} \\
&= -b\left[\mathbf{g}^T \mathbf{D}_0 \mathbf{g}\right] + b^2 \left[\mathbf{g}^T \mathbf{D}_0 (\kappa \mathbf{I}_3 + \mathbf{\Theta})^{-1} \mathbf{g}\mathbf{g}^T \mathbf{D}_0 (\kappa \mathbf{I}_3 + \mathbf{\Theta})^{-1} (\frac{\kappa}{2}\mathbf{I}_3 + \mathbf{\Theta})\mathbf{g}\right] - \ldots
\end{aligned}
\tag{10}
$$

First it shows that, as the concentration κ increases, the behavior of $\ln(S/S_0)$ becomes closer to linear in b, with $\ln(S/S_0) = -b\mathbf{g}^T \mathbf{D}_0 \mathbf{g}$ which corresponds to homogeneous Gaussian diffusion described by the tensor $\mathbf{D}_0$. The equations in (10) also show that, similarly to Kurtosis imaging, the asymmetric DIAMOND expression exhibits a positive b^2 term. This term, however, is balanced by other higher-order terms which prevent the model from numerically diverging as frequently observed with Kurtosis imaging and high b-values. More importantly, Kurtosis imaging focuses on estimating a dimensionless mathematical measure of deviation from Gaussian diffusion. Unfortunately, this deviation is not directly linked to biophysical mechanisms of the signal generation. Instead, asymmetric DIAMOND describes each compartment with a peak-shaped distribution of diffusion tensors, the shape of which is described via κ and $\mathbf{\Theta}$, *i.e.* via the axial and radial distribution concentrations $\kappa^{\parallel}$ and $\kappa^{\perp}$ with respect to the diffusion orientation. In contrast to Kurtosis imaging, the parameters $\kappa^{\parallel}$ and $\kappa^{\perp}$ capture a phenomenon that has a physical interpretation: the intra-compartment axial and radial heterogeneities, respectively, around the mean tensor $\mathbf{D}_0$ describing the compartment.

Other authors have considered distributions of tensors to model the diffusion profile in DW-MRI [6,7]. These approaches, however, correspond to voxel-based distributions of tensors; they conflate the signal arising from all the compartments and do not enable characterization of both the orientation and diffusivity of each compartment in each voxel. Moreover, spherical deconvolution based distribution models such as [6] rely on the definition of a pre-fixed fascicle response function, which is not known *a priori* and likely changes during brain maturation or disease, making longitudinal data analysis challenging. Instead of using a distribution of tensors to describe the voxel-wise diffusion profile, we propose to estimate a distribution of tensors for each compartment in each voxel. It enables characterization of both the orientation *and* diffusivities of each white matter fascicle in each voxel. Moreover, we propose to estimate the shape of the distribution so that the compartment heterogeneity can be quantified.

In this work, we focused on DWI acquisitions that can be achieved on a clinical scanner ($\delta = 30\,\mathrm{ms}, \Delta = 40\,\mathrm{ms}$) and considered a model in which intra- and extra-axonal diffusion arising from a white matter fascicle were both represented by a single non-central matrix-variate Gamma distribution. We showed that the shape of the distribution (*i.e.*, the amount of captured heterogeneity) was sensitive to changes in axonal dispersion and changes in axonal radius heterogeneity. With a single distribution per white matter fascicle, however, axonal dispersion and changes in axonal radius heterogeneity could not be disentangled, as expected. In future work we will use this new asymmetric distribution to investigate models that separately represent intra-axonal and extra-axonal diffusion for each white matter fascicle, so that the intra-axonal volume fraction can be estimated and axonal dispersion and axonal radius heterogeneity can be disentangled.

Acknowledgements. This work was supported by BCH TRP Innovator Award, Fondation Helaers (MT), Foulkes Foundation (MT), FRS-FNRS (GR) and by NIH grants R01 NS079788, R01 EB018988, U01 NS082320.

References

1. Assaf, Y., Basser, P.J.: Composite hindered and restricted model of diffusion (CHARMED) MR imaging of the human brain. Neuroimage **27**(1), 48–58 (2005)
2. Basser, P.J., Mattiello, J., LeBihan, D.: Estimation of the effective self-diffusion tensor from the NMR spin echo. J. Magn. Reson. B. **103**(3), 247–254 (1994)
3. Efron, B.: Estimating the error rate of a prediction rule: improvement on cross-validation. J. Am. Stat. Assoc. **78**(382), 316–331 (1983)
4. Gupta, A.K., Nagar, D.K.: Matrix Variate Distributions. Chapman & Hall/CRC, Boca Raton (2000)
5. Hall, M.G., Alexander, D.C.: Convergence and parameter choice for Monte-Carlo simulations of diffusion MRI. IEEE Trans. Med. Imaging **28**(9), 1354–1364 (2009)
6. Jian, B., Vemuri, B.C., Ozarslan, E., Carney, P.R., Mareci, T.H.: A novel tensor distribution model for the diffusion-weighted MR signal. Neuroimage **37**(1), 164–176 (2007)
7. Leow, A.D., Zhu, S., Zhan, L., McMahon, K., de Zubicaray, G.I., Meredith, M., Wright, M.J., Toga, A.W., Thompson, P.M.: The tensor distribution function. Magn. Reson. Med. **61**(1), 205–214 (2009)
8. Mollink, K., Kleinnijenhuis, M., Sotiropoulos, S.N., Cottaar, M., et al.: Exploring fibre orientation dispersion in the corpus callosum: comparison of diffusion MRI, polarized light imaging and histology. In: Proceedings of the 24th ISMRM (2016)
9. Muirhead, R.J.: Aspects of Multivariate Statistical Theory. Wiley, Hoboken (1982)
10. Panagiotaki, E., Schneider, T., Siow, B., Hall, M.G., Lythgoe, M.F., Alexander, D.C.: Compartment models of the diffusion MR signal in brain white matter: a taxonomy and comparison. Neuroimage **59**(3), 2241–2254 (2012)

11. Powell, M.J.D.: The BOBYQA algorithm for bound constrained optimization without derivatives. Technical report NA2009/06. Department of Applied Mathematics and Theoretical Physics, Cambridge, England (2009)
12. Scherrer, B., Schwartzman, A., Taquet, M., Sahin, M., Prabhu, S.P., Warfield, S.K.: Characterizing brain tissue by assessment of the distribution of anisotropic microstructural environments in diffusion-compartment imaging (DIAMOND). Magn. Reson. Med. **76**(3), 963–977 (2016)
13. Scherrer, B., Taquet, M., Warfield, S.K.: Reliable selection of the number of fascicles in diffusion images by estimation of the generalization error. In: Gee, J.C., Joshi, S., Pohl, K.M., Wells, W.M., Zöllei, L. (eds.) IPMI 2013. LNCS, vol. 7917, pp. 742–753. Springer, Heidelberg (2013). doi:10.1007/978-3-642-38868-2_62
14. Yablonskiy, D.A., Bretthorst, G.L., Ackerman, J.J.: Statistical model for diffusion attenuated MR signal. Magn. Reson. Med. **50**(4), 664–669 (2003)
15. Zhang, H., Schneider, T., Wheeler-Kingshott, C.A., Alexander, D.C.: NODDI: practical in vivo neurite orientation dispersion and density imaging of the human brain. Neuroimage **61**(4), 1000–1016 (2012)

Bayesian Dictionary Learning and Undersampled Multishell HARDI Reconstruction

Kratika Gupta and Suyash P. Awate[✉]

Computer Science and Engineering Department, Indian Institute of Technology (IIT)
Bombay, Mumbai, India
suyash@cse.iitb.ac.in

Abstract. High angular resolution diffusion imaging (HARDI) at higher b values leads to signal measurements having (exponentially) lower magnitudes, a strong Rician bias, and more corruptions from artifacts. Typical undersampled-HARDI reconstruction methods assume Gaussian noise models and limited/no regularization, leading to underestimated tract anisotropy and reduced ability to detect crossings. We propose novel *Bayesian frameworks* to model *Rician* statistics during *dictionary learning* and *reconstruction*. For dictionary learning, we propose *edge-preserving smoothness* priors on dictionary atoms. For reconstruction, we employ *sparsity-based multiscale smoothness* priors on the reconstructed image. In both frameworks, we propose kernel-based *non-local regularization* on dictionary coefficients and stronger sparsity via *quasi norms*. The results show improved dictionaries and reconstructions, over the state of the art.

Keywords: HARDI · Dictionary learning · Reconstruction · Bayesian estimation · Rician statistics · Non-local regularization · Quasi-norm sparsity

1 Introduction

High angular resolution diffusion imaging (HARDI) [1,20] acquires diffusion weighted (DW) magnetic resonance (MR) images using a large number of gradient directions (≥ 64) over multiple (≥ 2) shells, with b values ranging from 10^3 to $10^4 \, \text{s/mm}^2$. Multishell HARDI combines the advantages of (i) lower b values, giving higher signal-to-noise ratio (SNR), with (ii) higher b values, giving greater ability to resolve tract directions and narrow-angle crossings [18]. Reliable tracking of neural tracts is key in several applications, including neurosurgery and deep brain stimulation. To reduce scan time, the most effective scheme is to reduce the number of directions during acquisition.

With increasing b values, diffusion signals have exponentially lower magnitudes, thereby inevitably leading to measurements that exhibit strongly *Rician* noise, with significant bias effects. Typical methods for HARDI reconstruction,

S.P. Awate—Thanks to funding from IIT Bombay Seed Grant 14IRCCSG010.

M. Niethammer et al. (Eds.): IPMI 2017, LNCS 10265, pp. 453–465, 2017.
DOI: 10.1007/978-3-319-59050-9_36

including those based on dictionary learning [12,14] in HARDI (also in diffusion spectrum imaging [4]), assume Gaussian noise models, explicitly or implicitly, which leads to loss of contrast in the estimates of diffusion signals, or in the values of the orientation distribution function (ODF), over the directional domain. This leads to artificially inflated variability in tractography, reduction in the ability to detect crossings, and underestimation of generalized fractional anisotropy (GFA). In contrast, we propose a novel *Bayesian framework* to model Rician characteristics during *dictionary learning* and *reconstruction*.

Undersampled HARDI reconstruction needs *regularization* to avoid overfitting in the presence of noise and outliers resulting from several artifacts [13] dominating the low signal magnitudes. Typical regularization is limited to sparse modeling in analytical or data-driven bases (*not* both) and using spatial regularization through total variation (TV). We propose priors for *edge-preserving smoothness* on dictionary *atoms*, *multiscale smoothness* on images, and kernel-based *non-local regularization* and *quasi-norm* sparsity on dictionary coefficients.

We propose novel Bayesian frameworks for dictionary learning and reconstruction for HARDI. In both frameworks, we propose (i) to exploit the Rician noise model, (ii) a kernel-based non-local spatial regularizer on the image of coefficient vectors, which learns and exploits the manifold structure underlying the data, and (ii) a sparsity prior on the dictionary coefficients using a q-generalized Normal probability density function (PDF), for robustness. To handle noise/outliers during dictionary learning, we propose an edge-preserving smoothness prior on dictionary atoms in the directional domain. During reconstruction, we also propose multiscale image regularization through a wavelet-based sparsity prior, which is complementary to the dictionary prior and the non-local regularity on the coefficients. The results on simulated and brain HARDI show improvements from our likelihood and prior models over the state of the art.

2   Related Work

Early methods *model diffusion signals* using the analytical bases of spherical harmonics [5,6,11,19] or spherical ridgelets [15–17]. Other works [2,3,12] design dictionaries based on tensor or parametric models. Later methods [14] learn parametric dictionaries with L^1 sparsity constraints. To model unknown tract orientations, [12] expands the dictionary to include rotated atoms at the risk of overfitting, [2,3] explicitly optimize each atom's rotation at a high computational cost and the risk of local optima with corrupted data, [9] does *not* impose any rotation-invariant structure on the atoms, learning redundant atoms to capture different rotations, but at the risk of underfitting arbitrary tract orientations in new data. In contrast, we propose robust nonparametric dictionary learning in a Bayesian framework, using strong sparsity priors based on q-generalized Normal PDFs (to reduce overfitting because of noise/artifacts/model complexity in the form of dictionary size), non-local regularizers on the dictionary coefficients, and edge-preserving smoothness priors on the atoms. We couple the notions of a core dictionary, modeling rotation-invariant signal profiles, and an expanded dictionary with atoms that model arbitrary tract orientations.

An early work on HARDI denoising (*not* reconstruction) [7] advocates the Rician model. However, almost all works related to (i) dictionary learning in HARDI [9,10,14], and (ii) HARDI reconstruction from direction-undersampled, or fully-sampled but corrupted, magnitude images [5,6,8–12,14–17,19], assume Gaussian noise. In contrast, we exploit Rician statistics during dictionary learning and reconstruction. While typical dictionary-based reconstruction ignores spatial regularization [2,5,6,9,11,12,14,19], few methods used spatial regularization via TV [15–17]. We propose spatial regularization, during reconstruction, using (i) wavelets for DW images (modeling multiscale texture statistics, unlike TV) and (ii) non-local smoothing on the dictionary coefficients. We propose directional-domain regularization on atoms during dictionary learning.

3   Methods

3.1   A Generative Model for Multishell HARDI Signals

Let the HARDI acquisition employ S shells, with shell s comprising N_s gradient directions $\{g_{sn} \in \mathbb{R}^3 : \|g_{sn}\|_2 = 1\}_{n=1}^{N_s}$. Diffusion signal values are modeled as non-negative real [20]. Let f be an *uncorrupted signal* vector, where $f_{sn} \in \mathbb{R}_{\geq 0}$ be the nonnegative diffusion-signal value from shell s for gradient direction g_{sn}.

A Dictionary Model. Let a dictionary $\mathcal{D}$ comprise K uncorrupted multishell diffusion signals $\{d^k\}_{k=1}^K$ called *atoms*, with $d_{sn}^k \in \mathbb{R}_{\geq 0}$ as the value from shell s for gradient direction g_{sn}. We consider that the atoms are well aligned, such that the underlying principal directions of diffusion are similar, and call $\mathcal{D}$ the *core dictionary*. To be able to model arbitrary orientations of diffusion signals f in different brain regions and subjects, we create an *expanded dictionary* $\mathcal{D}^\Theta$, from $\mathcal{D}$, by using each core atom d^k in $\mathcal{D}$ to create multiple copies $\{d^{k\theta_r}\}_{r=1}^R$ by reorienting the diffusion signal d^k along a large set of directions $\{\theta_r\}_{r=1}^R$ spread roughly uniformly over a hemisphere. For some direction θ, let the associated rotation matrix be $R(\theta)$. Then, the signal at direction g in the reoriented atom is $d^{k\theta}(g) := d^k(R(\theta)^\top g)$ that we can obtain by Barycentric interpolation, on the spherical domain, using geodesic distances.

For simplicity, we fix the set of directions θ_r as the gradient directions g_{sn} for the shell s with the maximum number of directions N_s. Thus, the unknowns underlying the expanded dictionary are only the core atoms in dictionary $\mathcal{D}$. This strategy leads to fewer unknowns and tends to avoid data fragmentation and learning of redundant atoms that are only reoriented versions of each other (more in Sect. 3.2). Let c be the vector of coefficients used to represent f as a linear combination of the atoms $\{d^{k\theta_r}\}_{r=1}^R$, in turn represented via the core atoms $\{d^k\}_{k=1}^K$. Thus, $f = \mathcal{D}^\Theta c = \sum_{k=1}^K \sum_{r=1}^R c_{kr} d^{k\theta_r}$.

Rician Likelihood Model. The acquired diffusion signal h (magnitude images) is corrupted with independent and identically distributed (i.i.d.) noise. Given the uncorrupted diffusion signal f and the noise variance in the real and imaginary parts as σ^2 (σ^2 can be estimated reliably), the likelihood of observing noisy data

h is $P(h|f,\sigma) := \prod_{s=1}^{S} \prod_{n=1}^{N} \left(\frac{h_{sn}}{\sigma^2}\right) \exp\left(\frac{-(h_{sn}^2 + f_{sn}^2)}{2\sigma^2}\right) I_0\left(\frac{h_{sn}f_{sn}}{\sigma^2}\right)$, where $I_0(\cdot)$ is the modified Bessel function of the first kind with order zero.

Prior on Core-Dictionary $\mathcal{D}$ Atoms. Because of low SNR, even small corruptions, in the form of eddy-current distortions, geometric distortion due to magnetic susceptibility, echo-planar imaging artifacts, and motion artifacts [13], can lead to outliers in the data. To ensure robust dictionary learning, we impose an edge-preserving smoothness prior $P(d^k)$ on each atom d^k using a Markov random field (MRF) model. The prior on the core dictionary $\mathcal{D}$ is $P(\mathcal{D}) := \prod_{k=1}^{K} P(d_k)$. For the MRF model, we consider a neighborhood structure on the spherical domain of each shell where $\mathcal{N}_n$ gives the set of neighbors of direction n. Then, the PDF $P(d^k)$, upto a normalization constant, is $P(d^k) \propto \exp\left(\alpha \sum_{s=1}^{S} \sum_{n=1}^{N_s} \sum_{n' \in \mathcal{N}_n} w_{snn'} \|d_{sn}^k - d_{sn'}^k\|_{1,\epsilon}^1\right)$, where α controls the prior strength, $\|x\|_{q,\epsilon}^q := \sum_{k=1}^{K} \left(|x_k|^2 + \epsilon\right)^{q/2}$ is the q-th power of the ϵ-regularized L^q quasi-norm, and $w_{snn'} \in [0,1]$ weights the roughness penalty for the difference between atom values in directions g_{sn} and $g_{sn'}$. We set weights based on a von Mises-Fisher (vMF) kernel on the sphere: $w_{snn'} := \exp(\pi\langle g_{sn}, g_{sn'}\rangle)$.

Prior on Coefficients C. First, we impose nonnegativity on the coefficients. Second, to avoid overfitting, we want to ensure that very few atoms in the large-sized expanded dictionary $\mathcal{D}^\Theta$ are used during fitting. The standard sparsity prior is a Laplacian PDF that leads to the L^1-norm penalty on the coefficient vectors. We propose to strengthen the sparsity prior by replacing the Laplacian prior with the q-generalized Normal PDF $P(c) \propto \exp(-\beta\|c\|_q^q)$, where $\|c\|_q$ is the L^q quasi norm for $q \in (0,1)$. While this PDF reduces to the Laplace PDF for $q = 1$, when $q < 1$ it concentrates more mass near the origin and has longer tails than the Laplace PDF. The L^0 pseudo-norm is the limit of $\|c\|_q^q$ as $q \to 0$.

Third, if two diffusion signals f^i and f^j are similar, their coefficient vectors c^i and c^j should also be similar. This prior adds to the reliability of the fits. We encode this prior PDF in the form of a zero-mean multivariate Gaussian distribution on the coefficient matrix C. Specifically, if F is the data matrix with each column as a signal f^i, and if C is the coefficient matrix with each column as c^i, then the prior PDF on the coefficient matrix C is $P(C) \propto \exp(-0.5 \sum_{i=1}^{I} \sum_{j=1}^{I} \|c^i - c^j\|_2^2 \Omega_{ij})$, where the weight $\Omega_{ij} > 0$ is larger if the signals f^i and f^j are closer to each other. We design Ω_{ij} using a Mercer kernel that implicitly learns the *manifold structure* underlying the distribution of the signals f and then regularizes c^i based on the neighborhoods on the manifold. We use a Gaussian kernel to define $\Omega_{ij} := \exp(-0.5\|f^i - f^j\|_2^2/\upsilon)$, where we set υ to the mean of the squared distances between all given pairs of diffusion signals f^i and f^j. Thus, when all coefficients are nonnegative, the prior on C is $P(C) \propto \exp\left(-\sum_{i=1}^{I} \beta\|c^i\|_{q,\epsilon}^q - \gamma \sum_{i=1}^{I} \sum_{j=1}^{I'} \|c^i - c^j\|_2^2 \Omega_{ij}\right)$.

3.2 Bayesian Dictionary Learning

We formulate the problem of learning the core dictionary $\mathcal{D}$ from a sample of observed (corrupted) diffusion signals $H := \{h^i\}_{i=1}^I$, as a maximum-a-posteriori (MAP) Bayesian estimation problem for the posterior $P(\mathcal{D}, C|H)$. The optimal dictionary is $\mathcal{D}^* := \arg\max_{\mathcal{D}:\|d^k\|_2 \leq 1, \forall k} \left[\max_{C \succeq 0} P(H|\mathcal{D}^\Theta(\mathcal{D}), C)P(\mathcal{D})P(C)\right]$, where the norm constraint on atoms d^k prevents a trivial solution where all coefficients in C tend to zero, $C \succeq 0$ denotes the nonnegativity constraint $c_k^i \geq 0, \forall i, k$, the Rician likelihood $P(H|\mathcal{D}^\Theta(\mathcal{D}), C) := \prod_{i=1}^I P(h^i|\mathcal{D}^\Theta(\mathcal{D}), C)$, variables $\mathcal{D}$ and C are independent, $P(\mathcal{D})$ is the core-dictionary prior, and $P(C)$ is the coefficient-matrix prior. For learning the dictionary, we select only those (high-quality) voxels where the GFA is sufficiently high; this ignores brain voxels in the fluid regions and the gray matter.

After learning the core dictionary, we add *constant atoms* d^{K+s} to it, one for each shell s, to better model isotropic diffusion in the fluid and the gray matter.

Optimization. We propose a two-stage practical optimization strategy for the MAP estimation, avoiding local optima. While Stage I proposes a good initialization of the core dictionary $\mathcal{D}$ using a subset of the data, the Stage II refines the dictionary $\mathcal{D}$ using a larger dataset. In each stage, we solve MAP problems similar to the one described in this section.

Stage I collects signals at voxels in regions that have a single tract passing through them, e.g., corpus callosum, lateral corticospinal tract, etc. where the strongly anisotropic diffusion leads to higher contrast-to-noise ratios in the signal. To factor out arbitrary differences in (i) imaging coordinate-frame origins and poses across individuals, (ii) orientations of a specific tract across individuals, and (iii) orientations of different tracts within an individual, we reorient each diffusion signal to align it with a fixed signal that models prolate-tensor diffusion along direction $[1, 0, 0]^\top$. We rotationally align two diffusion signals defined on the spherical domain of gradient directions by minimizing the sum of squared residuals over the discretized spherical domain. The first stage does *not* create the expanded dictionary $\mathcal{D}^\Theta$, but uses $\mathcal{D}$ (*not* $\mathcal{D}^\Theta$) directly to model f. We use K-means to initialize d^k to the K cluster means. We set $q = 1$.

Stage II takes all the data, including diffusion signals that have tract crossings, uses the expanded dictionary $\mathcal{D}^\Theta$, initializes the core dictionary $\mathcal{D}$ with the one optimized in the previous stage, and then optimizes $\mathcal{D}$ via iterative gradient descent with adaptive step size. To prevent overfitting with the much larger size of the expanded dictionary $\mathcal{D}^\Theta$, we set $q \ll 1$ imposing stronger sparsity closer to L^0 sparsity. The learned $\mathcal{D}$ typically continues to have atoms without crossings.

3.3 Bayesian Reconstruction of Multishell HARDI

We propose a Bayesian formulation for reconstructing a multishell HARDI image U from multishell HARDI image data X that is undersampled in the number of directions in each shell. Let the anatomical image comprise V voxels. Let the fully-sampled HARDI acquisition employ S shells, with shell s comprising

N_s gradient directions. Let the undersampled HARDI acquisition X employ T shells, with shell t comprising N_t gradient directions; in this paper $T = S$. The matrix U is of dimension $V \times (\sum_{s=1}^{S} N_s)$. At voxel v in the image corresponding to shell s and direction n, the image value is $u_{snv} \in \mathbb{R}_{\geq 0}$. Let u_{sn} denote the spatial image of diffusion signal values for shell s and gradient direction g_{sn}. Let u_v denote the multishell diffusion signal at voxel v.

We reuse the dictionary-based generative model from in Sect. 3.1. Given the expanded dictionary $\mathcal{D}^{\Theta}$ and the direction-undersampled (magnitude) data X, we propose to estimate the underlying fully-sampled image U, along with the coefficients C, by maximizing the posterior $P(U, C | X, \mathcal{D}^{\Theta})$. The optimal MAP reconstruction is $U^* := \arg\max_U \left[\max_{C \geq 0} P(X|U) P(U|C, \mathcal{D}^{\Theta}) P(C) \right]$, where we know that data X is conditionally independent of $\mathcal{D}^{\Theta}$ and C given the image U, $P(X|U)$ is the Rician likelihood, $P(C)$ is the prior on the coefficient matrix C, and $P(U|C, \mathcal{D}^{\Theta})$ is the prior on the uncorrupted HARDI image U given C.

Rician Likelihood Model of Undersampled HARDI. The likelihood of X, which is a noisy and subsampled version of unknown image U, is:
$$P(X|U) := \prod_{t=1}^{T} \prod_{n=1}^{N_t} \prod_{v=1}^{V} \left(\frac{x_{tnv}}{\sigma^2} \right) \exp \left(\frac{-(x_{tnv}^2 + u_{tnv}^2)}{2\sigma^2} \right) I_0 \left(\frac{x_{tnv} u_{tnv}}{\sigma^2} \right).$$

Prior on HARDI Image U. We use two complementary types of prior information on the image U. We assume that, at each voxel v, the diffusion signal u_v has a close sparse representation in the expanded dictionary $\mathcal{D}^{\Theta}$. The signal u_v may deviate from the dictionary representation because of artifacts [13] that are non-trivial to model. We propose a simple but effective prior to penalize the squared residual between u_v and its sparse representation. In addition to the dictionary-based prior on u_v that models regularity over the directional domain, we enforce a complementary prior for multiscale spatial regularization based on an overcomplete wavelet frame. We enforce a prior on each diffusion-weighted image u_{sn} to have a sparse wavelet representation, by imposing a Laplacian prior on the vector of wavelet coefficients. Let $\mathcal{W}$ be an operator representing a wavelet transform (vectorized output) applied on a spatial image u_{sn}. Then, the effective prior on the image U, upto normalization constant, is
$$P(U|C, \mathcal{D}^{\Theta}) \propto \exp \left(-(1-\lambda) \sum_{s=1}^{S} \sum_{n=1}^{N_s} \|\mathcal{W} u_{sn}\|_{q,\epsilon}^q - \lambda \sum_{v=1}^{V} \|u_v - \mathcal{D}^{\Theta} c_v\|_2^2 \right).$$

Prior on Coefficients C. The prior $P(C)$ is the same as in Sect. 3.1. During reconstruction, $P(C)$ enforces *non-local regularity* on the image of coefficient vectors c_v, in addition to the manifold-based regularity described before.

Optimization. The MAP optimization uses alternating (projected) gradient descent, with adaptive step size. At each voxel v, we initialize u_v and c_v by independently fitting the dictionary $\mathcal{D}^{\Theta}$ to the undersampled data x_v.

4   Results and Discussion

We evaluate our Bayesian frameworks for dictionary learning and reconstruction on simulated and real-world data. We tune parameters $\alpha, \beta, \gamma, \lambda$, and q via cross validation. The relative root mean squared error (RRMSE) between vector y and a reference vector z is $\|y - z\|_2/\|z\|_2$. For Rician noise with parameter σ^2, SNR is the largest signal magnitude, over all voxels and directions, divided by σ.

(a) Baseline   (b) Rician+Reg.(**Proposed**) (c) Gaussian+Reg.   (d) Rician

Fig. 1. Bayesian dictionary learning: effect on atoms. Two example atoms learned from: (a) high-quality data (baseline); (b) high-noise data with Rician noise model with smoothness prior on atoms (**proposed**); (c) high-noise data with *Gaussian* noise model with smoothness prior on atoms; (d) high-noise data with Rician noise model *without* smoothness prior on atoms.

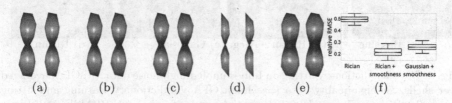

(a)   (b)   (c)   (d)   (e)   (f)

Fig. 2. Bayesian dictionary learning: effect on fits. (a) High-quality data. Example fits to high-noise data using a dictionary learned from: (b) high-quality data; (c) high-noise data with Rician noise model and smoothness prior (**proposed**); (d) high-noise data with Rician noise model *without* smoothness prior; (e) high-noise data with Gaussian noise model and smoothness prior. (f) RRMSE in fits via dictionaries learned with/without Rician noise model and smoothness prior.

Bayesian Dictionary Learning. We evaluate the effects of the Rician noise model and smoothness prior on atoms. We take 10^3 high-quality signals and learn a dictionary (Fig. 1(a)). Then, we corrupt the data with Rician noise to give SNRs of 7 and 5 for the 2 shells, and learn dictionaries again. Atoms learned without spatial smoothness on the atoms (Fig. 1(d)) get affected by the noise in the data. Indeed, to infer the original ODFs in the presence of high noise levels, without priors, huge sample sizes are necessary. With limited sample size and high noise, priors play an important role. Atoms learned using a Gaussian noise model with a smoothness prior (Fig. 1(c)) are unable to remove the Rician bias, leading to inflated (less sharp) ODFs, reducing GFA. Atoms learned using a Rician noise model coupled with a smoothness prior (Fig. 1(b)) are very close to atoms learned from high-quality data (Fig. 1(a)).

The dictionary learned with the Rician noise model and smoothness prior on the atoms leads to fits (Fig. 2(c)) that are very close to the high-quality data (Fig. 2(a)). Fits from the dictionary learned without the smoothness prior (Fig. 2(d)) or with the Gaussian noise model (Fig. 2(e)) are poor, either lacking smoothness or showing significant bias (less sharp ODFs). RRMSEs (Fig. 2(f)) for the fits are the lowest for our approach.

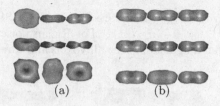

Fig. 3. Bayesian dictionary learning. *Core dictionary* $\mathcal{D}$ learned from high-noise data, with smoothness prior on atoms, with: (a) a Rician **(proposed)** and (b) a Gaussian noise model.

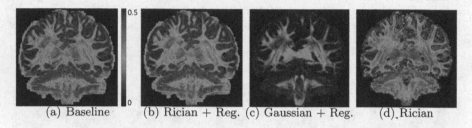

(a) Baseline   (b) Rician + Reg.   (c) Gaussian + Reg.   (d) Rician

Fig. 4. Bayesian dictionary fitting on fully-sampled high-noise data. (a) GFA, averaged over shells, for high-quality data (baseline). GFA via dictionary learning and fitting using: (b) Rician noise models with spatial regularity on U, C, RRMSE 0.01 **(proposed)**; (c) *Gaussian* models with spatial regularity, RRMSE 0.12; (d) Rician models *without* spatial regularity, RRMSE 0.11.

We learn the *core dictionary* $\mathcal{D}$ using the two-stage algorithm described in Sect. 3.2. We select diffusion signals from the white matter (inferred from the $b0$ image) having high GFA. This eliminates voxels (i) from the fluid and gray matter regions and (ii) that are severely corrupted with noise and/or artifacts. A majority of the selected diffusion signals exhibit a single tract or two tracts with crossing angle close to $\pi/2$, containing informative data. Recall that the *expanded-dictionary* $\mathcal{D}^\Theta$ allow combinations of rotated atoms in the core dictionary $\mathcal{D}$ to model crossings with many tracts and/or arbitrary crossing angles. $\mathcal{D}$ learned using the Rician noise model (Fig. 3(a)) learns atoms exhibiting sharper ODFs and clearer tract crossings. The Gaussian noise model is unable to "see through" the Rician bias in the data, leading to learned atoms (Fig. 3(b)) depicting significant Rician bias and a smaller variety of diffusion profiles.

The improved dictionary learning contributes to better fits to fully-sampled high-noise brain HARDI; we treat this as a 'reconstruction' problem (Sect. 3.3) with fully-sampled HARDI. Rician noise modeling (during dictionary learning and reconstruction) and spatial regularity on U and C (during reconstruction) leads to fits (Fig. 4(b)) with GFA values very close to the GFA computed for high-quality data (Fig. 4(a)). Gaussian noise modeling leads to much reduced GFA estimates (Fig. 4(c)) that are consistent with less-sharp ODF estimates. Rician noise modeling without spatial regularity on image U and coefficients C leads to fits (Fig. 4(d)) and GFA values that are susceptible to noise and lack spatial regularity, especially in/near the cortex.

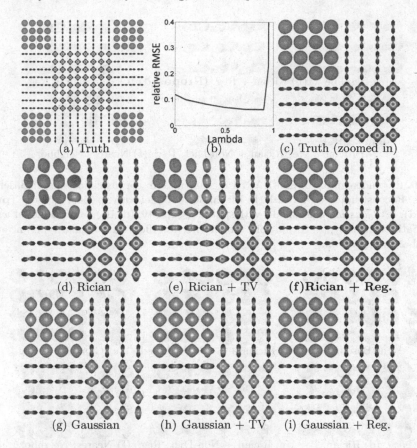

(a) Truth   **(b)**   **(c)** Truth (zoomed in)

(d) Rician   **(e)** Rician + TV   **(f)** Rician + Reg.

(g) Gaussian   **(h)** Gaussian + TV   **(i)** Gaussian + Reg.

Fig. 5. Undersampled high-noise HARDI reconstruction: simulated data. (a) Ground truth diffusion signals, in simulated phantom. We simulated 10× *undersampling* and SNRs 7 and 5 in 2 shells. (b) Our method's performance with different weights λ for the dictionary and wavelet prior. (c) True ODFs (zoomed top-left 8×8 region). Reconstructed ODFs (top-left 8×8 region) with *Rician* noise model (during dictionary learning and reconstruction): (d) without spatial regularization on U; (e) with TV prior on U; (f) with wavelet prior on U and non-local regularity on C **(proposed)**. Reconstructed ODFs (top-left 8×8 region) with *Gaussian* noise model (during dictionary learning and reconstruction): (d) without spatial regularization on U; (e) with TV prior on U; (f) with wavelet prior on U and non-local regularity on C.

Undersampled HARDI Reconstruction with Simulated Data. We simulate a phantom with a 16×16 voxel grid, 2 shells, and 81 gradient directions per shell. It comprises 2 crossing tracts (Fig. 5(a)). Figure 5 shows ODFs computed from the higher-b shell signals. We simulate 10× undersampling in gradient directions, acquiring 8 of 81 directions, per shell, spread roughly uniformly over the hemisphere. We introduce i.i.d. Rician noise with SNRs 7 and 5 for the 2 shells that mimics clinical acquisitions at higher b (e.g., $b \geq 1500 \, \text{s/mm}^2$).

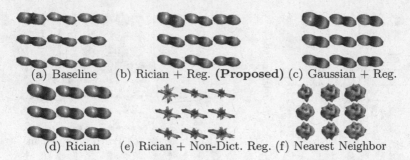

(a) Baseline   (b) Rician + Reg. **(Proposed)** (c) Gaussian + Reg.

(d) Rician   (e) Rician + Non-Dict. Reg. (f) Nearest Neighbor

Fig. 6. 6× undersampled brain HARDI reconstruction: corpus callosum. (a) Baseline ODFs. Reconstructed ODFs with (b) Rician noise model with spatial regularity (**proposed**); (c) *Gaussian* noise model with spatial regularity; (d) Rician noise model *without* spatial regularity; (e) Rician noise model with non-dictionary regularity; (f) nearest neighbor interpolation.

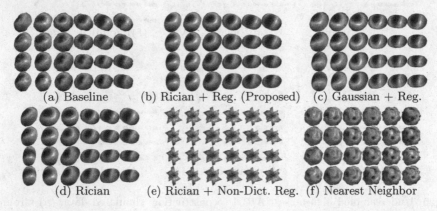

(a) Baseline   (b) Rician + Reg. (Proposed)   (c) Gaussian + Reg.

(d) Rician   (e) Rician + Non-Dict. Reg.   (f) Nearest Neighbor

Fig. 7. 6× undersampled brain HARDI reconstruction: tract crossing. (a) Baseline ODFs: bimodal ODFs in 3rd column. Reconstructions via: (b) Rician noise model with spatial regularity (**proposed**); (c) *Gaussian* model with spatial regularity; (d) Rician model *without* spatial regularity; (e) Rician model with non-dictionary-based regularity; (f) nearest neighbor interpolation.

We learn 2 (core) dictionaries $\mathcal{D}$, with 1 anisotropic atom (adding isotropic atoms), from fully-sampled noisy (training) data, using: (i) our method (Sect. 3.2) and (ii) an alternative method using a Gaussian noise model, on the atoms and coefficients. Our approaches of Bayesian dictionary learning (Sect. 3.2) and Bayesian reconstruction (Sect. 3.3) give results (Fig. 5(f)) that are very close to the ground truth (Fig. 5(c)). Our best results are obtained by coupling dictionary and wavelet regularization (Fig. 5(b)). Replacing multiscale wavelet-based spatial regularization with (single-scale) TV-based spatial regularization leads to poorer results (Fig. 5(e)) that show the imbalance between reconstructed ODF accuracy and spatial smoothness despite optimal parameter tuning. Eliminating the spatial regularization altogether leads to further degradation in results

(Fig. 5(d)) that show inaccurate and irregular ODF reconstructions, especially in the crossing region. Replacing the Rician noise model with a Gaussian (that is the current state of the art) leads to poor results (Fig. 5(g)–(i)), showing less-sharp ODFs in voxels with 1 and 2 tracts (stemming from the Rician bias).

Undersampled HARDI Reconstruction with Brain HARDI. We use high-quality fully-sampled 2-shell HARDI (magnitude) images with 90 gradient directions from the HCP dataset, treat them as baselines, and perform retrospective undersampling (6× reduced directions) and Rician noise corruption to mimic SNRs 7 and 5 for 2 shells.

In the corpus callosum, with single-tract voxels (Fig. 6), the ODFs produced by our approach of Rician noise modeling along with spatial regularity on U and C (Fig. 6(b)) are close to the baseline (Fig. 6(a)). Changing the noise model to Gaussian (Fig. 6(c)) reduces ODF sharpness. Eliminating spatial regularity negatively affects the ODFs (Fig. 6(d)). Eliminating dictionary-based regularity, and keeping only regularity terms related to wavelets and C, leads to poor ODFs because they are unable to fill in the data in the missing directions (Fig. 6(e)). Filling in data in missing directions, within a shell, using the acquired data at the nearest direction in that shell, leads to poor reconstructions at this high level of undersampling (Fig. 6(f)).

In a region with crossing tracts/bimodal ODFs (Fig. 7), our approach (Fig. 7(b)) gives ODFs closest to the baseline (Fig. 7(a)). The Gaussian model reduces the ability to model bimodal ODFs (Fig. 7(c)) because the Rician bias reduces the contrast in diffusion signal values over directions. Lack of spatial regularity (Fig. 7(d)) leads to more perturbations in ODF orientations, where the irregularity leads to less sharp ODFs in the crossing. Eliminating dictionary-based regularity or nearest-neighbor interpolation leads to poor ODFs (Fig. 7(e), (f)). The means and standard deviations of angular errors [14] (radians) for white-matter regions are: (i) Rician noise model with spatial regularity: 0.3(0.3) (proposed); (ii) Gaussian model, with spatial regularity: 0.5(0.4); (iii) Rician model, without spatial regularity: 0.4(0.4). The GFA from reconstructions using

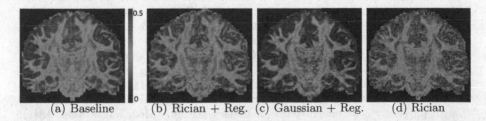

(a) Baseline   (b) Rician + Reg.   (c) Gaussian + Reg.   (d) Rician

Fig. 8. 6× undersampled brain HARDI reconstruction: GFA. GFA images, averaged over shells, for: (a) Baseline (high quality) data; (b) reconstruction using Rician noise model with spatial regularity **(proposed)**; (c) reconstruction using *Gaussian* noise models with spatial regularity; (d) reconstruction using Rician noise model *without* spatial regularity.

our approach (Fig. 8(b)) are closer to the truth (Fig. 8(a)) and more spatially regular. A Gaussian noise model leads to reduced GFA (Fig. 8(c)).

Conclusion. We proposed novel Bayesian frameworks for dictionary learning and undersampled reconstruction in HARDI, including Rician noise models (perhaps the first to do so). The Rician model yields sharper ODFs and improved accuracy in modeling crossings and estimating GFA. Our edge-preserving smoothness prior on dictionary atoms reduces the effect of high noise levels/artifacts in the data. Our spatial image priors via wavelets and non-local regularity (on coefficient vectors) improves over TV-based smoothness. The results using our models improve over the state of the art.

References

1. Alexander, D.: Multiple-fiber reconstruction algorithms for diffusion MRI. Ann. N. Y. Acad. Sci. **1064**, 113–133 (2005)
2. Aranda, R., Ramirez-Manzanares, A., Rivera, M.: Sparse and adaptive diffusion dictionary for recovering intra-voxel white matter structure. Med. Image Anal. **26**(1), 243–255 (2015)
3. Awate, S.P., DiBella, E.V.R.: Compressed sensing HARDI via rotation-invariant concise dictionaries, flexible k-space undersampling, and multiscale spatial regularity. In: IEEE International Symposium on Biomedical Imaging, pp. 9–12 (2013)
4. Bilgic, B., Setsompop, K., Cohen-Adad, J., Wedeen, V., Wald, L.L., Adalsteinsson, E.: Accelerated diffusion spectrum imaging with compressed sensing using adaptive dictionaries. In: Ayache, N., Delingette, H., Golland, P., Mori, K. (eds.) MICCAI 2012. LNCS, vol. 7512, pp. 1–9. Springer, Heidelberg (2012). doi:10.1007/978-3-642-33454-2_1
5. Cheng, J., Shen, D., Basser, P.J., Yap, P.-T.: Joint 6D k-q space compressed sensing for accelerated high angular resolution diffusion MRI. In: Ourselin, S., Alexander, D.C., Westin, C.-F., Cardoso, M.J. (eds.) IPMI 2015. LNCS, vol. 9123, pp. 782–793. Springer, Cham (2015). doi:10.1007/978-3-319-19992-4_62
6. Descoteaux, M., Deriche, R., LeBihan, D., Mangin, J.F., Poupon, C.: Multiple q-shell diffusion propagator imaging. Med. Image Anal. **15**, 603–621 (2011)
7. Descoteaux, M., Wiest-Daesslé, N., Prima, S., Barillot, C., Deriche, R.: Impact of Rician adapted non-local means filtering on HARDI. In: Metaxas, D., Axel, L., Fichtinger, G., Székely, G. (eds.) MICCAI 2008. LNCS, vol. 5242, pp. 122–130. Springer, Heidelberg (2008). doi:10.1007/978-3-540-85990-1_15
8. Duarte-Carvajalino, J., Lenglet, C., Xu, J., Yacoub, E., Ugurbil, K., Moeller, S., Carin, L., Sapiro, G.: Estimation of the CSA-ODF using Bayesian compressed sensing of multi-shell HARDI. Magn. Reson. Med. **72**(5), 1471–1485 (2014)
9. Gramfort, A., Poupon, C., Descoteaux, M.: Denoising and fast diffusion imaging with physically constrained sparse dictionary learning. Med. Image Anal. **18**(1), 36–49 (2014)
10. Gupta, K., Adlakha, D., Agarwal, V., Awate, S.P.: Regularized dictionary learning with robust sparsity fitting for compressed sensing multishell HARDI. In: Computational Diffusion MRI Workshop at MICCAI, pp. 1–12 (2016)
11. Jian, B., Vemuri, B.: A unified computational framework for deconvolution to reconstruct multiple fibers from diffusion weighted MRI. IEEE Trans. Med. Imag. **26**, 1464–1471 (2007)

12. Landman, B., Bogovic, J., Wan, H., ElShahaby, F., Bazin, P.L., Prince, J.: Resolution of crossing fibers with constrained compressed sensing using diffusion tensor MRI. NeuroImage **59**, 2175–2186 (2012)
13. Le-Bihan, D., Poupon, C., Amadon, A., Lethimonnier, F.: Artifacts and pitfalls in diffusion MRI. J. Magn. Reson. Imaging **24**, 478–488 (2006)
14. Merlet, S., Caruyer, E., Ghosh, A., Deriche, R.: A computational diffusion MRI and parametric dictionary learning framework for modeling the diffusion signal and its features. Med. Image Anal. **17**(7), 830–843 (2013)
15. Michailovich, O., Rathi, Y., Dolui, S.: Spatially regularized compressed sensing for high angular resolution diffusion imaging. IEEE TMI **30**, 1100–1115 (2011)
16. Ning, L., Setsompop, K., Michailovich, O., Makris, N., Shenton, M., Westin, C.F., Rathi, Y.: A joint compressed-sensing and super-resolution approach for very high-resolution diffusion imaging. NeuroImage **125**, 386–400 (2016)
17. Rathi, Y., Michailovich, O., Laun, F., Setsompop, K., Grant, P., Westin, C.F.: Multi-shell diffusion signal recovery from sparse measurements. Med. Image Anal. **18**(7), 1143–1156 (2014)
18. Scherrer, B., Warfield, S.: Why multiple b-values are required for multi-tensor models: evaluation with a constrained log-Euclidean model. In: IEEE ISBI, pp. 1389–1392 (2012)
19. Tristán-Vega, A., Westin, C.-F.: Probabilistic ODF estimation from reduced HARDI Data with sparse regularization. In: Fichtinger, G., Martel, A., Peters, T. (eds.) MICCAI 2011. LNCS, vol. 6892, pp. 182–190. Springer, Heidelberg (2011). doi:10.1007/978-3-642-23629-7_23
20. Tuch, D., Reese, T., Wiegell, M.: High angular resolution diffusion imaging reveals intravoxel white matter fiber heterogeneity. Magn. Reson. Med. **48**(4), 477–582 (2002)

Estimation of Tissue Microstructure Using a Deep Network Inspired by a Sparse Reconstruction Framework

Chuyang Ye[1,2]([✉])

[1] Brainnetome Center, Institute of Automation, Chinese Academy of Sciences,
Beijing, China
[2] National Laboratory of Pattern Recognition, Institute of Automation,
Chinese Academy of Sciences, Beijing, China
chuyang.ye@nlpr.ia.ac.cn

Abstract. *Diffusion magnetic resonance imaging* (dMRI) provides a unique tool for noninvasively probing the microstructure of the neuronal tissue. The NODDI model has been a popular approach to the estimation of tissue microstructure in many neuroscience studies. It represents the diffusion signals with three types of diffusion in tissue: intra-cellular, extra-cellular, and cerebrospinal fluid compartments. However, the original NODDI method uses a computationally expensive procedure to fit the model and could require a large number of diffusion gradients for accurate microstructure estimation, which may be impractical for clinical use. Therefore, efforts have been devoted to efficient and accurate NODDI microstructure estimation with a reduced number of diffusion gradients. In this work, we propose a deep network based approach to the NODDI microstructure estimation, which is named *Microstructure Estimation using a Deep Network* (MEDN). Motivated by the AMICO algorithm which accelerates the computation of NODDI parameters, we formulate the microstructure estimation problem in a dictionary-based framework. The proposed network comprises two cascaded stages. The first stage resembles the solution to a dictionary-based sparse reconstruction problem and the second stage computes the final microstructure using the output of the first stage. The weights in the two stages are jointly learned from training data, which is obtained from training dMRI scans with diffusion gradients that densely sample the *q*-space. The proposed method was applied to brain dMRI scans, where two shells each with 30 gradient directions (60 diffusion gradients in total) were used. Estimation accuracy with respect to the gold standard was measured and the results demonstrate that MEDN outperforms the competing algorithms.

Keywords: Diffusion MRI · NODDI · Microstructure · Deep network

1 Introduction

Diffusion magnetic resonance imaging (dMRI) provides a unique tool for noninvasively probing the microstructure of the neuronal tissue by capturing the

© Springer International Publishing AG 2017
M. Niethammer et al. (Eds.): IPMI 2017, LNCS 10265, pp. 466–477, 2017.
DOI: 10.1007/978-3-319-59050-9_37

displacement pattern of water molecules [8]. *Diffusion tensor imaging* (DTI) was first developed to model the anisotropy of water diffusion using a Gaussian model, where fractional anisotropy and mean diffusivity can be computed to describe tissue microstructure. More complex methods have been proposed for improved diffusion modeling using biophysical models consisting of different tissue compartments, such as CHARMED [2], ActiveAx [1], and NODDI [23].

Among the existing algorithms for microstructure estimation, the NODDI model has been a popular choice in a number of scientific studies, for example, on brain development [10] or pathological changes caused by diseases [9]. The NODDI model distinguishes three different types of diffusion in tissue, leading to the intra-cellular, extra-cellular, and *cerebrospinal fluid* (CSF) compartments [23]. By relating these compartments with observed diffusion signals, the parameters in the NODDI model are estimated with a maximum likelihood approach. The contribution of each compartment, the mean orientation of the intracellular compartment, and the orientation dispersion are then achieved, which give estimates of the tissue microstructural organization.

The NODDI model uses a computationally expensive procedure to fit the model, and thus requires powerful computer clusters and/or takes a long computation time [5]. To efficiently solve the NODDI model, a dictionary-based framework has been proposed in the AMICO algorithm [5], where the microstructure estimation is accelerated drastically. AMICO computes the mean orientation beforehand using DTI and estimates the CSF volume fraction, intra-cellular volume fraction, and orientation dispersion. First, it uses a dictionary that encodes discretized NODDI parameters to represent the diffusion signals. The *mixture fractions* (MFs) of the dictionary atoms can be estimated by solving a regularized least squares problem. The MF associated with the CSF atom provides an estimate of the CSF volume fraction. The other MFs, after normalization, linearly weight the discretized NODDI parameters to compute the rest of the microstructural properties. However, NODDI or AMICO could require a large number of diffusion gradients for accurate microstructure estimation, which may limit their clinical use. Thus, a multi-layer perceptron was used in [6] to estimate scalar quantities including the NODDI parameters with a reduced number of diffusion gradients.

Efficient and accurate NODDI microstructure estimation using the number of diffusion gradients that is clinically practical (for example, around 60) is still an open problem. In this work, we design a deep network to predict the NODDI microstructural properties. The method is named *Microstructure Estimation using a Deep Network* (MEDN). Because the mean orientation can be estimated accurately using the simple DTI model [5], we focus on the scalar NODDI parameters like [5]. Unlike [6], where a general multi-layer perceptron is used, the deep network in MEDN is designed specifically for the estimation of NODDI parameters. The proposed network structure is motivated by the AMICO [5] procedure and comprises two cascaded stages where all the weights are jointly learned for microstructure prediction. The first stage uses a network structure that unfolds an iterative process similar to iterative hard thresholding [4], and can solve a dictionary-based sparse reconstruction problem after the network weights are learned [20]. In the second stage, one of the output of the first stage corresponds to the CSF volume fraction; the other outputs are normalized and weighted to predict the intra-cellular volume fraction and orientation dispersion (after a transformation), where the weights are also learned. Like [6], for each dMRI dataset acquired with a fixed imaging protocol, one deep network is trained. To generate the training data, we use a strategy similar to [6], which requires training dMRI scans acquired with diffusion gradients that densely sample the q-space. The microstructure estimated by AMICO on the training images are then used to train the network, where the sum of the mean squared errors of the CSF volume fraction, intra-cellular volume fraction, and orientation dispersion is used as the loss function. The proposed method was evaluated on brain dMRI scans, where two shells each with 30 gradient directions were used, and the results demonstrate that MEDN outperforms the competitors.

2   Methods

2.1   Background: NODDI and AMICO for Tissue Microstructure Estimation

NODDI models the neuronal tissue with three types of microstructural environments, which are the intra-cellular, extra-cellular, and CSF compartments [23]. The water diffusion in each compartment has different distributions and thus different response functions to diffusion gradients. Suppose the number of diffusion gradients is K, the diffusion signal associated with the k-th ($k = 1, \ldots, K$) diffusion gradient at a voxel is S_k, and the signal without diffusion weighting is S_0. The normalized signal $y_k = S_k/S_0$ is modeled using the three compartments:

$$y_k = (1 - v_{\mathrm{iso}})(v_{\mathrm{ic}} A_{\mathrm{ic},k} + (1 - v_{\mathrm{ic}}) A_{\mathrm{ec},k}) + v_{\mathrm{iso}} A_{\mathrm{iso},k}, \tag{1}$$

where $A_{\mathrm{ic},k}$, $A_{\mathrm{ec},k}$, and $A_{\mathrm{iso},k}$ are the normalized signals of the intra-cellular, extra-cellular, and CSF compartments, respectively; v_{ic}, $1 - v_{\mathrm{ic}}$, and v_{iso} are the volume fractions of the intra-cellular, extra-cellular, and CSF compartments, respectively [23].

In NODDI, $A_{\mathrm{ic},k}$ is represented using a stick model, where the orientation $\boldsymbol{\mu}$ has a Watson distribution with a concentration parameter κ that can measure the *orientation dispersion* (OD) by

$$\mathrm{OD} = \frac{2}{\pi} \arctan(1/\kappa). \tag{2}$$

$A_{\mathrm{ec},k}$ is modeled as anisotropic Gaussian diffusion, which is dependent on both v_{ic} and κ. $A_{\mathrm{iso},k}$ is modeled as isotropic Gaussian diffusion with predetermined diffusivity. For the specific design of the signal models for these compartments, we refer readers to [23]. Using the diffusion signals associated with all K diffusion gradients, the parameters v_{ic}, κ, $\boldsymbol{\mu}$, and v_{iso} are estimated with a maximum likelihood approach [23], and OD is derived from κ according to Eq. (2)

The original nonlinear approach to the NODDI model fitting in [23] is very time-consuming and could cause practical problems for application to large cohorts [5]. Therefore, AMICO [5] is proposed to accelerate the estimation. It first decouples the estimation of mean orientations μ and the other scalar quantities, and computes μ using DTI. Then, the distinct water pools orientated in the direction μ can be accounted for using a linear dictionary-based formulation

$$y = \Phi_\mu f + \eta, \tag{3}$$

where $y = (y_1, \ldots, y_K)^T$ is the observed signal vector, Φ_μ is the dictionary, f is the MFs of the dictionary atoms, and η is noise. The dictionary is computed from a fixed set of discretized v_{ic} and κ. It can be written as $\Phi_\mu = [\Phi_\mu^{\mathrm{a}} | \Phi^{\mathrm{i}}]$, where $\Phi_\mu^{\mathrm{a}} \in \mathbb{R}^{K \times N_{\mathrm{a}}}$ comprises N_{a} columns of anisotropic signals of the coupled intra- and extra-cellular compartments corresponding to combinations of specific discretized v_{ic} and κ, and $\Phi^{\mathrm{i}} \in \mathbb{R}^{K \times 1}$ comprises the signal terms of a constant isotropic diffusion. The discretized v_{ic} and κ associated with the j-th column in Φ_μ^{a} are denoted by $\tilde{v}_{\mathrm{ic},j}$ and $\tilde{\kappa}_j$, respectively. AMICO uses 12 discretized v_{ic} and 12 discretized κ, leading to $N_{\mathrm{a}} = 144$ combinations. f can be denoted by $f = (f_1, \ldots, f_{N_{\mathrm{a}}}, f_{N_{\mathrm{a}}+1})^T$, where $f^{\mathrm{a}} = (f_1, \ldots, f_{N_{\mathrm{a}}})^T$ and $f^{\mathrm{i}} = f_{N_{\mathrm{a}}+1}$ are associated with Φ_μ^{a} and Φ^{i}, respectively.

The MFs are estimated by solving

$$\hat{f} = \arg\min_{f \geq 0} ||\Phi_\mu f - y||_2^2 + \alpha||f||_2^2 + \beta||f||_1, \tag{4}$$

where α and β are weights specified by users. Then, the NODDI parameters are computed from the MFs and discretized v_{ic} and κ as follows

$$v_{\mathrm{ic}} = \frac{\sum_{j=1}^{N_{\mathrm{a}}} \tilde{v}_{\mathrm{ic},j} \hat{f}_j}{\sum_{j=1}^{N_{\mathrm{a}}} \hat{f}_j}, \kappa = \frac{\sum_{j=1}^{N_{\mathrm{a}}} \tilde{\kappa}_j \hat{f}_j}{\sum_{j=1}^{N_{\mathrm{a}}} \hat{f}_j}, \text{ and } v_{\mathrm{iso}} = \hat{f}_{N_{\mathrm{a}}+1}, \tag{5}$$

and OD is computed from κ using Eq. (2). It is demonstrated in [5] that AMICO reduces the computational time by two orders of magnitude.

2.2   Tissue Microstructure Estimation Using a Deep Network

The deep network has been applied to many computer vision tasks [15], and in this work we explore its use in tissue microstructure estimation. The design of a deep network structure can be motivated in many ways, for example, by the organization of neurons in the brain [13] or by procedures performed by specific algorithms [7,20]. Our design of the network structure for microstructure estimation belongs to the latter category. As introduced in Sect. 2.1, AMICO consists of two steps: (1) solving a regularized least squares problem (see Eq. (4)) and (2) computing the NODDI parameters using the MFs and discretized parameters (see Eq. (5)). Motivated by these steps, we construct a deep network whose structure is similar to the AMICO procedure, while the weights in the network are learned instead of predetermined. The proposed network structure is shown in Fig. 1, which comprises two cascaded stages. The input and output of the network are indicated by the green and orange colors, respectively. The design is explained in detail in the following paragraphs.

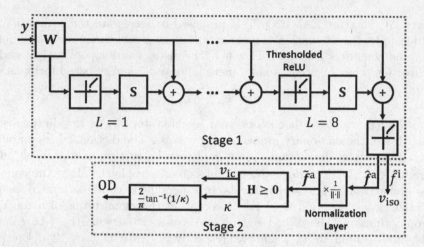

Fig. 1. The deep network designed for microstructure estimation. The input and output of the network are indicated by the green and orange colors, respectively. (Color figure online)

Stage One. The first stage takes the observed normalized diffusion signals y as input and seeks to solve a regularized least squares problem with learned parameters. We notice that in [5] the weight α is much smaller than β in Eq. (4), and setting $\alpha = 0$ can still achieve low estimation errors. Thus, we let $\alpha = 0$ and Eq. (4) becomes an ℓ_1-norm regularized least squares problem, which is an approximation of the (nonnegative) sparse reconstruction problem

$$\hat{f} = \arg\min_{f \geq 0} \|\boldsymbol{\Phi} f - y\|_2^2 + \beta \|f\|_0. \tag{6}$$

For convenience, here we have dropped the symbol μ. Conventionally, the sparse reconstruction problem can be solved using iterative hard thresholding (IHT) [4], which iteratively updates the estimate. Specifically, at iteration $t + 1$

$$f^{t+1} = h_\lambda(\mathbf{W}y + \mathbf{S}f^t), \tag{7}$$

where $\mathbf{W} = \boldsymbol{\Phi}^T$, $\mathbf{S} = \mathbf{I} - \boldsymbol{\Phi}^T\boldsymbol{\Phi}$, and $h_\lambda(\cdot)$ is a thresholding operator with a parameter $\lambda > 0$

$$[h_\lambda(\boldsymbol{a})]_i = \begin{cases} 0 & \text{if} \quad a_i < \lambda \\ a_i & \text{if} \quad a_i \geq \lambda \end{cases}. \tag{8}$$

Note that due to the constraint $f \geq 0$, $[h_\lambda(\boldsymbol{a})]_i$ is always zero when a_i is negative.

Motivated by the iterative process in IHT, a feed-forward network structure can be constructed by unfolding and truncating this process [20], which is indicated by the blue box in Fig. 1. The number of layers in this stage is eight, which lies in the range of the numbers used by previous works [17,20,21]. We assume

$\boldsymbol{f}^0 = 0$ and the thresholded *rectified linear unit* (ReLU) [12] corresponds to the operator $h_\lambda(\cdot)$ ($\lambda = 0.01$ in this work). The update of $\boldsymbol{f}$ according to Eq. (7) is completed after each thresholded ReLU. Here, instead of using $\mathbf{W}$ and $\mathbf{S}$ predetermined by $\boldsymbol{\Phi}$, $\mathbf{W} \in \mathbb{R}^{N \times K}$ and $\mathbf{S} \in \mathbb{R}^{N \times N}$ in the network are learned from training data, and the dimension N is to be specified by the users. Greater N leads to more weights to be learned in the network, and in this work we empirically set $N = 301$. Note that $\mathbf{S}$ is shared among layers, thus increasing the number of layers does not increase the number of weights to be learned.

It was demonstrated in [21] that learned layer-wise fixed weights could guarantee successful sparse reconstruction across a wider range of *restricted isometry property* (RIP) conditions than IHT. In addition, because usually we only seek to solve a problem where inputs are similar to the training data, the problem is smaller than a general sparse reconstruction problem for all possible inputs, and it is possible to use learned weights to achieve superior reconstruction [7].

Note that in the original AMICO framework, different $\boldsymbol{\Phi}_{\boldsymbol{\mu}}$ is needed for different $\boldsymbol{\mu}$. However, in this work we only construct one deep network for microstructure estimation for all possible $\boldsymbol{\mu}$, and it can be interpreted in the following way. The mean orientations can be discretized as well [14, 22], which gives a basis orientation set $\mathcal{U} = \{\tilde{\boldsymbol{\mu}}_i\}_{i=1}^{|\mathcal{U}|}$ ($|\mathcal{U}|$ is the cardinality of $\mathcal{U}$). Then, the dictionary matrix can be expanded to include the signal terms associated with the discretized $\boldsymbol{\mu}$, v_{ic}, and κ, so that $\boldsymbol{\Phi} = \left[\boldsymbol{\Phi}_{\tilde{\boldsymbol{\mu}}_1}^{\mathrm{a}} \big| \dots \big| \boldsymbol{\Phi}_{\tilde{\boldsymbol{\mu}}_{|\mathcal{U}|}}^{\mathrm{a}} \big| \boldsymbol{\Phi}^{\mathrm{i}}\right]$. The microstructure can still be computed from the MFs associated with $\boldsymbol{\Phi}$ using Eq. (5).

Stage Two. The second stage (indicated by the purple box in Fig. 1) computes the NODDI parameters using the output of the first stage. v_{iso} is immediately achieved from the entry $\hat{f}^{\mathrm{i}}$ in $\hat{\boldsymbol{f}}$ that corresponds to the CSF compartment. From Eq. (5), we see that v_{ic} and κ are computed by linearly transforming the normalized MFs of anisotropic diffusion compartments. Thus, the other entries $\hat{\boldsymbol{f}}^{\mathrm{a}}$ in $\hat{\boldsymbol{f}}$ are first normalized by the normalization layer in the second stage. Note that to ensure numerical stability, we use $\tilde{\boldsymbol{f}}^{\mathrm{a}} = (\hat{\boldsymbol{f}}^{\mathrm{a}} + \tau \mathbf{1})/\|\hat{\boldsymbol{f}}^{\mathrm{a}} + \tau \mathbf{1}\|_1$ for the normalization, where $\tau = 10^{-10}$. Then, the computation of v_{ic} and κ resembling Eq. (5) can be written in the matrix form

$$[v_{\mathrm{ic}} \ \kappa]^T = \mathbf{H}\tilde{\boldsymbol{f}}^{\mathrm{a}}, \tag{9}$$

where $\mathbf{H} \in \mathbb{R}^{2 \times (N-1)}$ contains the weights of $\tilde{\boldsymbol{f}}^{\mathrm{a}}$ and is to be learned. Because the discretized v_{ic} and κ in Eq. (5) are nonnegative, here we require each element in $\mathbf{H}$ to be nonnegative. OD is computed from κ using Eq. (2). The final outputs of the network are v_{ic}, v_{iso}, and OD.

2.3 Training and Evaluation

The weights in the two stages are learned jointly. We use the sum of the mean squared errors of v_{ic}, v_{iso}, and OD as the loss function and the Adam algorithm [11] as the optimizer, where the learning rate is 0.0001, the batch size is

128, and the number of epochs is 10. Similar to [6], 10% of the training samples were used as a validation set to prevent overfitting. The network is implemented using Keras[1].

We use a training strategy similar to [6]. Because the observed diffusion signals are dependent on the diffusion gradients used in the imaging protocol, for each dataset of dMRI scans that are acquired with a fixed set $\mathcal{G}$ of diffusion gradients, one deep network needs to be trained for microstructure prediction. Because ground truth microstructure is difficult to acquire, to generate training samples, training dMRI scans should be acquired with a set $\tilde{\mathcal{G}}$ of diffusion gradients that densely sample the q-space, where $\mathcal{G} \subseteq \tilde{\mathcal{G}}$. Each voxel in the training images represents a training sample, and the microstructure computed by AMICO on the training dMRI scans using all diffusion gradients $\tilde{\mathcal{G}}$ and the diffusion signals associated with $\mathcal{G}$ were used to train the network.

Using the trained network, tissue microstructure at each voxel on a test image can be estimated. To quantitatively evaluate the estimation performance, the gold standard should be obtained, with which estimation results are compared. Similar to the generation of training images, for each test dMRI scan with diffusion gradients $\mathcal{G}$, diffusion gradients $\tilde{\mathcal{G}}$ densely sampling the q-space were also applied to compute the gold standard of tissue microstructure using AMICO. Note that $\tilde{\mathcal{G}}$ was only used for computing the gold standard for evaluation, and was not used in the test phase. The mean absolute difference was used to compute the disagreement between the estimates and the gold standard.

3   Results

The proposed method was applied to brain dMRI for evaluation on a 16-core Linux machine. We randomly selected ten subjects from the Human Connectome Project (HCP) dataset [19]. The *diffusion weighted images* (DWIs) were acquired on a 3T MR scanner (ConnectomS, Siemens, Erlangen, Germany), where 270 diffusion gradients over three shells with b-values of 1000, 2000, and 3000 s/mm^2 were used. The resolution of the DWIs is 1.25 mm isotropic. Five subjects were randomly selected as training scans and the other five were used as test scans. For each training or test scan, 60 fixed diffusion gradients were selected as the diffusion gradients $\mathcal{G}$, and the normalized diffusion signals associated with $\mathcal{G}$ are the input to the network in the training or test phase, respectively. These 60 diffusion gradients resemble clinically achievable protocols. They consist of 30 gradient directions on each of the shell $b = 1000, 2000$ s/mm^2, and the gradient directions are approximately evenly distributed over the unit sphere. The full set of 270 diffusion gradients were used to compute the training and gold standard microstructure for the training and test scans, respectively.

The training process using the five training subjects took about 8.5 h. The overall training loss and validation loss in the training phase are shown in Fig. 2, together with the loss of each microstructure quantity. We can see that both the

---

[1] http://keras.io/.

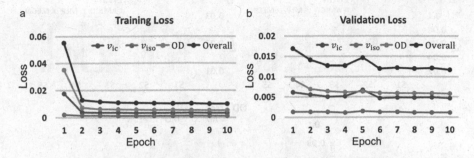

Fig. 2. The training and validation loss after each epoch in the training phase.

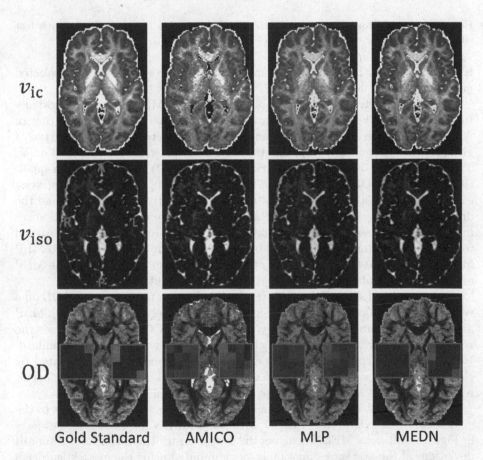

Fig. 3. Microstructure estimation of AMICO, MLP, and MEDN shown together with the gold standard on a representative subject. The orientation is indicated on the gold standard v_{iso} map (the left image in the middle row). The contrasts in the zoomed regions on the OD maps are enhanced with the same mapping.

474   C. Ye

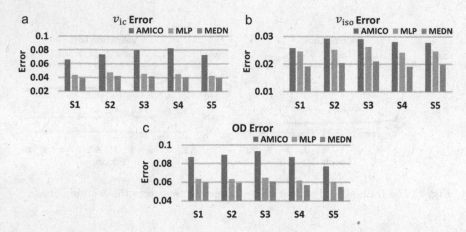

Fig. 4. Average errors of tissue microstructure estimation in the brain for each test subject (S1–S5): (a) v_{ic}, (b) v_{iso}, and (c) OD.

training loss and validation loss become stable after ten epochs with the selected parameters of the network.

The trained network was then applied to the test dMRI scans for microstructure prediction. The estimation accuracy of MEDN was compared with that of AMICO (using the implementation and default parameters provided at https://github.com/daducci/AMICO/) and the deep network structure proposed in [6]. The authors of [6] used a *multi-layer perceptron* (MLP) to predict scalar quantities including NODDI parameters. The MLP consists of three hidden layers, each comprising 150 hidden units with a ReLU [16] activation function, and the dropout fraction is 0.1; 10% of the training voxels were used as a validation set in the training phase. In our experiments, the weights in the MLP were learned from the same training samples used by MEDN. The input of AMICO and MLP for the test scans is the same as that of MEDN. For each test subject, both MLP and MEDN took about 30 min, and AMICO took about five hours.

Cross-sectional slices of the gold standard and estimated v_{ic}, v_{iso}, and OD on a representative subject are shown in Fig. 3 for qualitatively evaluation. Both MLP and MEDN produced a smoother v_{ic} map than AMICO (for example, see the regions pointed by the blue arrow), which better agrees with the gold standard. In the anterior corpus callosum (for example, the zoomed regions indicated by the green arrows) on the OD maps, the MEDN result is less noisy and better resembles the gold standard than the AMICO and MLP results.

The average microstructure estimation errors in the brain with respect to the gold standard are shown for AMICO, MLP, and MEDN for all five test subjects in Fig. 4. In all cases MEDN achieves the lowest error. The means and standard deviations of the average estimation errors computed using the five test subjects are shown in Fig. 5, and AMICO and MLP were compared with MEDN using a paired Student's t-test. The estimation error of MEDN is significantly smaller than that of AMICO and MLP for v_{ic}, v_{iso}, and OD. Compared with MLP which has the second best performance, MEDN reduces the mean errors of v_{ic}, v_{iso}, and OD by about 9%, 20%, and 7%, respectively.

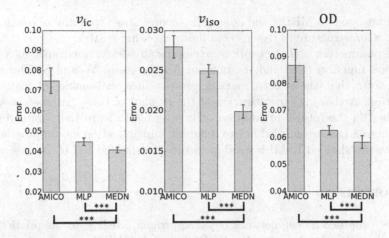

Fig. 5. Means and standard deviations of the average estimation errors in Fig. 4 computed using all five test subjects. MEDN was compared with AMICO and MLP using a paired Student's t-test, and asterisks indicate that the difference is significant ($^{***}p < 0.001$).

4   Discussion

The original NODDI model fitting approach in [23] can be very time-consuming. As reported in [5], the original NODDI computation took around 65 h on a dMRI scan at a resolution much lower than that of the HCP data used in this work. Thus, performing the original NODDI model fitting would be prohibitive for the experiments in this work. AMICO has been shown to produce results comparable to [23] and reduce the computational time by two orders of magnitude. Therefore, we used AMICO to compute the training data and gold standard of tissue microstructure.

The NODDI model can be improved by modeling anisotropic orientation dispersion that is widespread due to fiber bending and fanning [18]. In [18] the Bingham-NODDI model was proposed, which replaces the Watson distribution in NODDI with the Bingham distribution to allow estimation of anisotropic dispersion and thus introduces extra parameters. It is possible to formulate the Bingham-NODDI model in a dictionary-based framework like AMICO, where the dictionary atoms are computed using the Bingham distribution with its discretized parameters. Thus, the first stage in MEDN still applies, and the second stage needs to be adapted to compute additional microstructure descriptors modeled by Bingham-NODDI.

NODDI and AMICO only assume one fiber orientation in a voxel while brain regions can contain crossing fibers [3]. Thus, AMICOx was proposed in [3], which improves AMICO by expanding the dictionary to encode atoms corresponding to multiple precomputed fiber orientations. Since AMICOx also relies on solving a dictionary-based regularized least squares problem, we can still use the structure in the first stage in MEDN and adapt the second stage to compute orientation-specific microstructure in regions containing crossing tracts.

The parameters in the network were empirically determined, such as λ in the activation function $h_\lambda(\cdot)$ and the number N of rows in $\mathbf{W}$ and $\mathbf{S}$. The results demonstrate that the selected parameters produce reasonable microstructure estimation. A thorough investigation of the impact of these parameters will be performed in the future. In addition, it is possible to learn the parameter λ as well, where λ can be encoded in two different multiplication modules before and after the thresholded ReLU instead of in the thresholded ReLU [20].

5   Conclusion

We have proposed a deep network based approach, MEDN, to the prediction of tissue microstructure based on the NODDI model. MEDN comprises two stages, where the weights are learned jointly. The first stage resembles the solution to a sparse reconstruction problem and the second stage computes the microstructure using the output of the first stage. Results on brain dMRI data demonstrate that MEDN outperforms the competing methods.

Acknowledgement. This work is supported by NSFC 61601461. Data were provided by the Human Connectome Project, WU-Minn Consortium (Principal Investigators: David Van Essen and Kamil Ugurbil; 1U54MH091657).

References

1. Alexander, D.C., Hubbard, P.L., Hall, M.G., Moore, E.A., Ptito, M., Parker, G.J., Dyrby, T.B.: Orientationally invariant indices of axon diameter and density from diffusion MRI. NeuroImage **52**(4), 1374–1389 (2010)
2. Assaf, Y., Basser, P.J.: Composite hindered and restricted model of diffusion (CHARMED) MR imaging of the human brain. NeuroImage **27**(1), 48–58 (2005)
3. Auría, A., Romascano, D.P.R., Canales-Rodriguez, E., Wiaux, Y., Dirby, T.B., Alexander, D., Thiran, J.P., Daducci, A.: Accelerated microstructure imaging via convex optimisation for regions with multiple fibres (AMICOx). In: IEEE International Conference on Image Processing 2015, pp. 1673–1676. IEEE (2015)
4. Blumensath, T., Davies, M.E.: Iterative thresholding for sparse approximations. J. Fourier Anal. Appl. **14**(5–6), 629–654 (2008)
5. Daducci, A., Canales-Rodríguez, E.J., Zhang, H., Dyrby, T.B., Alexander, D.C., Thiran, J.P.: Accelerated Microstructure Imaging via Convex Optimization (AMICO) from diffusion MRI data. NeuroImage **105**, 32–44 (2015)
6. Golkov, V., Dosovitskiy, A., Sperl, J.I., Menzel, M.I., Czisch, M., Sämann, P., Brox, T., Cremers, D.: q-space deep learning: twelve-fold shorter and model-free diffusion MRI scans. IEEE Trans. Med. Imaging **35**(5), 1344–1351 (2016)
7. Gregor, K., LeCun, Y.: Learning fast approximations of sparse coding. In: International Conference on Machine Learning, pp. 399–406 (2010)
8. Johansen-Berg, H., Behrens, T.E.J.: Diffusion MRI: From Quantitative Measurement to in Vivo Neuroanatomy. Academic Press, Waltham (2013)

9. Kamagata, K., Hatano, T., Okuzumi, A., Motoi, Y., Abe, O., Shimoji, K., Kamiya, K., Suzuki, M., Hori, M., Kumamaru, K.K., Hattori, N., Aoki, S.: Neurite orientation dispersion and density imaging in the substantia nigra in idiopathic Parkinson disease. Eur. Radiol. **26**(8), 2567–2577 (2016)

10. Kelly, C.E., Thompson, D.K., Chen, J., Leemans, A., Adamson, C.L., Inder, T.E., Cheong, J.L., Doyle, L.W., Anderson, P.J.: Axon density and axon orientation dispersion in children born preterm. Hum. Brain Mapp. **37**(9), 3080–3102 (2016)

11. Kingma, D., Ba, J.: Adam: a method for stochastic optimization. arXiv preprint arXiv:1412.6980 (2014)

12. Konda, K., Memisevic, R., Krueger, D.: Zero-bias autoencoders and the benefits of co-adapting features. arXiv preprint arXiv:1402.3337 (2014)

13. Krizhevsky, A., Sutskever, I., Hinton, G.E.: ImageNet classification with deep convolutional neural networks. In: Advances in Neural Information Processing Systems, pp. 1097–1105 (2012)

14. Landman, B.A., Bogovic, J.A., Wan, H., ElShahaby, F.E.Z., Bazin, P.L., Prince, J.L.: Resolution of crossing fibers with constrained compressed sensing using diffusion tensor MRI. NeuroImage **59**(3), 2175–2186 (2012)

15. LeCun, Y., Bengio, Y., Hinton, G.: Deep learning. Nature **521**(7553), 436–444 (2015)

16. Nair, V., Hinton, G.E.: Rectified linear units improve restricted Boltzmann machines. In: Proceedings of the 27th International Conference on Machine Learning, pp. 807–814 (2010)

17. Sprechmann, P., Bronstein, A.M., Sapiro, G.: Learning efficient sparse and low rank models. IEEE Trans. Pattern Anal. Mach. Intell. **37**(9), 1821–1833 (2015)

18. Tariq, M., Schneider, T., Alexander, D.C., Wheeler-Kingshott, C.A.G., Zhang, H.: Bingham-NODDI: mapping anisotropic orientation dispersion of neurites using diffusion MRI. NeuroImage **133**, 207–223 (2016)

19. Van Essen, D.C., Smith, S.M., Barch, D.M., Behrens, T.E.J., Yacoub, E., Ugurbil, K.: The WU-Minn human connectome project: an overview. NeuroImage **80**, 62–79 (2013)

20. Wang, Z., Ling, Q., Huang, T.S.: Learning deep ℓ_0 encoders. In: AAAI Conference on Artificial Intelligence, pp. 2194–2200 (2016)

21. Xin, B., Wang, Y., Gao, W., Wipf, D.: Maximal sparsity with deep networks? arXiv preprint arXiv:1605.01636 (2016)

22. Ye, C., Zhuo, J., Gullapalli, R.P., Prince, J.L.: Estimation of fiber orientations using neighborhood information. Med. Image Anal. **32**, 243–256 (2016)

23. Zhang, H., Schneider, T., Wheeler-Kingshott, C.A., Alexander, D.C.: NODDI: practical in vivo neurite orientation dispersion and density imaging of the human brain. NeuroImage **61**(4), 1000–1016 (2012)

HFPRM: Hierarchical Functional Principal Regression Model for Diffusion Tensor Image Bundle Statistics

Jingwen Zhang[1], Chao Huang[1], Joseph G. Ibrahim[1], Shaili Jha[2],
Rebecca C. Knickmeyer[3], John H. Gilmore[3], Martin Styner[3],
and Hongtu Zhu[1,4(✉)]

[1] Department of Biostatistics, University of North Carolina at Chapel Hill,
Chapel Hill, USA
[2] Curriculum in Neurobiology, University of North Carolina at Chapel Hill,
Chapel Hill, USA
[3] Department of Psychiatry, University of North Carolina at Chapel Hill,
Chapel Hill, USA
[4] Department of Biostatistics, University of Texas MD Anderson Cancer Center,
Houston, USA
HZhu5@mdanderson.org

Abstract. Diffusion-weighted magnetic resonance imaging (MRI) provides a unique approach to understand the geometric structure of brain fiber bundles and to delineate the diffusion properties across subjects and time. It can be used to identify structural connectivity abnormalities and helps to diagnose brain-related disorders. The aim of this paper is to develop a novel, robust, and efficient dimensional reduction and regression framework, called hierarchical functional principal regression model (HFPRM), to effectively correlate high-dimensional fiber bundle statistics with a set of predictors of interest, such as age, diagnosis status, and genetic markers. The three key novelties of HFPRM include the simultaneous analysis of a large number of fiber bundles, the disentanglement of global and individual latent factors that characterizes between-tract correlation patterns, and a bi-level analysis on the predictor effects. Simulations are conducted to evaluate the finite sample performance of HFPRM. We have also applied HFPRM to a genome-wide association study to explore important genetic variants in neonatal white matter development.

Knickmeyer was partially supported by the National Institutes of Health grant MH083045.

Gilmore was partially supported by the National Institutes of Health grants MH064065, MH070890, and HD053000.

Styner was partially supported by the National Institutes of Health grant EB005149-01.

Zhu was partially supported by the National Institutes of Health grant MH086633, the National Science Foundation grants SES-1357666 and DMS-1407655, as well as a senior investigator grant from the Cancer Prevention Research Institute of Texas.

M. Niethammer et al. (Eds.): IPMI 2017, LNCS 10265, pp. 478–489, 2017.
DOI: 10.1007/978-3-319-59050-9_38

Keywords: Fiber bundle statistics · Varying coefficient model · Functional principal component analysis · Factor analysis · Imaging genetics

1   Introduction

Scientifically, investigation in the connectional organization of human brain and its variation across subjects is a critical step to understand the pathology of many neuro-related disorders. Diffusion-weighted MRI offers a non-invasive approach to study the tissue structure of white matter fiber bundles *in vivo*, including both the geometric shape and the diffusion properties [2,6,9,12,17,24,27]. Delineating diffusion statistics along fiber bundles may help identify structural connectivity abnormalities across different spatial-temporal scales. It could eventually inspire new approaches for disease preventions, diagnoses and clinical treatments.

Group analysis of fiber bundle statistics poses remarkable computational and mathematical challenges to existing statistical methods. The first challenge is to efficiently and simultaneously study multiple fiber bundles with heterogeneous geometric structures and variation patterns. The second challenge is to correlate fiber bundle statistics with a large number of covariates, such as millions of genetic markers. This challenge is motivated by the demand to carry out a genome-wide association study on fiber bundle statistics. Voxel-wise methods [21] and single tract analysis [8,26,28] suffer from performing massive multiple comparison adjustments, which would severely reduce detection power. The third challenge is to properly handle the potential correlation among multiple tracts and to disentangle tract-specific information from global information shared by a large portion of fiber bundles.

The aim of this paper is to develop a hierarchical functional principal regression model (HFPRM) framework to address the three challenges discussed above. HFPRM consists of three statistical models, including a varying coefficient model (VCM), a latent factor analysis (LFA) procedure, and a multivariate regression model (MRM). The path diagram of HFPRM is presented in Fig. 1. The VCM not only captures the functional structure of fiber bundle statistics for each single tract, but also maps the heterogeneous geometric structure of multiple fiber bundles onto a common coordinate system. The LFA is applied to characterize potential inter-tract correlation across multiple bundles. It allows us to explicitly identify both tract-specific and global latent signals. The integration of VCM and LFA dramatically reduces the dimension of fiber bundle statistics. Finally, using MRM, we are able to examine the effect of selected predictors on both global level and individual level.

In Sect. 2, we introduce the general framework of HFPRM and propose a two stage estimation procedure to study both global effect and individual tract effect. In Sects. 3 and 4, we use numerical simulations and a real data example to examine the finite sample performance of HFPRM. Section 5 concludes with some remarks.

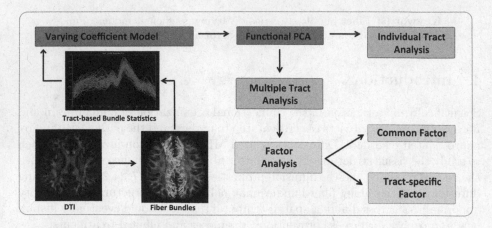

Fig. 1. A schematic overview of HFPRM

2   Methods

2.1   Data Structure

Suppose that we obtain a data set with clinical, genetic variables as well as DTI statistics along M fiber bundles from n subjects. For the m-th fiber bundle, $m = 1, \cdots, M$, we use $s_m \in [0, S_m]$ to denote the arc length of any point relative to a fixed end point, where S_m is the longest arc length on the tract. For the i-th subject where $i = 1, \cdots, n$, $y_{i,m}(s_m)$ denotes a specific diffusion statistics observed at arc-length s_m along the m-th tract, and $\boldsymbol{x}_i$ is a $q \times 1$ vector of covariates.

2.2   HFPRM

HFRPM is proposed to study the association between diffusion properties (e.g., FA, MD or RD) along M fiber bundles with a set of covariates, such as age, gender, and genetic markers. It consists of three key components, a varying coefficient model (VCM), a latent factor analysis (LFA) procedure, and a multivariate regression model (MRM).

The VCM describes the functional association between $\{y_{i,m}(s_m) : s_m \in [0, S_m]\}$ and $\boldsymbol{x}_i$ for a single tract. It admits the following form,

$$y_{i,m}(s_m) = \mu_m(s_m) + \eta_{i,m}(s_m) + e_{i,m}(s_m), \tag{1}$$

where $\mu_m(s_m)$ is the function of population mean, $\eta_{i,m}(s_m)$ is an individual function characterizing subject-specific spatial variations along the m-th tract, and $e_{i,m}(s_m)$ is the measurement error. Let $SP(0, \Sigma)$ represent a stochastic process with mean zero and covariance operator $\Sigma(s_m, s_m')$. It is assumed that $\eta_{i,m}(s_m)$ and $e_{i,m}(s_m)$ are mutually independent and identical copies of stochastic processes $SP(0, \Sigma_{\eta_m})$ and $SP(0, \Sigma_{e_m})$ respectively, in which $\Sigma_{e_m}(s_m, s_m') = \sigma_{e_m}^2(s_m)\mathbf{1}(s_m = s_m')$ and $\mathbf{1}(\cdot)$ is an indicator function.

The major challenge to simultaneously study M fiber bundles is the heterogenuity in their geometric structures. It is necessary to find a common coordinate system for $\{\eta_{i,m}(s_m)\}_{m=1}^M$. Specifically, we use functional principal component analysis (fPCA) to extract the key features in $\eta_{i,m}(s_m)$. Based on Mercer's theorem, $\Sigma_{\eta_m}(s_m, s'_m)$ admits a spectral decomposition as follows:

$$\Sigma_{\eta_m}(s_m, s'_m) = \sum_{d=1}^{+\infty} \lambda_{md}\phi_{md}(s_m)\phi_{md}(s'_m), \qquad (2)$$

where $\{\lambda_{md} \geq 0\}$ are eigenvalues in descending order with $\sum_{d=1}^{\infty} \lambda_{md} < \infty$ and $\{\phi_{md}(s_m)\}$ are the corresponding orthonormal eigenfunctions. Using Karhunen-Loeve expansion [13,16], $\eta_{im}(s_m)$ can be expressed as

$$\eta_{i,m}(s_m) = \sum_{d=1}^{+\infty} z_{i,md}\phi_{md}(s_m) \text{ with } z_{i,md} = \int_0^{S_m} \eta_{i,m}(s_m)\phi_{md}(s_m)ds_m. \quad (3)$$

Individual function $\eta_{i,m}(s_m)$ can then be equivalently represented by a set of functional principal component (fPC) scores $\{z_{i,md} : d = 1, \ldots, \infty\}$. In practice, a relatively small number of fPC scores would account for the majority of variation in $\eta_{i,m}(s)$. Therefore, we can approximate $\eta_{i,m}(s_m)$ by a finite vector $z_{i,m} = (z_{i,m1}, \ldots, z_{i,mD})^T$ of dimension D. For notational simplicity, it is assumed that D is the same across all M bundles. Now we use $z_{i,m}$ to integrate information across M bundles and denote z_i as a $p \times 1$ long vector that concatenates all $z_{i,m}$s together, where $p = DM$.

A LFA is then proposed to account for potential inter-tract correlation across multiple bundles. Specifically, z_i is assumed to have the following latent factor structure,

$$z_i = \Lambda f_i + u_i, \qquad (4)$$

where Λ is a $p \times L$ loading matrix and f_i and u_i, respectively, represent global and individual latent factors. When there exist homogeneous signal patterns across multiple fiber bundles, L is expected to be much smaller than p. Global factor f_i thus allows us to study the shared pattern in a low dimensional space. And tract-specific pattern can also be captured by each component in $u_i = (u_{i,1}, \cdots, u_{i,M})^T$.

Finally, a MLM is introduced to correlate the global and individual latent factors with covariate x_i,

$$f_i = B_f^T x_i + \epsilon_{f,i} \text{ and } u_{i,m} = B_{u_m}^T x_i + \epsilon_{u_m,i}, \text{ for } m = 1, \cdots, M, \qquad (5)$$

where B_f and B_{u_m} are, respectively, $q \times L$ and $q \times D$ coefficient matrices and $\epsilon_{f,i}$ and $\epsilon_{u_m,i}$ are residual terms. Using (5), we are able to perform a hierarchical analysis on both global level and individual level.

2.3   Estimation and Inference Procedure

In practice, diffusion statistics are observed on discrete grid points along each tract. For the m-th tract, assume $y_{i,m}(s_m)$ is observed on sample point set $\mathcal{S}_m = \{s_{m,1}, \ldots, s_{m,k}, \ldots, s_{m,K_m}\} \subset [0, S_m]$, we use the following two-stage procedure to estimate fPC scores $\mathbf{Z} = \{z_i\}_{1 \leq i \leq n}$, global factors $\mathbf{F} = \{f_i\}_{1 \leq i \leq n}$ and individual factors $\mathbf{U} = \{u_i\}_{1 \leq i \leq n}$.

- Stage I: For each tract, $\mu_m(s_m)$ and $\eta_{i,m}(s_m)$ are estimated from (1) and functional principal component analysis is applied to calculate $\hat{\phi}_{md}(s_m)$ and $\hat{z}_i$,
- Stage II: Perform factor analysis on $\hat{z}_i$ to extract global factor $\hat{f}_i$ and individual factor $\hat{u}_i$. Regression and hypothesis testing can then be applied on $\hat{f}_i$ and $\hat{u}_i$ respectively.

Details of the two stages are given below.

In Stage I, to estimate the mean curve from model (1), we apply the local linear kernel smoothing technique. $\mu_m(s_m)$ is first approximated by the following taylor expansion,

$$\mu_m(s_{m,k}) \approx \mu_m(s_m) + d\mu_m(s_m)(s_{m,k} - s_m). \tag{6}$$

Let $K(s)$ be a predetermined smoothing kernel and denote $K_h(s) = \frac{1}{h}K(\frac{s}{h})$ as the rescaled function with bandwidth h, $\hat{\mu}_m(s_m)$ and $d\hat{\mu}_m(s_m)$ can be estimated as the minimizers of the following weighted least square function,

$$\sum_{i=1}^{n} \sum_{k=1}^{K_m} [y_{i,m}(s_{m,k}) - \mu_m(s_m) - d\mu_m(s_m)(s_{m,k} - s_m)]^2 K_h(s_{m,k} - s_m), \tag{7}$$

and solution $\hat{\mu}_m(s_m)$ is smooth curve with local linearity. More complicated polynomial structure can be applied using higher order expansion if necessary.

Similarly, we expand individual function $\eta_{i,m}(s_m)$ for subject i as follows,

$$\eta_{i,m}(s_{m,k}) \approx \eta_{i,m}(s_m) + d\eta_{i,m}(s_m)(s_{m,k} - s_m). \tag{8}$$

The corresponding weighted least square function is given by,

$$\sum_{k=1}^{K_m} [y_{i,m}(s_{m,k}) - \hat{\mu}_m(s_{m,k}) - \eta_{i,m}(s_m) - d\eta_{i,m}(s_m)(s_{m,k} - s_m)]^2 K_h(s_{m,k} - s_m). \tag{9}$$

When smoothed individual functions are obtained as $\{\hat{\eta}_{i,m}(s_m)\}_{i=1}^{n}$, we can calculate the empirical covariance function $\hat{\Sigma}_{\eta_m}(s_m, s_m') = \frac{1}{n}\sum_{i=1}^{n} \hat{\eta}_{i,m}(s_m)\hat{\eta}_{i,m}(s_m')$. And eigenbases $\{\hat{\phi}_{md}(s_m)\}$ can be estimated from spectral decomposition,

$$\hat{\Sigma}_{\eta_m}(s_m, s_m') = \sum_d \hat{\lambda}_{md}\hat{\phi}_{md}(s_m)\hat{\phi}_{md}(s_m'). \tag{10}$$

Then individual random effect $\hat{\eta}_{i,m}(s_m)$ is projected onto basis functions $\{\hat{\phi}_{md}(s_m)\}$ to get functional PC scores,

$$\hat{z}_{i,md} = \sum_{k=1}^{K_m} \hat{\eta}_{i,m}(s_{k,m})\hat{\phi}_{md}(s_{k,m}). \tag{11}$$

There are several strategies to determine the number of fPCs to be extracted. For example, the analog of some model selection techniques have been generalized for this purpose, such as Akaike information criterion (AIC), Bayesian information criterion (BIC) [25] and cross-validation (CV) [20]. Alternatively, the percentage of explained variation has been widely used to give an appropriate cut-off in practice. Here, we choose D as the minimum number of fPCs that incorporates at least $V\%$ of total variation in each tract. When the optimal $D = D_m$ is different across tracts, the largest D_m will be used for all tracts.

In Stage II, a PCA-based factor analysis is performed. Let $\hat{\boldsymbol{\xi}}_1, \ldots, \hat{\boldsymbol{\xi}}_L$ be the first L eigenvectors of sample covariance matrix $\hat{\boldsymbol{\Sigma}}_{\mathbf{z}} = \frac{1}{n}\hat{\mathbf{Z}}^T\hat{\mathbf{Z}}$. The loading matrix, the global factors and the individual factors are estimated as,

$$\hat{\boldsymbol{\Lambda}} = \sqrt{p}(\hat{\boldsymbol{\xi}}_1, \ldots, \hat{\boldsymbol{\xi}}_L), \ \hat{\mathbf{F}} = \frac{1}{p}\hat{\mathbf{Z}}\hat{\boldsymbol{\Lambda}}, \text{ and } \hat{\mathbf{U}} = \hat{\mathbf{Z}} - \hat{\mathbf{F}}\hat{\boldsymbol{\Lambda}}^T \tag{12}$$

Finally, the MLM (5) is used to estimate regression coefficients. Standard test statistics, such as wald and score statistics, can be applied subsequently for inference purpose.

3 Simulations

In this section, numerical simulations are conducted to evaluate the proposed method. Particularly, we examine the performance of HFPRM to detect covariate effect in hypothesis testing.

3.1 Setup

11 fiber tracts with FA measure shown in Table 1 were selected from diffusion tensor tractography in UNC Early Human Brain Development Studies [7]. Functional responses were simulated from a vary coefficient model with fixed covariate effects,

$$y_{i,m}(s_m) = \mu_m(s_m) + \boldsymbol{\beta}_m(s_m)^T\boldsymbol{x}_i + \eta_{i,m}(s_m) + e_{i,m}(s_m), \tag{13}$$

where $i = 1, \cdots, n$ and $m = 1, \cdots, 11$, $\boldsymbol{\beta}(s_m)$ was a $q \times 1$ vector of coefficient functions along the $m-$th tract, covariates $\boldsymbol{x}_i = (x_{i1}, \cdots, x_{iq})^T$ were generated from $N(0,1)$ for continuous variables or from multinomial distribution with equal probabilities for categorical variables, $\eta_{i,m}(s_m)$ followed gaussian process $GP\{0, \Sigma_{\eta_m}\}$ and $e_{i,m}(s_m)$ followed $GP\{0, \Sigma_{e_m}\}$. Compared to model (1), the above equation directly specified the covariates as fixed effect. Sample size n

was set to be 100 and true parameters $(\boldsymbol{\beta}(s_m), \Sigma_{\eta_m}, \Sigma_{e_m})$ were estimated from real data using FADTTS [28].

To examine our method, the following two scenarios on $\boldsymbol{\beta}(s_m)^T x_i$ were simulated. In case I, the aim is to study shared effect of multiple tracts. Gender (G) and gestational age at birth (Gage) were included as covariates for all the 11 tracts,

$$y_{i,m}(s_m) = \mu_m(s_m) + c\beta_{m,1}(s_m)\text{Gage}_i + \beta_{m,2}(s_m)\text{G}_i + \eta_{i,m}(s_m) + e_{i,m}(s_m), \; \forall m,$$

in which we assumed $c = 0, 0.2, 0.4, 0.6$ and Gage effect was tested.

In case II, we want to examine a tract-specific effect. Birth weight (BW) was added as covariate to one particular tract, right uncinate fasciculus ($m = 11$), in addition to case I,

$$y_{i,m}(s_m) = \mu_m(s_m) + \beta_{m,1}(s_m)\text{Gage}_i + \beta_{m,2}(s_m)\text{G}_i + \eta_{i,m}(s_m) + e_{i,m}(s_m), \; m \leq 10,$$
$$y_{i,11}(s_m) = \mu_m(s_m) + \beta_{11,1}(s_m)\text{Gage}_i + \beta_{11,2}(s_m)\text{G}_i + c\beta_{11,3}(s_m)\text{BW}_i$$
$$+ \eta_{i,11}(s_m) + e_{i,11}(s_m),$$

where effect size c was set to take values $0, 0.5, 1, 1.5$ and the effect of BW was tested.

We applied HFPRM to the simulated dataset. The varying coefficient model (1) was first fitted to estimate individual functions. Functional principal components were then extracted such that at least 85% of total variation is included for each tract. In factor analysis, the first elbow point in the scree plot was taken as a cut-off to determine the number of global factors. In testing step, type I error and statistical power were calculated at significance level $\alpha = 0.05$ based on 1000 simulation replications. FADTTS was also applied on each single tract and the results were compared.

3.2   Results

In case I, the first five functional principal components were extracted for each tract and the first factor was identified as global factor. The rejection rates for global factor analysis and FADTTS on testing Gage effect are presented by Fig. 2(a). The global factor analysis is substantially more powerful than the single tract analysis when detecting commonly shared effect. Such results are expected since common effect tends to be accumulated in the global factor.

In case II, the first five functional principal components were extracted for each tract and the first two factors were identified as global factors. Figure 2(b) shows the rejection rates for global factor analysis, individual factor analysis and FADTTS on testing BW effect. As can be seen, individual factor analysis in HFPRM achieves comparable power to single tract analysis for detecting tract-specific effect.

4   Early Human Brain Development Study

To investigate how genetic factors influence brain structure in prenatal and early postnatal stage, we conducted a genome-wide association study on the fiber

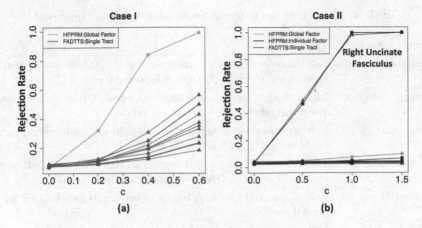

Fig. 2. Simulation result

bundle statistics in a unique cohort of infants. A total number of 662 neonatal twin subjects were taken from the UNC Early Brain Development Studies [7].

4.1 Data Acquisition and Preprocessing

MRI scans were acquired either on a 3T Siemens Allegra head-only scanner ($N = 566$) or on a 3T Siemens TIM Trio 3T scanner ($N = 96$). For the Allegra model, 339 diffusion weighted images were acquired by a single shot EPI DTI sequence with the following parameters: $TR/TE = 5200/73$ ms, voxel resolution $= 2 \times 2 \times 2$ mm^3, 6 non-collinear directions with $b = 1000$ s/mm^2 and 1 baseline image with $b = 0$. To improve the signal-to-noise ratio, five scans were repeated and averaged. For the remaining subjects scanned on Allegra, DWI was acquired with the following parameters: $TR/TE = 7680/82$ ms, voxel resolution $= 2 \times 2 \times 2$ mm^3, 42 non-collinear directions with diffusion gradients of $b = 1000$ s/mm^2 in addition to 7 baseline images. For the Trio model, DWIs were acquired using a similar protocol to that of the 42 direction Allegra model with $TR/TE = 7200/83$ ms. Quality control was applied on raw DWIs using DTIPrep [18], and FSL [11,22] was performed for skull stripping and brain masking. We used a weighted least squares method [8] to estimate diffusion tensors and followed the UNC-Utah NA-MIC framework [23] to create a study-specific atlas. Subsequently, a total number of 44 fiber tracts listed in Table 1 were reconstructed in the atlas space using a streamline algorithm [5]. For each subject, four scalar diffusion properties, FA, MD, AD and RD, were then calculated at each location along each tract using neighboring diffusion tensors.

Genotyping of single nucleotide polymorphisms (SNPs) was conducted on Affymetrix Axiom genome-wide LAT Array. Samples with call rates less than 95%, outliers for homozygosity, ancestry outliers and unexpected relatedness were excluded from the study. We also removed genetic markers with Hardy-Weinberg equilibrium p-value less than 10^{-8}, call rate less than 95% and

Table 1. List of fiber tracts in simulation and real data experiment

Bundle group	Tract segments
Arcuate fasciculus	Left fronto-parietal, right fronto-parietal, left fronto-temporal*, right fronto-temporal*, right temporo-parietal
Corpus callosum	Motor body*, occipital splenium, parietal body*, premotor body, rostrum*, genu*, temporal tapetum*
Cingulum	Left premotor, left cingulate gyrus, right cingulate gyrus, right hippocampal, right prefrontal cortex
Corticothalamic	left motor, right motor, left premotor, right premotor, left parietal, right parietal, left prefrontal, right prefrontal
CorticoFugal	Left motor, right motor, left parietal, right parietal, left prefrontal cortex,
Others	Left fornix, right fornix, left inferior fronto-occipital fasciculi, right inferior fronto-occipital fasciculi, left inferior longitudinal fasciculi*, right inferior longitudinal fasciculi*, left medial lemniscus, right medial lemniscus, left optic, right optic, left superior longitudinal fasciculus, right superior longitudinal fasciculus, left uncinate fasciculus*, right uncinate fasciculus*

*Selected tracts for simulation study

Mendelian error rate larger than 10%. Population stratification was assessed using PCA [19]. Imputation was performed with MaCH-Admix [15] using 1000G reference panel [3]. To evaluate the quality of imputed SNPs, we computed the mean R^2 under varying minor allele frequency (MAF) categories and selected R^2 cutoffs as described in [14]. SNPs with MAF less than 0.01 were excluded from imputed dataset. Eventually, 472 twin subjects (32 MZ pairs, 75 DZ pairs and 259 singletons or unpaired twin subjects) and 8,538,562 genetic markers were retained for further analysis.

4.2   Data Analysis

In this experiment, we chose to focus on the fractional anisotropy (FA) measure. FA quantifies the extent of local directional water diffusion and partially reflects the degree of bundle maturation in premature brains [4]. To eliminate the heterogeneity in variance among different tracts, $y_{i,m}(s_m)$ was rescaled by the total standard deviation along the tract. For the twin study, ACE model was fitted in (5) to account for correlation within twin pairs. Seven variables were added as covariates, including gestational age at birth, gender, DTI direction, scanner type and the first three genetic principal component to adjust for population stratification.

4.3   Results

In functional PCA, the first 5 functional principal components were extracted for each tract to include at least 70% of variation. Figure 3(a) shows the scree plot in factor analysis and the elbow point is located at factor 2. Therefore, the first factor is identified as the global factor. We then performed GWAS on the global factor. The result is visualized by Fig. 3(b). In the Manhattan plot, we observed a significant region in anaplastic lymphoma kinase (ALK) gene on chromosome 2. The ALK gene is a neuronal orphan receptor tyrosine kinase that plays an important role in the nervous system development [1], and is highly expressed in the neonatal brain [10]. As a comparison, we also performed association analysis for top hit rs66556850 on each single tract. The result is presented by Fig. 3(c). A number of tracts have relatively small pvalue yet not small enough to be detected by a single tract GWAS. It indicates that the global factor analysis is more powerful to detect commonly shared genetic effect than single tract analysis.

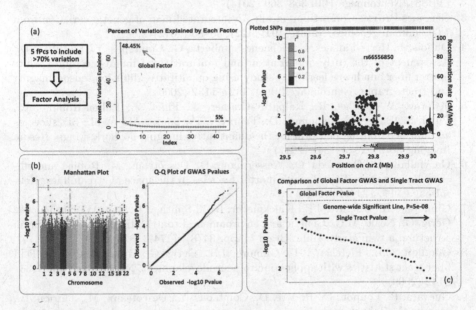

Fig. 3. Real data analysis result: (a) Functional PCA and factor analysis. (b) Visualization of GWAS result of the global factor. (c) A comparison between global factor analysis and single tract analysis on marker rs66556850, the $-\log_{10}p$ value in the association test is plotted. The majority of pvalues in single tract analysis are around $10^{-2} \sim 10^{-6}$.

5   Conclusion

We have developed a hierarchical functional principal regression model (HFPRM) to efficiently conduct joint analysis on diffusion statistics from multiple neurofiber bundles. A varying coefficient model is introduced and functional PCA is applied to capture major tract variation. Factor analysis is then adopted to extract key features at both global level and individual level. Finally, standard estimation and testing procedures can be applied to study global effect and tract-specific effect. Simulation results demonstrated that HFPRM is powerful to detect common effect shared by multiple tracts. HFPRM has also been successfully applied to a genome-wide association study on neonatal twins. We are able to identify some important genetic variants related to early childhood brain development that were ignored by single tract analysis.

References

1. National Center for Biotechnology Information. https://www.ncbi.nlm.nih.gov/gene/238
2. Bach, M., Laun, F.B., Leemans, A., Tax, C.M., Biessels, G.J., Stieltjes, B., Maier-Hein, K.H.: Methodological considerations on tract-based spatial statistics (TBSS). Neuroimage 100, 358–369 (2014)
3. Genomes Project Consortium, et al.: An integrated map of genetic variation from 1,092 human genomes. Nature 491(7422), 56–65 (2012)
4. Dubois, J., Hertz-Pannier, L., Dehaene-Lambertz, G., Cointepas, Y., Le Bihan, D.: Assessment of the early organization and maturation of infants' cerebral white matter fiber bundles: a feasibility study using quantitative diffusion tensor imaging and tractography. Neuroimage 30(4), 1121–1132 (2006)
5. Fedorov, A., Beichel, R., Kalpathy-Cramer, J., Finet, J., Fillion-Robin, J.C., Pujol, S., Bauer, C., Jennings, D., Fennessy, F., Sonka, M., et al.: 3D slicer as an image computing platform for the quantitative imaging network. Magn. Reson. Imaging 30(9), 1323–1341 (2012)
6. Garyfallidis, E., Ocegueda, O., Wassermann, D., Descoteaux, M.: Robust and efficient linear registration of white-matter fascicles in the space of streamlines. NeuroImage 117, 124–140 (2015)
7. Gilmore, J.H., Schmitt, J.E., Knickmeyer, R.C., Smith, J.K., Lin, W., Styner, M., Gerig, G., Neale, M.C.: Genetic and environmental contributions to neonatal brain structure: a twin study. Hum. Brain Mapp. 31(8), 1174–1182 (2010)
8. Goodlett, C.B., Fletcher, P.T., Gilmore, J.H., Gerig, G.: Group analysis of DTI fiber tract statistics with application to neurodevelopment. NeuroImage 45, S133–S142 (2009)
9. Guevara, P., Poupon, C., Rivière, D., Cointepas, Y., Descoteaux, M., Thirion, B., Mangin, J.: Robust clustering of massive tractography datasets. NeuroImage 54(3), 1975–1993 (2011)
10. Iwahara, T., Fujimoto, J., Wen, D., Cupples, R., Bucay, N., Arakawa, T., Mori, S., Ratzkin, B., Yamamoto, T.: Molecular characterization of ALK, a receptor tyrosine kinase expressed specifically in the nervous system. Oncogene 14(4), 439–449 (1997)
11. Jenkinson, M., Beckmann, C.F., Behrens, T.E., Woolrich, M.W., Smith, S.M.: FSL. Neuroimage 62(2), 782–790 (2012)
12. Jin, Y., Shi, Y., Zhan, L., Gutman, B.A., de Zubicaray, G.I., McMahon, K.L., Wright, M.J., Toga, A.W., Thompson, P.M.: Automatic clustering of white matter fibers in brain diffusion mri with an application to genetics. NeuroImage 100, 75–90 (2014)
13. Karhunen, K.: Zur Spektraltheorie stochastischer Prozesse. Ann. Acad. Sci. Finnicae Ser. A 1, 34 (1946)

14. Liu, E.Y., Buyske, S., Aragaki, A.K., Peters, U., Boerwinkle, E., Carlson, C., Carty, C., Crawford, D.C., Haessler, J., Hindorff, L.A., et al.: Genotype imputation of metabochipsnps using a study-specific reference panel of 4,000 haplotypes in african americans from the women's health initiative. Genet. Epidemiol. **36**(2), 107–117 (2012)
15. Liu, E.Y., Li, M., Wang, W., Li, Y.: Mach-admix: genotype imputation for admixed populations. Genet. Epidemiol. **37**(1), 25–37 (2013)
16. Loève, M.: Fonctions aléatoires à décomposition orthogonale exponentielle. La Revue Scientifique **84**, 159–162 (1946)
17. O'Donnell, L.J., Westin, C.F., Golby, A.J.: Tract-based morphometry for white matter group analysis. NeuroImage **45**, 832–844 (2009)
18. Oguz, I., Farzinfar, M., Matsui, J., Budin, F., Liu, Z., Gerig, G., Johnson, H.J., Styner, M.A.: DTIPrep: quality control of diffusion-weighted images. Front. Neuroinform. **8**, 4 (2014)
19. Price, A.L., Patterson, N.J., Plenge, R.M., Weinblatt, M.E., Shadick, N.A., Reich, D.: Principal components analysis corrects for stratification in genome-wide association studies. Nat. Genet. **38**(8), 904–909 (2006)
20. Rice, J.A., Silverman, B.W.: Estimating the mean and covariance structure non-parametrically when the data are curves. J. R. Stat. Soc. Ser. B (Methodol.) **53**, 233–243 (1991). JSTOR
21. Smith, S.M., Jenkinson, M., Johansen-Berg, H., Rueckert, D., Nichols, T.E., Mackay, C.E., Watkins, K.E., Ciccarelli, O., Cader, M.Z., Matthews, P.M., et al.: Tract-based spatial statistics: voxelwise analysis of multi-subject diffusion data. Neuroimage **31**(4), 1487–1505 (2006)
22. Smith, S.M., Jenkinson, M., Woolrich, M.W., Beckmann, C.F., Behrens, T.E., Johansen-Berg, H., Bannister, P.R., De Luca, M., Drobnjak, I., Flitney, D.E., et al.: Advances in functional and structural mr image analysis and implementation as FSL. Neuroimage **23**, S208–S219 (2004)
23. Verde, A.R., Budin, F., Berger, J.B., Gupta, A., Farzinfar, M., Kaiser, A., Ahn, M., Johnson, H.J., Matsui, J., Hazlett, H.C., et al.: UNC-Utah NA-MIC framework for DTI fiber tract analysis. Front. Neuroinform. **7**, 51 (2014)
24. Wedeen, V.J., Rosene, D.L., Wang, R., Dai, G., Mortazavi, F., Hagmann, P., Kaas, J.H., Tseng, W.Y.I.: The geometric structure of the brain fiber pathways. Science **335**(6076), 1628–1634 (2012)
25. Yao, F., Müller, H.G., Wang, J.L.: Functional data analysis for sparse longitudinal data. J. Am. Stat. Assoc. **100**(470), 577–590 (2005)
26. Yuan, Y., Gilmore, J.H., Geng, X., Martin, S., Chen, K., Wang, J.I., Zhu, H.: FMEM: functional mixed effects modeling for the analysis of longitudinal white matter tract data. NeuroImage **84**, 753–764 (2014)
27. Yushkevich, P.A., Zhang, H., Simon, T.J., Gee, J.C.: Structure-specific statistical mapping of white matter tracts. NeuroImage **41**, 448–461 (2008)
28. Zhu, H., Kong, L., Li, R., Styner, M., Gerig, G., Lin, W., Gilmore, J.H.: FADTTS: functional analysis of diffusion tensor tract statistics. NeuroImage **56**(3), 1412–1425 (2011)

Quantitative Imaging

Orthotropic Thin Shell Elasticity Estimation for Surface Registration

Qingyu Zhao[1]([✉]), Stephen Pizer[1,2], Ron Alterovitz[1], Marc Niethammer[1], and Julian Rosenman[1,2]

[1] Computer Science, UNC Chapel Hill, Chapel Hill, NC, USA
zenyo@cs.unc.edu
[2] Radiation Oncology, UNC Chapel Hill, Chapel Hill, NC, USA

Abstract. Elastic physical models have been widely used to regularize deformations in different medical object registration tasks. Traditional approaches usually assume uniform isotropic tissue elasticity (a constant regularization weight) across the whole domain, which contradicts human tissue elasticity being not only inhomogeneous but also anisotropic. We focus on producing more physically realistic deformations for the task of surface registration. We model the surface as an orthotropic elastic thin shell, and we propose a novel statistical framework to estimate inhomogeneous and anisotropic shell elasticity parameters only from a group of known surface deformations. With this framework we show that a joint estimation of within-patient surface deformations and the shell elasticity parameters can improve groupwise registration accuracy. The method is tested in the context of endoscopic reconstruction-surface registration.

1 Introduction

A popular way of solving medical image registration problems is to formulate an optimization that minimizes a weighted sum of two energy terms: data mismatch and the *regularity* of the deformation that deforms one data item to the other. In particular, the latter term has been formulated from different standpoints, one of which is to use physical energy derived from an *elastic model* to regularize deformations [1]. Even though some other methods [2–4] have also produced reasonable results via different regularization formulations, the elasticity-model-based idea is particularly appealing because in many medical applications anatomical deformations are indeed elastic processes caused by muscles or other forces.

The key to realistic physical modeling is to apply proper elasticity parameters. As a matter of fact, human tissue elasticity is both *inhomogeneous* (different tissue types show different stiffness) [5] and *anisotropic* (e.g., different stiffness along and across the tissue fiber direction) [6]. However, traditional registration approaches simply assume a spatially constant elasticity parameter (the single regularization weight), which makes the physical modeling unrealistic. Therefore, the use of elasticity models in registration currently becomes more of a motivational concept than the seeking of truly physical deformations. The above

© Springer International Publishing AG 2017
M. Niethammer et al. (Eds.): IPMI 2017, LNCS 10265, pp. 493–504, 2017.
DOI: 10.1007/978-3-319-59050-9_39

argument motivates research interest in studying spatially varying tissue elasticity, not only for registration, but also for simulation [7] and pathology analysis [8]. However, most approaches for non-uniform elasticity estimation have to use a sophisticated mechanical system equipped with a force generation/measurement capability, which is often unavailable in a common registration setting.

In this paper, we propose a statistical framework that can estimate spatially varying anisotropic elasticity parameters only using a set of known material deformations. In particular, we focus on studying a physical model for registration of anatomic surfaces that have deformed within a patient. We first propose to model the surface as an orthotropic elastic thin shell. To be specific, *orthotropy* is a special kind of anisotropy that can characterize different material stiffness along different directions, but the orthotropic model has fewer parameters than arbitrary anisotropy. Next we show that with some proper prior knowledge, spatially inhomogeneous and orthotropic elasticity parameters can be estimated from a set of known shell (surface) deformations via a novel *maximum-a-posteriori* (MAP) optimization. We finally show that with this statistical framework we can improve the groupwise surface registration accuracy by a joint estimation of surface deformations and shell elasticity parameters.

We test this framework in the context of endoscopy 3D reconstruction, the goal of which is to produce a 3D reconstruction surface from multiple endoscopic movie frames. Since the tissue is constantly deforming during endoscopy, a key step of this reconstruction is to register all the single-frame 3D reconstruction surfaces into a unified surface to account for the aforementioned deformations across frames. We show that our elasticity estimation framework is able to retrieve insightful tissue elastic properties from the data and in turn to improve this groupwise registration.

1.1 Related Work

Closely related to our work is a research branch known as *spatially-varying registration*, the idea of which is to let regularization strength be dependent on location. This can be modeled by spatially-varying diffusion [9], non-stationary Gaussian processes [10] or applying a non-stationary metric in the LDDMM setting [11]. Despite their theoretical appeal, those methods explore the problem mostly from the computational aspect and lack physical motivation, and they also don't handle the anisotropic situation. The notion of spatially-varying registration has been also used in elastic models [12,13], but the elasticity parameters have to be manually chosen for known segmented regions.

Automatic elasticity estimation has been studied in different medical applications [6,14]. With tissue displacements and external forces taken as known values, the elasticity can be computed directly as an inverse problem of the Finite Element Method (FEM). Elastography is another widely used non-invasive procedure for determining local elastic properties, but it either requires a force exertion/measurement device or a vibration actuation mechanism [15], which is often not available in other imaging modalities.

Therefore, *modality-independent* and purely *image-based* approaches are desired and have been under investigation for several years. Miga et al. [5] introduced registration-based elastography to estimate tissue stiffness of an object given two images of it undergoing an elastic deformation. Risholm et al. [16] extended this approach by forming a probabilistic model over the registration parameters and inhomogeneous isotropic elasticity parameters. While our framework is related to theirs, ours is different by incorporating anisotropy and by applying the model to surface data.

In a broader context, *Statistical Shape Analysis* seeks a statistical distribution or a low dimensional subspace, called a shape space, for describing a given set of shapes (or shape deformations). Most existing approaches [17,18] construct the shape space by constraining the shape's global appearance, such as deformation vector fields, point positions or normal directions. Our framework provides an alternative perspective in the sense that it recovers the underlying physical reason that can best explain the given shape deformations.

2   Orthotropic Thin Shell

Thin shells are special 3D structures bounded by two curved surfaces (Fig. 1a), where the distance between the surfaces (thickness) is small in comparison with other body dimensions (width). Due to this high width-to-thickness ratio, the behavior of a thin shell can be characterized by its middle surface $\mathcal{M}$, the locus of points that lie at equal distances from the two bounding surfaces. In this situation, out-of-plane strain can be neglected, and the elastic model is reduced to 2D. The 2D linear *Hooke's law* for arbitrary anisotropy reads

$$\sigma = [\sigma_{xx}, \sigma_{yy}, \sigma_{xy}]^T = C[\varepsilon_{xx}, \varepsilon_{yy}, \varepsilon_{xy}]^T = C\varepsilon, \tag{1}$$

where σ and ε are the *local* in-plane stress and strain tensors parameterized on the tangent plane of the middle surface $\mathcal{M}$, and C is a 3×3 positive definite matrix, called a *stiffness matrix*, characterizing *local* elasticity.

For a thin shell, it can be shown that the *local* strain ε can be classified into the stretching strain φ and bending strain κ, where the relationship between ε and $\{\varphi, \kappa\}$ follows the *Love-Kirchhoff hypothesis* [19,20]. The *local* deformation energy is approximated by the function W:

$$W(\varphi, \kappa, C) = \lambda_s \varphi^T C \varphi + \lambda_b \kappa^T C \kappa, \tag{2}$$

where $\varphi = [\varphi_{xx}, \varphi_{yy}, \varphi_{xy}]^T$ is the tangential Cauchy-Green strain tensor characterizing local stretching, $\kappa = [\kappa_{xx}, \kappa_{yy}, \kappa_{xy}]^T$ is the shape operator difference characterizing local bending (local curvature change), and $\{\lambda_s, \lambda_b\}$ are the global mixing weights determined by shell thickness.

Orthotropic material is a special type of anisotropic material. For an orthotropic shell, the anisotropy on the tangent plane is symmetric w.r.t. two orthogonal axes, known as the *natural axes*. This leads to a simplified stiffness

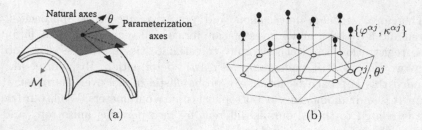

Fig. 1. (a) A thin shell model. (b) A Gaussian MRF model with nodes (white) defined on the dual graph (blue) of a triangle mesh. Node j (triangle $\mathcal{T}^j$) is associated with unknown variables (C^j, θ^j) and a set of observed variables $\{\varphi^{\alpha j}, \kappa^{\alpha j} | \alpha = 1 \dots N\}$ (Color figure online)

matrix in the following form when σ and ε are parameterized under this natural-axes coordinate system:

$$
C = \begin{bmatrix} c_1 & c_2 & 0 \\ c_2 & c_3 & 0 \\ 0 & 0 & c_4 \end{bmatrix} = \frac{1}{1 - \nu_{xy}\nu_{yx}} \begin{bmatrix} E_x & \nu_{vu}E_x & 0 \\ \nu_{xy}E_y & E_y & 0 \\ 0 & 0 & 2G_{xy}(1 - \nu_{xy}\nu_{yx}) \end{bmatrix}, \quad (3)
$$

where $\{E_x, E_y\}$ are the Young's moduli along the natural axes, $\{\nu_{xy}, \nu_{yx}\}$ are the Poisson's ratios, and G_{xy} is the shear modulus. In the following text, we will use C to denote such a simplified matrix, called the *canonical orthotropic stiffness matrix*. We denote the space of such matrices as $\mathbf{SPD}_C$.

Rotation of Frame. When σ and ε are parameterized under an arbitrary orthogonal frame (Fig. 1a) instead of rotated into the natural axes, we have the following relationship,

$$
\begin{bmatrix} \varepsilon_{xx} & \varepsilon_{xy} \\ \varepsilon_{xy} & \varepsilon_{yy} \end{bmatrix} = \begin{bmatrix} cos(\theta) & sin(\theta) \\ -sin(\theta) & cos(\theta) \end{bmatrix} \begin{bmatrix} \varepsilon'_{xx} & \varepsilon'_{xy} \\ \varepsilon'_{xy} & \varepsilon'_{yy} \end{bmatrix} \begin{bmatrix} cos(\theta) & -sin(\theta) \\ sin(\theta) & cos(\theta) \end{bmatrix}, \quad (4)
$$

where $\{\varepsilon'_{\alpha\beta}\}$ is the strain tensor parameterized under an arbitrary orthogonal frame and θ is the rotation angle between the two frames, known as the *canonical angle*. The same rotational relationship applies for σ. Combining with Eq. 1, the stiffness matrix under an arbitrary frame is $C' = R^{-1}CR$, where

$$
R = \begin{bmatrix} cos(\theta)^2 & sin(\theta)^2 & 2cos(\theta)sin(\theta) \\ sin(\theta)^2 & cos(\theta)^2 & -2cos(\theta)sin(\theta) \\ -cos(\theta)sin(\theta) & cos(\theta)sin(\theta) & cos(\theta)^2 - sin(\theta)^2 \end{bmatrix}. \quad (5)
$$

In other words, C and θ uniquely determines the *local* orthotropic stiffness matrix parameterized under an arbitrary frame.

The orthotropic elasticity model has shown its effectiveness in modeling 3D soft tissues in the situations where the stiffness is usually different in a direction parallel to the fibers than in the transverse directions [6,7]. We adapt this model to the essentially 2D situation of the physical thin shell model Zhao et al. [21] proposed for surface registration.

3 Elasticity Estimation via MAP

We assume some observed material deformations are the realization of tissue elasticity of a single patient. Then a common way to estimate elasticity parameters is to solve an inverse problem given such deformations and external force measurements. However, when only the material deformations are available, the parameter estimation can be highly ill-posed. Therefore, we opt for energy-based models that are commonly used in statistical mechanics. In these models high probability states are associated with low energy configurations. Here we propose a *Physical-Energy-Based Markov Random Field* (MRF) model to estimate the elasticity parameters from a probabilistic point of view.

Problem Statement. With some abuse of notation we use $\mathcal{M}$ to represent both a shell and its middle surface domain. Given a reference shell $\mathcal{M}$ and a set of N example deformations $\mathcal{D} = \{\mathcal{D}^\alpha : \mathcal{M} \to \mathbb{R}^3 | \alpha = 1 \dots N\}$, our goal is to find the canonical orthotropic stiffness matrix function $\mathbf{C} : \mathcal{M} \to \mathbf{SPD}_C$ and the canonical angle function $\boldsymbol{\theta} : \mathcal{M} \to \mathbf{S}^1$, namely the orthotropic elasticity parameters of every location on the shell. To simplify the problem, we start off by discretizing the continuous shell $\mathcal{M}$ to a triangle-mesh $\{\mathcal{T}^j | j = 1 \dots M\}$ with M triangles. We associate each triangle $\mathcal{T}^j$ with its own local elasticity parameters (C^j, θ^j). Each deformation $\mathcal{D}^\alpha$ is then reparameterized locally on the tangent planes (triangles). In other words, each triangle $\mathcal{T}^j$ has its own local stretching strain $\varphi^{\alpha j}$ and bending strain $\kappa^{\alpha j}$. Finally, the goal is to estimate the set of elasticity parameters $(\mathbf{C}, \boldsymbol{\theta}) = \{C^j, \theta^j\}$ given the set of local strains $\{\varphi^{\alpha j}, \kappa^{\alpha j}\}$.

The MRF Model. Our idea is that the elasticity parameters that "best fit" the observed deformations should yield small total elastic deformation energy. Meanwhile, we assume the parameters should vary smoothly across the shell. Finally, due to the scale ambiguity caused by the lack of external force measurements [8,16], we assign the parameters with a prior to avoid the trivial solution (similar to [8,16], we compute parameters relative to the prior).

We build an MRF model on the dual graph of the triangle mesh as shown in Fig. 1b. Each node on the graph represents the elasticity parameters associated with the underlying triangle. We want to find $(\mathbf{C}, \boldsymbol{\theta})$ to maximize the posterior distribution $p(\mathbf{C}, \boldsymbol{\theta} | \mathcal{D})$:

$$p(\mathbf{C}, \boldsymbol{\theta} | \mathcal{D}) \propto p(\mathcal{D} | \mathbf{C}, \boldsymbol{\theta}) p(\mathbf{C}, \boldsymbol{\theta}). \tag{6}$$

The likelihood $p(\mathcal{D} | \mathbf{C}, \boldsymbol{\theta})$ is associated with the total deformation energy of all example deformations. Assuming local deformation energy follows independent Boltzmann distributions, we design our the likelihood as the following:

$$p(\mathcal{D} | \mathbf{C}, \boldsymbol{\theta}) = \prod_\alpha \prod_j p(\varphi^{\alpha j}, \kappa^{\alpha j} | C^j, \theta^j) \propto \prod_\alpha \prod_j \exp(-W(\varphi^{\alpha j}, \kappa^{\alpha j}, C^j, \theta^j)) \tag{7}$$

Consider the prior distribution of $(\mathbf{C}, \boldsymbol{\theta}) = \{C^j, \theta^j\}$, the second term of Eq. 6. Following the idea from Gaussian MRFs, each node has its own per-node prior function ψ_j, and each edge has an edge potential function ψ_{jk}:

$$p(\mathbf{C}, \boldsymbol{\theta}) \propto \prod_j \psi_j(C^j) \prod_{j,k} \psi_{jk}(C^j, \theta^j, C^k, \theta^k). \tag{8}$$

The ψ_{jk} function models the spatial smoothness nature of the shell's orthotropic property by penalizing the difference of stiffness matrices between neighbouring nodes and the smoothness of the natural-axes direction field. We assume $\mathbf{C}$ and θ are independent and design

$$\psi_{jk}(C^j, \theta^j, C^k, \theta^k) \propto \exp(-d(C^j, C^k)^2) \cdot \exp(-(p_{jk}(\theta^j) - \theta^k)^2), \tag{9}$$

where $d(\cdot, \cdot)$ is a proper distance metric for $\mathbf{SPD}_C$. We use the Log-Euclidean metric [22] for its computational convenience. $p(\cdot)$ is the Levi-Civita parallel transport operation [23] that transports a vector associated with θ_j from $\mathcal{T}^j$ to the neighbouring triangle $\mathcal{T}^k$.

For the per-node prior function ψ_j, we assume anisotropy is distributed in a Gaussian sense with the isotropic case being the mean situation. Therefore, given an isotropic prior Young's modulus E and Poisson's ratio ν, we design $\psi_j(C^j) \propto exp(-d(C^j, \bar{C})^2)$, where $\bar{C}$ is the commonly used isotropic stiffness matrix derived from E and ν. Finally, we optimize the negative log posterior in the following form:

$$\begin{aligned}
-\log p(\mathbf{C}, \boldsymbol{\theta}|\mathcal{D}) = \sum_{j,k}[\lambda_1 d(C^j, C^k)^2 + \lambda_2 (p_{jk}(\theta^j) - \theta^k)^2] + \\
\sum_\alpha \sum_j W(\epsilon^{\alpha j}, \kappa^{\alpha j}, C^j, \theta^j) + \sum_j \lambda_3 d(C^j, \bar{C})^2
\end{aligned} \tag{10}$$

where the λ parameters are the global weights.

4   Joint Estimation of Registration and Elasticity

In many groupwise registration analysis [24], both the material deformations and elasticity parameters are unknown variables. Formally, we want to investigate the joint probability of the group of deformations $\mathcal{D}$ and elasticity parameters $(\mathbf{C}, \boldsymbol{\theta})$, given a reference shell $\mathcal{M}$ and its many deformed version $\{\mathcal{M}^\alpha | i = \alpha \ldots N\}$. A common approach is to treat one set of variables, e.g., $(\mathbf{C}, \boldsymbol{\theta})$, as latent variables and perform an *Expectation-Maximization* algorithm to estimate the posterior

$$p(\mathcal{D}|\mathcal{M}, \{\mathcal{M}^i | i = 1 \ldots N\}) = \int_{\mathbf{C}, \boldsymbol{\theta}} p(\mathcal{D}, \mathbf{C}, \boldsymbol{\theta}|\mathcal{M}, \{\mathcal{M}^i | i = 1 \ldots N\}). \tag{11}$$

In this study, we opt for a simple *alternating optimization* algorithm that uses the mode over the $(\mathbf{C}, \boldsymbol{\theta})$ parameters to approximate the posterior for computational simplicity.

Our alternating optimization approach iterates between the following steps:

1. *Input*: a reference shell $\mathcal{M}$ and a set of deformed shells $\{\mathcal{M}^\alpha | \alpha = 1 \ldots N\}$. The elasticity parameters are initialized to be $\bar{C}$ everywhere.

2. With the current estimate of $(\mathbf{C}, \boldsymbol{\theta})$, perform MAP on

$$p(\mathcal{D}|\mathbf{C}, \boldsymbol{\theta}, \mathcal{M}, \{\mathcal{M}^\alpha | \alpha = 1 \dots N\}) = \prod_{\alpha=1}^{N} p(\mathcal{D}^\alpha | \mathbf{C}, \boldsymbol{\theta}, \mathcal{M}, \mathcal{M}^\alpha) \qquad (12)$$

This step is essentially a set of independent pairwise surface registrations between $(\mathcal{M}, \mathcal{M}^\alpha)$ with inhomogeneous and orthotropic energy as the deformation regularization. We adopt the Thin Shell Demons method [21] to accomplish this step. It uses curvature-based geometric features to drive the deformation and allows thin-shell-based elastic regularization.

3. Using the framework in Sect. 3, perform MAP on $p(\mathbf{C}, \boldsymbol{\theta}|\mathcal{D}, \mathcal{M})$ with the deformations estimated from Step 2 to update the elasticity parameter.
4. Iterate to Step 2 until convergence.

5 Experiments

Proof of Concept. In this experiment we tested on a toy example the capability of elasticity parameter estimation from known deformations without any registration involved. We mainly investigated the estimation accuracy of the canonical angle and the two Young's moduli, which are the three most important parameters in characterizing local orthotropy. A bar-shaped surface shown in Fig. 2a was manually assigned ground truth elasticity parameters (Fig. 2b), including both the orthotropic canonical stiffness matrices and natural axes directions. The bar is more elastic at the center (inhomogeneity) and more elastic along the vertical direction (orthotropy). The other elasticity parameters were set to satisfy $\nu_{xy}\nu_{yx} = 0.25^2$ and $G_{xy} = 2k\,Pa$. We created 20 synthetic deformations to the bar (Fig. 2c) by first fixing its two ends at random positions as boundary constraints and then optimizing Eq. 7 to solve for the deformations using ground truth elasticity. We tested our framework introduced in Sect. 3 to estimate the elasticity parameters from this set of simulated deformations. The weighting parameters $\{\lambda_1 = 1, \lambda_2 = 10, \lambda_3 = 0.1\}$ were chosen empirically to best fit this toy problem. We found that the natural axes first have to be accurate to yield meaningful anisotropy, so we set a larger λ_2 to regularize the vector field. Other model parameters $\{\lambda_s = 80, \lambda_b = 10\}$ and the isotropic prior $\{E = 2k\,Pa, \nu = 0.25\}$ were chosen the same as in [24]. Figure 2d shows the two estimated Young's moduli and the estimated natural axes directions. The average canonical angle error is $0.74°$, which shows we can successfully estimate the natural axes directions. Figure 2e shows that with the estimated orthotropic elasticity parameters the simulated deformation is more accurate in the sense that the center-elastic part has a larger bending effect than the one simulated from isotropic elasticity under the same boundary constraints.

Synthetic Head-and-Neck Data. We tested joint registration and elasticity parameter estimation with synthetic deformations on 5 real patients' head-and-neck CT data. In particular, a pharyngeal surface (Fig. 3a) from the pharynx down to the vocal cord was segmented from a 3D CT image. Each surface

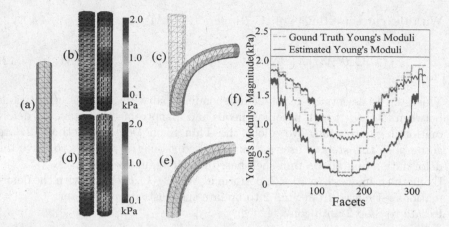

Fig. 2. (a) A reference bar-shaped surface. (b) The two ground truth Young's moduli are respectively color-coded across the surface. Red regions indicate smaller Young's moduli (more elastic). Each local Young's modulus is associated with a natural axis direction (black vector fields) (c) A deformed surface derived from ground truth elasticity. Red regions are the fixed boundary constraints. (d) Estimated Young's moduli and the associated estimates of natural axes. (e) Deformed surfaces derived from ground truth elasticity (blue wireframe), estimated elasticity (gray surface) and isotropic elasticity (red frame). (f) The two ground truth Young's moduli (the orange curves) and the two estimated Young's moduli (the blue curves) on all faces. (Color figure online)

has about 6k facets. We manually assigned ground truth orthotropic elasticity parameters and natural axes directions to the reference surface to reflect known anatomical facts: the epiglottis being stiffer than the vallecula and the pharyngeal wall being more elastic cross-sectionally (Fig. 3b). Similar to the previous example, we simulated 20 synthetic deformations to each patient's surface by assigning 20 manually constructed boundary conditions. These deformations include the expansion/compression of the pharyngeal wall and the opening/closing of the larynx. These deformations were also used as ground truth deformations for testing the accuracy of the later registration. We tuned down λ_1 to 0.1 to avoid overly smoothing the estimation. All the other algorithm parameters were kept the same.

To further test the elasticity estimation framework, we first estimated the elasticity parameters directly from the ground truth deformations (not for the registration purpose). Figure 3c shows that the general pattern of the two Young's moduli and the natural axes can be reasonably recovered, but the scale difference with the ground truth suggests our method only recovers parameters up to a scale relative to the prior isotropic elasticity. Moreover, the elasticity-smoothness term in Eq. 10 tends to yield blurred estimation. Due to these artifacts, the average error over all facets for the two Young's moduli are 0.41 kPa and 0.38 kPa respectively. The average canonical angle error is 12°.

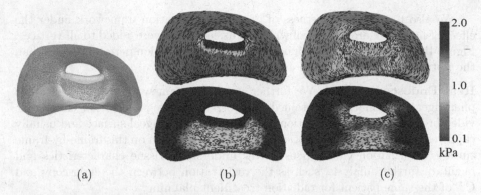

Fig. 3. (a) A pharyngeal CT segmentation surface (gray surface) and one of its synthetic deformations (red wireframe). (b) Ground truth Young's Moduli along the two natural axes. The epiglottis (blue region in the top figure) is set to be stiffer than the vallecula (yellow region in the bottom figure). (c) Estimated elasticity using ground truth deformations. (Color figure online)

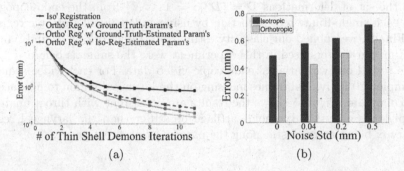

Fig. 4. (a) Registration accuracy over registration iterations under different options. (b) Final registration accuracy under different levels of noise.

To test joint estimation accuracy, we performed one iteration of the framework introduced in Sect. 4. To be specific, we first performed 20 independent registrations between the reference surface and the 20 deformed surfaces using isotropic elasticity, followed by an elasticity estimation using the 20 resulting deformations. This gives us estimated orthotropic elasticity across the reference surface for a second round of registrations. Figure 4a gives accuracy measurement under different registration options. The error is computed as the average per-vertex Euclidean distance error (compared against the aforementioned ground truth deformations) over all vertices and all 3 patients. Note that the x-axis in Fig. 4a denotes the iterations within the Thin Shell Demons [21] registration, not to be confused with the overall joint estimation iteration discussed in Sect. 4. The 2nd-round orthotropic registration (blue curve) performs better than the isotropic registration (black). Meanwhile, it is only slightly worse than using orthotropic elasticity estimated directly from ground truth deformations. This means that further elasticity update won't improve the results too much.

We also tested the robustness of this joint estimation framework under the effect of noise. Different levels of white Gaussian noise were added to all vertices. Figure 4b shows that the 2nd-round orthotropic registration performs better than the isotropic registration in all 4 cases.

Real Endoscopic Data. We further used our framework to investigate the pharyngeal deformations contained in live nasopharyngoscopy. An endoscopic video provides direct visualization of a patient's pharyngeal surface and usually captures its rich swallowing motion. Elasticity estimation on this frame-by-frame surface deformation can help us better understand tissue characteristics and facilitate further analysis, such as the registration between the endoscopy and CT of the same patient for radiation treatment planning.

We first reconstructed a surface model from the video as the reference surface $\mathcal{M}$. This reconstructed surface, called an endoscopogram, was computed by first applying Shape-from-Motion-and-Shading (SfMS) [25] to produce a set of N single-frame reconstructions $\{\mathcal{M}^\alpha | \alpha = 1 \dots N\}$ and then fusing $\{\mathcal{M}^\alpha | \alpha = 1 \dots N\}$ into a unified and complete surface $\mathcal{M}$ [24]. Next, we computed the set of deformations $\mathcal{D} = \{\mathcal{D}^\alpha | \alpha = 1 \dots N\}$ from the endoscopogram $\mathcal{M}$ to each single-frame reconstruction by using independent isotropic registration. Finally, we applied our elasticity estimation framework on $\mathcal{D}$ and $\mathcal{M}$. The algorithm parameters used in this experiment were the same as before.

We tested on two patients' endoscopic video data. For each video sequence we sampled 20 individual frames focusing on the laryngeal region to produce the endoscopogram. Figure 5 shows the results are consistent with throat anatomy: the epiglottis and the arytenoid cartilage be stiffer than the laryngeal region, the larynx being more elastic along the patient axial direction.

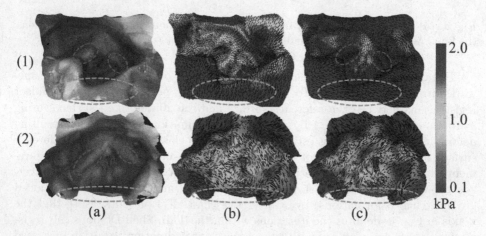

Fig. 5. (a) Endoscopogram surfaces reconstructed from video. Red circles indicate the arytenoid cartilage. Green circles indicate the epiglottis. (b) and (c) Estimated Young's moduli and the associated natural axes. (Color figure online)

6   Discussion

We have introduced a statistical framework to estimate inhomogeneous and anisotropic elasticity parameters of a thin shell structure from a set of its known deformations. We have shown that an MAP analysis on a novel MRF-based probability distribution can automatically recover both the orthotropic stiffness matrix and natural axes directions of every location on the shell. We have also shown that this framework can be further used as a part in a joint registration and elasticity estimation framework. Both the elasticity estimation framework and the joint estimation framework can be helpful in studying within-patient deformations of anatomical surfaces. Despite the promising results shown in our experiments, we still have to address the following concerns in future work:

1. In many situations anatomical surfaces are deformed by the underlying muscles, so it is not appropriate to simply model the surface as a shell structure. We should generalize our framework to the 3D volume situation.
2. Model parameters selection needs to be further studied.
3. In several real endoscopic cases, real tissue deformations were dominated by other non-physical deformations (e.g. reconstruction errors). The applicability of our framework in this situation needs to be further examined.

Acknowledgement. This work was supported by NIH grant R01 CA158925. We thank Dr. Bhisham Chera from the Department of Radiation Oncology for providing the endoscopy data.

References

1. Bajcsy, R., Kovačič, S.: Multiresolution elastic matching. Comput. Vis. Graph. Image Process. **46**(1), 1–21 (1989)
2. Christensen, G., Rabbitt, R., Miller, M.: Deformable templates using large deformation kinematics. Comput. Vis. Graph. Image Process. **5**(10), 1435–1447 (1996)
3. Thirion, J.: Image matching as a diffusion process: an analogy with Maxwells demons. Med. Image Anal. **2**(3), 243–260 (1998)
4. Beg, M., Miller, M., Trouvé, A., Younes, L.: Computing large deformation metric mappings via geodesic flows of diffeomorphisms. Int. J. Comput. Vis. **61**(2), 139–157 (2005)
5. Miga, M.: A new approach to elastography using mutual information and finite elements. Phys. Med. Biol. **48**(4), 467–480 (2003)
6. Kroon, M., Holzapfel, G.A.: Estimation of the distributions of anisotropic, elastic properties and wall stresses of saccular cerebral aneurysms by inverse analysis. Proc. R. Soc. Lond. A: Math. Phys. Eng. Sci. **464**(2092), 807–825 (2008)
7. Schneider, R., Faust, G., Hindenlang, U., Helwig, P.: Inhomogeneous, orthotropic material model for the cortical structure of long bones modeled on the basis of clinical CT or density data. Comput. Methods Appl. Mech. Eng. **198**(27–29), 2167–2174 (2009)
8. Yang, S., Jojic, V., Lian, J., Chen, R., Zhu, H., Lin, M.C.: Classification of prostate cancer grades and t-stages based on tissue elasticity using medical image analysis. In: Ourselin, S., Joskowicz, L., Sabuncu, M.R., Unal, G., Wells, W. (eds.) MICCAI 2016. LNCS, vol. 9900, pp. 627–635. Springer, Cham (2016). doi:10.1007/978-3-319-46720-7_73

9. Freiman, M., Voss, S.D., Warfield, S.K.: Demons registration with local affine adaptive regularization: application to registration of abdominal structures. In: IEEE International Symposium on Biomedical Imaging, pp. 1219–1222 (2011)
10. Gerig, T., Shahim, K., Reyes, M., Vetter, T., Lüthi, M.: Spatially varying registration using gaussian processes. In: Golland, P., Hata, N., Barillot, C., Hornegger, J., Howe, R. (eds.) MICCAI 2014. LNCS, vol. 8674, pp. 413–420. Springer, Cham (2014). doi:10.1007/978-3-319-10470-6_52
11. Vialard, F.-X., Risser, L.: Spatially-varying metric learning for diffeomorphic image registration: a variational framework. In: Golland, P., Hata, N., Barillot, C., Hornegger, J., Howe, R. (eds.) MICCAI 2014. LNCS, vol. 8673, pp. 227–234. Springer, Cham (2014). doi:10.1007/978-3-319-10404-1_29
12. Davatzikos, C.: Spatial transformation and registration of brain images using elastically deformable models. Comput. Methods Appl. Mech. Eng. **66**(2), 207–222 (1997)
13. Alterovitz, R., Goldberg, K., Pouliot, J., Hsu, I.C.J., Kim, Y., Noworolski, S.M., Kurhanewicz, J.: Registration of MR prostate images with biomechanical modeling and nonlinear parameter estimation. Med. Phys. **33**(2), 446–454 (2006)
14. Misra, S., Ramesh, R., Okamura, A.: Modelling of non-linear elastic tissues for surgical simulation. Comput. Methods Appl. Mech. Eng. **13**(6), 811–818 (2010)
15. Green, M., Geng, G., Qin, E., Sinkus, R., Gandevia, S., Bilston, L.: Measuring anisotropic muscle stiffness properties using elastography. NMR Biomed. **26**(11), 1387–1394 (2013)
16. Risholm, P., Ross, J., Washko, G.R., Wells, W.M.: Probabilistic elastography: estimating lung elasticity. In: Székely, G., Hahn, H.K. (eds.) IPMI 2011. LNCS, vol. 6801, pp. 699–710. Springer, Heidelberg (2011). doi:10.1007/978-3-642-22092-0_57
17. Bauer, M., Bruveris, M., Michor, P.W.: Overview of the geometries of shape spaces and diffeomorphism groups. J. Math. Imaging Vis. **50**(1), 60–97 (2014)
18. Schulz, J., Pizer, S.M., Marron, J., Godtliebsen, F.: Nonlinear hypothesis testing of geometrical object properties of shapes applied to Hippocampi. J. Math. Imaging Vis. **54**(1), 15–34 (2015)
19. Ventsel, E., Krauthammer, T.: Thin Plates and Shells: Theory: Analysis, and Applications. CRC Press, Boca Raton (2001)
20. Gingold, Y., Secord, A., Han, J.Y., Grinspun, E., Zorin, D.: A discrete modelfor inelastic deformation of thin shells. Technical report, Courant Institute of Mathematical Sciences (2004)
21. Zhao, Q., Price, J.T., Pizer, S., Niethammer, M., Alterovitz, R., Rosenman, J.: Surface registration in the presence of topology changes and missing patches. In: Medical Image Understanding and Analysis, pp. 8–13 (2015)
22. Arsigny, V., Fillard, P., Pennec, X., Ayache, N.: Log-euclidean metrics for fast and simple calculus on diffusion tensors. Phys. Med. Biol. **56**(2), 411–421 (2006)
23. Crane, K., Desbrun, M., Schröder, P.: Trivial connections on discrete surfaces. In: Symposium on Geometry Processing, vol. 29 (2010)
24. Zhao, Q., Price, T., Pizer, S., Niethammer, M., Alterovitz, R., Rosenman, J.: The endoscopogram: a 3D model reconstructed from endoscopic video frames. In: Ourselin, S., Joskowicz, L., Sabuncu, M.R., Unal, G., Wells, W. (eds.) MICCAI 2016. LNCS, vol. 9900, pp. 439–447. Springer, Cham (2016). doi:10.1007/978-3-319-46720-7_51
25. Price, T., Zhao, Q., Rosenman, J., Pizer, S., Frahm, J.M.: Shape from motion and shading in uncontrolled environments. Technical report, Department of Computer Science, University of North Carolina at Chapel Hill (2016)

Direct Estimation of Regional Wall Thicknesses via Residual Recurrent Neural Network

Wufeng Xue, Ilanit Ben Nachum, Sachin Pandey, James Warrington,
Stephanie Leung, and Shuo Li[⊠]

Department of Medical Imaging, Western University, London, ON, Canada
xwolfs@hotmail.com, slishuo@gmail.com

Abstract. Accurate estimation of regional wall thicknesses (RWT) of left ventricular (LV) myocardium from cardiac MR sequences is of significant importance for identification and diagnosis of cardiac disease. Existing RWT estimation still relies on segmentation of LV myocardium, which requires strong prior information and user interaction. No work has been devoted into direct estimation of RWT from cardiac MR images due to the diverse shapes and structures for various subjects and cardiac diseases, as well as the complex regional deformation of LV myocardium during the systole and diastole phases of the cardiac cycle. In this paper, we present a newly proposed Residual Recurrent Neural Network (ResRNN) that fully leverages the spatial and temporal dynamics of LV myocardium to achieve accurate frame-wise RWT estimation. Our ResRNN comprises two paths: (1) a feed forward convolution neural network (CNN) for effective and robust CNN embedding learning of various cardiac images and preliminary estimation of RWT from each frame itself independently, and (2) a recurrent neural network (RNN) for further improving the estimation by modeling spatial and temporal dynamics of LV myocardium. For the RNN path, we design for cardiac sequences a Circle-RNN to eliminate the effect of null hidden input for the first time-step. Our ResRNN is capable of obtaining accurate estimation of cardiac RWT with Mean Absolute Error of 1.44 mm (less than 1-pixel error) when validated on cardiac MR sequences of 145 subjects, evidencing its great potential in clinical cardiac function assessment.

Keywords: Regional wall thickness · Residual recurrent neural network · Spatial dependency · Temporal dependency · Circle-RNN

1 Introduction

Estimation of regional wall thicknesses (RWT) of left ventricle (LV) myocardium is of significant importance for early identification and diagnosis of cardiac disease [8,12,15]. Figure 1 demonstrates the RWT to be estimated for a short-axis view cardiac image. A traditional way for RWT estimation is to segment the LV myocardium from other structures first and then measure the corresponding RWT of each region. However, existing segmentation methods for cardiac

© Springer International Publishing AG 2017
M. Niethammer et al. (Eds.): IPMI 2017, LNCS 10265, pp. 505–516, 2017.
DOI: 10.1007/978-3-319-59050-9_40

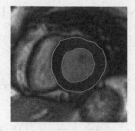 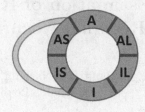

Fig. 1. Illustration of RWT for short-axis view cardiac MR image. Left: cardiac image with the contours of myocardium delineated. Right: the 6 segments model for mid-slice cardiac left ventricle. A: anterior; AS: anterospetal; IS: inferoseptal; I: inferior; IL: inferolateral; AL: anterolateral.

images [3,12,13] require strong prior information and user interaction to obtain reliable results, which may hinder them from efficient clinical application. An alternative way is to circumvent this segmentation step and estimate RWT from cardiac images directly. Direct estimation of cardiac volumes [1,2,17,18,20–22] have achieved great success in recent years, while direct estimation of RWT has never been explored due to the diversity of cardiac shape and structures for various subjects and various diseases, as well as the complication of regional myocardium deformation through the cardiac cycle.

In this work, we provide a method to estimate the frame-wise RWT from cardiac MR sequences through a newly proposed Residual Recurrent Neural Network (ResRNN). This ResRNN contains two paths: (1) a CNN path for low dimension embedding to robustly represent cardiac images of diverse structures, and preliminary estimation of RWT independently from the embedding of each frame itself, and (2) an RNN path for residual estimation from neighboring frames by leveraging the temporal and spatial dynamic deformation in cardiac sequences simultaneously. In the RNN path, a temporal RNN is applied to the features of temporally neighboring frames for modeling the complex long-range temporal dependencies, and another spatial RNN is applied to the predicted results of spatially neighboring wall thicknesses for modeling the mutual dependencies among these wall thicknesses. For the RNN module, a new Circle-RNN is designed to eliminate the effect of null initial hidden states by characterizing the periodicity of cardiac sequences and the circular spatial layout of cardiac RWT. With image represented by the CNN embeddings, the dynamic deformation of myocardium and the diversity of cardiac shape are well captured by the temporal and spatial RNN, thus leading to accurate estimation of RWT.

1.1   Related Work

Segmentation-Based and Direct Methods for Cardiac Volumes Estimation. Currently, the most related work to RWT estimation is cardiac volumes estimation, which falls into two categories: segmentation-based methods [3,12, 13] and direct methods [1,2,17,18,20–22]. Segmentation-based methods rely on the premise of cardiac segmentation, which is still a great challenge due to the diverse structure of cardiac image and therefore requires strong prior information and user interaction [3,12,13].

To circumvent these limitations, direct methods without segmentation have grown in popularity in cardiac volumes estimation [1,2,17,18,20–22]. In these methods, hand-crafted features extracted from cardiac images are fed into regression models such as random forest (RF), adaptive K-clustering RF (AKRF), Bayesian model, and neural networks, to predict cardiac volumes. The employed features include Bhattacharyya coefficient between image distributions [1,2], appearance features [18], multiple low level image features [21], as well as features from multiscale convolutional deep belief network (MCDNB) [22] and supervised descriptor learning (SDL) [20]. Although these methods obtained effective performance, two limitations still exist: (1) they followed two separated phases, i.e., *feature extraction+volumes regression*, and no feedback exists between them to make them compatible with each other; (2) neither the temporal dependencies nor the spatial dependencies are taken into account, while the dependencies are important for dynamic modeling of cardiac sequence. In the present work, we provide an elegant solution for direct RWT estimation with an end-to-end architecture that respects both temporal and spatial dependencies.

Recurrent Neural Network. Recurrent neural network, especially when the long short-term memory units (LSTM) are deployed, is specialized in long-range temporal dynamic modeling and spatial context modeling. Promising results have been achieved by RNN in a wide spectrum of applications including language modeling [19], object recognition [11], visual recognition and description [5,10], and also medical image analysis [9,14,16]. In the work of cardiac image segmentation [14], an RNN was employed to capture the spatial changes of cardiac structure (represented as low dimensional CNN embeddings) in cardiac sequences. In [9], an RNN with LSTM was employed to model the temporal dependencies in cardiac MR sequences to identify the end-diastole and end-systole frames across a cardiac cycle. In [16], an RNN was trained to describe the contexts of detected disease in Chest X-Rays. These methods only explored one of the spatial or temporal dependencies while in cardiac sequences, both are important for robust dynamic modeling.

To fully explore the dependencies that exist in cardiac sequences during RWT estimation, two RNN modules are deployed in our work accounting for the temporal and spatial dependencies simultaneously. Besides, we propose a Circle-RNN for periodic cardiac sequences to better serve this aim, avoiding the effect of the null initial hidden input in existing RNN.

1.2 Contributions

The contributions of our work include:

- An effective end-to-end method that has great potential in clinical cardiac function assessment is proposed for direct cardiac RWT estimation, which has never been investigated previously.

- The newly proposed two-path ResRNN endows the network with abilities to robustly represent complex cardiac structure, and effectively model the capricious spatial and temporal dynamic deformation.
- The temporal RNN that accounts for the temporal deformation of the cardiac shape, and the spatial RNN that accounts for the smoothness of the LV myocardium shape, enable ResRNN to estimate collaboratively RWT of all frames and all regions by leveraging the temporal and spatial dependencies in cardiac MR sequences, rather than to estimate independently each cardiac RWT from a single image.
- A Circle-RNN designed for characterizing the periodicity of cardiac sequences and the circular spatial layout of cardiac RWT is proposed to eliminate the effect of the null hidden input for the first time step, to incorporate both the future and the past information in the dynamic modeling, and to treat every frame in the sequence with equally long-term dependencies.

2 RWT Estimation via ResRNN

2.1 Problem Formulation

For a set of cardiac MR sequences $\mathcal{X} = \{X_f^s\}$, where $s = 1 \cdots S$ indexes the subject and $f = 1 \cdots F$ indexes the frame in a cardiac cycle, we aim to estimate the frame-wise values of RWT $\mathcal{Y} = \{y_{f,l}^s\}$ for all the frames, where $l = 1 \cdots 6$ indexes the spatial location of each RWT (see Fig. 1, from IS to AS in counter-clockwise order). We consider in this work the mid-cavity of LV myocardium in short axis view, which is divided into six segments according to the AHA 17 segments model [4]. The objective function can be formulated as:

$$\min_{\theta} \frac{1}{2S \times F} \sum_f \sum_s \|y_f^s - \mathbf{Q}(X_f^s|\theta)\|_2^2 + \lambda \mathcal{R}(\theta) \tag{1}$$

where $\mathbf{Q}$ is the network, θ is the parameter vector to be learned, and $\mathcal{R}(\theta)$ regularizes the parameter vector.

2.2 Overview of the Proposed Method

To estimate the frame-wise RWT from cardiac MR sequence, we build a new architecture of network: ResRNN. As shown in Fig. 2, two paths are included in ResRNN: with the CNN path $\mathbf{Q_{CNN}}$, each frame in the sequence is independently processed by the CNN network, forming a low dimensional embedding of the cardiac images, from which the RWT is preliminarily estimated with another fully-connected layer; with the RNN path $\mathbf{Q_{RNN}}$, two RNN modules are deployed to model the temporal dependencies between neighboring frames and the spatial dependencies between neighboring RWTs, so as to further correct the residual of the preliminary estimation. The RNN path shares the same CNN embedding with the CNN path. The final RWT estimation is computed as:

$$\mathbf{Q}(X_f^s|\theta) = \mathbf{Q}_{CNN}(X_f^s|\theta) + \mathbf{Q}_{RNN}(X_f^s|\theta) \tag{2}$$

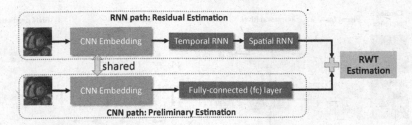

Fig. 2. Overview of ResRNN. A CNN path (the lower part) is employed to learn CNN embedding for the cardiac image and further obtain a preliminary estimation of RWT from these features. An RNN path (the upper part) is employed to model the temporal and spatial dependencies based on the CNN embedding of the cardiac sequences to estimate the residual of the preliminary estimation.

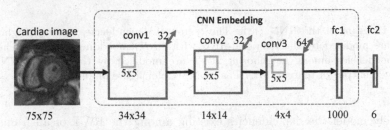

Fig. 3. Diagram of the CNN path. Each convolution layer (conv) is followed by a rectified linear unit (ReLU) layer and a max-pooling layer. The CNN embedding part represents the cardiac image as a low dimensional feature vector, which is shared by both the CNN and RNN paths.

2.3 Preliminary Estimation with the CNN Path

The diagram of our CNN path is shown in Fig. 3. Three convolution (conv1 $\sim$ 3) and one fully-connected (fc1) layers are deployed to obtain the low dimensional CNN embedding e_f^s of cardiac images. The second fully-connected layer (fc2) estimates a preliminary results $y_f^{s,CNN}$ of RWT from the CNN embeddings.

$$y_f^{s,CNN} = \theta_{fc2:w} e_f^s + \theta_{fc2:b} \tag{3}$$

where $\theta_{fc2:w}$ and $\theta_{fc2:b}$ are the weight matrix and bias of the fc2 layer.

As a feed forward neural network, the CNN path bears a notable limitation that it relies on the assumption of independence among samples, which does not hold for cardiac sequence. The dependencies among cardiac sequences have to be modeled to further reduce the residual of the CNN estimation.

2.4 Residual Estimation with the RNN Path

The diagram of the RNN path is shown in Fig. 4. Based on the CNN embedding obtained with the CNN path, temporal and spatial RNN are employed to

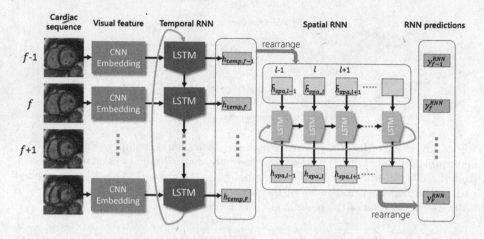

Fig. 4. Diagram of the RNN path. The temporal dependencies among neighboring frames are modeled by the temporal-RNN with CNN embedding as input. The spatial dependencies among neighboring RWT are modeled by the spatial-RNN with rearranged output of temporal-RNN as input. (Color figure online)

effectively model the dependencies existing among the RWT of all frames. In this section, we first introduce the memory unit LSTM that we use in the RNN path, and then describe the temporal and spatial RNN.

LSTM. In order to learn the long-term dynamics in sequential data and avoid the gradient vanishing/exploding problem in traditional RNN, LSTM unit [6], as shown in Fig. 5, was introduced into RNN. The input gate, output gate, forget gate and the memory cell allow the network to learn when to forget previous hidden states and when to update current hidden states given current input. This strategy enables LSTM to adaptively memorize and access information

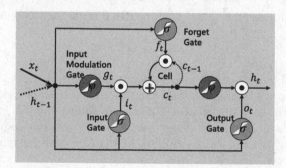

Fig. 5. A diagram of LSTM unit in RNN, which is capable of adaptively modeling dynamic deformations in cardiac sequences due to the input gate, forget gate, and output gate.

long term ago. The LSTM computations for time step t given the current input x_t, the previous hidden states h_{t-1} and memory states c_{t-1}, are as follows [6]:

$$
\begin{aligned}
i_t &= \sigma(W_{xi}x_t + W_{hi}h_{t-1} + b_i) \\
f_t &= \sigma(W_{xf}x_t + W_{hf}h_{t-1} + b_f) \\
o_t &= \sigma(W_{xo}x_t + W_{ho}h_{t-1} + b_o) \\
g_t &= \varphi(W_{xc}x_t + W_{hc}h_{t-1} + b_c) \\
c_t &= f_t \odot c_{t-1} + i_t \odot g_t \\
h_t &= o_t \odot \varphi(c_t)
\end{aligned}
\tag{4}
$$

where $\sigma(\cdot)$ and $\varphi(\cdot)$ are element-wise sigmoid and hyperbolic tangent non-linearity functions, $\odot$ are element-wise product. The first three equations map the current input and previous hidden states to the input gate i_t, the forget gate f_t and the output gate o_t, to adaptively control the information flow. Ws are the weight matrices to be learned and bs are the corresponding bias terms.

Temporal RNN and Spatial RNN. With CNN embedding e_f^s, we first deploy a temporal RNN with the frame index in a cardiac sequences as time step to predict the values of RWT $h_{temp,f}^s \in \mathcal{R}^6$ for each frame f taking account of the dependencies between neighboring frames (See *Temporal RNN* in Fig. 4).

$$
h_{temp,f}^s = LSTM(e_f^s, h_{temp,f-1}^s), f = 1 \ldots F
\tag{5}
$$

Based on the predicted of temporal RNN, we again deploy a spatial RNN with spatial location as time step to predict RWT $h_{spa,l}^s \in \mathcal{R}^F$ of one specific location l for all the frames in the sequences (See *Spatial RNN* in Fig. 4). We rearrange column vectors $[h_{temp,1}^s, h_{temp,2}^s, \ldots, h_{temp,F}^s]$ to row vectors $[\hat{h}_{spa,1}^{s,T}; \hat{h}_{spa,2}^{s,T}, \ldots, \hat{h}_{spa,6}^{s,T}]$. Then we have

$$
h_{spa,l}^s = LSTM(\hat{h}_{spa,l}^s, h_{spa,l-1}^s), l = 1 \ldots 6
\tag{6}
$$

By rearranging these row vectors $[h_{spa,1}^{s,T}; h_{spa,2}^{s,T}; \ldots, h_{spa,6}^{s,T}]$ back to column vectors $[y_1^{s,RNN}, y_2^{s,RNN}, \ldots, y_F^{s,RNN}]$, we get the RNN predictions for frame-wise RWT.

Circle-RNN. As can be seen from Eqs. 5 and 6, three limitations exist for RNN: (1) for the first time step ($f = 1$ or $l = 1$), there is no value for previous hidden units, which influences the prediction of the first frame; (2) only past information can be used to determine the output of current time step, while future information is also equally important; (3) for the first few time steps, long-term dependency model can not be well built from the limited past information, leading to unfair treatment of different frames.

We provide an elegant solution to overcome these limitations for cardiac MR sequence: Circle-RNN, which connects the output of the last frame to the hidden

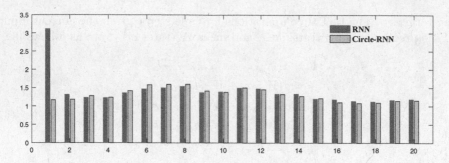

Fig. 6. Average estimation error (mm) of different frames by RNN and Circle-RNN for cardiac RWT. Only temporal RNN is employed here for comparison. The estimation error for the first frame is clearly reduced by Circle-RNN.

input of the first frame, as the red arrows show in Fig. 4. Within Circle-RNN, Eqs. 5 and 6 become:

$$h^s_{temp,f} = LSTM(e^s_f, h^s_{temp,mod(f-1-1,F)+1}), f = 1 \dots F \qquad (7)$$

$$h^s_{spa,l} = LSTM(\hat{h}^s_{spa,l}, h^s_{spa,mod(l-1-1,6)+1}), l = 1 \dots 6 \qquad (8)$$

where $mod(a, b)$ computes the modulus. Circle-RNN can be easily optimized with the BPTT algorithm [6]. To avoid infinite information loop within this Circle-RNN, we introduce a parameter *depth* to control how many rounds the information flow in our Circle-RNN. Figure 6 shows the error reduction of Circle-RNN over RNN when predicting cardiac RWT from the CNN embedding with only temporal RNN employed.

3 Experiments

3.1 Dataset and Implementations

A dataset of short-axis cine MR images paired with manually obtained ground truth values of RWT is constructed to evaluate the performance of our method, which includes 2900 images from 145 subjects. These subjects are collected from 3 hospitals affiliated with two health care centers and 2 vendors (GE and Siemens). Each subject contains 20 frames throughout a cardiac cycle. In each frame, the middle slice is selected following the standard AHA prescriptions [4] for validation of the proposed cardiac RWT estimation method. The ground truth values of RWT are manually obtained for each image.

In our experiments, two landmarks, i.e., junctions of the right ventricular wall with the left ventricular, are manually marked for each cardiac image to provide reference for ROI cropping and the LV myocardial segments division. The cropped images are resized to dimension of 80×80. All values of RWT are normalized to the range of [0,1] according to the image dimension (80). Five-fold cross validation is employed for performance evaluation and comparison. Mean

Table 1. Estimation error comparison of CNN, RNN and ResRNN for cardiac RWT estimation in terms of MAE (Mean±standard deviation) (mm). WT-IS means wall thickness for the inferoseptal segment of myocardium, similar for the rest. Best results are highlighted in bold.

Method	CNN	RNN (plain)	RNN (circle)	ResRNN (plain)	**ResRNN (circle)**
WT-IS	1.28 ± 1.10	1.30 ± 1.11	1.31 ± 1.04	1.26 ± 1.15	$\mathbf{1.22 \pm 1.02}$
WT-I	1.56 ± 1.27	1.60 ± 1.28	1.54 ± 1.26	1.55 ± 1.24	$\mathbf{1.47 \pm 1.22}$
WT-IL	1.81 ± 1.51	1.99 ± 1.66	1.86 ± 1.60	1.80 ± 1.48	$\mathbf{1.78 \pm 1.53}$
WT-AL	1.64 ± 1.30	1.70 ± 1.42	1.66 ± 1.35	$\mathbf{1.60 \pm 1.29}$	1.60 ± 1.31
WT-A	1.35 ± 1.09	1.36 ± 1.18	1.30 ± 1.09	1.40 ± 1.20	$\mathbf{1.31 \pm 1.08}$
WT-AS	1.26 ± 0.80	1.39 ± 1.06	1.29 ± 1.01	1.34 ± 1.10	$\mathbf{1.25 \pm 0.97}$
Average	1.49 ± 0.76	1.56 ± 0.83	1.49 ± 0.80	1.49 ± 0.81	$\mathbf{1.44 \pm 0.74}$

absolute error (MAE) between estimation and the ground truth is computed to evaluate the performance. The network is implemented by Caffe [7] with SGD solver. Learning rate and weight decay are set to (0.05, 0.0005). 'step' learning policy is employed with gamma and step size being (0.5, 2500) and momentum 0.9. The depth of Circle-RNN is set as the number of time steps, i.e., 20 for the temporal RNN and 6 for the spatial RNN. Data augmentation is conducted by randomly cropping images of size 75×75 from the original image.

3.2 Performance Comparison: ResRNN vs. CNN and RNN

The advantages of the proposed ResRNN are firstly demonstrated by comparing performance of three different network architectures: (1) CNN, i.e. the CNN path as shown in Fig. 3; (2) RNN, i.e. the RNN path as shown in Fig. 4, and (3) the proposed ResRNN. For RNN and ResRNN, both the original RNN (the plain RNN) and Circle-RNN are employed for comparison.

From the average estimation error shown in Table 1, we can observe the followings. (1) The two-path ResRNN outperforms CNN and RNN, with either plain or circle RNN deployed, which can be ascribed to the complementarity of the preliminary estimation from each frame itself and the residual estimation that modeling the dependencies of cardiac sequence. (2) When Circle-RNN, rather than the plain RNN, is deployed, lower estimation error can be obtained by RNN or ResRNN, due to the fact that Circle-RNN is capable of memorizing useful cardiac dynamic information for the first time step. In the following experiments, Circle-RNN is deployed in ResRNN.

3.3 Performance Comparison: ResRNN vs. State-of-the-Art

To demonstrate the advantages of our proposed method over segmentation based [3] and two-phase direct methods [20–22], we apply these methods to our database for cardiac RWT estimation. For the direct methods, the same five-fold cross-validation protocol is used. As can be observed in Table 2 and Fig. 7, the

Table 2. Estimation error comparison of the proposed ResRNN with segmentation based method and existing direct methods for RWT estimation in terms of MAE (Mean± standard deviation) (mm). Best results are highlighted in bold.

Method	Max Flow [3]	Multi-features+RF [21]	SDL+AKRF [20]	MCDBN+RF [22]	ResRNN
WT-IS	1.53 ± 1.73	1.70 ± 1.47	1.98 ± 1.58	1.78 ± 1.40	$\mathbf{1.22 \pm 1.02}$
WT-I	3.23 ± 2.83	1.71 ± 1.34	1.67 ± 1.40	1.68 ± 1.41	$\mathbf{1.47 \pm 1.22}$
WT-IL	4.15 ± 3.17	1.97 ± 1.54	1.88 ± 1.63	1.92 ± 1.45	$\mathbf{1.78 \pm 1.53}$
WT-AL	5.08 ± 3.95	1.82 ± 1.41	1.87 ± 1.55	1.66 ± 1.20	$\mathbf{1.60 \pm 1.31}$
WT-A	3.47 ± 3.25	1.55 ± 1.33	1.65 ± 1.45	$\mathbf{1.20 \pm 1.01}$	1.31 ± 1.08
WT-AS	1.76 ± 1.80	1.68 ± 1.43	2.04 ± 1.59	1.63 ± 1.23	$\mathbf{1.25 \pm 0.97}$
Average	3.21 ± 1.98	1.73 ± 0.97	1.85 ± 1.03	1.65 ± 0.77	$\mathbf{1.44 \pm 0.74}$

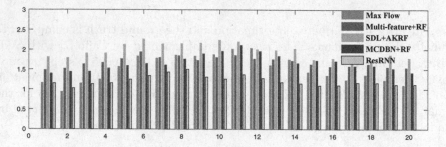

Fig. 7. Average frame-wise estimation error (mm) of WT-IS over all subjects for ResRNN and all other competitors. The proposed ResRNN delivers clearly lower estimation error than other methods.

proposed ResRNN demonstrates great advantages over existing segmentation-based and two-phase direct methods for cardiac RWT estimation.

From Table 2, we can see that the proposed ResRNN estimates cardiac RWT with high accuracy (average MAE of 1.44 mm) and outperforms all competitors. Specifically, it outperforms the Max Flow method with 55.14% MAE reduction. Note that Max Flow obtained high dice metric of 0.9182 for LV cavity segmentation when applied to our database. In fact, the dependency on manual segmentation of the first frame makes the estimation error of Max Flow increase as the estimated frame is far from the first frame within the cardiac cycle (see the frame-wise estimation error of Max Flow in Fig. 7). ResRNN outperforms the best of the direct methods (MCDBN+RF [22]) with a clear error reduction: 12.73%. Within the two-phase framework, the hand-crafted multifeatures, the features obtained by supervised learning, and MCDBN features employed in existing methods all fail to beat ResRNN, which evidences the benefits of the network architecture in ResRNN over the two-phase direct methods. Figure 7 also shows that ResRNN estimates each frame with consistently lower MAE.

Besides, we can draw that all the deep neural network based methods in Table 1 outperform existing two-phase direct methods in Table 2. This further confirms the argument that independent feature extraction and regression cannot make the two phases maximumly compatible with each other. The end-to-end learning procedure of neural network integrates both phases together and leads to clearly improved performance.

4   Conclusions

In this paper, we propose an effective network architecture ResRNN for the task of cardiac RWT estimation, which has never been explored before. In ResRNN, a CNN path is employed to estimate from each cardiac image independently the preliminary results of RWT, and an RNN path is employed to compensate the residual of CNN estimations with temporal and spatial dependencies being accounted by Circle-RNN. Validation on a data set of cardiac MR sequences from 145 subjects demonstrates that the proposed ResRNN is capable of estimating cardiac RWT values with performance better than state-of-the-art methods, and is of great potential in clinical cardiac function assessment.

References

1. Afshin, M., Ayed, I.B., Islam, A., Goela, A., Peters, T.M., Li, S.: Global assessment of cardiac function using image statistics in MRI. In: Ayache, N., Delingette, H., Golland, P., Mori, K. (eds.) MICCAI 2012. LNCS, vol. 7511, pp. 535–543. Springer, Heidelberg (2012). doi:10.1007/978-3-642-33418-4_66
2. Afshin, M., Ben Ayed, I., Punithakumar, K., Law, M., Islam, A., Goela, A., Peters, T.M., Li, S.: Regional assessment of cardiac left ventricular myocardial function via MRI statistical features. IEEE Trans. Med. Imaging **33**(2), 481–494 (2014)
3. Ayed, I.B., Chen, H.M., Punithakumar, K., Ross, I., Li, S.: Max-flow segmentation of the left ventricle by recovering subject-specific distributions via a bound of the bhattacharyya measure. Med. Image Anal. **16**(1), 87–100 (2012)
4. Cerqueira, M.D., Weissman, N.J., Dilsizian, V., Jacobs, A.K., Kaul, S., Laskey, W.K., Pennell, D.J., Rumberger, J.A., Ryan, T., Verani, M.S., et al.: Standardized myocardial segmentation and nomenclature for tomographic imaging of the heart a statement for healthcare professionals from the cardiac imaging committee of the council on clinical cardiology of the american heart association. Circulation **105**(4), 539–542 (2002)
5. Donahue, J., Anne Hendricks, L., Guadarrama, S., Rohrbach, M., Venugopalan, S., Saenko, K., Darrell, T.: Long-term recurrent convolutional networks for visual recognition and description. In: IEEE CVPR, pp. 2625–2634 (2015)
6. Graves, A.: Supervised sequence labelling. In: Graves, A. (ed.) Supervised Sequence Labelling with Recurrent Neural Networks. SCI, vol. 385, pp. 5–13. Springer, Heidelberg (2012). doi:10.1007/978-3-642-24797-2_2
7. Jia, Y., Shelhamer, E., Donahue, J., Karayev, S., Long, J., Girshick, R., Guadarrama, S., Darrell, T.: Caffe: convolutional architecture for fast feature embedding. In: ACM International Conference on Multimedia, pp. 675–678. ACM (2014)

8. Kawel, N., Turkbey, E.B., Carr, J.J., Eng, J., Gomes, A.S., Hundley, W.G., Johnson, C., Masri, S.C., Prince, M.R., van der Geest, R.J., et al.: Normal left ventricular myocardial thickness for middle-aged and older subjects with steady-state free precession cardiac magnetic resonance the multi-ethnic study of atherosclerosis. Circ.: Cardiovasc. Imaging **5**(4), 500–508 (2012)

9. Kong, B., Zhan, Y., Shin, M., Denny, T., Zhang, S.: Recognizing end-diastole and end-systole frames via deep temporal regression network. In: Ourselin, S., Joskowicz, L., Sabuncu, M.R., Unal, G., Wells, W. (eds.) MICCAI 2016. LNCS, vol. 9902, pp. 264–272. Springer, Cham (2016). doi:10.1007/978-3-319-46726-9_31

10. Li, Y., Lan, C., Xing, J., Zeng, W., Yuan, C., Liu, J.: Online human action detection using joint classification-regression recurrent neural networks. In: Leibe, B., Matas, J., Sebe, N., Welling, M. (eds.) ECCV 2016. LNCS, vol. 9911, pp. 203–220. Springer, Cham (2016). doi:10.1007/978-3-319-46478-7_13

11. Liang, X., Shen, X., Xiang, D., Feng, J., Lin, L., Yan, S.: Semantic object parsing with local-global long short-term memory. arXiv preprint arXiv:1511.04510 (2015)

12. Peng, P., Lekadir, K., Gooya, A., Shao, L., Petersen, S.E., Frangi, A.F.: A review of heart chamber segmentation for structural and functional analysis using cardiac magnetic resonance imaging. Magn. Reson. Mater. Phys. Biol. Med. **29**(2), 155–195 (2016)

13. Petitjean, C., Dacher, J.N.: A review of segmentation methods in short axis cardiac MR images. Med. Image Anal. **15**(2), 169–184 (2011)

14. Poudel, R.P., Lamata, P., Montana, G.: Recurrent fully convolutional neural networks for multi-slice MRI cardiac segmentation. arXiv preprint arXiv:1608.03974 (2016)

15. Puntmann, V.O., Gebker, R., Duckett, S., Mirelis, J., Schnackenburg, B., Graefe, M., Razavi, R., Fleck, E., Nagel, E.: Left ventricular chamber dimensions and wall thickness by cardiovascular magnetic resonance: comparison with transthoracic echocardiography. Eur. Heart J.-Cardiovasc. Imaging **14**(3), 240–246 (2013)

16. Shin, H.C., Roberts, K., Lu, L., Demner-Fushman, D., Yao, J., Summers, R.M.: Learning to read chest x-rays: recurrent neural cascade model for automated image annotation. arXiv preprint arXiv:1603.08486 (2016)

17. Wang, H., et al.: Prediction of clinical information from cardiac MRI using manifold learning. In: van Assen, H., Bovendeerd, P., Delhaas, T. (eds.) FIMH 2015. LNCS, vol. 9126, pp. 91–98. Springer, Cham (2015). doi:10.1007/978-3-319-20309-6_11

18. Wang, Z., Ben Salah, M., Gu, B., Islam, A., Goela, A., Li, S.: Direct estimation of cardiac biventricular volumes with an adapted Bayesian formulation. IEEE Trans. Biomed. Eng. **61**(4), 1251–1260 (2014)

19. Zhang, X., Lu, L., Lapata, M.: Tree recurrent neural networks with application to language modeling. arXiv preprint arXiv:1511.00060 (2015)

20. Zhen, X., Islam, A., Bhaduri, M., Chan, I., Li, S.: Direct and simultaneous four-chamber volume estimation by multi-output regression. In: Navab, N., Hornegger, J., Wells, W.M., Frangi, A.F. (eds.) MICCAI 2015. LNCS, vol. 9349, pp. 669–676. Springer, Cham (2015). doi:10.1007/978-3-319-24553-9_82

21. Zhen, X., Wang, Z., Islam, A., Bhaduri, M., Chan, I., Li, S.: Direct estimation of cardiac bi-ventricular volumes with regression forests. In: Golland, P., Hata, N., Barillot, C., Hornegger, J., Howe, R. (eds.) MICCAI 2014. LNCS, vol. 8674, pp. 586–593. Springer, Cham (2014). doi:10.1007/978-3-319-10470-6_73

22. Zhen, X., Wang, Z., Islam, A., Bhaduri, M., Chan, I., Li, S.: Multi-scale deep networks and regression forests for direct bi-ventricular volume estimation. Med. Image Anal. **30**, 120–129 (2016)

Multi-class Image Segmentation in Fluorescence Microscopy Using Polytrees

Hamid Fehri[1,2,3,4]($\boxtimes$), Ali Gooya[1,4], Simon A. Johnston[2,3],
and Alejandro F. Frangi[1,4]

[1] Center for Computational Imaging Simulation Technologies in Biomedicine
(CISTIB), The University of Sheffield, Sheffield, UK
h.fehri@sheffield.ac.uk
[2] Bateson Centre, University of Sheffield, Sheffield, UK
[3] Department of Infection, Immunity and Cardiovascular Disease, Medical School,
University of Sheffield, Sheffield, UK
[4] Department of Electronic and Electrical Engineering, Faculty of Engineering,
The University of Sheffield, Sheffield, UK

Abstract. Multi-class segmentation is a crucial step in cell image analysis. This process becomes challenging when little information is available for recognising cells from the background, due to their poor discriminative features. To alleviate this, directed acyclic graphs such as trees have been proposed to model top-down statistical dependencies as a prior for improved image segmentation. However, using trees, modelling the relations between labels of multiple classes becomes difficult. To overcome this limitation, we propose a polytree graphical model that captures label proximity relations more naturally compared to tree based approaches. A novel recursive mechanism based on two-pass message passing is developed to efficiently calculate closed form posteriors of graph nodes on the polytree. The algorithm is evaluated using simulated data, synthetic images and real fluorescence microscopy images. Our method achieves Dice scores of 94.5% and 98% on macrophage and seed classes, respectively, outperforming GMM based classifiers.

1 Introduction

Macrophages are cells that play vital roles within the immune system. They recognise invasions to body and combat their agents and are also involved in healing processes. Studying these cells in depth requires quantification of their behaviour in their interactions with other cells and proteins, which needs segmentation of cells in microscopy images. One instance of such studies is the segmentation of nuclear and surface areas of mice macrophages in fluorescence microscopy images [9], which defines a multi-class segmentation problem addressed here. The challenges are more highlighted when limited information is available for recognition of each area, due to the low quality of images and/or complexity of shapes. In these cases, quality of segmentation is subject to improvement by employing inter-object relations.

© Springer International Publishing AG 2017
M. Niethammer et al. (Eds.): IPMI 2017, LNCS 10265, pp. 517–528, 2017.
DOI: 10.1007/978-3-319-59050-9_41

Segmentation can be a primary step for cell, and in general, object count-ing. Although not directly considered in this paper, two categories of counting methods exist: first category recognises cells using detection based algorithms [6], while the other one estimates density based on regression [1]. Former approaches perform based on a prior segmentation or detection of individual cells, while the latter do not rely on individual object detection and rather take a holistic app-roach towards counting and have been proven to be more efficient. Inspired by the counting application outlined in [1], our segmentation method is capable of extracting the image foreground as the union of subregions having different labels. The segmented foreground can be further used for efficient recognition of individual cells and their nuclei through post processing steps.

Graphical models are tools for modelling associative relations between objects. The key aspect of these models is that the label of each node is deter-mined based on both its own attributes as well as attributes of other nodes con-nected to it through graph edges. This way, not only all the relevant information is incorporated in inferring the labels, but also label configuration constraints can be effectively projected on the model and be used during the inference. For instance, Chen et al. [5] employed graphical models to incorporate nuclear positions with boundary information for yeast cell segmentation. In a broader context of application, Uzunbas et al. [12] used an interactive graphical-model-based approach which seeks user's input for nodes with uncertain labels and learns from mislabelled nodes. Another instance is the use of graphical models for combining appearance models with shape priors for retinal segmentation [11].

Two types of graphical models have been used for image segmentation. Markov Random Fields have weighted edges indicating the degree of dependen-cies between variables. These models require iterative procedures for estimating the hidden random variables and are therefore computationally demanding [4] and only approximate solutions are achievable for them [7]. On the other hand, Bayesian Networks (BNs) have directed edges that show how random variables depend on each other. Laferte et al. [8] proposed an efficient posterior calcu-lation algorithm for nodes on a tree BN using message passing. Tree BNs are models in which there is only one route between any two nodes, and each node (except the root node) has exactly one parent node. Despite the efficiency of their proposed model, it lacks the ability to model complex multi-label config-uration constraints. More specifically, the tree model proposed in [8] is capable of modelling two-wise constraints between nodes and thus suitable for binary image segmentation. However, many applications, such as cell/nuclei segmenta-tion involve more complex constraints due to the presence of multiple classes.

In this paper, we introduce the application of polytree based BNs to image segmentation. Polytree BNs share features such as existence of a unique route between each two nodes on the graph with their tree relatives, however, each node in a polytree can have more than one parent. In comparison to tree graph-ical models, polytrees can model more complex label proximity relations on the graph (three-wise and more, based on the number of parent nodes) more nat-urally to achieve a potentially better image segmentation. This paper presents a tractable and efficient inference algorithm on BN polytrees for the first time.

The proposed algorithm calculates closed form posteriors through two successive bottom-up and top-down inference passes on the polytree. The method is evaluated by ancestral sampling on arbitrary graphs, and applied on synthetic and real microscopy images to segment macrophages and nuclei (seeds) from background. However, we anticipate that more general applications of polytrees using the proposed inference algorithm.

2 Method

Here, the procedure of using our proposed graphical model for image segmentation is presented. First, a polytree is generated for the image by grouping similar pixels and regarding them as nodes of the graph. Next, the parameters of the likelihood functions are trained and labels of the nodes are inferred. Finally, the segmented image is constructed based on the optimal labels on the graph.

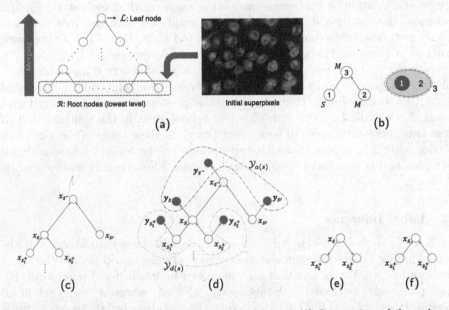

Fig. 1. Graph generation and inference on the polytree. (a) Generation of the polytree for the sample image. (b) Symbolic process of node merging for a synthetic macrophage with a seed. (c) Presenting the notation for nodes connected to an internal node s of the graph. (d) Graphical representation of ascendant, $\mathcal{Y}_{a(s)}$, and descendant, $\mathcal{Y}_{d(s)}$, observation nodes. Edge directions on cliques in conventional directed tree graphical models and the proposed polytree structure are shown in figures (e) and (f), respectively. (Color figure online)

2.1 Graph Generation

The graph is generated by firstly grouping pixels into locally coherent areas (superpixels), each representing a single root node (Fig. 1a). We use the SEEDS algorithm [2], which refines the initial grid of identically block shaped superpixels into more coherent ones. The two most similar superpixels are then recursively merged to generate nodes in higher levels of the hierarchical graph, as follows.

Firstly, for each superpixel at the finest level, one (root) node in the lowest level of the graph is created (see Fig. 1a). Each two nodes that achieve the highest score in a similarity metric are then merged to create a new node. The new node corresponds to the union of image regions attached to its two lower level descendant nodes. We define the similarity metric as a superposition of distances using spatial and intensity features of the superpixels. A vector β is introduced to adjust contributions of each of these features in the similarity metric. The choice of β is investigated in Sect. 3.3. After each merging step, the new node and all the other *orphan* nodes, are assessed with the similarity metric to recognise candidate nodes for the subsequent merging step. Region merging is continued until only two orphan nodes remain in the graph, which are eventually merged to create the leaf node that corresponds to the whole image (Fig. 1a). It is worth mentioning that since two nodes are merged at each step of graph evolution, the resulting structure is a binary graph; i.e. each non-root node has exactly two descendent nodes directly connected to it. We call this three-wise structure a *clique* and denote it by $parent1 - child - parent2$.

Once the graph is generated for the image, a set of observed and latent variables are assigned to nodes to define of the inference problem, which is presented in the next section. Figure 1b shows a symbolic process of merging for a cell with a seed. Nodes 1 and 2 align with blue and yellow areas in the synthetic cell. If these two nodes are chosen to be merged based on their value in the similarity metric, node 3 is generated which corresponds to the union of blue and yellow areas and is annotated by the dashed ellipse. This clique is represented by $1 - 3 - 2$.

2.2   Label Inference

Let $\mathbb{X} = \{x_s\}$ and $\mathbb{Y} = \{y_s\}$ denote sets of labels (latent variables) and the corresponding observed features at nodes, respectively, and $\mathcal{G}$ denote the set of nodes and edges. We assume that each node can be labelled as background (B), macrophage (M) or seed (S). Equivalently, $x_s \in \Lambda$, where Λ is the set of all possible labels, $\Lambda = \{B, M, S\}$. Following the notation of [8], for an internal node (neither in the lowest level nor the leaf node) s in the graph, s^-, s^+ and s' denote nodes in higher, lower and same layers, respectively (Fig. 1c).

Figure 1e shows the structure of a clique in conventional trees [8], where graph edges are oriented accordingly from the root node s to the leaves s_1^+, s_2^+. For this configuration, the joint probability factorises into probabilities of 1-1 child-parent constraints, as $p(\mathbb{X}) = p(x_{s_1^+}|x_s)p(x_{s_2^+}|x_s)p(x_s)$. The limitation of this structure is that constraints can only be enforced on individual child-parent connections. This factorisation implies that label of each node is dependant on the label of its parent node on the hierarchy. However, many applications such as multi-class cell segmentation require to enforce three-wise prior constraints to ensure the expected clique configurations occur in the model. For instance, in our case of three possible classes of B, M and S, we expect to see an M node having one M and one S parent nodes, as depicted in Fig. 1b. In the conventional structures, this prior knowledge is projected on the model through setting the probabilities $p(x_{s_i^+} = S | x_s = M)$ and $p(x_{s_i^+} = M | x_s = M)$ to non-zero values. However, enforcing the former constraint also makes $S - M - S$ cliques feasible, even though they are not acceptable based on the nature of the problem. This example shows the shortcoming of conventional directed tree models.

To overcome this limitation, we propose the use of another type of hierarchical graphical models with reverse edge orientations, as depicted in Fig. 1f, called *polytrees* [3]. In a polytree, each node at the lowest graph level (finest image resolution) is a root (in contrast to the single root node in conventional tree graphs) and there is only one leaf node (see Fig. 1a). This subtle yet *effective* change replaces 1-1 child-parent constraints with three-wise constraints on the cliques. The joint probability in this case is factorised as $p(\mathbb{X}) = p(x_s | x_{s_1^+}, x_{s_2^+}) p(x_{s_1^+}) p(x_{s_2^+})$, in which the term $p(x_s | x_{s_1^+}, x_{s_2^+})$ enforces the constraint on the clique. Using this configuration, the example structure of Fig. 1b requires setting the constraint $p(x_s = M | x_{s_1^+} = S, x_{s_2^+} = M)$ to be nonzero. However, in contrast to the previous structure, enforcing this constraint does not give rise to the emergence of physically infeasible clique structures.

We now derive equations governing the posterior probabilities of graph nodes. Given the observed data $\mathbb{Y}$, finding the best segmentation is equivalent to inferring the best configuration of labels $\mathbb{X}$ for the graph. Bayesian inference associates the most probable label from the set of possible labels Λ, given all observations:

$$\forall s \in \mathcal{G}, \hat{x}_s = \arg \max_{x_s \in \Lambda} p(x_s | \mathbb{Y}) \tag{1}$$

As the dependencies of nodes' labels have been revised in the proposed graph structure, a new set of equations are derived to calculate the closed-form posterior probabilities at each node. The inference algorithm on the polytree calculates the posteriors in two passes. These two consist of a pass from the leaf to the roots, (*top-down* pass), and from the roots to the leaf (*bottom-up* pass).

Probability of a node's label x_s, given all data $\mathbb{Y}$, is computed by marginalising the probability of the clique over two parent nodes s_1^+ and s_2^+ given $\mathbb{Y}$ and is called *joint posterior*.

$$p(x_s | \mathbb{Y}) = \sum_{x_{s_1^+}, x_{s_2^+}} p(x_s, x_{s_1^+}, x_{s_2^+} | \mathbb{Y}) \tag{2}$$

Here, three-wise constraints on cliques appear in the posterior calculation. Using the D-separation rule [10], the joint posterior is expanded as follows:

$$\begin{aligned} p(x_s, x_{s_1^+}, x_{s_2^+} | \mathbb{Y}) &= p(x_s | x_{s_1^+}, x_{s_2^+}, \mathbb{Y}) p(x_{s_1^+}, x_{s_2^+} | \mathbb{Y}) \\ &= p(x_s | x_{s_1^+}, x_{s_2^+}, \mathcal{Y}_{a(s)}) p(x_{s_1^+}, x_{s_2^+} | \mathcal{Y}_{a(s_1^+, s_2^+)}, \mathcal{Y}_{d(s_1^+, s_2^+)}) \end{aligned} \tag{3}$$

where $\mathcal{Y}_{a(.)}$ and $\mathcal{Y}_{d(.)}$ refer to the set of observation nodes of the ascendant and descendant nodes, respectively. For each node s (or a set of nodes $\mathcal{S}$) ascendant nodes refer to the set of all nodes that are connected to s ($\mathcal{S}$) through edges with inward directions. Similarly, descendant nodes include the nodes that are connected to node s ($\mathcal{S}$) through outward oriented graph edges. The union of ascendant and descendant observation nodes constructs the set of all observations (see Fig. 1d for a graphical explanation).

We first elaborate the term $p(x_s|x_{s_1^+}, x_{s_2^+}, \mathcal{Y}_{a(s)})$ on the right-hand side of Eq. 3. This term enforces posteriors of infeasible configurations to zero, as it is a product of the joint probability of a child node and its two parent nodes.

$$p(x_s|x_{s_1^+}, x_{s_2^+}, \mathcal{Y}_{a(s)}) = \frac{p(x_s, x_{s_1^+}, x_{s_2^+}|\mathcal{Y}_{a(s)})}{\sum_{x'_s} p(x'_s, x_{s_1^+}, x_{s_2^+}|\mathcal{Y}_{a(s)})} \tag{4}$$

Using D-separation rule, the nominator becomes:

$$\begin{aligned} p(x_s, x_{s_1^+}, x_{s_2^+}|\mathcal{Y}_{a(s)}) &= p(x_{s_1^+}, x_{s_2^+}|x_s)p(x_s|\mathcal{Y}_{a(s)}) \\ &= \frac{p(x_s, x_{s_1^+}, x_{s_2^+})}{p(x_s)} p(x_s|\mathcal{Y}_{a(s)}). \end{aligned} \tag{5}$$

Term $p(x_s, x_{s_1^+}, x_{s_2^+})$ in Eq. 5 controls the occurrence of feasible and infeasible configurations on the graph, by being set to zero and nonzero values for them, respectively. Term $p(x_s|\mathcal{Y}_{a(s)})$ in Eq. 5 is the posterior of node s having given observations of all its ascendant nodes as well as its own observation. This *top-down posterior* is expanded as:

$$p(x_s|\mathcal{Y}_{a(s)}) \propto \sum_{x_{s^-}, x_{s'}} p(\boldsymbol{y}_s|x_s)p(\boldsymbol{y}_{s'}|x_{s'})p(x_{s'}|\mathcal{Y}_{d(s')})\frac{p(x_s, x_{s'}, x_{s^-})}{p(x_{s^-})p(x_{s'})}p(x_{s^-}|\mathcal{Y}_{a(s^-)}) \tag{6}$$

Equation 6 indicates that having calculated the likelihood probabilities $p(\boldsymbol{y}_s|x_s)$ and $p(\boldsymbol{y}_{s'}|x_{s'})$ and the posterior $p(x_{s'}|\mathcal{Y}_{d(s')})$, the top-down posterior of node s is calculated based on top-down posterior of node s^-. This implies that a top-down recursion calculates the top-down posteriors for all nodes.

On the other hand, term $p(x_{s_1^+}, x_{s_2^+}|\mathcal{Y}_{a(s_1^+, s_2^+)}, \mathcal{Y}_{d(s_1^+, s_2^+)})$ on the right-hand side of Eq. 3 is factorised by several usages of D-separation rule. This factorisation separates parts that are calculated from ascendant and descendant nodes.

$$\begin{aligned} p(x_{s_1^+}, x_{s_2^+}|\mathcal{Y}_{a(s_1^+, s_2^+)}, \mathcal{Y}_{d(s_1^+, s_2^+)}) &\propto p(\mathcal{Y}_{a(s_1^+, s_2^+)}, \mathcal{Y}_{d(s_1^+, s_2^+)}|x_{s_1^+}, x_{s_2^+})p(x_{s_1^+}, x_{s_2^+}) \\ &= p(\mathcal{Y}_{a(s_1^+, s_2^+)}|x_{s_1^+}, x_{s_2^+})p(\mathcal{Y}_{d(s_1^+, s_2^+)}|x_{s_1^+}, x_{s_2^+})p(x_{s_1^+}, x_{s_2^+}) \\ &= p(\mathcal{Y}_{a(s_1^+, s_2^+)}|x_{s_1^+}, x_{s_2^+})p(\mathcal{Y}_{d(s_1^+)}|x_{s_1^+})p(\mathcal{Y}_{d(s_2^+)}|x_{s_2^+})p(x_{s_1^+}, x_{s_2^+}) \\ &\propto p(x_{s_1^+}, x_{s_2^+}|\mathcal{Y}_{a(s_1^+, s_2^+)})\frac{p(x_{s_1^+}|\mathcal{Y}_{d(s_1^+)})}{p(x_{s_1^+})}\frac{p(x_{s_2^+}|\mathcal{Y}_{d(s_2^+)})}{p(x_{s_2^+})} \end{aligned} \tag{7}$$

Similar to Eq. 6, term $p(x_{s_1^+}, x_{s_2^+}|\mathcal{Y}_{a(s_1^+, s_2^+)})$ on the right-hand side of Eq. 7 is calculated through a top-down recursion as below.

$$p(x_{s_1^+}, x_{s_2^+}|\mathcal{Y}_{a(s_1^+, s_2^+)}) \propto \sum_{x_s} p(\boldsymbol{y}_{s_1^+}|x_{s_1^+})p(\boldsymbol{y}_{s_2^+}|x_{s_2^+})p(x_{s_1^+}, x_{s_2^+}|x_s)p(x_s|\mathcal{Y}_{a(s)}) \tag{8}$$

Using a definition similar to that of top-down posterior, terms $p(x_{s_1^+}|\mathcal{Y}_{d(s_1^+)})$ and $p(x_{s_2^+}|\mathcal{Y}_{d(s_2^+)})$ in Eq. 7 are called *bottom-up* posteriors as they are calculated based on posteriors of their descendant nodes. For each node s in the graph, the bottom-up posterior is written as

$$p(x_s|\mathcal{Y}_{d(s)}) \propto \sum_{x_{s_1^+}, x_{s_2^+}} p(\boldsymbol{y}_{s_1^+}|x_{s_1^+})p(\boldsymbol{y}_{s_2^+}|x_{s_2^+})$$
$$p(x_{s_1^+}|\mathcal{Y}_{d(s_1^+)})p(x_{s_2^+}|\mathcal{Y}_{d(s_2^+)})p(x_s|x_{s_1^+}, x_{s_2^+}) \tag{9}$$

Derivations of Eqs. 6, 8 and 9 are not included due to the shortage of space.

Making use of Eqs. 3, 4, 5 and 7 the node's posterior in Eq. 2 given all the observations is written as follows.

$$p(x_s|\mathbb{Y}) \propto \sum_{x_{s_1^+}, x_{s_2^+}} \frac{p(x_s, x_{s_1^+}, x_{s_2^+}|\mathcal{Y}_{a(s)})}{\sum_{x'_s} p(x'_s, x_{s_1^+}, x_{s_2^+}|\mathcal{Y}_{a(s)})}$$
$$p(x_{s_1^+}, x_{s_2^+}|\mathcal{Y}_{a(s_1^+, s_2^+)}) \frac{p(x_{s_1^+}|\mathcal{Y}_{d(s_1^+)})}{p(x_{s_1^+})} \frac{p(x_{s_2^+}|\mathcal{Y}_{d(s_2^+)})}{p(x_{s_2^+})} \tag{10}$$

Equation 10 calculates the posterior at each node s using three marginal posteriors $p(x_s, x_{s_1^+}, x_{s_2^+}|\mathcal{Y}_{a(s)})$, $p(x_{s_1^+}, x_{s_2^+}|\mathcal{Y}_{a(s_1^+, s_2^+)})$ and $p(x_s|\mathcal{Y}_{d(s)})$, in Eqs. 5, 8 and 9. Each of these terms are calculated through either top-down or bottom-up recursions. The inference is summarised in Algorithm 1. Note that $\mathcal{R}$ and $\mathcal{L}$ denote the set of root nodes and the leaf node in the graph, respectively.

3 Results

3.1 Validation of the Inference Algorithm in a Two-Class Labelling Problem

To assess the performance of the core inference algorithm, regardless of the problem it is applied to, ancestral sampling was used [3]. This technique, which is applied to generative models, mimics the creation of the observed data by generating sets of *fantasy* data. In this case, the model is a perfect representation of the observed data. Using the generated fantasy data as the observed data and comparing the inferred labels with the sampled values gives a measure for the method performance.

Consider we aim to draw a sample $\hat{x}_1, \hat{x}_2, \ldots, \hat{x}_N$ from the joint distribution $p(\mathbb{X}, \mathbb{Y})$. The graph consists of N nodes and x_N denotes the only leaf node in the graph. To draw this sample, we start from the root nodes by taking samples $\hat{x}_s$ from the probability distribution $p(x_s)\big|_{s \in \mathcal{R}}$ for all root nodes. Visiting the internal nodes in an upward recursion, we draw a sample $\hat{x}_s$ from the conditional distribution $p(x_s|x_{s_1^+}, x_{s_2^+})$, for which the parent labels $x_{s_1^+}$ and $x_{s_2^+}$ have been sampled in the previous stages. Once we have sampled from the leaf node of the graph, x_N, we will have obtained a sample from the joint distribution $p(\mathbb{X}, \mathbb{Y})$.

Algorithm 1. Label inference on polytree directed graphical model

---

☐ **Preliminary pass.** This initial upward recursion computes prior marginals for each node. $p(x_s | x_{s_1^+}, x_{s_2^+})$ are parameters set based on the nature of problem the model is representing.

for all $s \in \mathcal{R}$ **do**

$\quad p(x_s) = \frac{1}{|A|}$

end for

for all $s \notin \mathcal{R}$ **do**

$\quad p(x_s) = \sum_{x_{s_1^+}, x_{s_1^+}} p(x_s | x_{s_1^+}, x_{s_2^+}) p(x_{s_1^+}) p(x_{s_2^+})$

$\quad p(x_{s_1^+}, x_{s_2^+} | x_s) = \frac{p(x_s | x_{s_1^+}, x_{s_2^+}) p(x_{s_1^+}) p(x_{s_2^+})}{p(x_s)}$

end for

△ **Bottom-up pass.** Upward recursion for calculating bottom-up posteriors of nodes.

for all $s \in \mathcal{R}$ **do**

$\quad p(x_s | \mathcal{Y}_{d(s)}) = p(x_s)$

end for

for all $s \notin \mathcal{R}$ **do**

$\quad p(x_s | \mathcal{Y}_{d(s)}) \propto \sum_{x_{s_1^+}, x_{s_2^+}} p(\boldsymbol{y}_{s_1^+} | x_{s_1^+}) p(\boldsymbol{y}_{s_2^+} | x_{s_2^+}) p(x_{s_1^+} | \mathcal{Y}_{d(s_1^+)}) p(x_{s_2^+} | \mathcal{Y}_{d(s_2^+)}) p(x_s | x_{s_1^+}, x_{s_2^+})$

end for

▽ **Top-down pass.** Downward recursion for calculating top-down posteriors and calculation of complete posteriors from marginal posteriors.

if $s = \mathcal{L}$ **then**

$\quad p(x_s | \mathcal{Y}_{a(s)}) = p(x_s | \boldsymbol{y}_s) \propto p(\boldsymbol{y}_s | x_s) p(x_s)$

end if

for all $s \neq \mathcal{L}$ **do**

$\quad p(x_s | \mathcal{Y}_{a(s)}) \propto \sum_{x_{s_-}, x_{s'}} p(\boldsymbol{y}_s | x_s) p(\boldsymbol{y}_{s'} | x_{s'}) p(x_{s'} | \mathcal{Y}_{d(s')}) \frac{p(x_s, x_{s'} | x_{s_-})}{p(x_{s'})} p(x_{s_-} | \mathcal{Y}_{a(s_-)})$

$\quad p(x_s, x_{s_1^+}, x_{s_2^+} | \mathcal{Y}_{a(s)}) = p(x_{s_1^+}, x_{s_2^+} | x_s) p(x_s | \mathcal{Y}_{a(s)})$

$\quad p(x_{s_1^+}, x_{s_2^+} | \mathcal{Y}_{a(s_1^+, s_2^+)}) \propto \sum_{x_s} p(\boldsymbol{y}_{s_1^+} | x_{s_1^+}) p(\boldsymbol{y}_{s_2^+} | x_{s_2^+}) p(x_{s_1^+}, x_{s_2^+} | x_s) p(x_s | \mathcal{Y}_{a(s)})$

end for

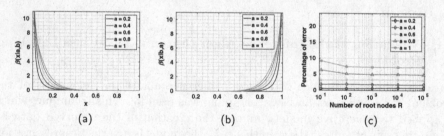

(a)   (b)   (c)

Fig. 2. Likelihood distribution functions and their effect on ancestral sampling inference accuracy. (a) and (b) show β distributions chosen as class-conditional likelihood functions in the ancestral sampling. b value was fixed and curves correspond to values of a from 0.2 to 1. (c) Percentage of wrongly inferred labels using ancestral sampling.

In this section only, we considered two classes for latent variables x_s and selecting y_s from the continuous range $[0, 1]$ and beta distributions were used as class conditional likelihood functions, $p(y_s | x_s)$. Labels done for different numbers of root nodes ranging from 10 to 100000 (leading to 19 to 199999 nodes in total as the graph is binary) and for different selectivities of the likelihood functions, controlled by parameters of β distributions. Figure 2a and b show beta distributions for different values of parameter a. Figure 2c depicts percentage of nodes with wrongly inferred labels for different numbers of nodes in the graph and for different beta distributions. This experiment verifies the correctness of the developed derivations and also indicates that more selective likelihood distribution functions result in higher inference accuracies. The best accuracy was achieved for $a = 0.2$ with the average error of 0.30%.

3.2   Validation of the Algorithm on a Synthetic Image

The method was evaluated on a synthetic image containing two types of objects. A multi-scale first and second order derivative based invariant features have been utilized here. The segmentation results were compared to those of using Gaussian Mixture Models (GMMs). Yellow and blue areas in the synthetic image represent macrophages and seeds, respectively (chosen to be similar to the real image dataset). At each node, median of intensity across the superpixel was utilised as feature. Random noise was added to these features. Random noise was added to feature values of each node, which were median of node's intensity.

Segmentation was done for different noise levels added to the synthetic image. Figure 3 shows the synthetic image and its segmentation results for four cases of 0%, 30%, 60% and 65% of noise amplitudes, in each row, respectively. First column depicts the input image and second and third columns show results of segmentation for GMM and the proposed method, respectively. Dice scores of segmentations for GMM and the proposed method are shown in Fig. 4a. It can be seen that the proposed algorithm is more robust to intensive additive noise compared to GMM.

3.3   Applying the Method to Multi-class Cell Segmentation

We applied the proposed method to the image set BBBC020 from the Broad Bioimage Benchmark Collection [9] including 20 two-channel fluorescent microscopy images with ground truth annotations and compared the results with GMM. Multi-scale first and second derivatives of the image were calculated and a 10-dimensional feature vector y_s containing median of feature values over the node's region was created for each node s. Class-conditional distribution functions were considered to be Gaussian and their parameters were trained by feeding the algorithm with a few samples of manually segmented cells. Figure 5 shows three samples from the image dataset (first column) that were segmented using GMM classifier (second column) and the proposed method (third column). Dice scores of using the two methods on the dataset of real images are depicted in Fig. 4b. Segmentation results and the Dice scores indicate that the proposed method segments the images more accurately, which is due to considering semantically meaningful relationships between labels of nodes.

In graph generation, the β vector, used for similarity metric, consists of uniform weights (set as one) over intensity and β weighted spatial features (barycenters of the superpixels). To select a suitable value for β, we run a 5-fold

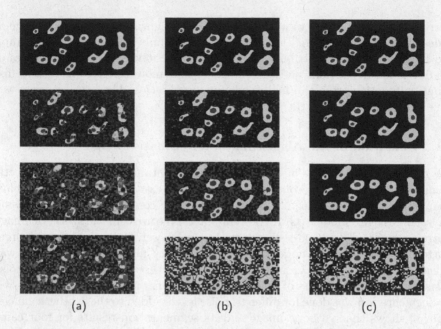

Fig. 3. Segmentation of the synthetic image for different random noise levels using GMM and the proposed method. Rows of column (a) correspond to images, with 0%, 30%, 60% and 65% (of maximum image intensity levels), respectively. (b) and (c) show results of segmentation using GMM and the proposed method for the input images of the first column, respectively. Last row illustrates the case where the proposed method cannot handle the added noise. (Color figure online)

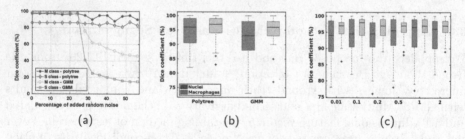

Fig. 4. Dice accuracies of segmentation for the proposed method and Gaussian Mixture Model (GMM). (a) Dice score for segmentation of two classes of objects, M and S, for the proposed method and GMM for different amounts of random noise added to the synthetic image. The proposed method shows more robustness to noise. (b) Accuracy of segmenting bone-marrow macrophages dataset for macrophage surface and the seeds for the proposed method and GMM. (c) Effect of β vector used in graph generation on segmentation accuracy. Horizontal axis shows the ratio of weights of intensity features to those of spatial features.

crossvalidation experiment where we learn the Gaussian likelihoods from training sets and measure the Dice score on the test set. Figure 4c shows how the choice of this parameter affects segmentation results. Based on this, we chose $\beta = 0.1$.

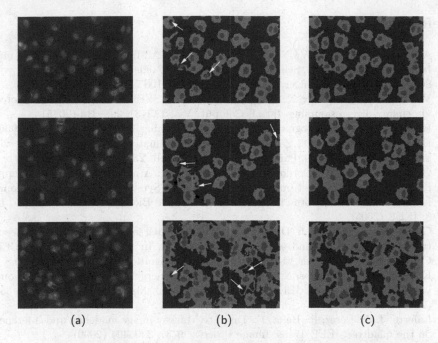

Fig. 5. Segmentation results for 3 samples from the image dataset. Column (a) shows real image samples. Columns (b) and (c) show segmentation results for GMM and the proposed method, respectively. Red arrows point to areas of the cell or the seeds that were not recognised by GMM, while the proposed algorithm segmented them correctly. (Color figure online)

4   Conclusion

We proposed polytree based directed graphical models for multi-class cell segmentation. A non-iterative algorithm was derived for inferring labels of nodes on polytree that calculates closed form posteriors through two successive bottom-up and top-down recursions. The derived recursive inference algorithm is novel and contributes to the state-of-the-art from methodological perspective. The method was evaluated by ancestral sampling on the graph level, in addition to segmentation of cell surfaces and seeds in synthetic and real microscopy images. This study was focused on the application of the proposed method to image segmentation and three-wise constraints. However, the designed formulation can be straightforwardly used for more complex applications where more complicated constraints are required to be projected on the model.

Acknowledgments. This work was supported by MRC fellowship (MR/J009156/1) and the Krebs Institute fellowship. Alejandro F. Frangi is partially funded by BBSRC through grant BB/M01021X/1.

References

1. Arteta, C., Lempitsky, V., Noble, J.A., Zisserman, A.: Interactive object counting. In: Fleet, D., Pajdla, T., Schiele, B., Tuytelaars, T. (eds.) ECCV 2014. LNCS, vol. 8691, pp. 504–518. Springer, Cham (2014). doi:10.1007/978-3-319-10578-9_33
2. Van den Bergh, M., Boix, X., Roig, G., Van Gool, L.: SEEDS: superpixels extracted via energy-driven sampling. Int. J. Comput. Vis. 111(3), 298–314 (2015)
3. Bishop, C.: Pattern Recognition and Machine Learning. Springer, New York (2006)
4. Boykov, Y., Veksler, O., Zabih, R.: Fast approximate energy minimization via graph cuts. IEEE Trans. Pattern Anal. Mach. Intell. 23(11), 1222–1239 (2001)
5. Chen, S.C., Zhao, T., Gordon, G.J., Murphy, R.F.: A novel graphical model approach to segmenting cell images. In: 2006 IEEE Symposium on Computational Intelligence and Bioinformatics and Computational Biology, CIBCB 2006, pp. 1–8. IEEE (2006)
6. Girshick, R., Donahue, J., Darrell, T., Malik, J.: Rich feature hierarchies for accurate object detection and semantic segmentation. In: Proceedings of the IEEE Conference on Computer Vision and Pattern Recognition, pp. 580–587 (2014)
7. Komodakis, N., Paragios, N., Tziritas, G.: MRF energy minimization and beyond via dual decomposition. IEEE Trans. Pattern Anal. Mach. Intell. 33(3), 531–552 (2011)
8. Laferté, J.M., Pérez, P., Heitz, F.: Discrete Markov image modeling and inference on the quadtree. IEEE Trans. Image Process. 9(3), 390–404 (2000)
9. Ljosa, V., Sokolnicki, K.L., Carpenter, A.E.: Annotated high-throughput microscopy image sets for validation. Nat. Methods 9(7), 637 (2012)
10. Pearl, J.: Probabilistic Reasoning in Intelligent Systems: Networks of Plausible Inference. Morgan Kaufmann, Burlington (2014)
11. Rathke, F., Schmidt, S., Schnörr, C.: Probabilistic intra-retinal layer segmentation in 3-D OCT images using global shape regularization. Med. Image Anal. 18(5), 781–794 (2014)
12. Uzunbas, M.G., Chen, C., Metaxas, D.: An efficient conditional random field approach for automatic and interactive neuron segmentation. Med. Image Anal. 27, 31–44 (2016)

Direct Estimation of Spinal Cobb Angles by Structured Multi-output Regression

Haoliang Sun[1,2], Xiantong Zhen[2], Chris Bailey[3], Parham Rasoulinejad[3], Yilong Yin[1(✉)], and Shuo Li[2]

[1] Shandong University, Jinan, China
ylyin@sdu.edu.cn
[2] The University of Western Ontario, London, ON, Canada
[3] London Health Sciences Center, London, ON, Canada

Abstract. The Cobb angle that quantitatively evaluates the spinal curvature plays an important role in the scoliosis diagnosis and treatment. Conventional measurement of these angles suffers from huge variability and low reliability due to intensive manual intervention. However, since there exist high ambiguity and variability around boundaries of vertebrae, it is challenging to obtain Cobb angles automatically. In this paper, we formulate the estimation of the Cobb angles from spinal X-rays as a multi-output regression task. We propose structured support vector regression (S^2VR) to jointly estimate Cobb angles and landmarks of the spine in X-rays in one single framework. The proposed S^2VR can faithfully handle the nonlinear relationship between input images and quantitative outputs, while explicitly capturing the intrinsic correlation of outputs. We introduce the manifold regularization to exploit the geometry of the output space. We propose learning the kernel in S^2VR by kernel alignment to enhance its discriminative ability. The proposed method is evaluated on the spinal X-rays dataset of 439 scoliosis subjects, which achieves the inspiring correlation coefficient of 92.76% with ground truth obtained manually by human experts and outperforms two baseline methods. Our method achieves the direct estimation of Cobb angles with high accuracy, indicating its great potential in clinical use.

1 Introduction

Cobb angles are widely used for scoliosis diagnosis and treatment decisions in clinical routine. Scoliosis is a structural, lateral, rotated curvature of the spine, which especially arises in children at or around puberty and leads to disability [1]. For clinical examination of scoliosis, the radiography (X-ray) is the most common imaging technique with the cheap acquisition and less time cost [2]. Cobb angles (Fig. 1(a)) derived from a posteroanterior (back to front) X-ray and manually measured by selecting the most tilted vertebra at the top and bottom of the spine respect to the horizontal line are faithfully used to quantify the magnitude of spinal deformities [3].

However, conventional manual measurement involves the heavy intervention of identifying the vertebrae and measuring angles, it suffers from huge variability

© Springer International Publishing AG 2017
M. Niethammer et al. (Eds.): IPMI 2017, LNCS 10265, pp. 529–540, 2017.
DOI: 10.1007/978-3-319-59050-9_42

and high unreliability while being labor-intensive. The accuracy of measurement is affected by many factors, such as the selection of vertebrae, the bias of different observers and inaccurate protractors.

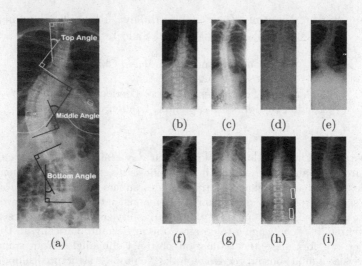

Fig. 1. It is challenging to measure three Cobb angles in (a) due to high ambiguity and variability in scoliosis X-rays from different subjects (a)–(i).

It is challenging to estimate Cobb angles automatically due to the high ambiguity and variability of X-rays. As shown in Fig. 1, large anatomical variability and low tissue contrast can lead to the complexity of identification of interesting vertebrae and further measurement. Active contour model [4], customized filter [5] and charged-particle model [6] were used for localizing vertebrae. Angles are computed from the slope of these vertebrae. Although these methods can derive the Cobb angles automatically, they suffer from the complexity of multiple processing stages, which is computationally expensive. Moreover, segmentation for multiple objects of all vertebrae is extremely challenging, especially in spinal X-rays with variant structures and ambiguous boundaries.

Without filtering or segmentation, direct estimation methods [7–11] based on statistical learning, which achieves the great success of large-scale image data recently, have the potential for Cobb angles estimation. Compared with conventional segmentation methods, such as variational models [12], direct estimation methods characterize the relationship between the appearance of images and high-level semantic concepts via supervised learning, which enables efficient computation and compact structure modeling. By exploring data statistics, direct methods are robust and can handle fuzzy boundaries and region heterogeneity.

The estimation of the Cobb angles can benefit from the prediction of coordinates of landmarks. Due to the ambiguity and variability of spinal images, it is challenging to obtain the angles separately. Intuitively, the Cobb angles closely correspond to the spinal shape which can be substantially characterized by landmarks. In this paper, we train the model by minimizing the loss with respect to both the Cobb angles and all coordinates of landmarks simultaneously, which demonstrates the robustness of our method. In contrast to existing direct methods [7–10], the proposed method jointly estimates landmarks and Cobb angles, which not only improves the prediction accuracy but also provides an intuitive validation of angle estimation for the radiologist.

Although existing direct methods achieved great success, their direct application to our task suffers from three major limitations. First, these methods fail to explicitly characterize the correlations among outputs, which is essential for discriminative learning. Second, they neglect the intrinsic geometry of the distribution of output values, which would result in the non-smooth solution and then has a negative effect on the angle estimation. Third, the kernel parameters, e.g., the bandwidth, are usually set manually, which does not guarantee to be optimal for different applications.

In this paper, we propose structured support vector regression (S^2VR) to directly predict the Cobb angles and landmarks of a spine from its X-ray. In comparison to conventional support vector regression (SVR), the S^2VR accomplishes of nonlinear mapping and explicit correlation modeling in one single framework. In particular, the nonlinear mapping handles the relationship between input images and high-level outputs (angles and landmarks), while the explicit correlation modeling captures the correlations among outputs.

In summary, our work contributes to the following aspects:

- We achieve the jointly automatic estimation of Cobb angles and spinal landmarks by multi-output regression, which is essential for the evaluation of spinal curvature from radiography directly.
- We propose a novel multi-output regression model called S^2VR, which can simultaneously handle the nonlinear input-output relationship and intrinsic inter-output correlation. The framework is endowed with great generality which enables wide applications for other measurement estimation.
- We introduce a manifold regularizer into the framework by exploring the geometry structure of the output space, which enables smooth solutions.
- To improve the performance, we propose to learn the kernels by using kernel target alignment, which increase the discriminative ability of the kernels.

2 Methodology

The proposed structured support vector regression (S^2VR) directly estimates the Cobb angles and coordinates of landmarks by formulating the prediction as a multi-output regression task. S^2VR consists of nonlinear mapping process and explicit correlation learning stage. The manifold regularization is introduced to explore the intrinsic geometry of the output space. Since our method is built on support vector regression, we learn the kernel based on kernel target alignment.

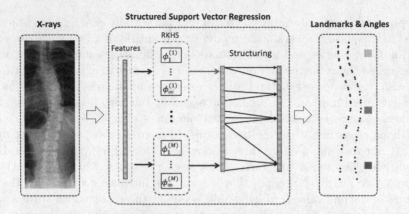

Fig. 2. The framework of the structured support vector regression (S^2VR).

2.1 Structured Support Vector Regression

Within the proposed S^2VR, we extract image features of a X-ray that denoted as $\mathbf{x}_i \in \mathbb{R}^d$. The coordinates and angles are represented by $\mathbf{y}_i \in \mathbb{R}^q$ and $\mathbf{y}_i = [h_1, \ldots, h_c, v_1, \ldots v_c, a_1, a_2, a_3]$, c is the number of landmarks, h_i and v_i are the horizontal and vertical axises of i-th landmark point. In addition, the number of Cobb angles is 3, thus, $q = 2c + 3$. The regression task is to predict the coordinates and the Cobb angles from the input features. The framework of S^2VR is illustrated in Fig. 2.

SVR for Nonlinear Input-Output Relationship Learning. Support vector regression (SVR) has been widely used to handle complex nonlinear relationships. Its effectiveness is guaranteed by the sparseness of solutions. The SVR model takes the following optimization formulation:

$$\arg \min L(W, \mathbf{b}) = \frac{1}{2}\|W\|^2 + \tau \sum_{i=1}^{N} \nu(u_i) \qquad (1)$$

where

$$\nu(u_i) = \begin{cases} 0 & u_i < \varepsilon \\ (u_i - \varepsilon)^2 & u_i \geq \varepsilon \end{cases}, \qquad (2)$$

$u_i = \|\mathbf{y}_i - f_p(\mathbf{x}_i)\|^2$, $f_p(\mathbf{x}_i) = W\phi(\mathbf{x}_i) + \mathbf{b}$, $\|\cdot\|$ is ℓ^2-norm, $\phi : \mathbb{R}^d \to \mathbb{R}^H$ is a nonlinear transformation to a higher H-dimensional space, $W \in \mathbb{R}^{q \times H}$, $\mathbf{b} \in \mathbb{R}^q$, $\phi(\mathbf{x}_i) \in \mathbb{R}^H$, $\mathbf{y}_i \in \mathbb{R}^q$, τ and N denote a positive constant of the tuning parameter and the number of training samples, respectively.

S^2VR for Explicit Inter-output Correlation Learning. We introduce a structure matrix $S, S \in \mathbb{R}^{q \times q}$ to capture the intrinsic correlations of outputs (angles and landmarks). The prediction model becomes $f(\mathbf{x}_i) = S(W\phi(\mathbf{x}_i) + \mathbf{b})$ and the S^2VR model can be defined as:

$$L(W, \mathbf{b}, S) = \frac{1}{2}\|W\|^2 + \tau \sum_{i=1}^{N} \nu(u_i) + \lambda \|S^\top\|_{2,1}, \tag{3}$$

where $u_i = \|\mathbf{y}_i - f(\mathbf{x}_i)\|$, $\|S\|_{2,1} = \sum_{i=1}^{q} \sqrt{\sum_{j=1}^{q} S_{ij}^2}$ and λ is the tuning parameter.

Advantages: The appealing property of structure matrix S via $\ell_{2,1}$-norm regularization is to encourage multiple outputs to share the similar sparsity patterns of parameters. Therefore, the structure, such as spatial correlations which share similar specific patterns, can be captured for the robust prediction of angles and coordinates.

Manifold Regularization for S^2VR. To further improve the performance of the proposed algorithm, we consider incorporating a manifold regularization [13] term based on a graph Laplacian to model the local geometrical structure of the output space. It has been shown that learning performance can be significantly enhanced if the geometrical structure is exploited and the local invariance is considered.

We adopt the loss function with the additional regularization as:

$$L(W, \mathbf{b}, S) = \frac{1}{2}\|W\|^2 + \frac{\gamma}{2}\mathrm{Tr}(FGF^\top) + \tau \sum_{i=1}^{n} \nu(u_i) + \lambda \|S^\top\|_{2,1}, \tag{4}$$

where $G \in \mathbb{R}^{N \times N}$ is the graph Laplacian matrix [14] and $F = [f(\mathbf{x}_1), \ldots, f(\mathbf{x}_N)]^\top$.

Here we select the unnormalized graph Laplacian matrix given by $G = \hat{D} - E$ to represent the labels $\mathbf{y}_i|_{i=1:N}$ of data in form of the similarity graph. We simply connect all points with positive similarity with each other, and we weight all edges by E_{ij}. The similarity function is the Gaussian function $E_{ij} = \exp(-\|\mathbf{y}_i - \mathbf{y}_j\|^2/(2\rho^2))$, where the parameter ρ is the width of the function. $\hat{D}$ is the diagonal matrix given by $\hat{D}_{ii} = \sum_{j=1}^{N} E_{ij}$.

Advantages: The manifold regularization exploits the geometry of the distribution of output data. In particular, due to the high ambiguity and variability of image appearance, distributions of input features and output angles (landmarks) could be inconsistent in estimation. Therefore, by leveraging the strength of manifold regularization, we ensure the smoothness of solution with respect to the output space.

2.2   Kernelization

Since the relationship between inputs of image features and outputs of angles (landmarks) is complex and highly nonlinear, we kernelize the (4) to conduct nonlinear regression.

Kernel S^{2}VR. Before kernelizaiton, we rewrite (4) in term of traces:

$$L(W, \mathbf{b}, S) = \frac{1}{2} \mathrm{Tr}(W^\top W) + \frac{\gamma}{2} \mathrm{Tr}(FGF^\top) + \tau \, \mathrm{Tr}(UE^\top E) + \lambda \|S^\top\|_{2,1}, \quad (5)$$

where $E = [\mathbf{e}_1, \ldots, \mathbf{e}_N]$, $\mathbf{e}_i = \mathbf{y}_i - S(W\phi(\mathbf{x}_i)) + \mathbf{b})$, and U is the diagonal matrix given by

$$U_{ii} = \begin{cases} 0 & u_i < \varepsilon \\ 1 & u_i \geq \varepsilon \end{cases}. \quad (6)$$

Assume that the mapping function $\phi(\mathbf{x}_i)$ is in some RKHS of infinite dimensionality. According to the Representer Theorem [15], $W = \boldsymbol{\beta}\boldsymbol{\Phi}^\top(X)$, where $\boldsymbol{\beta} \in \mathbb{R}^{q \times N}$ and $X = [\mathbf{x}_1, \ldots, \mathbf{x}_N]$. The kernel matrix is defined as $K = \boldsymbol{\Phi}^\top(X)\boldsymbol{\Phi}(X)$. We rewrite (5) with the kernel version:

$$Q(\boldsymbol{\beta}, S) = \frac{1}{2} \mathrm{Tr}(\boldsymbol{\beta}K\boldsymbol{\beta}^\top) + \frac{\gamma}{2} \mathrm{Tr}(S\boldsymbol{\beta}KGK\boldsymbol{\beta}^\top S^\top) + \frac{1}{2} \mathrm{Tr}(UE^\top E) + \lambda \|S^\top\|_{2,1}, \quad (7)$$

where

$$E = Y - S\boldsymbol{\beta}K. \quad (8)$$

Discriminant Kernel Learning. We focus on learning a cone combination of given base kernels $K_z|_{z=1:Z}$ to obtain an efficient kernel. Therefore, for the summation formulation of $K = \sum_{z=1}^{Z} \mu_z K_z$, we propose learning the weight coefficients $\boldsymbol{\mu}$ associated with basic kernels by kernel alignment, which has shown great effectiveness in learning the optimal combination of multiple kernels [16, 17].

Kernel alignment is proposed to align an input kernel K to a target kernel K_T by maximizing the similarity between them, which offers a best-suited way to obtain the weight coefficients $\boldsymbol{\mu}$. We now introduce the kernel alignment formulation to learn the kernel in S^{2}VR. We would like to maximize the alignment $A(K_{\boldsymbol{\mu}}, K_T)$ between the target kernel matrix K_T and the kernel $K_{\boldsymbol{\mu}}$. The optimization problem can be formulated as

$$\boldsymbol{\mu}^* = \arg\max A(K_{\boldsymbol{\mu}}, K_T) = \arg\max \frac{\mathrm{Tr}(K_{\boldsymbol{\mu}}K_T)}{\sqrt{\mathrm{Tr}(K_T K_T)\,\mathrm{Tr}(K_{\boldsymbol{\mu}}K_{\boldsymbol{\mu}})}}. \quad (9)$$

The target kernel matrix K_T is constructed by defining the target kernel $K_T = Y^\top Y$, where $Y = [\mathbf{y}_1, \ldots, \mathbf{y}_N]$.

The objective function in (9) can be equivalently rewritten as follows:

$$\boldsymbol{\mu}^* = \arg\max_{\|\boldsymbol{\mu}\|=1, \boldsymbol{\mu} \geq 0} \frac{\boldsymbol{\mu}^\top \boldsymbol{\alpha}\boldsymbol{\alpha}^\top \boldsymbol{\mu}}{\boldsymbol{\mu}^\top V \boldsymbol{\mu}} \quad (10)$$

where $\|\boldsymbol{\mu}\| = 1$ is a regularization term, $\boldsymbol{\mu} \geq 0$ guarantees the positive definiteness, for $i, j \in \{1, \cdots, Z\}$, $\boldsymbol{\alpha}$ is defined by $\alpha_i = \mathrm{Tr}(K_i K_T)$ and the matrix V is defined by $V_{ij} = \mathrm{Tr}(K_i K_j)$. By following [18], we resort to a more efficient quadratic programming problem to solve (10).

Advantages: The kernels in S^2VR are learned in a supervised way via kernel alignment, which increases the discriminative ability of the kernels. Also, it is efficient that parameters in kernel functions are learned automatically rather than tuned by cross validation.

2.3   Alternating Optimization

S^2VR is efficiently optimized by using a new alternating optimization method. The proposed method is fast, whose convergence is theoretically analyzed. Minimization (7) can be decomposed into two sub-problems with respect to the kernel coefficients β and the structure matrix S.

Fixing S, the minimization problem with respect to β can be optimized by iteratively reweighted least squares (IRWLS) [19]. We construct a quadratic approximation of (5) about u_i:

$$Q(W, \mathbf{b}) = \frac{1}{2} \operatorname{Tr}(W^\top W) + \frac{\gamma}{2} \operatorname{Tr}(FGF^\top) + \frac{1}{2} \operatorname{Tr}(DE^\top E) + \tau T, \quad (11)$$

where D is the diagonal matrix given by

$$D_{ii} = \frac{\tau}{u_i} \left. \frac{dL(u)}{du} \right|_{u_i} = \begin{cases} 0 & u_i < \varepsilon \\ \frac{2\tau(u_i - \varepsilon)}{u_i} & u_i \geq \varepsilon \end{cases} \quad (12)$$

and τT is a sum of constant terms that do not depend either on W or $\mathbf{b}$. We modify (11) in the kernel version:

$$Q(\beta) = \frac{1}{2} \operatorname{Tr}(\beta K \beta^\top) + \frac{\gamma}{2} \operatorname{Tr}(S\beta KLK\beta^\top S^\top) + \frac{1}{2} \operatorname{Tr}(DE^\top E) + \tau T, \quad (13)$$

where $E = Y - S\beta K$. To obtain β, we can equate its gradient to zero:

$$\frac{\partial Q}{\partial \beta} = \beta K - \gamma S^\top S\beta KGK - S^\top (Y - S\beta K)DK = 0, \quad (14)$$

$$(S^\top S)^{-1} \beta + \beta K(\gamma G + D) = S^{-1} YD. \quad (15)$$

It is the standard Sylvester equation ($A\beta + \beta B = C$, where $A = (S^\top S)^{-1}$, $B = K(\gamma G + D)$ and $C = S^{-1} YD$).

We minimize (13) by constructing a descending direction using the optimal solution of (15), and the next step solution is computed by a line search algorithm [18]. Inspired by the IRWLS, we propose the adapted IRWLS procedure summarized in Algorithm 1.

Given fixed β, the derivative of (7) respect to S is computed as:

$$\frac{\partial Q}{\partial S} = 2\lambda SP - \tau(Y - S\beta K)D(\beta K)^\top + \gamma S\beta KGK\beta^\top = 0 \quad (16)$$

$$S = \tau Y DK\beta^\top \left(2\lambda P + \tau \beta KDK\beta^\top + \gamma \beta KGK\beta^\top \right)^{-1}, \quad (17)$$

Algorithm 1. Adapted IRWLS

1: Initialization: set $k = 0$, compute D^k using (12)
2: **repeat**
3:     Compute β^k in (15) by using the Sylvester equation, and denote it as β^ℓ. Get the descending direction as $\Delta^k = \beta^\ell - \beta^k$.
4:     Update $\beta^{k+1} = \beta^k + \eta^k \Delta^k$, and the step size η^k is computed by using the backtracking algorithm.
5:     Obtain D^{k+1}.
6:     Set $k = k + 1$.
7: **until** Convergence

Algorithm 2. Iteratively Computing S

1: Initialization: set $k = 0$
2: **repeat**
3:     Compute the diagonal matrix P^k.
4:     Update S^{k+1} using (17).
5:     Set $k = k + 1$.
6: **until** Convergence

---

where S is a diagonal matrix with $P_{jj} = \frac{1}{2\|S_j\|_2}$, $P \in \mathbb{R}^{q \times q}$ and S_j is the column vector of S.

We compute the derivative of S using (17). The calculation of P is based on S. Therefore, the new S is computed by using the current S. The procedure is summarized in Algorithm 2. Therefore, minimization (7) can be solved by alternatively optimizing β and S.

Proof of Convergence: The fast convergence for optimization ensures the efficiency of our method. We provide the theoretical analysis with rigorous proof for the convergence of the optimization algorithm. Since the optimization is conducted in an alternating iterative way, we first prove the convergence for the adapted IRWLS procedure for optimizing β.

Theorem 1. $Q(\beta)$ *in* (13) *bounds together all outputs and monotonically decreases in each iteration of Algorithm* 1

Proof. The proof can be referred to the proof of Appendix in [19].

Now that the convergence for the adapted IRWLS procedure is guaranteed in Theorem 1, the following theorem shows the convergence of the alternating iterative method.

Theorem 2. $Q(\beta, S)$ *in* (7) *is bounded from below and monotonically decreases with each alternating iterative optimization step for β and S.*

Proof. Due to the sum formation of $Q(\beta, S)$ in (13), we have the bound of $Q(\beta, S) \geq 0$. Let $\beta^{(t)}$ and $S^{(t)}$ denote β and S in the t-th iteration respectively. Then, $\beta^{(t)}$ and $S^{(t)}$ are computed by $\beta^{(t)} \leftarrow \arg\min_\beta Q(\beta, S^{(t-1)})$ and

$S^{(t)} \leftarrow \arg\min_S Q(\boldsymbol{\beta}^{(t-1)}, S)$. Since $Q(\boldsymbol{\beta}, S^{(t-1)}) \geq Q(\boldsymbol{\beta}, S^{(t)})$ has been proved in [20], we obtain the following inequality:

$$\cdots \geq Q(\boldsymbol{\beta}^{(t-1)}, S^{(t-1)}) \geq Q(\boldsymbol{\beta}^{(t)}, S^{(t-1)}) \geq Q(\boldsymbol{\beta}^{(t)}, S^{(t)}) \geq \cdots . \quad (18)$$

$Q(\boldsymbol{\beta}^{(t)}, S^{(t)})$ is monotonically decreasing as $t \to +\infty$. Therefore, the convergence of the optimization of $Q(\boldsymbol{\beta}, S)$ is proved.

2.4 Prediction

In the testing stage, given a new input $\mathbf{x}^{(t)}$, the predicted angles and landmarks are given by $\hat{\mathbf{y}}^{(t)} = S\boldsymbol{\beta}K^{(t)}$, where $K^{(t)} = \sum_{z=1}^{Z} \mu_z K_z^{(t)}$, $K_z^{(t)} = \boldsymbol{\Phi}^{\top}(\hat{X})\phi(\mathbf{x}^{(t)})$ and $\hat{X}$ is the matrix composed of the support vectors.

3 Experiments

S^2VR has been validated on the spinal X-ray dataset with a large number of subjects. Extensive experiments show that our method with significant effectiveness consistently outperforms the baseline methods, which can be practically used in clinical scoliosis analysis.

3.1 Datasets and Implementation Details

The posteroanterior spinal X-ray dataset is composed of 439 samples from different individuals. Since the cervical vertebrae (the vertebrae of the neck) are seldom involved in spinal deformity [21], we select 17 vertebrae composed of the thoracic spine and lumbar spine for spinal shape characterization. And each vertebra is located by four landmarks with respect to four corners. The landmarks of a spine consist of $c = 68$ points which are annotated manually, while the Cobb angles with 3 values (from top to bottom: TA, MA, BA) are measured by human experts. We choose histogram of oriented gradient (HOG) descriptor [22] as the input of the model due to its strength in local representation. The Gaussian Kernel is selected as the basic kernel and the σ parameter is in the range of $[0.1, 1]$. Our model has been validated using the leave-one-out cross validation scheme.

3.2 Results

The S^2VR achieves desirable performance on the spinal X-ray dataset and demonstrates great effectiveness for the Cobb angle estimation and landmark detection. We show the qualitative results of landmark detection in Fig. 3. We also compare with two baseline methods, which shows the strength of our method on the spinal curvature analysis.

Comparison. As demonstrated in Table 1, we compare with two baseline methods, i.e. support vector regression (SVR) [19], shape regression machine (SRM)

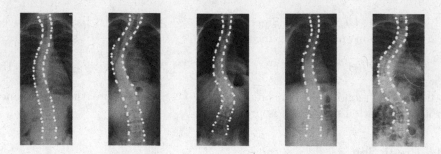

Fig. 3. Our method overcomes huge variations and high ambiguities and achieves high accuracy in landmark detection.

[23] about the relative root mean squared error (RRMSE) and the correlation coefficient, which shows the effectiveness of our method. For vectors of the length of l, let $\hat{y}, y, \bar{Y}$ denotes the ground truth, the estimated vector, the mean of target variable Y over train data, respectively, the RRMSE is defined as

$$R_r = \frac{\sum_{i=1}^{l} \hat{y}_i - y_i}{\sum_{i=1}^{l} \bar{Y}_i - y_i}. \tag{19}$$

The S^2VR achieves the lowest average RRMSE of 21.63 and the highest correlation coefficient of 92.76. Since there are strong correlations between outputs, explicit correlation learning in the S^2VR can faithfully exploit the structure information for a better result. Also, the learned and more robust kernel is powerful enough to handle the correspondence between the image appearance and high-level semantic concepts. We also compare the separated prediction with joint prediction. As shown in two tables, the joint prediction consistently outperforms than the separated one.

Table 1. The comparison of the average RRMSE (%) and the correlation coefficient (%) of three angles.

Method	Average RRMSE (%)		Correlation Coefficient (%)	
	Angles	Angles & Landmarks	Angles	Angles & Landmarks
SVR [19]	25.01	23.72	90.83	91.95
SRM [23]	24.83	23.35	91.30	92.13
S^2VR (Ours)	23.69	21.63	91.94	92.76

Effectiveness. The effectiveness of the proposed method is demonstrated by the outstanding performance on the spinal X-ray dataset. The estimated Cobb angles by the proposed method are compared with those by manual measurement. The correlations between estimated angles and ground truth are depicted in Fig. 4, respectively. The proposed method achieves a correlation coefficient of 0.923 for the middle angle and can yield 0.884 and 0.902 for the rest two angles.

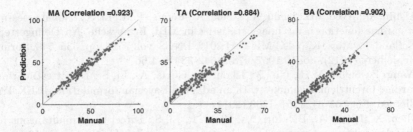

Fig. 4. The correlation coefficients between three angles predicted by the proposed method and ground truth for the MA, TA and BA, respectively. The method achieves a high correlation coefficient with manual measurement.

4 Conclusion

In this paper, we propose structured support vector regression (S^2VR) to directly predict the Cobb angles and landmarks in spinal X-rays from image features. The proposed S^2VR consists of non-linear mapping and explicit structure modeling, which can handle the highly nonlinear relationship between features and quantitative evaluation parameters and explicitly learn the inter-output corrections. Moreover, the manifold regularization is introduced for the smooth solution. To obtain a discriminative kernel, we propose to learn the kernel in S^2VR by kernel target alignment, which can leverage the strength of supervised kernel learning. Extensive experiments on the spinal X-ray dataset show the great effectiveness of our method compared with two baseline methods.

Acknowledgments. The work is supported by NSFC Joint Fund with Guangdong under Key Project No. U1201258, National Natural Science Foundation of China under Grant No. 61573219, and the Fostering Project of Dominant Discipline and Talent Team of Shandong Province Higher Education Institutions.

References

1. Weinstein, S.L., Dolan, L.A., Cheng, J.C., Danielsson, A., Morcuende, J.A.: Adolescent idiopathic scoliosis. Lancet **371**(9623), 1527–1537 (2008)
2. Greiner, K.A.: Adolescent idiopathic scoliosis: radiologic decision-making. Am. Fam. Phys. **65**(9), 1817–1822 (2002)
3. Vrtovec, T., Pernuš, F., Likar, B.: A review of methods for quantitative evaluation of spinal curvature. Eur. Spine J. **18**(5), 593–607 (2009)
4. Anitha, H., Prabhu, G.: Automatic quantification of spinal curvature in scoliotic radiograph using image processing. J. Med. Syst. **36**(3), 1943–1951 (2012)
5. Anitha, H., Karunakar, A., Dinesh, K.: Automatic extraction of vertebral endplates from scoliotic radiographs using customized filter. Biomed. Eng. Lett. **4**(2), 158–165 (2014)
6. Sardjono, T.A., Wilkinson, M.H., Veldhuizen, A.G., van Ooijen, P.M., Purnama, K.E., Verkerke, G.J.: Automatic Cobb angle determination from radiographic images. Spine **38**(20), 1256–1262 (2013)

7. Afshin, M., Ayed, I.B., Islam, A., Goela, A., Peters, T.M., Li, S.: Global assessment of cardiac function using image statistics in MRI. In: Ayache, N., Delingette, H., Golland, P., Mori, K. (eds.) MICCAI 2012. LNCS, vol. 7511, pp. 535–543. Springer, Heidelberg (2012). doi:10.1007/978-3-642-33418-4_66

8. Wang, Z., Salah, M.B., Gu, B., Islam, A., Goela, A., Li, S.: Direct estimation of cardiac biventricular volumes with an adapted Bayesian formulation. IEEE Trans. Biomed. Eng. **61**(4), 1251–1260 (2014)

9. Zhen, X., Islam, A., Bhaduri, M., Chan, I., Li, S.: Direct and simultaneous four-chamber volume estimation by multi-output regression. In: Navab, N., Hornegger, J., Wells, W.M., Frangi, A.F. (eds.) MICCAI 2015. LNCS, vol. 9349, pp. 669–676. Springer, Cham (2015). doi:10.1007/978-3-319-24553-9_82

10. Zhen, X., Wang, Z., Islam, A., Bhaduri, M., Chan, I., Li, S.: Multi-scale deep networks and regression forests for direct bi-ventricular volume estimation. Med. Image Anal. **30**, 120–129 (2016)

11. Zhen, X., Zhang, H., Islam, A., Bhaduri, M., Chan, I., Li, S.: Direct and simultaneous estimation of cardiac four chamber volumes by multioutput sparse regression. Med. Image Anal. **36**, 184–196 (2017)

12. Mumford, D., Shah, J.: Optimal approximations by piecewise smooth functions and associated variational problems. Commun. Pure Appl. Math. **42**(5), 577–685 (1989)

13. Belkin, M., Niyogi, P., Sindhwani, V.: Manifold regularization: a geometric framework for learning from labeled and unlabeled examples. J. Mach. Learn. Res. **7**, 2399–2434 (2006)

14. Von Luxburg, U.: A tutorial on spectral clustering. Stat. Comput. **17**(4), 395–416 (2007)

15. Kimeldorf, G.S., Wahba, G.: A correspondence between Bayesian estimation on stochastic processes and smoothing by splines. Ann. Math. Stat. **41**(2), 495–502 (1970)

16. Cristianini, N., Shawe-Taylor, J., Elisseeff, A., Kandola, J.S.: On kernel-target alignment. In: NIPS, pp. 367–373 (2002)

17. Cortes, C., Mohri, M., Rostamizadeh, A.: Two-stage learning kernel algorithms. In: ICML, pp. 239–246 (2010)

18. Wright, J.N.S.J.: Numerical optimization

19. Sánchez-Fernández, M., de Prado-Cumplido, M., Arenas-García, J., Pérez-Cruz, F.: SVM multiregression for nonlinear channel estimation in multiple-input multiple-output systems. IEEE Trans. Signal Process. **52**(8), 2298–2307 (2004)

20. Nie, F., Huang, H., Cai, X., Ding, C.H.: Efficient and robust feature selection via joint 2, 1-norms minimization. In: NIPS, pp. 1813–1821 (2010)

21. Spinal Deformity Study Group, Radiographic Measurement Manual, Medtronic Sofamor Danek USA (2008)

22. Dalal, N., Triggs, B.: Histograms of oriented gradients for human detection. In: CVPR, vol. 1, pp. 886–893, IEEE (2005)

23. Zhou, S.K.: Shape regression machine and efficient segmentation of left ventricle endocardium from 2D B-mode echocardiogram. Med. Image Anal. **14**(4), 563–581 (2010)

Imaging Genomics

Identifying Associations Between Brain Imaging Phenotypes and Genetic Factors via a Novel Structured SCCA Approach

Lei Du[1], Tuo Zhang[1], Kefei Liu[2], Jingwen Yan[2], Xiaohui Yao[2], Shannon L. Risacher[2], Andrew J. Saykin[2], Junwei Han[1], Lei Guo[1], Li Shen[2(✉)], and for the Alzheimer's Disease Neuroimaging Initiative

[1] School of Automation, Northwestern Polytechnical University, Xi'an, China
dulei@nwpu.edu.cn
[2] Radiology and Imaging Sciences, Indiana University School of Medicine, Indianapolis, IN, USA
shenli@iu.edu

Abstract. Brain imaging genetics attracts more and more attention since it can reveal associations between genetic factors and the structures or functions of human brain. Sparse canonical correlation analysis (SCCA) is a powerful bi-multivariate association identification technique in imaging genetics. There have been many SCCA methods which could capture different types of structured imaging genetic relationships. These methods either use the group lasso to recover the group structure, or employ the graph/network guided fused lasso to find out the network structure. However, the group lasso methods have limitation in generalization because of the incomplete or unavailable prior knowledge in real world. The graph/network guided methods are sensitive to the sign of the sample correlation which may be incorrectly estimated. We introduce a new SCCA model using a novel graph guided pairwise group lasso penalty, and propose an efficient optimization algorithm. The proposed method has a strong upper bound for the grouping effect for both positively and negatively correlated variables. We show that our method performs better than or equally to two state-of-the-art SCCA methods on both synthetic and real neuroimaging genetics data. In particular, our method identifies stronger canonical correlations and captures better canonical loading profiles, showing its promise for revealing biologically meaningful imaging genetic associations.

L. Shen—This work was supported by NSFC under Grant 61602384, and the Fundamental Research Funds for the Central Universities under Grant 3102016OQD0065. This work was also supported by NIH R01 EB022574, R01 LM011360, U01 AG024904, P30 AG10133, R01 AG19771, UL1 TR001108, R01 AG 042437, R01 AG046171, and R01 AG040770, by DoD W81XWH-14-2-0151, W81XWH-13-1-0259, W81XWH-12-2-0012, and NCAA 14132004.
Data used in preparation of this article were obtained from the Alzheimer's Disease Neuroimaging Initiative (ADNI) database (adni.loni.usc.edu). As such, the investigators within the ADNI contributed to the design and implementation of ADNI and/or provided data but did not participate in analysis or writing of this report. A complete listing of ADNI investigators can be found at: http://adni.loni.usc.edu/wp-content/uploads/how_to_apply/ADNI_Acknowledgement_List.pdf.

© Springer International Publishing AG 2017
M. Niethammer et al. (Eds.): IPMI 2017, LNCS 10265, pp. 543–555, 2017.
DOI: 10.1007/978-3-319-59050-9_43

1   Introduction

In recent years, brain imaging genetics becomes a popular research topic in biomedical and bioinformatics studies. Brain imaging genetics refers to the study of modeling and understanding how genetic factors influence the structure or function of human brain using the imaging measurements as the quantitative endophenotype [11–13]. Both the genetic factors, such as the single nucleotide polymorphisms (SNPs), and the imaging measurements such as the imaging quantitative traits (QTs) are multivariate. Therefore, discovering meaningful bi-multivariate associations is an important task in brain imaging genetics.

Equipped with feature selection, sparse canonical correlation analysis (SCCA) gains tremendous attention for its powerful ability in bi-multivariate association identification. There are many SCCA methods using different types of shrinkage techniques. The ℓ_1-norm penalty and its variants are widely used, but they only pursuit individual level sparsity [8,16]. In biomedical studies, the genetic biomarkers usually function simultaneously other than individually [14]. This is also the case for the imaging measurements. Therefore, the structure level sparsity, such as the group structure or the graph/network structure, is of great interest and importance in brain imaging genetics [14,15].

To capture the high-level structure information, several different structure-aware penalties have been proposed. There are roughly two kinds of structured SCCA methods according to their different penalties [4]. The first kind of SCCA methods consider the group information using the group lasso regularizer, which is an intra-group ℓ_2-norm and inter-group ℓ_1-norm [1,6]. The group lasso tends to assign equal weights for those variables in a same group, and each group will be selected or not as a whole [18]. To our knowledge, this type of SCCA methods require the priori knowledge to define the group structure. This limits their applications as it is hard to obtain precise priori knowledge in real biological studies [4]. The second kind of SCCA methods rebuild the structure information via the graph guided or network guided penalty [2–6]. These SCCA methods can capture the structure information using any available priori knowledge. Moreover, they can also recover the structure information based on the input data [4]. Three types of graph guided penalties have been used: (1) the graph guided fused lasso penalty and its variants [1,3,7], (2) the correlation sign based graph guided fused ℓ_2-norm penalty [2], and (3) the improved GraphNet based penalty [4]. Du et $al.$ [4] has shown that the first two types of graph guided penalties could introduce estimation bias because of the sign of the correlations can be wrongly calculated. The reason could be that the sign of the correlations can be easily changed when removing a fraction of the data or perturbing the data as in bootstrap or sub-sampling. The improved GraphNet utilizes ℓ_2-norm with respect to the structure penalty terms, which may not produce desirable sparse results at structure level.

Inspired by the success of group lasso in group selection, we consider a case where each group is made up of only two variables. Both variables will be extracted together with similar or equal weights. Interestingly, this novel group lasso can be used in data-driven mode where no priori knowledge is provided.

We call it graph guided pairwise group lasso (GGL) which bridges the gap between the group lasso and graph guided penalties. We then propose a new graph guided pairwise group lasso based sparse canonical correlation analysis model (GGL-SCCA) with intention to recover the structure information automatically. The proposed SCCA method is sample correlation sign independent and it is robust to those existing SCCA methods using graph guided penalty. We also propose an efficient optimization algorithm to solve the problem. Besides, we also provide a quantitative upper bound for the grouping effect of our method to demonstrate its structure identifying ability. Compared with the state-of-art SCCA methods such as NS-SCCA [2] and AGN-SCCA [4], GGL-SCCA can not only obtain higher or equal and more stable correlation coefficients than the competing methods, but also find out cleaner canonical loading patterns on both synthetic data and real imaging genetic data.

2   The Graph Guided Pairwise Group Lasso

Throughout this paper, we denote a vector as the boldface lowercase letter, and a matrix is denoted by a boldface uppercase one. The Euclidean norm of vector $\mathbf{u}$ is $||\mathbf{u}||$. Let $\mathbf{X} = [\mathbf{x}^1; \ldots; \mathbf{x}^n]^T \subseteq \mathbb{R}^p$ and $\mathbf{Y} = [\mathbf{y}^1; \ldots; \mathbf{y}^n]^T \subseteq \mathbb{R}^q$ be the SNP data and the QT data from the same participants.

We have known that the group lasso tends to extract a subset of the features. However, it depends on the priori knowledge and there is no overlap between groups. The graph guided fused lasso overcomes this limitation, but it requires the sign of the sample correlations to be defined in advance. This will introduce undesirable estimation bias [17]. In this paper, we introduce the graph guided pairwise group lasso penalty by taking advantage of both group lasso and graph guided fused lasso. The GGL penalty is defined as,

$$\Omega_{\mathrm{GGL}}(\mathbf{u}) = \sum_{(i,j)\in E} \sqrt{u_i^2 + u_j^2} \tag{1}$$

where E is the edge set of the graph where those highly correlated features are connected.

The GGL penalty has the following two merits. First, if there is no priori knowledge, every pairwise term will be included to encourage $|u_i| \approx |u_j|$ which is guaranteed by the pairwise ℓ_2-norm. This holds for both positively and negatively correlated features, which will be demonstrated later in Theorem 1. Second, if some priori knowledge such as the pathway information about genetic markers is provided, the whole penalty will be guided by the pathway information. This will encourage $|u_i| = |u_j|$ no matter whether they are positively or negatively correlated. Therefore, the two genetic markers have very high probability to be selected simultaneously. The same results hold for the imaging measurements if we have the brain connectivity pattern such as the human connectome.

3   Method

3.1   GGL-SCCA Model and Optimization

We then propose the GGL-SCCA model,

$$\min_{\mathbf{u},\mathbf{v}} -\mathbf{u}^T\mathbf{X}^T\mathbf{Y}\mathbf{v} \tag{2}$$

$$s.t.\ ||\mathbf{Xu}||^2 \leq 1, ||\mathbf{Yv}||^2 \leq 1, \Omega_{\mathrm{GGL}}(\mathbf{u}) \leq c_1, \Omega_{\mathrm{GGL}}(\mathbf{v}) \leq c_2$$

where $\Omega_{\mathrm{GGL}}(\mathbf{u})$ and $\Omega_{\mathrm{GGL}}(\mathbf{v})$ are the GGL penalty to assure structure informa-tion. Of note, we use $||\mathbf{Xu}||^2 \leq 1$ instead of $||\mathbf{u}||^2 \leq 1$ to accommodate the in-set covariance $\mathbf{X}^T\mathbf{X}$ which can improve the model performance [6].

In order to solve this problem, we write the objective function of GGL-SCCA into matrix form using the Lagrange method,

$$\mathcal{L}(\mathbf{u},\mathbf{v}) = -\mathbf{u}^T\mathbf{X}^T\mathbf{Y}\mathbf{v} + \frac{\gamma_1}{2}||\mathbf{Xu}||^2 + \frac{\gamma_2}{2}||\mathbf{Yv}||^2 + \lambda_1\Omega_{\mathrm{GGL}}(\mathbf{u}) + \lambda_2\Omega_{\mathrm{GGL}}(\mathbf{v}) \tag{3}$$

We approximate the objective function by a quadratic function. Obviously, the first term $\mathbf{u}^T\mathbf{X}^T\mathbf{Y}\mathbf{v}$ is bilinear and biconvex in $\mathbf{u}$ and $\mathbf{v}$. We then show the quadratic expression of the GGL term. Let $\mathbf{u}^t$ and $\mathbf{u}^{t+1}$ be the estimation at steps t and $t+1$ respectively, the first-order Taylor expansion of term $\sqrt{u_i^2 + u_j^2}$ regarding $u_i^2 + u_j^2$ is,

$$\sqrt{(u_i^{t+1})^2 + (u_j^{t+1})^2} \approx \sqrt{(u_i^t)^2 + (u_j^t)^2}$$

$$+ \frac{1}{2\sqrt{(u_i^t)^2 + (u_j^t)^2}}(((u_i^{t+1})^2 + (u_j^{t+1})^2) - ((u_i^t)^2 + (u_j^t)^2))$$

$$= \frac{(u_i^{t+1})^2}{2\sqrt{(u_i^t)^2 + (u_j^t)^2}} + C \tag{4}$$

where $C = \sqrt{(u_i^t)^2 + (u_j^t)^2} + \frac{(u_j^{t+1})^2 - ((u_i^t)^2 + (u_j^t)^2)}{2\sqrt{(u_i^t)^2 + (u_j^t)^2}}$. From the point of view of optimization, the term C makes no contribution towards optimizing u_i.[1]

Then the GGL penalty can be simplified,

$$\Omega_{\mathrm{GGL}}(\mathbf{u}) \approx \sum_i \sum_j \frac{(u_i^{t+1})^2}{2\sqrt{(u_i^t)^2 + (u_j^t)^2}} + C^* \tag{5}$$

with C^* being the sum of C across all pairwise penalty terms. Therefore, the GGL penalty is quadratically expressed.

---

[1] Each u_i can be solved with u_j's ($j \neq i$) fixed (i.e., we use u_j^t to approximate u_j^{t+1} in C), thus u_j's do not contribute to the optimization of u_i [9].

Algorithm 1. The GGL-SCCA algorithm

Require:
    $\mathbf{X} = [\mathbf{x}_1, ..., \mathbf{x}_n]^T$, $\mathbf{Y} = [\mathbf{y}_1, ..., \mathbf{y}_n]^T$
Ensure:
    Canonical loadings $\mathbf{u}$ and $\mathbf{v}$.
1: Initialize $\mathbf{u} \in \mathbb{R}^{p \times 1}$, $\mathbf{v} \in \mathbb{R}^{q \times 1}$;
2: **while** not convergence **do**
3:    Update the diagonal matrix $\mathbf{D}_1$ by taking derivative of Eq. (5);
4:    Solve $\mathbf{u}$ according to Eq. (8);
5:    Update the diagonal matrix $\mathbf{D}_2$ by taking derivative of Eq. (5);
6:    Solve $\mathbf{v}$ according to Eq. (9);
7: **end while**
8: Scale $\mathbf{u}$ so that $\|\mathbf{X}\mathbf{u}\|_2^2 = 1$, and $\mathbf{v}$ so that $\|\mathbf{Y}\mathbf{v}\|_2^2 = 1$.

Now the objective function conveys to a quadratic function, and there exists a closed-form solution. Since GGL-SCCA is biconvex in $\mathbf{u}$ and $\mathbf{v}$, we take the derivative with respect to them respectively. The solution to the Eq. (3) satisfies,

$$0 \in -\mathbf{X}^T\mathbf{Y}\mathbf{v} + (\lambda_1\mathbf{D}_1 + \gamma_1\mathbf{X}^T\mathbf{X})\mathbf{u}, \tag{6}$$

$$0 \in -\mathbf{Y}^T\mathbf{X}\mathbf{u} + (\lambda_2\mathbf{D}_2 + \gamma_2\mathbf{Y}^T\mathbf{Y})\mathbf{v}, \tag{7}$$

where $\mathbf{D}_1$ can be deduced from the previous step's value of $\mathbf{u}$ according to Eq. (5). $\mathbf{D}_2$ can be computed similarly. Therefore, $\mathbf{D}_1$ is a diagonal matrix with the k_1-th element being $\sum_{i,i \neq k_1} \frac{1}{\sqrt{u_{k_1}^2 + u_i^2}}$ ($k_1 \in [1, p]$), and $\mathbf{D}_2$ is a diagonal matrix with the k_2-th element being $\sum_{j,j \neq k_2} \frac{1}{\sqrt{v_{k_2}^2 + v_j^2}}$ ($k_2 \in [1, q]$).[2]

Therefore, $\mathbf{u}$ and $\mathbf{v}$ have the closed-form updating expressions,

$$\mathbf{u}^{t+1} = (\lambda_1\mathbf{D}_1^t + \gamma_1\mathbf{X}^T\mathbf{X})^{-1}\mathbf{X}^T\mathbf{Y}\mathbf{v}^t, \tag{8}$$

$$\mathbf{v}^{t+1} = (\lambda_2\mathbf{D}_2^t + \gamma_2\mathbf{Y}^T\mathbf{Y})^{-1}\mathbf{Y}^T\mathbf{X}\mathbf{u}^{t+1}. \tag{9}$$

We have known that GGL-SCCA model is biconvex with respect to $\mathbf{u}$ and $\mathbf{v}$ respectively. Then the Alternate Convex Search (ACS) method which is designed to solve the biconvex problem can be employed [10]. According to the ACS method, we address our SCCA model via alternative optimization by updating $\mathbf{u}$ and $\mathbf{v}$ alternatively. The procedure of the GGL-SCCA is shown in Algorithm 1. In every iteration, $\mathbf{u}$ and $\mathbf{v}$ are updated in turn till the algorithm converges or reaches a predefined stopping condition.

---

[2] Note that an element of diagonal matrix $\mathbf{D}_1$ will nonexist if $\sqrt{u_i^2 + u_{k_1}^2} = 0$. We handle this issue by regularizing it as $\sqrt{u_i^2 + u_{k_1}^2 + \zeta}$ with ζ being a tiny positive number. Then the objective function regarding $\mathbf{u}$ becomes $\tilde{\mathcal{L}}(\mathbf{u}) = \sum_{i=1}^{p}(-u_i\mathbf{x}_i^T\mathbf{Y}\mathbf{v} + \lambda_1\sum_{k_1}\sqrt{u_i^2 + u_{k_1}^2 + \zeta} + \frac{\gamma_1}{2}\|\mathbf{x}_i u_i\|_2^2)$. We can prove that $\tilde{\mathcal{L}}(\mathbf{u})$ will reduce to the original problem (3) when ζ approaching zero. Likewise, $\sqrt{v_j^2 + v_{k_2}^2} = 0$ can be regularized by the same method.

3.2   The Grouping Effect

In structured learning, a method that can estimate equal or similar values for a group of variables is more desirable [4,19]. This is called grouping effect and of great importance. We have the following theorem with respect to the grouping effects of the GGL-SCCA method.

Theorem 1. *Given two views of data* $\mathbf{X}$ *and* $\mathbf{Y}$, *and the tuned parameters* (λ, γ). *Let* $\mathbf{u}^*$ *be the solution to our SCCA problem. For the sake of simplicity, we assume there are only two features, e.g.* u_i *and* u_j, *are connected on the graph. Let* ρ_{ij} *be their sample correlation. Then the optimal* $\mathbf{u}^*$ *satisfies,*

$$|u_i^* - u_j^*| \leq \frac{(1+\gamma_1)\sqrt{u_i^{*2} + u_j^{*2}}}{\lambda_1}\sqrt{2(1-\rho_{ij})}, \;\; if \;\; \rho_{ij} \geq 0,$$

$$|u_i^* + u_j^*| \leq \frac{(1+\gamma_1)\sqrt{u_i^{*2} + u_j^{*2}}}{\lambda_1}\sqrt{2(1+\rho_{ij})}, \;\; if \;\; \rho_{ij} < 0.$$

$$(10)$$

Proof. (1) We first prove the inequations when $\rho_{ij} \geq 0$ indicating features being positively correlated. We have the following two equations,

$$\frac{\partial \mathcal{L}}{\partial u_i} = \lambda_1 D_{1,i} u_i^* + \gamma_1 \mathbf{x}_i^T \mathbf{X} \mathbf{u} = \mathbf{x}_i^T \mathbf{Y} \mathbf{v}, \;\; \frac{\partial \mathcal{L}}{\partial u_j} = \lambda_1 D_{1,j} u_j^* + \gamma_1 \mathbf{x}_j^T \mathbf{X} \mathbf{u} = \mathbf{x}_j^T \mathbf{Y} \mathbf{v}. \quad (11)$$

Given u_i and u_j are the only connected features, we have $D_{1,i} = D_{1,j} = \frac{1}{\sqrt{u_i^2 + u_j^2}}$. Then we arrive at

$$\frac{\lambda_1}{\sqrt{u_i^{*2} + u_j^{*2}}} u_i^* = \mathbf{x}_i^T \mathbf{Y} \mathbf{v} - \gamma_1 \mathbf{x}_i^T \mathbf{X} \mathbf{u}, \;\; \frac{\lambda_1}{\sqrt{u_i^{*2} + u_j^{*2}}} u_j^* = \mathbf{x}_j^T \mathbf{Y} \mathbf{v} - \gamma_1 \mathbf{x}_j^T \mathbf{X} \mathbf{u}. \quad (12)$$

Subtracting these two equations, we have

$$\frac{\lambda_1}{\sqrt{u_i^{*2} + u_j^{*2}}} (u_i^* - u_j^*) = (\mathbf{x}_i - \mathbf{x}_j)^T (\mathbf{Y}\mathbf{v} - \gamma_1 \mathbf{X}\mathbf{u}) \quad (13)$$

Taking ℓ_2-norm on both sides, we arrive at

$$\frac{\lambda_1}{\sqrt{u_i^{*2} + u_j^{*2}}} |u_i^* - u_j^*| = ||\mathbf{x}_i - \mathbf{x}_j|| \; ||\mathbf{Y}\mathbf{v} - \gamma_1 \mathbf{X}\mathbf{u}|| = ||\mathbf{x}_i - \mathbf{x}_j||\sqrt{||\mathbf{Y}\mathbf{v}|| - 2\gamma_1 \mathbf{u}^\top \mathbf{X}^\top \mathbf{Y}\mathbf{v} + \gamma^2 ||\mathbf{X}\mathbf{u}||}$$

$$(14)$$

Using $||\mathbf{x}_i - \mathbf{x}_j|| = \sqrt{2(1-\rho_{ij})}$, $||\mathbf{X}\mathbf{u}|| \leq 1$, $||\mathbf{Y}\mathbf{v}|| \leq 1$ and $-\mathbf{u}^T \mathbf{X}^T \mathbf{Y}\mathbf{v} \leq 1$, we obtain the upper bound

$$|u_i^* - u_j^*| \leq \frac{(1+\gamma_1)\sqrt{u_i^{*2} + u_j^{*2}}}{\lambda_1}\sqrt{2(1-\rho_{ij})}. \quad (15)$$

(2) If $\rho_{ij} < 0$, it is clear that $\text{sign}(u_i) = -\text{sign}(u_j)$. By adding both equations in Eq. (12) instead of subtracting them, we finally arrive at,

$$|u_i^* + u_j^*| \leq \frac{(1 + \gamma_1)\sqrt{u_i^{*2} + u_j^{*2}}}{\lambda_1}\sqrt{2(1 + \rho_{ij})}. \qquad (16)$$

Note that GGL-SCCA model is symmetric about **u** and **v**, we can obtain the same upper bound of grouping effect for canonical weights **v**.

The Theorem 1 provides a qualitative theoretical description of the bound for both differences and sums of the coefficients. The bound between two coefficients directly depends on their correlation. If $\rho_{ij} \geq 0$, a higher correlation between two variables makes sure a smaller difference between their estimated coefficients. If $\rho_{ij} < 0$, a smaller value assures a smaller sum between their coefficients. This implies that the two coefficients will be approximate in amplitude. Therefore, the GGL-SCCA is capable of capture structure information no matter whether those features are positively or negatively correlated.

3.3   The Complexity Analysis

In Algorithm 1, Steps 2–7 are repeated until convergence. In each iteration, Step 3 is easy to calculate as $\mathbf{D}_1$ can be computed via matrix manipulation to avoid time consuming loop. This is the same case for Step 5. Step 4 and Step 6 are the key steps, and we compute them via solving a system of linear equations with quadratic complexity instead of computing the matrix inverse with cubic complexity. This can reduce the computation burden greatly. Step 8 is a rescale steps and very simple to calculate. Therefore, the algorithm runs fast and efficiently.

In this study, we terminate Algorithm 1 when either of the two conditions satisfies, $\max\{|\delta| \mid \delta \in (\mathbf{u}_{t+1} - \mathbf{u}_t)\} \leq \epsilon$ and $\max\{|\delta| \mid \delta \in (\mathbf{v}_{t+1} - \mathbf{v}_t)\} \leq \epsilon$, where ϵ is a desirable estimation error. We chose $\epsilon = 10^{-5}$ empirically from experiments in this paper.

4   Experimental Study

4.1   Experimental Setup

We compare GGL-SCCA with two structure-aware SCCA methods. The first one is the network guided fused lasso based SCCA (NS-SCCA) which takes the sample correlation signs into consideration [2]. The second method is the AGN-SCCA which uses the absolute value based GraphNet to penalize those correlated variables [4]. These two methods are different in both modeling and optimizing techniques, and is deemed to be among the best structured SCCA methods by now.

We tune the parameters based on the following considerations to reduce time consumption. (1) According to Theorem 1, $\lambda_{i=1,2}$ and $\gamma_{i=1,2}$ contribute to the grouping effect oppositely. (2) The grouping effect is more sensitive to $\lambda_{i=1,2}$ than to $\gamma_{i=1,2}$. Therefore, we fix $\gamma_{i=1,2}$ to a moderate constant, and let $\gamma_{i=1,2} = 10$ in this paper. Finally, we have only two parameters $\lambda_{i=1,2}$ to be tuned and optimally tune them via a grid search from a moderate range 10^{-2} to 10^2 through nested five-fold cross-validation to make sure efficiency. The parameters that generate the highest correlation coefficients are used.

4.2   Results on Simulation Data

Four different data sets with different properties are generated in this study. We also set the number of observations be smaller than the number of features to simulate a large p small n problem. The details of the data sets are as follows. Firstly, $\mathbf{u}$ and $\mathbf{v}$ are generated according to the predefined structure. Secondly, a latent variable $\mathbf{z} \sim N(\mathbf{0}, \mathbf{I}_{n \times n})$ is generated. And thirdly, $\mathbf{X}$ is created by $\mathbf{x}_i \sim N(z_i \mathbf{u}, \sum_x)$, where $(\sum_x)_{jk} = \exp^{-|u_j - u_k|}$. Similarly, $\mathbf{Y}$ with the entry: $\mathbf{y}_i \sim N(z_i \mathbf{v}, \sum_y)$, where $(\sum_y)_{jk} = \exp^{-|v_j - v_k|}$ is created. During this procedure, the true signals and the correlation strengths of the data are all distinct to assure diversity. This setup can make a thorough comparison.

We apply GGL-SCCA, NS-SCCA and AGN-SCCA to all four data sets. The true and estimated canonical loadings $\mathbf{u}$ and $\mathbf{v}$ are shown in Fig. 1. We observe that both GGL-SCCA and AGN-SCCA identify similar canonical loading profiles that are consistent to the ground truth across all data sets. NS-SCCA produces too many signals which are not so perfect to the ground truth. In addition, we also show the estimated correlation coefficients on both the training and testing sets calculated using the trained SCCA models in Table 1 (Left). The results show that GGL-SCCA obtains highest scores on both training and testing sets. Its testing result is only inferior to the NS-SCCA on the second data. The results implies that GGL-SCCA has better training performance and generalization ability than those benchmarks. The area under ROC (AUC) shown

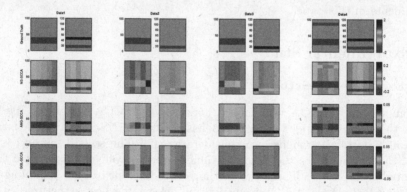

Fig. 1. Canonical loadings estimated on synthetic data. The first row is the ground truth, and each remaining row corresponds to a SCCA method: (1) NS-SCCA, (2) AGN-SCCA, and (3) GGL-SCCA. For each method, the estimated weights of $\mathbf{u}$ are shown on the left panel, and those of $\mathbf{v}$ are shown on the right.

Table 1. Performance comparison on synthetic data. Training and testing correlation coefficients (mean ± std) of 5-fold cross-validation are shown for NS-SCCA, AGN-SCCA and GGL-SCCA. The best value are shown in boldface. The AUC (area under the curve) values (mean ± std) of canonical loadings are also shown.

Data set	Training correlation coefficients			Area under ROC (AUC): u		
	NS-SCCA	AGN-SCCA	GGL-SCCA	NS-SCCA	AGN-SCCA	GGL-SCCA
Data1	0.39 ± 0.07	0.53 ± 0.10	**0.60 ± 0.07**	1.00 ± 0.00	1.00 ± 0.00	1.00 ± 0.00
Data2	0.31 ± 0.08	0.35 ± 0.08	**0.48 ± 0.08**	0.20 ± 0.45	0.60 ± 0.55	0.60 ± 0.55
Data3	0.20 ± 0.07	0.29 ± 0.07	**0.40 ± 0.07**	0.20 ± 0.45	0.80 ± 0.45	1.00 ± 0.00
Data4	0.44 ± 0.08	0.44 ± 0.07	**0.50 ± 0.05**	1.00 ± 0.00	1.00 ± 0.00	0.93 ± 0.15
	Testing correlation coefficients			Area under ROC (AUC): v		
Data1	0.42 ± 0.10	0.60 ± 0.10	**0.62 ± 0.23**	1.00 ± 0.00	0.96 ± 0.09	1.00 ± 0.00
Data2	**0.25 ± 0.18**	0.21 ± 0.14	0.22 ± 0.08	0.20 ± 0.45	0.80 ± 0.45	1.00 ± 0.00
Data3	0.28 ± 0.19	0.33 ± 0.24	**0.43 ± 0.21**	0.20 ± 0.45	1.00 ± 0.00	1.00 ± 0.00
Data4	0.25 ± 0.10	0.32 ± 0.24	**0.44 ± 0.24**	1.00 ± 0.00	1.00 ± 0.00	1.00 ± 0.00

in Table 1 (Right) indicates the sensitivity and specificity. It reveals that GGL-SCCA outperforms the competing methods as it holds the highest values for the most times. In summary, the simulation results demonstrate that GGL-SCCA could identify not only stronger testing associations but also more better signals on these diversified data sets.

4.3   Results on Real Neuroimaging Genetics Data

The real imaging genetics data used in the preparation of this article were obtained from the Alzheimer's Disease Neuroimaging Initiative (ADNI) database (adni.loni.usc.edu). The ADNI was launched in 2003 as a public private partnership, led by Principal Investigator Michael W. Weiner, MD. One primary goal of ADNI is to test whether serial magnetic resonance imaging (MRI), positron emission tomography (PET), other biological markers, and clinical and neuropsychological assessment can be combined to measure the progression of mild cognitive impairment (MCI) and early Alzheimers disease (AD). For up-to-date information, please refer to www.adni-info.org.

Table 2. Participant characteristics.

	HC	MCI	AD
Num	196	343	28
Gender (M/F)	102/94	203/140	18/10
Handedness (R/L)	178/18	309/34	23/5
Age (mean ± std)	74.77 ± 5.39	71.92 ± 7.47	75.23 ± 10.66
Education (mean ± std)	15.61 ± 2.74	15.99 ± 2.75	15.61 ± 2.74

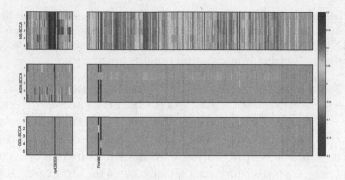

Fig. 2. Canonical loadings estimated on real imaging genetics data set. Each row corresponds to a SCCA method: (1) NS-SCCA, (2) AGN-SCCA, and (3) GGL-SCCA. For each method, the estimated weights of **u** are shown on the left panel, and those of **v** are shown on the right.

We use the genotyping and baseline amyloid imaging data (preprocessed [11C] Florbetapir PET scans) contributed by 567 non-Hispanic Caucasian participants (Table 2). The amyloid imaging data used in this study are downloaded from LONI (adni.loni.usc.edu). Preprocessing is conducted to format this imaging data, and we finally generate 191 ROI level mean amyloid measurements in which the ROIs are defined by the MarsBaR AAL atlas [4]. The genotyping data includes 58 candidate SNP markers from the AD-related genes, such as the *APOE* gene. The aim is to evaluate the associations between the SNP data and the amyloid data, as well as which SNPs and amyloid measurements are correlated in this AD cohort.

All three SCCA methods are performed on the real neuroimaging genetics data. Shown in Fig. 2 are the canonical loadings obtained from the training data, where the relevant imaging measurements and genetic markers are exhibited. It is clear that GGL-SCCA identifies two relevant ROIs and one SNPs for easy interpretation due to the novel GGL penalty. The two strongest imaging measurements come from the right frontal region, which are positively correlated with SNP rs429358, a confirmed AD related allele in *APOE* e4. The AGN-SCCA identifies similar results to our method, which however has many interfering signals for the genetic markers. The NS-SCCA finds out too many imaging signals that are very hard to interpret. To give a clear view, we map the canonical loadings regarding the imaging measurements of GGL-SCCA onto the brain. Figure 3 clearly shows that our method only highlights a small region of the whole brain. Moreover, we present the training and testing correlations in Table 3. GGL-SCCA obtains the highest values on both training set and testing set. Although AGN-SCCA has the same *mean* on training data, its *standard deviation* is larger than GGL-SCCA. Moreover, GGL-SCCA obtains better testing results than both competing methods. This implies that GGL-SCCA is more stable and has better generalization ability than AGN-SCCA and NS-SCCA. The results on this real data demonstrate that GGL-SCCA has better

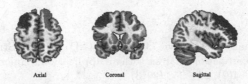

Axial   Coronal   Sagittal

Fig. 3. Mapping averaged canonical loading **v** of GGL-SCCA onto the brain.

Table 3. Performance comparison on real data. Training and testing correlation coefficients (each fold and mean ± std) of 5-fold cross-validation are shown for NS-SCCA, AGN-SCCA and GGL-SCCA. The best mean ± std is shown in boldface.

Method	Training results					mean ± std	Testing results					mean ± std
NS-SCCA	0.41	0.40	0.43	0.39	0.41	0.41 ± 0.01	0.37	0.41	0.23	0.43	0.37	0.36 ± 0.08
AGN-SCCA	0.49	0.43	0.52	0.49	0.51	0.49 ± 0.03	0.48	0.46	0.33	0.55	0.43	0.45 ± 0.08
GGL-SCCA	0.48	0.48	0.52	0.46	0.49	**0.49 ± 0.02**	0.51	0.45	0.34	0.55	0.47	**0.46 ± 0.08**

bi-multivariate identification ability than the benchmark methods. The strong association between the frontal morphometry and the *APOE* in AD cohort, indicating GGL-SCCA's promising and potential power in identifying biologically meaningful imaging genetic associations.

5   Conclusions

We have proposed a novel graph guided pairwise group lasso (GGL) based SCCA method (GGL-SCCA) to identify associations between brain imaging measurements and genetic factors. The existing group lasso based methods [1,6] were dependent on the priori knowledge which was not always available. The graph/netwrok guided fused lasso based approaches [2–6] only focus on the positively correlated variables, or depended on the signs of the sample correlation which were sensitive to the partition of the data. Our SCCA method combines the merits of group lasso and the graph/network guided fused lasso, which is independent to not only the signs of the sample correlation, but also the priori knowledge. Moreover, our method can also incorporate the priori knowledge to recover specific structures.

We have compared GGL-SCCA with two state-of-the-art structured SCCA methods on both synthetic data and real imaging genetic data. The results on the synthetic data show that GGL-SCCA performs better than both NS-SCCA and AGN-SCCA across all data sets. The results on real data show that, GGL-SCCA not only reports better canonical correlation values than the competing methods, but also obtains more accurate and cleaner canonical loading patterns. GGL-SCCA finds out a strong associations between the superior frontal morphometry and the *APOE* e4 SNP, revealing its power in brain imaging genetics. In this paper, we merely use the graph guided pairwise group lasso penalty to induce structured sparsity. In the future work, we will incorporate lasso into the model to assure additional sparsity, and incorporate the priori knowledge to evaluate the performance of GGL-SCCA.

References

1. Chen, J., Bushman, F.D., Lewis, J.D., Wu, G.D., Li, H.: Structure-constrained sparse canonical correlation analysis with an application to microbiome data analysis. Biostatistics **14**(2), 244–258 (2013)
2. Chen, X., Liu, H.: An efficient optimization algorithm for structured sparse CCA, with applications to eQTL mapping. Stat. Biosci. **4**(1), 3–26 (2012)
3. Chen, X., Liu, H., Carbonell, J.G.: Structured sparse canonical correlation analysis. In: AISTATS (2012)
4. Du, L., Huang, H., Yan, J., Kim, S., Risacher, S.L., Inlow, M., Moore, J.H., Saykin, A.J., Shen, L.: Structured sparse canonical correlation analysis for brain imaging genetics: an improved GraphNet method. Bioinformatics **32**(10), 1544–1551 (2016)
5. Du, L., Huang, H., Yan, J., Kim, S., Risacher, S.L., Inlow, M., Moore, J.H., Saykin, A.J., Shen, L.: Structured sparse CCA for brain imaging genetics via graph OSCAR. BMC Syst. Biol. **10**(Suppl. 3), 335–345 (2016)
6. Du, L., et al.: A novel structure-aware sparse learning algorithm for brain imaging genetics. In: Golland, P., Hata, N., Barillot, C., Hornegger, J., Howe, R. (eds.) MICCAI 2014. LNCS, vol. 8675, pp. 329–336. Springer, Cham (2014). doi:10.1007/978-3-319-10443-0_42
7. Du, L., et al.: GN-SCCA: GraphNet based sparse canonical correlation analysis for brain imaging genetics. In: Guo, Y., Friston, K., Aldo, F., Hill, S., Peng, H. (eds.) BIH 2015. LNCS, vol. 9250, pp. 275–284. Springer, Cham (2015). doi:10.1007/978-3-319-23344-4_27
8. Du, L., Zhang, T., Liu, K., Yao, X., Yan, J., Risacher, S.L., Guo, L., Saykin, A.J., Shen, L.: Sparse canonical correlation analysis via truncated ℓ_1-norm with application to brain imaging genetics. In: BIBM, pp. 707–711. IEEE Computer Society (2016)
9. Friedman, J.H., Hastie, T., Hofling, H., Tibshirani, R.: Pathwise coordinate optimization. Ann. Appl. Stat. **1**(2), 302–332 (2007)
10. Gorski, J., Pfeuffer, F., Klamroth, K.: Biconvex sets and optimization with biconvex functions: a survey and extensions. Math. Methods Oper. Res. **66**(3), 373–407 (2007)
11. Kim, S., Swaminathan, S., Inlow, M., Risacher, S.L., Nho, K., Shen, L., Foroud, T.M., Petersen, R.C., Aisen, P.S., Soares, H., et al.: Influence of genetic variation on plasma protein levels in older adults using a multi-analyte panel. PLoS One **8**(7), e70269 (2013)
12. Potkin, S.G., Turner, J.A., Guffanti, G., Lakatos, A., Torri, F., Keator, D.B., Macciardi, F.: Genome-wide strategies for discovering genetic influences on cognition and cognitive disorders: methodological considerations. Cognit. Neuropsychiatry **14**(4–5), 391–418 (2009)
13. Saykin, A.J., Shen, L., Yao, X., Kim, S., Nho, K., Risacher, S.L., Ramanan, V.K., Foroud, T.M., Faber, K.M., Sarwar, N., et al.: Genetic studies of quantitative MCI and AD phenotypes in ADNI: progress, opportunities, and plans. Alzheimer's Dement. **11**(7), 792–814 (2015)
14. Shen, L., Kim, S., Risacher, S.L., Nho, K., Swaminathan, S., West, J.D., Foroud, T., Pankratz, N., Moore, J.H., Sloan, C.D., et al.: Whole genome association study of brain-wide imaging phenotypes for identifying quantitative trait loci in MCI and AD: a study of the ADNI cohort. Neuroimage **53**(3), 1051–1063 (2010)

15. Shen, L., Thompson, P.M., Potkin, S.G., Bertram, L., Farrer, L.A., Foroud, T.M., Green, R.C., Hu, X., Huentelman, M.J., Kim, S., et al.: Genetic analysis of quantitative phenotypes in AD and MCI: imaging, cognition and biomarkers. Brain Imaging Behav. **8**(2), 183–207 (2014)
16. Witten, D.M., Tibshirani, R., Hastie, T.: A penalized matrix decomposition, with applications to sparse principal components and canonical correlation analysis. Biostatistics **10**(3), 515–534 (2009)
17. Yang, S., Yuan, L., Lai, Y.C., Shen, X., Wonka, P., Ye, J.: Feature grouping and selection over an undirected graph. In: KDD, pp. 922–930. ACM (2012)
18. Yuan, M., Lin, Y.: Model selection and estimation in regression with grouped variables. J. Royal Stat. Soc.: Ser. B (Stat. Methodol.) **68**(1), 49–67 (2006)
19. Zou, H., Hastie, T.: Regularization and variable selection via the elastic net. J. Royal Stat. Soc.: Ser. B (Stat. Methodol.) **67**(2), 301–320 (2005)

Image Registration

Frequency Diffeomorphisms for Efficient Image Registration

Miaomiao Zhang[1(✉)], Ruizhi Liao[1], Adrian V. Dalca[1], Esra A. Turk[2],
Jie Luo[2], P. Ellen Grant[2], and Polina Golland[1]

[1] Computer Science and Artificial Intelligence Laboratory, MIT, Cambridge, USA
miao86@csail.mit.edu, bonny1986@gmail.com
[2] Boston Children's Hospital, Harvard Medical School, Boston, USA

Abstract. This paper presents an efficient algorithm for large deformation diffeomorphic metric mapping (LDDMM) with geodesic shooting for image registration. We introduce a novel finite dimensional Fourier representation of diffeomorphic deformations based on the key fact that the high frequency components of a diffeomorphism remain stationary throughout the integration process when computing the deformation associated with smooth velocity fields. We show that manipulating high dimensional diffeomorphisms can be carried out entirely in the bandlimited space by integrating the nonstationary low frequency components of the displacement field. This insight substantially reduces the computational cost of the registration problem. Experimental results show that our method is significantly faster than the state-of-the-art diffeomorphic image registration methods while producing equally accurate alignment. We demonstrate our algorithm in two different applications of image registration: neuroimaging and in-utero imaging.

1 Introduction

Diffeomorphisms have been widely used in the field of image registration [6, 7], atlas-based image segmentation [4,10], and anatomical shape analysis [14, 22]. In this paper, we focus on a time-varying velocity field representation for diffeomorphisms as it supplies a distance metric that is critical to statistical analysis of anatomical shapes, for instance, by least squares, geodesic regression, or principal modes detection [13,16,22].

In spite of the advantages of supporting Riemannian metrics in LDDMM, the extremely high computational cost and large memory footprint of the current implementations has limited the use of time-varying velocity representations in important applications that require computational efficiency. The original LDDMM optimization performs gradient decent on the entire time-varying velocity field that is defined on a dense image grid. Since a geodesic is uniquely determined by its initial conditions on the velocity field, the geodesic shooting algorithm has been shown to reduce the computational complexity and improve optimization landscape by manipulating the initial velocity via the geodesic evolution equations [20]. FLASH (finite dimensional Lie algebras for shooting) [23]

© Springer International Publishing AG 2017
M. Niethammer et al. (Eds.): IPMI 2017, LNCS 10265, pp. 559–570, 2017.
DOI: 10.1007/978-3-319-59050-9_44

is a recent variant of LDDMM with geodesic shooting that employs a low dimensional bandlimited representation of the initial velocity field to further improve the convergence and efficiency of the optimization. The algorithm still maps the velocity fields from the low dimensional Fourier space back to the full image domain to perform forward integration at each iteration [23]. The computational complexity of this step thus dominates the entire procedure of diffeomorphic image registration.

Previous works that aimed to improve diffeomorphic representations have reduced the high degrees of freedom available to represent the velocity fields, but not the diffeomorphisms themselves. In this paper, we adopt the low dimensional representation of the tangent space of diffeomorphisms [23] and propose an efficient way to compute diffeomorphisms in the bandlimited space, thus further reducing the computational complexity of image registration. Our approach is based on the important insight that only the low frequency components of the diffeomorphisms vary over time when integrating a bandlimited velocity field to obtain the deformation. Since the optimization of image registration can be directly solved by advecting the inverse of diffeomorphisms [17], we propose a novel Fourier representation of the deformation in the inverse coordinate system that is computed entirely in the low dimensional bandlimited space. The theoretical tools developed in this paper are broadly applicable to other parametrization of diffeomorphic transformations, such as stationary velocity fields [2,3,19]. To evaluate the proposed algorithm, we perform image registration of real 3D MR images and show that the accuracy of the propagated segmentations is comparable to that obtained via the state-of-the-art diffeomorphic image registration methods, while the runtime and the memory demands are dramatically lower for our method. We demonstrate the method in the context of atlas-based segmentation of brain images and of temporal alignment of in-utero MRI scans.

2   Background

Before introducing our development, we provide a brief overview of continuous diffeomorphisms endowed with metrics on vector fields [6,21] and of the finite dimensional Fourier representation of the tangent space of diffeomorphisms [23].

Given an open and bounded d-dimensional domain $\Omega \subset \mathbb{R}^d$, we use $\text{Diff}(\Omega)$ to denote a space of continuous differentiable and inverse differentiable mappings of Ω onto itself. The distance metric between the identity element e and any diffeomorphism ϕ

$$\text{dist}(e, \phi) = \int_0^1 (\mathcal{L}v_t, v_t) \, dt \tag{1}$$

depends on the time-varying Eulerian velocity field v_t ($t \in [0, 1]$) in the tangent space of diffeomorphisms $V = T\text{Diff}(\Omega)$. Here $\mathcal{L} : V \to V^*$ is a symmetric, positive-definite differential operator, e.g., discrete Laplacian, with its inverse $\mathcal{K} : V^* \to V$, and $m_t \in V^*$ is a momentum vector that lies in the dual space V^* such that $m_t = \mathcal{L}v_t$ and $v_t = \mathcal{K}m_t$.

The path of deformation fields ϕ_t parametrized by $t \in [0,1]$ is generated by

$$\frac{d\phi_t}{dt} = v_t \circ \phi_t, \tag{2}$$

where $\circ$ is a composition operator. The inverse mapping of ϕ_t is defined via

$$\frac{d\phi_t^{-1}}{dt} = -D\phi_t^{-1} \cdot v_t, \tag{3}$$

where D is the $d \times d$ Jacobian matrix at each voxel and $\cdot$ is an element-wise multiplication.

The geodesic shooting algorithm estimates the initial velocity at $t = 0$ and relies on the fact that a geodesic path of transformations ϕ_t and its inverse ϕ_t^{-1} with a given initial condition v_0 can be uniquely determined through integrating the Euler-Poincaré differential equation (EPDiff) [1,12] as

$$\frac{\partial v_t}{\partial t} = -\mathcal{K}\left[(Dv_t)^T m_t + Dm_t\, v_t + m_t\, \mathrm{div}(v_t)\right], \tag{4}$$

where div is the divergence operator and $\mathcal{K}$ is a smoothing operator that guarantees the smoothness of the velocity fields.

2.1   Fourier Representation of Velocity Fields

Let $f : \mathbb{R}^d \to \mathbb{R}$ be a real-valued function. The Fourier transform $\mathcal{F}$ of f is given by

$$\mathcal{F}[f](\xi_1, \dots, \xi_d) = \int_{\mathbb{R}^d} f(x_1, \dots, x_d)e^{-2\pi i(x_1\xi_1 + \dots + x_d\xi_d)}\, dx_1, \dots, dx_d, \tag{5}$$

where $(\xi_1, \dots, \xi_d)$ is a d-dimensional frequency vector. The inverse Fourier transform $\mathcal{F}^{-1}$ of a discretized Fourier signal $\tilde{f}$

$$\mathcal{F}^{-1}[\tilde{f}](x_1, \dots, x_d) = \sum_{\xi_1, \dots, \xi_d} \tilde{f}(\xi_1, \dots, \xi_d)e^{2\pi i(\xi_1 x_1 + \dots + \xi_d x_d)} \tag{6}$$

is an approximation of the original signal f. To ensure that $\tilde{f}$ represents a real-valued vector field in the spatial domain, we require $\tilde{f}(\xi_1, \dots, \xi_d) = \tilde{f}^*(-\xi_1, \dots, -\xi_d)$, where $*$ denotes the complex conjugate. When working with vector-valued functions of diffeomorphisms ϕ and velocity fields v, we apply the Fourier transform to each vector component separately.

Since $\mathcal{K}$ is a smoothing operator that suppresses high frequencies in the Fourier domain, the geodesic evolution Eq. (4) suggests that the velocity field v_t can be represented efficiently as a bandlimited signal in Fourier space. Let $\tilde{V}$ denote the discrete Fourier space of velocity fields. As shown in [23], for any two elements $\tilde{v}, \tilde{w} \in \tilde{V}$, the distance metric at identity $\tilde{e}$ is defined as

$$\langle \tilde{u}, \tilde{v} \rangle_{\tilde{V}} = \int (\tilde{\mathcal{L}}\tilde{v}(\xi), \tilde{w}(\xi))d\xi,$$

where $\tilde{\mathcal{L}} : \tilde{V} \mapsto \tilde{V}^*$ is the Fourier transform of a commonly used Laplacian operator $(-\alpha\Delta + e)^c$, with a positive weight parameter α and a smoothness parameter c, i.e.,

$$\tilde{\mathcal{L}}(\xi_1, \ldots, \xi_d) = \left[-2\alpha \sum_{j=1}^{d} (\cos(2\pi\xi_j) - 1) + 1 \right]^c.$$

The Fourier representation of the inverse operator $\mathcal{K} : \tilde{V}^* \mapsto \tilde{V}$ is equal to $\tilde{\mathcal{K}}(\xi_1, \ldots, \xi_d) = \tilde{\mathcal{L}}^{-1}(\xi_1, \ldots, \xi_d)$.

Therefore, the geodesic shooting Eq. (4) can be efficiently computed in a low dimensional bandlimited velocity space:

$$\frac{\partial \tilde{v}_t}{\partial t} = -\tilde{\mathcal{K}} \left[(\tilde{D}\tilde{v}_t)^T \star \tilde{m}_t + \tilde{\nabla} \cdot (\tilde{m}_t \otimes \tilde{v}_t) \right], \tag{7}$$

where $\star$ is the truncated matrix-vector field auto-correlation and $\tilde{D}\tilde{v}_t$ is a tensor product $\tilde{D} \otimes \tilde{v}_t$ with $\tilde{D}(\xi_1, \ldots, \xi_d) = (i\sin(2\pi\xi_1), \ldots, i\sin(2\pi\xi_d))$ representing the Fourier frequencies of a central difference Jacobian matrix D. Operator $\tilde{\nabla}\cdot$ is the discrete divergence of a vector field $\tilde{v}$, which is computed as the sum of the Fourier coefficients of the central difference operator $\tilde{D}$ along each dimension, i.e., $\tilde{\nabla} \cdot (\xi_1, \ldots, \xi_d) = \sum_{j=1}^{d} i\sin(2\pi\xi_j)$.

3   Frequency Diffeomorphisms and Signal Decomposition

While geodesic shooting in the Fourier space (7) is efficient, integrating the ordinary differential Eq. (2) to compute the corresponding diffeomorphism from a velocity field remains computationally intensive. To address this problem, we introduce a Fourier representation of diffeomorphisms that is simple and easy to manipulate in the bandlimited space. The proposed representation promises improved computational efficiency of any algorithm that requires generation of diffeomorphisms from velocity fields.

Analogous to the continuous inverse flow in (3), we define a sequence of time-dependent inverse diffeomorphisms ϕ_t^{-1} in the Fourier domain that consequently generates a path of geodesic flow. Because that the pointwise multiplication of two vector fields in the spatial domain corresponds to convolution in the Fourier domain, we can easily compute the multiplication of a square matrix and a vector field in the Fourier domain as a single convolution for each row of the matrix.

Let $\widetilde{\mathrm{Diff}}(\Omega)$ denote the space of Fourier representations of diffeomorphisms. To simplify the notation, we use $\psi \triangleq \phi^{-1}$ in the remainder of this section. Given time-dependent velocity field $\tilde{v}_t \in \tilde{V}$, the diffeomorphism $\tilde{\psi}_t \in \widetilde{\mathrm{Diff}}(\Omega)$ in the finite-dimensional Fourier domain can be computed as

$$\frac{d\tilde{\psi}_t}{dt} = -\tilde{D}\tilde{\psi}_t * \tilde{v}_t, \tag{8}$$

where $*$ is a circular convolution with zero padding to avoid aliasing. To prevent the domain from growing infinity, we truncate the output of the convolution in each dimension to a suitable finite set.

Representing diffeomorphisms entirely in the Fourier space eliminates the effort of converting their associated velocity fields back and forth from the Fourier domain to the spatial domain. While current implementations of computing a diffeomorphism in (3) have complexity $O(N^d)$ on a full image grid of linear size N, the complexity of naively integrating (8) is $O(N^d \log N)$ if the convolution operator is implemented via fast Fourier transform (FFT) [18]. Here we show how to reduce the complexity of (8) via frequency decomposition of the deformations.

In particular, we consider a representation $\tilde{\psi} = \tilde{e} + \tilde{u}$, where $\tilde{e}$ is the Fourier transform of the identity transformation, and $\tilde{u}$ is the Fourier transform of the displacement field. We can now isolate the frequency response of the identity transformation in (8) as follows:

$$\frac{d\tilde{\psi}_t}{dt} = -\tilde{D}(\tilde{e} + \tilde{u}_t) * \tilde{v}_t = -\tilde{D}\tilde{e} * \tilde{v}_t - \tilde{D}\tilde{u}_t * \tilde{v}_t. \tag{9}$$

Since $De \cdot v_t = v_t$ in the spatial domain, we have

$$\tilde{D}\tilde{e} * \tilde{v}_t = \mathcal{F}(De \cdot v_t) = \mathcal{F}(v_t) = \tilde{v}_t. \tag{10}$$

Substituting (10) into (9), we arrive at

$$\frac{d\tilde{\psi}_t}{dt} = -\tilde{v}_t - \tilde{D}\tilde{u}_t * \tilde{v}_t \quad \text{with} \quad \tilde{\psi}_0 = \tilde{e}, \qquad \text{or}$$

$$\tilde{u}_t = -\int_0^t \tilde{v}_\tau + \tilde{D}\tilde{u}_\tau * \tilde{v}_\tau \, d\tau \quad \text{with} \quad \tilde{u}_0 = 0. \tag{11}$$

Importantly, we observe that the high frequency components of the diffeomorphisms that come from the initial condition $\tilde{\psi}_0 = \tilde{e}$ remain unchanged, and only low frequency components vary throughout the integration. Moreover, the evolution scheme for geodesic shooting in the Fourier domain (7) indeed maintains $\tilde{v}_t$ as a bandlimited signal. The truncated convolution operation does not introduce high frequencies if the displacement $\tilde{u}_t$ is also bandlimited. Figure 1 illustrates a 1D example of the integration (11).

The initial condition $\tilde{\psi}_0 = \tilde{e}$ corresponds to $\tilde{u}_0 = 0$. We first integrate (11) for bandlimited low frequency components of the signal and then add the high frequency components back. Therefore we have

$$\text{for } \xi \leqslant \eta, \ \tilde{u}_t(\xi) = -\int_0^t \tilde{v}_\tau(\xi) + \tilde{D}\tilde{u}_\tau(\xi) * \tilde{v}_\tau(\xi) \, d\tau,$$

$$\text{for } \xi > \eta, \ \tilde{u}_t(\xi) = 0, \tag{12}$$

where $\xi = (\xi_1, \ldots, \xi_d)$ and $\eta = (\eta_1, \ldots, \eta_d)$ is the vector of upper bounds on the frequency in the bandlimited representation of ψ.

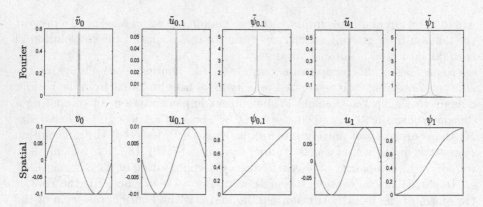

Fig. 1. A 1D example of an initial velocity v_0 as a sinusoid function and the resulting displacement field u_t and diffeomorphism ψ_t at $t = 0.1$ and $t = 1$. Both Fourier (red) and spatial (blue) representations are shown. (Color figure online)

3.1   Frequency Diffeomorphisms for Image Registration

In this section, we present a diffeomorphic image registration algorithm based on geodesic shooting that is carried out entirely in the Fourier space.

Let S be the source image and T be the target image defined on a torus domain $\Gamma = \mathbb{R}^d/\mathbb{Z}^d$ ($S(x), T(x) : \Gamma \to \mathbb{R}$). The problem of diffeomorphic image registration is to find the shortest path of diffeomorphisms $\psi_t \in \text{Diff}(\Gamma) : \Gamma \to \Gamma, t \in [0, 1]$ such that $S \circ \psi_1$ is similar to T, where $\circ$ is a composition operator that resamples S by the smooth mapping ψ_1. LDDMM with geodesic shooting [20] leads to a gradient decent optimization of an explicit energy function

$$E(v_0) = \frac{\lambda}{2} \, \text{dist}(S \circ \psi_1, T) + \frac{1}{2} \|v_0\|_V^2 \tag{13}$$

under the constraints (2) and (4). The distance function $\text{dist}(\cdot, \cdot)$ measures the dissimilarity between images. Commonly used distance metrics include sum-of-squared difference (L^2-norm) of image intensities, normalized cross correlation (NCC), and mutual information (MI). Here $\lambda > 0$ is a weight parameter.

The energy function in the finite-dimensional Fourier space can be equivalently formulated as

$$E(\tilde{v}_0) = \frac{\lambda}{2} \, \text{dist}(S \circ \psi_1, T) + \frac{1}{2} \|\tilde{v}_0\|_{\tilde{V}}^2 \tag{14}$$

with the new constraints (7) and (8).

We use a gradient decent algorithm on the initial velocity $\tilde{v}_0$ to estimate the path of diffeomorphic flow $\{\tilde{\psi}_t\}$ entirely in the bandlimited space. Beginning with the initialization $\tilde{v}_0 = 0$, the gradient of the energy (14) is computed via two steps below:

1. Compute the gradient $\nabla_{\tilde{v}_1} E$ of the energy (14) at $t = 1$. This requires integrating both the diffeomorphism $\tilde{\psi}_t$ and the velocity field $\tilde{v}_t$ forward in time, and then mapping $\tilde{\psi}_1$ to the spatial domain to obtain ψ_1. Formally,

$$\nabla_{\tilde{v}_1} E = \mathcal{K} \mathcal{F} \left(\frac{\partial \operatorname{dist}(S \circ \psi_1, T)}{\partial (S \circ \psi_1)} \cdot \nabla(S \circ \psi_1) \right). \qquad (15)$$

2. Bring the gradient $\nabla_{\tilde{v}_1} E$ in (15) back to $t = 0$ by reduced adjoint Jacobi field equations [8,23]. Integrate the reduced adjoint Jacobi field equations

$$\frac{d\hat{v}}{dt} = -\operatorname{ad}_{\tilde{v}}^{\dagger} \hat{h}, \qquad \frac{d\hat{h}}{dt} = -\hat{v} - \operatorname{ad}_{\tilde{v}} \hat{h} + \operatorname{ad}_{\hat{h}}^{\dagger} \tilde{v} \qquad (16)$$

in $\tilde{V}$ to get the gradient update $\nabla_{\tilde{v}_0} E$, where $\operatorname{ad}^{\dagger}$ is an adjoint operator and $\hat{v}, \hat{h} \in \tilde{V}$ are introduced adjoint variables.

The algorithm is summarized below.

Algorithm 1. Frequency diffeomorphisms for image registration

---

Input: source image S, target image T.
Initialize $\tilde{v}_0 = 0$.
repeat
    (a) Integrate (7) to compute $\tilde{v}_t$ at discrete time points $t = [0, \ldots, 1]$.
    (b) Integrate (8) to generate $\tilde{\psi}_t$.
    (c_i) Convert $\tilde{\psi}_1$ back to the spatial domain to transport the source image S.
    (c_{ii}) Compute the gradient $\nabla_{\tilde{v}_1} E$ (15) at time point $t = 1$.
    (d) Integrate $\nabla_{\tilde{v}_1} E$ backward in time via (16) to obtain $\nabla_{\tilde{v}_0} E$.
    (e) Update $\tilde{v}_0 \leftarrow \tilde{v}_0 - \delta \nabla_{\tilde{v}_0} E$, where δ is the step size.
until convergence

Computational Complexity. It has previously been shown that the complexity of steps (a) and (d) is $O(Tn^d)$, where T is the number of time steps in the integration and n is the truncated dimension in the bandlimited space. The complexity of the current methods for computing diffeomorphisms in the high-dimensional image space via (2) is $O(TN^d)$. In contrast, our algorithm reduces the complexity of this step to $O(Tn^d)$ (step (b)). To transport the images and measure the image dissimilarity at $t = 1$, we convert the transformation $\tilde{\psi}_1$ into the spatial domain via FFT ($O(N^d \log N)$) (step (c_i)). While the theoretical complexity of FFT is higher than

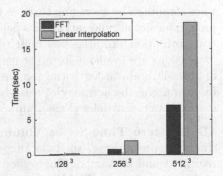

Fig. 2. Exact run-time of FFT (blue) and linear interpolation (yellow). (Color figure online)

the complexity of computing $S \circ \psi_1^{-1}$, which is $O(N^d)$, its empirical runtime for N a power of 2 is quite low by comparison. Figure 2 reports the empirical runtime of FFT and of linear interpolation for different image grid sizes ($N = 2^7, 2^8, 2^9$) as used by the current methods and ours to transport S. We note that the linear interpolation requires more than twice the amount of time than that of FFT.

4   Experimental Evaluation

To evaluate the proposed approach, we perform registration-based segmentation and examine the resulting segmentation accuracy, runtime and memory consumption of the algorithm. We compare the proposed method with the diffeomorphic demons implementation in ANTS software package [5] and the state-of-the-art fast geodesic shooting for LDDMM method FLASH [23] (downloaded from: https://bitbucket.org/FlashC/flashc). In all experiments, we set $\alpha = 1.5, c = 3.0, \lambda = 1.0e4$ and $T = 10$ for the time integration. A normalized cross correlation (NCC) metric for image dissimilarity and a multi-resolution optimization scheme with three levels are used in all three methods. To evaluate volume overlap between the propagated segmentation A and the manual segmentation B for each structure, we compute the Dice Similarity Coefficient $DSC(A, B) = 2(|A| \cap |B|)/(|A| + |B|)$ where $\cap$ denotes an intersection of two regions.

4.1   Data

We evaluate the method on 3D brain MRI scans [9] and 4D in-utero MRI time series [11].

3D Brain MRI. Thirty six brain MRI scans (T1-weighted MP-RAGE) were acquired in normal subjects and patients with Alzhimer's disease across a broad age range. The MRI images are of dimension 256^3, 1 mm isotropic voxels and were computed by averaging three or four scans. All scans underwent skull stripping, intensity normalization, bias field correction, and co-registration with affine transformation. An atlas was built from 20 images as a reference. Manual segmentations are available for all scans in the set. We perform image registration of the 3D brain atlas to the remaining 16 subjects. We evaluate registration by examining the accuracy of atlas-based delineations for white matter (WM), cortex (Cor), ventricles (Vent), hippocampus (Hipp), and caudate (Caud).

4D In-Utero Time-Series Volumetric MRI. Ten pregnant women (three singleton pregnancies, six twin pregnancies, and one triplet pregnancy) were recruited and consented. Single-shot GRE-EPI image series were acquired for each woman on a 3T MR scanner (Skyra Siemens, 18-channel body and 12-channel spine receive arrays, 3×3 mm^2 in-plane resolution, 3 mm slice thickness, interleaved slice acquisition, TR $= 5.8 - 8$ s, TE $= 32 - 36$ ms, FA $= 90°$). Odd and even slices of each volume were resampled onto an isotropic 3 mm^3 image grid to reduce the effects of interleaved acquisition. Each series includes

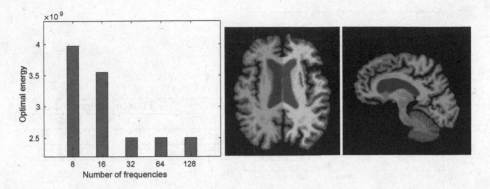

Fig. 3. Left: average final energy for different values of the truncated dimension $n = 8, 16, \ldots, 128$. Right: example propagated segmentation with 35 structures obtained by our method. 2D slices are shown for visualization only, all computations are carried out fully in 3D.

around 300 3D volumes. The placentae (total of 10) and fetal brains (total of 18) were manually delineated in the reference template and in five additional volumes in each series. When applying our method to in-utero MRI, we use it as part of sequential registration of the consecutive frames in the scan series. Each series requires about 300 consecutive image registration steps over time.

4.2   Results

3D Brain MRI. Figure 3 reports the total energy (14) averaged over 16 test images for different values of truncated dimension $n = 8, 16, \cdots, 128$. Our method arrives at the same solution at $n = 32$ and higher. For the remainder of this section, we use $n = 32$ to illustrate the results. An example segmentation obtained by our algorithm is also illustrated in Fig. 3. Figure 4 reports the volume overlap of segmentations for our method and the two baseline algorithms. All three algorithms produce comparable segmentation accuracy. The difference is not statistically significant in a paired t-test for each labelled structure ($p = 0.369$). Our algorithm has substantially lower computational cost than ANTS and FLASH. Figure 4 also provides runtime and memory consumption across all methods.

4D In-Utero Time-Series Volumetric MRI. Similar to the previous experiment, we cross-validated the optimal truncated dimension n at different scales and set $n = 16$ for the 4D in-utero time series. Once all the volumes in the series are aligned, we transform the manual segmentations in the first volume to other volumes in each series by using the estimated deformations. Figure 5 illustrates results for an example case from the study. We observe that the delineations achieved by transferring manual segmentations from the reference frame to the coordinate system of the target frame 25 align fairly well with the manual segmentations. Figure 6 reports segmentation volume overlap for the fetal brains

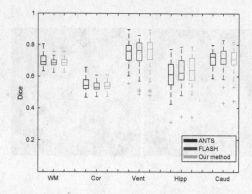

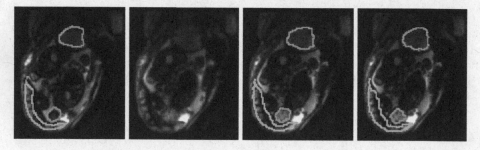

Fig. 4. Left: volume overlap between atlas-based and manual segmentations for five important regions (white matter, cortex, ventricles, hippocampus, and caudate) estimated via ANTS (black), FLASH (blue), and our method (red). Right: Runtime and memory consumption per image for all three methods. (Color figure online)

Model	Time(h)	Memory(MB)
ANTS	2.1	4885
FLASH	0.5	3375
Our method	**0.3**	**3083**

Fig. 5. An example case from the in-utero MRI study. Left to right: source with manual segmentation, deformed source, target with manual segmentation, and target with propagated segmentations for the fetal brains (green) and placenta (pink). 2D slices of axial view are shown for visualization only, all computations are carried out fully in 3D. (Color figure online)

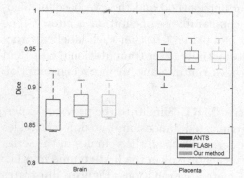

Model	Time(h)	Memory(MB)
ANTS	96.75	253.62
FLASH	37.75	109.52
Our method	**27.00**	**67.32**

Fig. 6. Left: volume overlap between transferred and manual segmentations of fetal brains and placenta averaged over all subjects. Statistics are reported for ANTS (black), FLASH (blue), and our method (red). Right: Runtime and memory consumption of 300 registrations for all three algorithms. (Color figure online)

and placenta, as well as the time and memory consumption for our method and the two baseline algorithms. Again, our algorithm achieves comparable results (paired t-test $p = 0.4671$) while offering significant improvements in computational efficiency.

5 Conclusion

We presented an efficient way to compute diffeomorphisms in the setting of LDDMM with geodesic shooting for image registration. Our method is the first to represent diffeomorphisms in the Fourier space, which provides a way to compute transformations from the associated velocity fields entirely in the low dimensional bandlimited space. This approach reduces the computational cost of the algorithms without loss in accuracy. The theoretical tools employed in this work are not only broadly applicable to other representations of diffeomorphic transformations such as stationary velocity fields, but also to the standard path optimization strategy in the original LDDMM. Our method can be naturally interpreted as operating with the left-invariant metric on the space of diffeomorphisms [15], which accepts spatially-varying smoothing kernels in special image registration scenarios where different regularizations are required at different locations. Future research will explore more of numerical analysis, as well as its theoretical connection and implications for diffeomorphic image registration.

Acknowledgments. This work was supported by NIH NIBIB NAC P41EB015902, NIH NINDS R01NS086905, NIH NICHD U01HD087211, and Wistron Corporation.

References

1. Arnol'd, V.I.: Sur la géométrie différentielle des groupes de Lie de dimension infinie et ses applications à l'hydrodynamique des fluides parfaits. Ann. Inst. Fourier **16**, 319–361 (1966)
2. Arsigny, V., Commowick, O., Pennec, X., Ayache, N.: A log-Euclidean framework for statistics on diffeomorphisms. In: Larsen, R., Nielsen, M., Sporring, J. (eds.) MICCAI 2006. LNCS, vol. 4190, pp. 924–931. Springer, Heidelberg (2006). doi:10. 1007/11866565_113
3. Ashburner, J.: A fast diffeomorphic image registration algorithm. Neuroimage **38**(1), 95–113 (2007)
4. Ashburner, J., Friston, K.J.: Unified segmentation. Neuroimage **26**(3), 839–851 (2005)
5. Avants, B.B., Epstein, C.L., Grossman, M., Gee, J.C.: Symmetric diffeomorphic image registration with cross-correlation: evaluating automated labeling of elderly and neurodegenerative brain. Med. Image Anal. **12**(1), 26–41 (2008)
6. Beg, M., Miller, M., Trouvé, A., Younes, L.: Computing large deformation metric mappings via geodesic flows of diffeomorphisms. Int. J. Comput. Vis. **61**(2), 139–157 (2005)
7. Christensen, G.E., Rabbitt, R.D., Miller, M.I.: Deformable templates using large deformation kinematics. IEEE Tran. Image Process. **5**(10), 1435–1447 (1996)

8. Francesco, B.: Invariant affine connections and controllability on lie groups. Technical report for Geometric Mechanics, California Institute of Technology (1995)
9. Johnson, K.A., Jones, K., Holman, B.L., Becker, J.A., Spiers, P.A., Satlin, A., Albert, M.S.: Preclinical prediction of Alzheimer's disease using spect. Neurology 50(6), 1563–1571 (1998)
10. Joshi, S., Davis, B., Jomier, M., Gerig, G.: Unbiased diffeomorphic atlas construction for computational anatomy. NeuroImage 23(Supplement 1), 151–160 (2004)
11. Liao, R., Turk, E.A., Zhang, M., Luo, J., Grant, P.E., Adalsteinsson, E., Golland, P.: Temporal registration in in-utero volumetric MRI time series. In: Ourselin, S., Joskowicz, L., Sabuncu, M.R., Unal, G., Wells, W. (eds.) MICCAI 2016. LNCS, vol. 9902, pp. 54–62. Springer, Cham (2016). doi:10.1007/978-3-319-46726-9_7
12. Miller, M.I., Trouvé, A., Younes, L.: Geodesic shooting for computational anatomy. J. Math. Imaging Vis. 24(2), 209–228 (2006)
13. Niethammer, M., Huang, Y., Vialard, F.-X.: Geodesic regression for image time-series. In: Fichtinger, G., Martel, A., Peters, T. (eds.) MICCAI 2011. LNCS, vol. 6892, pp. 655–662. Springer, Heidelberg (2011). doi:10.1007/978-3-642-23629-7_80
14. Qiu, A., Younes, L., Miller, M.I.: Principal component based diffeomorphic surface mapping. Med. Imaging IEEE Trans. 31(2), 302–311 (2012)
15. Schmah, T., Risser, L., Vialard, F.X.: Diffeomorphic image matching with left-invariant metrics. In: Chang, D.E., Holm, D.D., Patrick, G., Ratiu, T. (eds.) Geometry, Mechanics, and Dynamics, pp. 373–392. Springer, New york (2015)
16. Singh, N., Fletcher, P.T., Preston, J.S., Ha, L., King, R., Marron, J.S., Wiener, M., Joshi, S.: Multivariate statistical analysis of deformation momenta relating anatomical shape to neuropsychological measures. In: Jiang, T., Navab, N., Pluim, J.P.W., Viergever, M.A. (eds.) MICCAI 2010. LNCS, vol. 6363, pp. 529–537. Springer, Heidelberg (2010). doi:10.1007/978-3-642-15711-0_66
17. Singh, N., Vialard, F.X., Niethammer, M.: Splines for diffeomorphisms. Med. Image Anal. 25(1), 56–71 (2015)
18. Van Loan, C.: Computational Frameworks for the Fast Fourier Transform, vol. 10. SIAM, Philadelphia (1992)
19. Vercauteren, T., Pennec, X., Perchant, A., Ayache, N.: Diffeomorphic demons: efficient non-parametric image registration. NeuroImage 45(1), S61–S72 (2009)
20. Vialard, F.X., Risser, L., Rueckert, D., Cotter, C.J.: Diffeomorphic 3D image registration via geodesic shooting using an efficient adjoint calculation. Int. J. Comput. Vis. 97, 229–241 (2012)
21. Younes, L., Arrate, F., Miller, M.: Evolutions equations in computational anatomy. NeuroImage 45(1S1), 40–50 (2009)
22. Zhang, M., Fletcher, P.T.: Bayesian principal geodesic analysis in diffeomorphic image registration. In: Golland, P., Hata, N., Barillot, C., Hornegger, J., Howe, R. (eds.) MICCAI 2014. LNCS, vol. 8675, pp. 121–128. Springer, Cham (2014). doi:10.1007/978-3-319-10443-0_16
23. Zhang, M., Fletcher, P.T.: Finite-dimensional lie algebras for fast diffeomorphic image registration. In: Ourselin, S., Alexander, D.C., Westin, C.-F., Cardoso, M.J. (eds.) IPMI 2015. LNCS, vol. 9123, pp. 249–260. Springer, Cham (2015). doi:10.1007/978-3-319-19992-4_19

A Stochastic Large Deformation Model for Computational Anatomy

Alexis Arnaudon[1], Darryl D. Holm[1], Akshay Pai[2], and Stefan Sommer[2(✉)]

[1] Depatment of Mathematics Imperial College London, SW7 2AZ London, UK
[2] Department of Computer Science (DIKU), University of Copenhagen, Copenhagen, Denmark
sommer@di.ku.dk

Abstract. In the study of shapes of human organs using computational anatomy, variations are found to arise from inter-subject anatomical differences, disease-specific effects, and measurement noise. This paper introduces a stochastic model for incorporating random variations into the Large Deformation Diffeomorphic Metric Mapping (LDDMM) framework. By accounting for randomness in a particular setup which is crafted to fit the geometrical properties of LDDMM, we formulate the template estimation problem for landmarks with noise and give two methods for efficiently estimating the parameters of the noise fields from a prescribed data set. One method directly approximates the time evolution of the variance of each landmark by a finite set of differential equations, and the other is based on an Expectation-Maximisation algorithm. In the second method, the evaluation of the data likelihood is achieved without registering the landmarks, by applying bridge sampling using a stochastically perturbed version of the large deformation gradient flow algorithm. The method and the estimation algorithms are experimentally validated on synthetic examples and shape data of human corpora callosa.

Keywords: Computational anatomy · Stochastic processes · Large deformations · LDDMM

1 Introduction

Computational anatomy (CA) concerns the modelling and computational analysis of shapes of human organs. In CA, observed shapes or images of shapes exhibit variations due to multiple factors, such as inter-subject anatomical differences, disease-specific effects, and measurement noise. These variations in anatomy occur naturally over all populations and they must be handled in cross-sectional studies. In addition, neurodegenerative diseases such as Alzheimer's disease can cause temporal shape changes as the disease progresses. Finally, image acquisition and processing algorithms for extracting shape information can cause measurement variation in the estimated shapes. While variation can be incorporated into shape models via different approaches, e.g. via random initial conditions as

© Springer International Publishing AG 2017
M. Niethammer et al. (Eds.): IPMI 2017, LNCS 10265, pp. 571–582, 2017.
DOI: 10.1007/978-3-319-59050-9_45

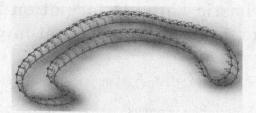

Fig. 1. Sample from bridge process (green lines) conditioned on two corpus callosum shapes (blue). The landmarks are influenced by noise with spatial correlation structure determined by the noise fields σ_l. The bridge is constructed by integrating the perturbed gradient flow described in Sect. 4.3. The shaded background indicates the shape variations in the transition distribution of the stochastic model. (Color figure online)

in the random orbit model [12] or in a mixed-effects setting [1], most models specify random variation relative to a base object, usually a template, and they involve some form of linearization. Here we will model these variations by inserting stochasticity directly into the nonlinear dynamics of shape transformations using Large Deformation Diffeomorphic Metric Mapping (LDDMM) [16]. In this paper, we use the approach of [2], based on the stochastic fluid models of [8], to introduce a model for incorporating stochastic variation into the shape deformation paths. This approach is particularly designed to be compatible with four geometric properties of LDDMM. Namely, (1) the noise is right-invariant in the same way as the LDDMM metric is right-invariant. (2) Evolution equations arise as extremal paths for a stochastic variational principle. (3) The Euler-Poincaré (EPDiff) equations in the deterministic case have stochastic versions. (4) Remarkably, the momentum maps arising via reduction by symmetry, and used to reduce dimensionality from the infinite-dimensional diffeomorphism group to finite-dimensional shape spaces, such as landmarks in deterministic LDDMM, still persist in this stochastic geometric setting. On top of that, our method permits a total control on the spatial correlation of the noise, independently of for example the data structure or the number of landmarks.

Plan. After a description of large deformation models in Sect. 2 and the LDDMM framework, we discuss the model of [2] in the CA context and use it to develop the stochastic equations for the landmark trajectories in Sect. 3. We then formulate two approaches for estimating the noise fields and initial momentum from prescribed data in Sect. 4. The first approach is a deterministic approximation of the Fokker-Planck equation with matching of moments of the probability distribution. The second is an Energy-Maximization (EM) algorithm which requires sampling of diffusion bridges to estimate data likelihood by sampling bridges without registering or matching the landmarks. From the bridge simulation scheme, we obtain (see Fig. 1) a stochastic version of the large deformation gradient flow algorithm, see e.g. [16]. Finally, we validate the approach in experiments on synthetic and real data in Sect. 5 before.

2   Background

This section briefly reviews large deformation shape modelling and LDDMM, referring to the monograph [16] for full details. A shape, defined as either a subset $s \subset \mathbb{R}^d$, $d = 2, 3$, or an image $I : \mathbb{R}^d \to \mathbb{R}$ can be modified by warping the domain $\mathbb{R}^d$ under the action of a diffeomorphism $\varphi : \mathbb{R}^d \to \mathbb{R}^d$. The diffeomorphism φ naturally acts on the left on a shape s by $\varphi.s = \varphi(s)$. For images, a left-action is obtained by letting $\varphi.I = I \circ \varphi^{-1}$. Changes in shape are then represented by an element $\varphi \in G_V \subset \mathrm{Diff}(\mathbb{R}^d)$ in the diffeomorphism group. The subset G_V is obtained as endpoints of flows

$$\partial_t \varphi_t(x) = v_t \circ \varphi_t(x), \ t \in [0, T] \tag{1}$$

where $v_t \in V$ is a time-dependent vector field contained in a space $V \subset \mathfrak{X}(\mathbb{R}^d)$. V is typically a reproducing kernel Hilbert space (RKHS) with inner product $\langle \cdot, \cdot \rangle_V$ defined in terms of a reproducing kernel $K_V : \mathbb{R}^d \times \mathbb{R}^d \to \mathbb{R}^{d \times d}$ and with corresponding momentum operator $L_V : V \to L^2$. Under reasonable assumptions, the RKHS structure defines a Riemannian metric on G_V by right-invariance, i.e. by defining $\langle v_\varphi, w_\varphi \rangle_\varphi = \langle v_\varphi \circ \varphi^{-1}, w_\varphi \circ \varphi^{-1} \rangle_V$ for tangent vectors $v_\varphi, w_\varphi \in T_\varphi G_V$. The corresponding Riemannian metric is

$$d_{G_V}(\varphi, \psi)^2 = \min_{v_t, \varphi_0 = \varphi, \varphi_1 = \psi} \int_0^T \|v_t\|_{\varphi_t}^2 dt \tag{2}$$

where φ_t evolves according to (1). Elements of G_V act on shapes, and d_{G_V} descends to shape spaces by $d_S(s_1, s_2) = \min_{\varphi.s_1 = s_2} d_{G_V}(\mathrm{Id}, \varphi)$ and similarly for images. Shapes can be matched by finding a minimising φ in this equation. In inexact matching of shapes, the distance is weighted against a dissimilarity measure. For images, the inexact matching problem becomes $\varphi_{\min} = \mathrm{argmin}\, E(I_1, I_2, \varphi)$, where $E(I_1, I_2, \varphi) = d_{G_V}(\mathrm{Id}, \varphi)^2 + \lambda S(\varphi.I_1, I_2)$. Here $\lambda > 0$ controls the dissimilarity penalty, and S is the dissimilarity measure, e.g. the L^2 difference $S(I_1, I_2) = \int_{\mathbb{R}^d} |I_1(x) - I_2(x)|^2 dx$. Optimal paths in the LDDMM framework satisfy the EPDiff equation $\partial_t m = -\mathrm{ad}_u^* m$, where $m = L_V u$ and ad^* is the coadjoint action on the dual of the Lie algebra of vector fields on the plane, see [9] for more details.

For a set of N landmarks $\mathbf{q} \in \mathbb{R}^{dN}$ at positions $q_1, \ldots, q_N \in \mathbb{R}^d$ with momentum $\mathbf{p} = (p_1, \cdots, p_N) \in \mathbb{R}^{dN}$, the singular momentum map of [9] is given by $m(x, t) = \sum_i p_i(t)\delta(\mathbf{x} - \mathbf{q}_i(t))$. The corresponding deformation velocity can be written as $u(x, t) = K_V * m = \sum_i p_i K_V(x - q_i)$. The ODE for the positions and momentum are the canonical Hamiltonian equations $\dot{\mathbf{q}}_i = \frac{\partial h}{\partial \mathbf{p}_i}$ and $\dot{\mathbf{p}}_i = -\frac{\partial h}{\partial \mathbf{q}_i}$, with Hamiltonian $h(p, q) = \frac{1}{2} \sum_{i,j=1}^N p_i \cdot p_j K_V(q_i - q_j)$. In 1D, these equations go back to the dynamics of singular solutions of the Camassa-Holm equation [4].

3   Stochastic Landmark Dynamics

Stochastic differential equations (SDEs) have previously been considered in context of LDDMM by [5, 14, 15]. More recently [11] introduced a stochastic landmark model with dissipation in the momentum equation which corresponds to a

Langevin equation. This allowed then to use the technology of statistical mechanics and Gibbs measure to study this stochastic system. We will use here the stochastic model of [2], based on the fluid models of [8]. The noise is introduced in the reconstruction relation (1) with J fields $\sigma_l : \mathbb{R}^d \to V$ as

$$d\varphi_t \circ \varphi_t^{-1}(x) = v_t(x)dt + \sum_{l=1}^{J} \sigma_l(x) \circ dW_t^l. \qquad (3)$$

The symbol d denotes stochastic evolution and ($\circ$), when adjacent to the process dW_t^l, means stochastic integrals are interpreted in the Stratonovich sense. Given a realisation of the noise, we impose the stochastic dynamics (3) and seek the φ_t that minimises the cost functional in (2). A short computation gives the stochastic EPDiff equation $dm + \text{ad}_v^* m dt + \sum_i \text{ad}_{\sigma_i}^* m \circ dW_t^i = 0$. The landmarks can be introduced and their stochastic ODE dynamics are given by

$$
\begin{aligned}
d\mathbf{q}_i &= \frac{\partial h}{\partial \mathbf{p}_i} dt + \sum_{l=1}^{J} \sigma_l(\mathbf{q}_i) \circ dW_t^l \\
d\mathbf{p}_i &= -\frac{\partial h}{\partial \mathbf{q}_i} dt - \sum_{l=1}^{J} \frac{\partial}{\partial \mathbf{q}_i} \left(\mathbf{p}_i \cdot \sigma_l(\mathbf{q}_i) \right) \circ dW_t^l.
\end{aligned}
\qquad (4)
$$

This is a Hamiltonian stochastic process in the sense of Bismut [3], where the stochastic extensions of the Hamiltonian, or stochastic potentials, are the momentum maps $\Phi_l(\mathbf{q}, \mathbf{p}) = \sum_i \mathbf{p}_i \cdot \sigma_l(\mathbf{q}_i)$ whose Hamilton equations generate the cotangent lift of the stochastic infinitesimal transformations of the landmark paths. In the following, we will only consider exact landmark matching, and refer to [2] for more details about the derivation of these equations which also includes the case of inexact matching. The noise can be seen as almost additive in the position equation, and it couples to the momentum with the gradient of the field $\sigma_l(\mathbf{q}_i)$ in the momentum equation. This last term ensures that the solution corresponds to a stochastic path in the diffeomorphism group. By comparison with previous works such as [11,14,15], this model has its noise amplitudes σ_l fixed to the domain, and not to each landmark. The noise is relative to a Eulerian frame and is right-invariant similar to the metric. Notice that the present approach is different from random initial conditions such as studied in [17].

3.1   The Fokker-Planck Equation

For each time t, we will denote the transition probability density by $\mathbb{P}(\mathbf{q}, \mathbf{p}, t)$, a function $\mathbb{P} : \mathbb{R}^{2dN} \to \mathbb{R}$ which integrates to 1 and represents the probability of finding the stochastic process at a given position in the phase space. For a given initial distribution $\mathbb{P}_0$, it is possible to compute the partial differential equation which governs the evolution of $\mathbb{P}$ in time. With the Hamiltonian bracket $\{F, G\}_{\text{can}} = \sum_i \frac{\partial F}{\partial q_i} \frac{\partial G}{\partial p_i} - \sum_i \frac{\partial F}{\partial p_i} \frac{\partial G}{\partial q_i}$, we compute the Fokker-Planck equation

$$\frac{d}{dt} \mathbb{P} = \{\mathbb{P}, h\}_{\text{can}} + \frac{1}{2} \sum_{l=1}^{J} \{\Phi_l, \{\Phi_l, \mathbb{P}\}_{\text{can}}\}_{\text{can}}. \qquad (5)$$

The right-hand side of this equation has two parts, the first is an advection with first order derivatives of $\mathbb{P}$, arising from the deterministic Hamiltonian dynamics of the landmarks. The second part is a diffusion term with second order derivatives of $\mathbb{P}$ which arises only from the noise. This is the term which will describe the error in each landmark path subject to noise.

3.2   Equivalent Formulation with 'Lagrangian Noise'

The covariance between the stochastic displacements $d\mathbf{q}_i$, $d\mathbf{q}_j$ conditioned on the position of two landmarks $\mathbf{q}_i$, $\mathbf{q}_j$ may be computed as

$$\text{Cov}(d\mathbf{q}_i|\mathbf{q}_i, d\mathbf{q}_j|\mathbf{q}_j) = \sum_l \sigma_l(\mathbf{q}_i|\mathbf{q}_i)\sigma_l(\mathbf{q}_j|\mathbf{q}_j)\text{Var}(dW_t^l),$$

where $\text{Var}(dW_t^l)$ is the variance of the l-th Brownian motion dW_t^l. Thus, for a finite time discretization of the process in Itô form and an increment $\Delta = [t_1, t_2]$, $\text{Cov}(\Delta\mathbf{q}_i|\mathbf{q}_i, \Delta\mathbf{q}_j|\mathbf{q}_j) = \sum_l \sigma_l(\mathbf{q}_i|\mathbf{q}_i)\sigma_l(\mathbf{q}_j|\mathbf{q}_j)(t_2-t_1)$. The stochastic differential $d\mathbf{q}$ can therefore formally be viewed as a Gaussian process on $\mathbb{R}^d$. The $dN \times dN$ matrix $\sigma^2(\mathbf{q}) = \sum_l [\sigma_l(\mathbf{q}_i)\sigma_l(\mathbf{q}_j)]_j^i$ is symmetric. If $\sigma^2(\mathbf{q})$ is positive definite, we let $K(\mathbf{q})$ be a square root, i.e. $\sigma^2(\mathbf{q}) = K(\mathbf{q})K(\mathbf{q})^T$. The following stochastic landmark dynamics is then equivalent to the original dynamics (4)

$$
\begin{aligned}
d\mathbf{q}_i &= \frac{\partial h}{\partial \mathbf{p}_i}dt + \sum_{j,\alpha} K(\mathbf{q})_{j,\alpha}^i \circ dW_t^j \\
d\mathbf{p}_i &= -\frac{\partial h}{\partial \mathbf{q}_i}dt - \sum_{j,\alpha} \frac{\partial}{\partial \mathbf{q}_i}\left(\mathbf{p}_i \cdot K(\mathbf{q})_{j,\alpha}^i\right) \circ dW_t^{j,\alpha},
\end{aligned}
\tag{6}
$$

where j runs on the landmarks and α the spatial dimensions. Note that in (6), $W_t \in \mathbb{R}^{dN}$ as compared to $\mathbb{R}^J$ previously. With this approach, instead of starting with the spatial noise fields $\sigma_1, \ldots, \sigma_J$, we can specify the stochastic system directly in terms of the matrix $K(\mathbf{q})$. One natural choice is to set $[K(\mathbf{q})]_j^i = \text{Id}_d k(\mathbf{q}_i - \mathbf{q}_j)$ for some scalar kernel k and where Id_d is the $d \times d$ identity matrix. The possible reduction in dimensionality of the noise from J to dN has computational benefits that we will exploit in the following.

4   Estimation of Noise and Initial Conditions

We now aim for estimating a set of parameters for the model from N sets of observed landmarks $\mathbf{q}_1, \ldots, \mathbf{q}_N$ at time T. The parameters can be both parameters for the noise fields as described below and the initial landmark configuration $\mathbf{q}_0$ and momentum $\mathbf{p}_0$. The initial configuration $\mathbf{q}_0$ can be considered an estimated template of the dataset. The template will be optimal in the sense of reproducing the moments of the distribution or in being fitted by maximum likelihood. We use spatial noise fields $\sigma_1, \ldots, \sigma_J$ of the form

$$\sigma_l^\alpha(\mathbf{q}_i) = \lambda_l^\alpha k(\|\mathbf{q}_i - \delta_l\|),\tag{7}$$

where $\lambda_l \in \mathbb{R}^d$ is the spacial direction of the noise σ_l, δ_l its centre, and the kernel k is either Gaussian $k(x) = e^{-x^2/(2r_l^2)}$ or cubic B-spline $k(x) = S_3(x/r_l)$ with scale r_l. The Gaussian kernels simplify calculations of the moment equations. The B-spline representation has the advantage of providing a partition of unity when used in a grid. The model is not limited to this set of noise functions.

4.1 Matching of Moments

Our first method relies on the Fokker-Planck equation of the landmarks and aims at minimising the cost functional

$$C(\langle \mathbf{p} \rangle (0), \lambda_l) = \frac{1}{\gamma_1} \|\langle \mathbf{q} \rangle_T - \langle \mathbf{q} \rangle (1)\|^2 + \frac{1}{\gamma_2} \|\Delta_2 \langle \mathbf{qq} \rangle_T - \Delta_2 \langle \mathbf{qq} \rangle (1)\|^2, \quad (8)$$

where $\langle \mathbf{p} \rangle (0)$ is the initial mean momentum, $\langle \mathbf{q} \rangle (1)$ the final mean position, $\langle \mathbf{q} \rangle_T$ the target sample mean position estimated from the observed landmarks, $\Delta_2 \langle \mathbf{qq} \rangle_T$ the centred sample covariance of the observations, $\Delta_2 \langle \mathbf{qq} \rangle (1)$ the centered final covariance, and γ_1, γ_2 two parameters. The covariances are in components $\Delta_2 \langle q_i^\alpha q_j^\beta \rangle$ and are 2×2 matrices if $i = j$. For the norm, we used a normalised norm for each landmark such that they contribute equally in the sum. More explicitly, we have $\langle q_i^\alpha \rangle (t) := \int q_i^\alpha \mathbb{P}(\mathbf{q}, \mathbf{p}, t) d\mathbf{q} d\mathbf{p}$, and $\Delta_2 \langle q_i^\alpha q_j^\beta \rangle :=$ $\langle q_i^\alpha \rangle \langle q_i^\beta \rangle - \langle q_i^\alpha q_j^\beta \rangle$. This cost functional corresponds to the error in matching the mean and covariance of the final probability density $\mathbb{P}(\mathbf{q}, \mathbf{p}, T)$.

It is not possible to solve the Fokker-Planck equation; so we will derive a set of ODEs that approximates the evolution of the mean and covariance by applying the standard cluster expansion method of quantum mechanics to the probability distribution, see [2] for the equations. The expected values of the higher-order products are approximated by only the $\Delta_2 \langle q_i^\alpha q_j^\beta \rangle$ and $\langle q_i^\alpha \rangle$ variables, upon neglecting higher-order correlations such as $\Delta_3 \langle q_i^\alpha q_j^\beta q_k^\beta \rangle$. In order to capture the effect of the noise in the momentum equation, the other correlations such as $\Delta_2 \langle p_i^\alpha q_j^\beta \rangle$ and $\Delta_2 \langle p_i^\alpha p_j^\beta \rangle$ must be taken into account. Their equations of motion are directly computed by taking the derivative in the definition of the correlation. For simplicity, we have used Gaussian kernels for both the Hamiltonian and noise fields so that derivatives have simple forms, and we have approximated $\langle \sigma_l(\mathbf{q}) \rangle \approx \sigma_l(\langle \mathbf{q} \rangle)$. Higher-order corrections of this approximation are possible, but they would not result in significantly better results in practice. To avoid local minima in the minimization of (8), we use a global optimisation method based on genetic algorithms, the differential evolution method [13].

4.2 Maximum Likelihood

We derive a method for parameter estimation using maximum likelihood (ML). Upon assuming the landmark observations are independent, the likelihood for the set of unknown parameters θ satisfies $\mathcal{L}_k(\mathbf{q}_1, \ldots, \mathbf{q}_N; \theta) = \prod_{i=1}^N \mathbb{P}(\mathbf{q}_i, T; \theta)$ where $\mathbb{P}(\mathbf{q}, T; \theta)$ is the transition density at $\mathbf{q}$ marginalized over $\mathbf{p}$ and with parameters θ. We will denote by $P(\mathbf{q}, \mathbf{p}; \theta)$ the law of the corresponding process.

An ML estimate of θ is then $\hat{\theta} \in \mathrm{argmax}_\theta \, \mathcal{L}(\mathbf{q}_1, \ldots, \mathbf{q}_N; \theta)$. The classic EM algorithm [7] finds parameter estimates θ_l converging to a $\hat{\theta}$ by iterating the following two steps:

(E) Compute expected log-likelihood using parameter estimate θ_{l-1}:

$$Q(\theta|\theta_{l-1}) = \sum_{i=1}^{N} \mathbb{E}_{P_{(\mathbf{q},\mathbf{p};\theta_{l-1})}} (\log \mathbb{P}(\mathbf{q}, \mathbf{p}; \theta|\mathbf{q}_i)). \tag{9}$$

(M) Update the parameter estimate $\theta_l = \mathrm{argmax}_\theta \, Q(\theta|\theta_{l-1})$.

We now describe a method for obtaining an approximation of Eq. (9).

4.3 Stochastically Perturbed Gradient Flow

The landmark trajectory $\mathbf{q}_i(t)$ for $t \in (0, T)$ and momentum $\mathbf{p}_i(t)$ for $t \in (0, T]$ can be considered the missing data for estimating the parameters θ. The conditional expectation in (9) amounts to marginalizing out the noise when finding the expected log-likelihood of the data. We approximate this by sampling diffusion bridges, i.e. producing sample paths conditioned on hitting $\mathbf{q}_i$ at time T. In [6,10], a guidance scheme is constructed that modifies a general diffusion process for a generic variable $\mathbf{x}$ conditioned on hitting a point $\mathbf{v}$ at time T by adding a term of the form $\frac{\mathbf{x}-\mathbf{v}}{T-t} dt$ to the SDE. This scheme allows sample based approximation of $\mathbb{E}_{\mathbf{x}}(f(\mathbf{x})|\mathbf{v})$ for functions f of the stochastic process $\mathbf{x}$ by the formula $\mathbb{E}_{\mathbf{x}}(f(\mathbf{x})|\mathbf{v}) = C_{\mathbf{v}}\mathbb{E}_{\mathbf{y}}(f(\mathbf{y})\phi_{\mathbf{v}}(\mathbf{y}))$ for the modified process $\mathbf{y}$ with a $\mathbf{v}$-dependent constant $C_{\mathbf{v}}$ and a path-dependent correction factor $\phi_{\mathbf{v}}(\mathbf{y})$. We need to modify this scheme for our application because the diffusion field $\Sigma(\mathbf{q}, \mathbf{p})$ in (4) may not be invertible as required in the scheme of [6,10]. A scheme based on the pseudo-inverse $\Sigma^\dagger$ can be derived, but it is computationally infeasible for high-dimensional problems. Instead, we construct the following landmark guidance scheme for the modified variables $\hat{\mathbf{q}}, \hat{\mathbf{p}}$

$$\begin{pmatrix} d\hat{\mathbf{q}} \\ d\hat{\mathbf{p}} \end{pmatrix} = \tilde{b}(\hat{\mathbf{q}}, \hat{\mathbf{p}})dt - \frac{\Sigma^2(\hat{\mathbf{q}}, \hat{\mathbf{p}})(\varphi_{T-t}(\hat{\mathbf{q}}, \hat{\mathbf{p}}) - \mathbf{v})}{T-t} dt + \Sigma(\hat{\mathbf{q}}, \hat{\mathbf{p}})dW. \tag{10}$$

$\tilde{b}$ is a bounded approximation of the drift term in (4) with the Itô correction; $\varphi_{T-t}(\hat{\mathbf{q}}, \hat{\mathbf{p}})$ is an approximation of the landmark position at time T, given their position at time t; and $\Sigma^2 := \Sigma\Sigma^T$. The boundedness condition together with appropriate conditions on Σ is necessary to show that $\lim_{t \to T} \hat{\mathbf{q}} = \mathbf{v}$ but it is not needed in practice. As in [6], we can compute the correction factor $\phi_{\mathbf{v}}$ for the modified process (10). Because of the multiplication on Σ^2, the correction factor does not depend on the inverse or pseudo-inverse of Σ and the scheme is thus computationally much more efficient.

Interestingly, the forcing term of (10) is a time-rescaled gradient flow. This can already be seen in the original scheme of [6] by noticing that $(\mathbf{y} - \mathbf{v}) = \nabla_{\mathbf{y}} \frac{1}{2}\|\mathbf{y} - \mathbf{v}\|^2$ has the form of a gradient flow. Here, with appropriate conditions on the noise fields $\Sigma(\mathbf{q}, \mathbf{p})$, we can define an admissible norm $\|\mathbf{v}\|_\Sigma^2 := \langle v, \Sigma^2 v \rangle$. The forcing term in (10) is then a derivative of a gradient flow for the norm $\|\varphi_{T-t}(\hat{\mathbf{q}}, \hat{\mathbf{p}}) - \mathbf{v}\|_\Sigma^2$ in the $\mathbf{q}$ variable. The gradient is taken with respect to the predicted endpoint $\varphi_{T-t}(\hat{\mathbf{q}}, \hat{\mathbf{p}})$ and it couples to the $\mathbf{p}$ variable through Σ^2. The flow is time rescaled with $t \to \frac{1}{2}(T-t)^2$, $dt \to (t-T)\,dt$, $\Sigma \to \sqrt{T-t}\,\Sigma$ and $dW \to \sqrt{T-t}\,dW$. This rescaling slows down the time when the original time t is close to T. This makes sure that the system has enough time to converge and reach the target $\mathbf{v}$. Deterministic gradient flows are used in greedy matching algorithms using the LDDMM right-invariant metric as described in e.g. [16]. With the present stochastic flow, sampling (10) allows efficient evaluation of the Q-function in EM and a similar evaluation of the data likelihood. In both cases, no matching or registration of the data is needed.

5   Numerical Examples

5.1   Synthetic Test Case

This synthetic test case addresses matching between two ellipses discretized by 5 landmarks. We used a low number of landmarks here in order to have readable pictures. (The algorithms scale well and are not limited by the number of landmarks.) For the noise fields σ_l, we use a grid of 4 by 4 Gaussian noise fields in the region $[-0.4, 0.4]^2$ with a fixed scale $r_l = 0.085$ corresponding to the distance between the grid points. For testing purposes, we let the bottom 8 of the noise fields have larger amplitude λ_l in the x direction, and the top 8 fields have larger amplitudes in the y direction. With these parameters, we produced 5000 sample landmark configurations from the model to estimate the sample mean and covariance of the landmarks at the final simulation time $T = 1$. On the left panel of Fig. 2, we display the result of the moment algorithm. In black are shown the density and variance in black ellipses as well as the original fields σ_l with the correct parameters. The estimated parameters λ_l of the noise fields σ_l after running the differential evolution algorithm are shown in blue. The algorithm performs the estimation given only the final sample mean and covariance of the sampled landmarks. The result is in good agreement for the final variances and shows small differences for the estimation of the parameters of the fields σ_l. The differences arise from three sources: the approximation used in the moment evolution; errors in the estimation of sample mean and variance; and the error in the solution of the minimisation algorithm. The minimisation algorithm may not have found the global minimum, but it did converge, as shown on the right panel of Fig. 2 where we display the value of the cost for each iteration of the genetic algorithm. Standard derivative-based algorithms would typically be caught in non-optimal local minima and thereby give worse results.

5.2   Stochastic Gradient Flows

We consider matching two ellipses using the stochastically perturbed gradient flow discussed in Sect. 4.3. In Fig. 3 (left), the initial set of landmarks $\mathbf{q}_0$ is

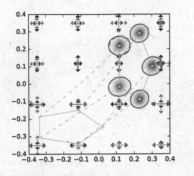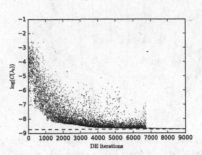

Fig. 2. (left) Estimation of the noise amplitude (blue arrows) using only the final variance of the landmark (black ellipses). The landmarks trajectories (dashed green) have initial positions on the bottom left and the final mean position is indicated with green dots. The amplitudes λ_l of the noise fields are represented by arrows (black: original data, blue: estimated data). We used the parameters $\alpha = 0.4$, $r_l = 0.085$, $\Delta t = 0.001$. (right) The convergence of the genetic algorithm which minimises the cost functional. For the last 2000 points we used a gradient descent algorithm to improve the result. (Color figure online)

displayed along the stochastic path that is pulled by the gradient term to target set $\mathbf{v}$. The guidance is computed from the predicted endpoint $\varphi_{T-t}(\mathbf{q}(t), \mathbf{p}(t))$. The prediction and the guidance term is shown at $t = T/4$. The guidance attraction in (10) becomes increasingly strong with time as $t \rightarrow T$. This enforces $\mathbf{q}(t) \rightarrow \mathbf{v}$.

Compared to the scheme of [6], the use of the function φ_{T-t} to predict the endpoint from $(\mathbf{q}(t), \mathbf{p}(t))$ removes much of the coupling between the momentum $\mathbf{p}$ and the guidance term. Without φ_{T-t}, the scheme would guide based solely on the difference $\mathbf{v} - \mathbf{q}(t)$. However, this would result in the scheme overshooting the target and producing samples of very low probability. The Σ^2 term on the guidance makes the scheme computationally feasible since the inverse of Σ^2 is not needed in the computation of the correction factor.

5.3 Corpus Callosum Variation and Template Estimation

From a dataset of 65 corpus callosum shapes represented by 77 2D landmarks $\mathbf{q}_{i,k}$, $i = 1, \ldots, 77$, $k = 1, \ldots, 65$ evenly distributed along the shape outline, here we aim at estimating the template $\mathbf{q}_0$ and noise correlation represented in this case by a correlation matrix K. The parameters of the model are $\theta = (\mathbf{q}_0, (\lambda_l^0, \lambda_l^1))$. For the MLE, we use the 'Lagrangian' scheme with components of the spatial correlation matrix $k(\mathbf{q}_i, \mathbf{q}_j) = \mathrm{diag}(\lambda_j^0, \lambda_j^1) S_3(\|\mathbf{q}_i - \mathbf{q}_j\|^2/r)$. The range r is $r = \mathrm{mean}_{ijk} \|\mathbf{q}_{i,k} - \mathbf{q}_{j,k}\|^2$. We initialize $\mathbf{q}_0$ with the Euclidean mean and run the EM algorithm for estimation of θ until convergence. The evolution of the variances $(\lambda_l^0, \lambda_l^1)$ is plotted in the right panel of Fig. 4. On the left panel of Fig. 4 shows the estimated template $\mathbf{q}_0$. The variance magnitude $(\lambda_l^0, \lambda_l^1)$ is

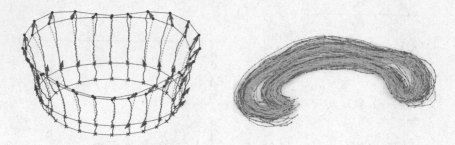

Fig. 3. (left) Stochastic gradient flow with guidance terms. At each time step t with landmarks $\mathbf{q}(t)$ (green line+crosses), a prediction $\varphi_{T-t}(\mathbf{q}(t), \mathbf{p}(t))$ of the endpoint configuration is computed (green line+dots). From the prediction, the difference $\mathbf{v} - \mathbf{q}(t)$ to the target $\mathbf{v}$ (red arrows) is multiplied on Σ^2 and back transported to $\mathbf{q}(t)$ giving the correction term (green arrows). (right) The set of 65 corpora callosa shapes. Landmarks are evenly distributed along the outline of each shape. (Color figure online)

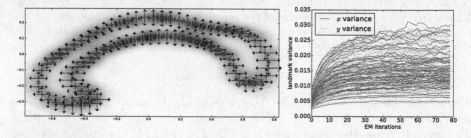

Fig. 4. (left) Estimated template $\mathbf{q}_0$ from the corpus callosum shapes with variance magnitude given by arrow length at each landmark. Sample noise covariances of each landmark of the original dataset plotted over each landmark (ellipsis). The background is shaded with a smoothed histogram of the observed landmark positions. (right) Convergence of all variance parameters $(\lambda_l^0, \lambda_l^1)$ is shown as a function of EM iterations.

plotted with arrows on each landmark and can be compared with the landmark-wise empirical variance from the dataset. The variance specified by $(\lambda_l^0, \lambda_l^1)$ is axis-aligned, and results in differences when the eigenvalues of the empirical variance are not axis-aligned.

This experiment is repeated in Fig. 5 with moment matching algorithm but with several differences of the model. First, the noise fields are the original spatially fixed Gaussian σ_l represented by red arrows. We also allow λ_l to be non-axis aligned and we placed them at the position of every 4 landmarks. We then applied the genetic algorithms using only the landmarks at the same position as the noise fields, fixing the initial momenta to 0 and the initial position to the mean positions of the landmarks. In addition to its rapid convergence, as shown in the right panel of Fig. 5, the global minimisation algorithm also gave a reliable estimate of the final variance for all the landmarks, even when fewer landmarks and noise fields were used.

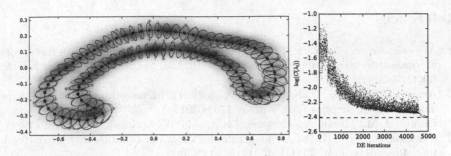

Fig. 5. (left) Corpus Callosum estimation with moment matching and setup as in Fig. 2 with parameters: $\alpha = 0.1$, $r_l = 0.1$, $\Delta t = 0.01$. We divided by 4 the number of landmarks and placed the σ at the same position. We ran the genetic algorithm to find the best set of parameters λ_l which reproduce the variance for this small set of landmarks. We used all the landmarks to compare the final estimated variance in blue with the observed variance in black. The σ fields are represented by red arrows. (right) Convergence of the differential evolution algorithm, as in Fig. (2). (Color figure online)

6   Conclusion and Open Problems

We have presented and implemented a model for large deformation stochastic variations in computational anatomy. The extremal paths are governed by stochastic EPDiff equations which arise from a right-invariant stochastic variational principle, and admit reduction from the diffeomorphism group to lower dimensional shape spaces (landmarks). We have shown that accurate estimation of the noise fields of the model can be achieved either by approximating the Fokker-Planck equations with a finite set of moments, or by Monte Carlo sampling and EM-estimation. We have derived and implemented the methods in both cases. The second approach introduces the concept of stochastically perturbed gradient flows for data likelihood evaluation. It can be hypothesised that shape evolution of human organs under the influence of diseases do not follow smooth geodesics as in conventional models used in computational anatomy, but rather it exhibits stochastic variations in shape as the disease progresses. The approaches presented enable modelling of such variations. We expect to test this hypothesis on additional shape spaces and with multiple time point longitudinal shape datasets in future work.

Acknowledgements. We are grateful to M. Bruveris, M. Bauer, N. Ganaba C. Tronci and T. Tyranowski for helpful discussions of this material. AA acknowledges partial support from an Imperial College London Roth Award. AA and DH are partially supported by the European Research Council Advanced Grant 267382 FCCA held by DH. DH is also grateful for support from EPSRC Grant EP/N023781/1. SS is partially supported by the CSGB Centre for Stochastic Geometry and Advanced Bioimaging funded by a grant from the Villum foundation.

References

1. Allassonnière, S., Amit, Y., Trouvé, A.: Towards a coherent statistical framework for dense deformable template estimation. J. R. Stat. Soc.: Ser. B (Stat. Methodol.) **69**(1), 3–29 (2007)
2. Arnaudon, A., Holm, D., Sommer, S.: A geometric framework for stochastic shape analysis. arXiv preprint (2017). arXiv:1703.09971
3. Bismut, J.-M.: Mécanique Aléatoire. LNM, vol. 866. Springer, Heidelberg (1981)
4. Camassa, R., Holm, D.D.: An integrable shallow water equation with peaked solitons. Phys. Rev. Lett. **71**(11), 1661–1664 (1993)
5. Cotter, C.J., Cotter, S.L., Vialard, F.X.: Bayesian data assimilation in shape registration. Inverse Probl. **29**(4), 045011 (2013)
6. Delyon, B., Hu, Y.: Simulation of conditioned diffusion and application to parameter estimation. Stoch. Process. Appl. **116**(11), 1660–1675 (2006)
7. Dempster, A.P., Laird, N.M., Rubin, D.B.: Maximum likelihood from incomplete data via the EM algorithm. JRSS Ser. B **39**(1), 1–38 (1977)
8. Holm, D.D.: Variational principles for stochastic fluid dynamics. Proc. R. Soc. Lond. A: Math. Phys. Eng. Sci. **471**(2176), 20140963 (2015)
9. Holm, D.D., Marsden, J.E.: Momentum maps and measure-valued solutions (peakons, filaments, and sheets) for the EDiff equation. In: Marsden, J.E., Ratiu, T.S., et al. (eds.) The Breadth of Symplectic and Poisson Geometry, pp. 203–235. Springer, Heidelberg (2005)
10. Marchand, J.L.: Conditioning diffusions with respect to partial observations. arXiv (2011). arXiv:1105.1608
11. Marsland, S., Shardlow, T.: Langevin equations for landmark image registration with uncertainty. arXiv preprint (2016). arXiv:1605.09276
12. Miller, M., Banerjee, A., Christensen, G., Joshi, S., Khaneja, N., Grenander, U., Matejic, L.: Statistical methods in computational anatomy. Stat. Methods Med. Res. **6**(3), 267–299 (1997)
13. Storn, R., Price, K.: Differential evolution-a simple and efficient heuristic for global optimization over continuous spaces. J. Glob. Optim. **11**(4), 341–359 (1997)
14. Trouvé, A., Vialard, F.X.: Shape splines and stochastic shape evolutions: a second order point of view. Q. Appl. Math. **70**(2), 219–251 (2012)
15. Vialard, F.X.: Extension to infinite dimensions of a stochastic second-order model associated with shape splines. Stoch. Process. Appl. **123**(6), 2110–2157 (2013)
16. Younes, L.: Shapes and Diffeomorphisms. Springer, Heidelberg (2010)
17. Zhang, M., Singh, N., Fletcher, P.T.: Bayesian estimation of regularization and atlas building in diffeomorphic image registration. In: Gee, J.C., Joshi, S., Pohl, K.M., Wells, W.M., Zöllei, L. (eds.) IPMI 2013. LNCS, vol. 7917, pp. 37–48. Springer, Heidelberg (2013). doi:10.1007/978-3-642-38868-2_4

Symmetric Interleaved Geodesic Shooting in Diffeomorphisms

Greg M. Fleishman[1,2]($\boxtimes$), P. Thomas Fletcher[3], and Paul M. Thompson[2]

[1] Department of Bioengineering, UC Los Angeles, Los Angeles, USA
gfleishman@ucla.edu
[2] Imaging Genetics Center, LONI, Univeristy of Southern California,
Los Angeles, USA
[3] Scientific Computing and Imaging Institute, University of Utah, Salt Lake, USA

Abstract. Many nonlinear registration algorithms are subject to an asymmetry with respect to the order of image inputs. Often, one image is considered the moving image while the other is fixed. Hence, the moving image is subject to additional interpolation relative to the fixed image. Further, the fixed image is in a way represented by the deformed moving image; any noise or artifacts present in the moving image are thus retained in this representation. This asymmetry has even been shown to result in bias in various forms of registration derived measurements. These problems are particularly evident in the geodesic shooting in diffeomorphisms context, where a continuous time geodesic model of image deformation is on the orbit of the moving image. Were the images input in the opposite order, the model would lie on the orbit of the other image. This paper presents a symmetrical formulation of the geodesic shooting in diffeomorphisms model with an accompanying algorithm that treats the intensity and gradient information in both images in nearly an equal way. After formulating the algorithm, we validate in a set of longitudinal 3D brain MRI pairs that the transformations the symmetrical algorithm produces are indeed significantly more robust to switching the order of image inputs than traditional geodesic shooting.

1 Introduction

Many nonlinear registration models treat one of the two input images as a moving template and the other as a fixed target. If the inputs are called I and J, this often appears in general image matching functionals as $\mathcal{D}(\phi^{IJ} \cdot I, J)$, where only I is warped (and thus interpolated) by the transformation ϕ^{IJ} (the superscript indicates the direction of the warp, *from I onto J*). If the images are given to the model in the opposite order, then J becomes the moving image and is warped by a transformation ϕ^{JI}. Idealistically, it is reasonable to expect that ϕ^{IJ} and ϕ^{JI} should have an inverse relationship; indeed ϕ^{IJ} maps the coordinate system of image I to that of J and ϕ^{JI} maps the coordinate system of image J to that of I. Further, both transformations were learned from the same two images, implicit to which should be only one optimal difference in form. This

© Springer International Publishing AG 2017
M. Niethammer et al. (Eds.): IPMI 2017, LNCS 10265, pp. 583–593, 2017.
DOI: 10.1007/978-3-319-59050-9_46

is particularly true in the case of diffeomorphic models wherein the existence of an inverse transformation is theoretically guaranteed. It is also particularly true in the case of longitudinal registrations, where a single ground truth deformation indeed exists. However, due to several approximations that occur when transcribing a continuous domain theory to a discrete domain implementation, and additionally due to the independent noise present in both I and J, this idealistic expectation does not hold in practice. That is, $\phi^{IJ} \circ \phi^{JI}$ may deviate from identity substantially.

For studies that extract biological information from deformations obtained by nonlinear registration (such as size and shape differences in a cross sectional study or growth/atrophy in a longitudinal study), this asymmetry implies that results may be influenced by the experimenters' choice of which image is moving and which is static. Worse yet, for the particular case of atrophy measurement in longitudinal studies, it has been shown that this asymmetry manifests as a bias to either over or underestimate atrophy for all subjects [13]. Even for subjects with severe neurodegenerative disease, annual atrophy is small relative to the volume of a typical image voxel (often below 10% relative volume loss) [7,8,11]. Hence, this bias can substantially impact study results and must be addressed carefully.

Asymmetry bias *has* been addressed for several specific nonlinear registration models. The Symmetric Normalization (SyN) algorithm proposed by Avants et al. [2] reformulates traditional LDDMM [4] such that the residual is computed at the halfway point along the path of deformations connecting the images. Consequently, both I and J are deformed when optimizing deformations. The SyN algorithm is the basis for non-linear registration in the popular software package ANTs, however in most cases the theoretical guarantees of SyN are compromised in favor of speed by using a so called greedy version [3]. The SyN algorithm is formulated in the traditional LDDMM context and has not been generalized to the case of geodesic shooting.

An older body of work exists investigating symmetry constraints for elastic and fluid registrations [1,5] wherein symmetry is explicitly enforced through priors on the deformation fields. This differs from both SyN and the method proposed in this paper, which both assume symmetry is implicit to the transformation model and construct algorithms that specifically enforce and rely on that symmetry.

We are specifically interested in the geodesic shooting model from the LDDMM framework [9,12]. Geodesic shooting in diffeomorphisms (GSID) learns not only a deformation ϕ^{IJ} mapping $I \to J$, but a continuous time flow of diffeomorphisms ϕ_t^{IJ} that smoothly warps I onto J. ϕ_t^{IJ} is a fully generative model and can be solved for any value of t, hence ϕ_t^{IJ} can interpolate and extrapolate the primary mode of deformation evident in the image pair. Consequently, the model of tissue deformation $\phi_t^{IJ} \cdot I$ is entirely on the orbit (with respect to the group action of diffeomorphisms) of the image I, which is distinct from the orbit $\phi_t^{JI} \cdot J$ that would be obtained from the symmetric problem. Hence, asymmetry bias manifests prominently in GSID in that any noise or artifacts in image I are encoded permanently into the model.

GSID does offer an intrinsic solution to this problem if the moving image is considered a template (simply initialized at I) whose intensity values are allowed to update. For example in [10] it is proposed that at every iteration, after the deformation model is updated, the moving image is also updated to be a weighted average of I and $\phi_{1,0}^{IJ,-1} \cdot J$, that is, J *pulled back* onto I by the appropriate inverse transformation. Ideally, this combines the intensity information in both I and J at corresponding locations to reduce the effect of noise and obtain a model that is more representative of the intensity characteristics of both images. However, it is important to remember that the model is fit by a gradient descent algorithm and the transformations ϕ_t^{IJ} are initialized to identity and the template is initialized to I. After the first iteration, the template will simply be the average of the unwarped I and J. This may force the optimization into a local minimum where intensity averaging at every voxel is preferable to deforming the image. Indeed in general, to average intensities between I and J properly, one needs a good correspondence, but to learn the correspondence without asymmetry bias, one needs the intensity average template. This renders optimization challenging.

Below, we present a symmetric version of GSID that does not require intensity averaging of the images and performs only a negligible amount of work beyond that of asymmetric GSID. The method exploits the intensity values of both I and J equally throughout optimization, and we show empirically that it results in deformations more robust to changing the order of the input images.

2 Methods

Background: Geodesic Shooting in Diffeomorphisms: A complete discussion of the GSID model is beyond the scope of this paper; for a thorough discussion of the following equations see [6,12]. For moving image I and fixed image J, GSID fits a geodesic flow of diffeomorphisms ϕ_t for $t \in [0,1]$, which is fully parameterized by an initial scalar momentum field P_0, such that the following objective function is minimal:

$$E(P_0) = \frac{1}{\sigma^2} \langle P_0 \nabla I, K(P_0 \nabla I) \rangle_{L_2} + \| I \circ \phi_1^{-1} - J \|^2 \qquad (1)$$

An initial momentum P_0 provides the initial conditions for the EPdiff equation(s), which govern the time evolution of the momentum and moving image:

$$\begin{cases} \partial_t I + \nabla I \cdot v = 0 \\ \partial_t P + \nabla \cdot (Pv) = 0 \\ v + K(P\nabla I) = 0 \end{cases} \qquad (2)$$

The third equation states the relationship between momentum and velocity, where K plays the role of an inertia; K is a smoothing kernel and $K(w)$ is taken to mean the convolution of vector field w with K. The path of diffeomorphisms ϕ_t is constructed from $v(x,t)$ according to the ODE:

$$\begin{cases} \partial_t \phi_t = v_t(\phi) \\ \phi_0 = \text{Id} \end{cases} \qquad (3)$$

This yields the geodesic path of diffeomorphisms ϕ_t, where the end point ϕ_1 is used to match I and J. The diffeomorphisms ϕ_t are inverted by solving the advection equation on the inverse diffeomorphism:

$$\partial_t \phi_t^{-1} + D\phi_t^{-1} v = 0 \tag{4}$$

to obtain ϕ_t^{-1}. The matching residual $J - I \circ \phi_1^{-1}$, which resides in the coordinate system of J, must be brought back to the coordinate system of I while respecting the geodesicity of the whole path ϕ_t. This is done by integrating the adjoint system backwards in time with initial conditions $\hat{I}_1 = J - I \circ \phi_1^{-1}$ and $\hat{P}_1 = 0$:

$$\begin{cases} \partial_t \hat{I} + \nabla \cdot (v\hat{I}) + \nabla \cdot (P\hat{v}) = 0 \\ \partial_t \hat{P} + v \cdot \nabla \hat{P} - \nabla I \cdot \hat{v} = 0 \\ \hat{v} + K(\hat{I}\nabla I - P\nabla \hat{P}) = 0 \end{cases} \tag{5}$$

The solution to the adjoint system together with the initial momentum and initial image gradient are sufficient to obtain the gradient of (1) with respect to P_0 which may be used to update P_0 in a steepest descent optimization:

$$P_0^{k+1} = P_0^k - \epsilon\left(\nabla I \cdot K(P_0^k \nabla I) - \hat{P}_0^k\right) \tag{6}$$

for some well chosen step size (or line search) ϵ.

Algorithm 1. GSID

input: Images I and J to be registered
output: Initial momentum P_0
Initialization: Let $P_0 = 0$

1. Given P_0, solve the forward system: eqs. (2), (3), and (4)
2. Let $\hat{I}_1 = J - I \circ \phi_1^{-1}$ and $\hat{P}_1 = 0$
3. Solve the backward system (5)
4. Update the momentum with eqn (6) and repeat from step 1

Hence optimization of a GSID model proceeds according to the GSID algorithm detailed in Algorithm 1. For brevity we have omitted several details that are nonetheless essential for implementation, see [12] for a very thorough reference. Notice that in this model, I is always the moving image. As a result, when $I \circ \phi_1^{-1}$ and J are compared, $I \circ \phi_1^{-1}$ has undergone one additional interpolation relative to J. Further, the model of image deformation $\phi_t \cdot I$ does not include any intensity information from image J. These asymmetries are the result of the arbitrary decision to assign I to be the moving image and J the fixed image. Hence, we would like to reformulate the model to eliminate this bias.

Symmetric Interleaved Geodesic Shooting in Diffeomorphisms: Objective function (1) is for moving image I and fixed image J, which we denote $I \to J$. The associated variables P_t^{IJ}, v_t^{IJ}, ϕ_t^{IJ}, and $\phi_t^{IJ,-1}$ are defined for $t \in [0,1]$. Consider the analogous objective function for the reciprocal problem $J \to I$, and let its associated variables P_s^{JI}, v_s^{JI}, ϕ_s^{JI}, and $\phi_s^{JI,-1}$ be defined for $s \in [0,1]$. We construct a new objective function as the half sum of (1) and the reciprocal analogue of (1):

$$E(P_{t=0}, P_{s=0}) = \frac{1}{2\sigma^2} \langle P_{t=0}^{IJ} \nabla I, K(P_{t=0}^{IJ} \nabla I) \rangle_{L_2} + \frac{1}{2} \| I \circ \phi_{t=1}^{IJ,-1} - J \|^2 + \qquad (7)$$
$$\frac{1}{2\sigma^2} \langle P_{s=0}^{JI} \nabla J, K(P_{s=0}^{JI} \nabla J) \rangle_{L_2} + \frac{1}{2} \| J \circ \phi_{s=1}^{JI,-1} - I \|^2.$$

Were we to augment this function with the EPdiff constraints for the $I \to J$ problem, and take the first variation with respect to $P_{t=0}^{IJ}$, we would arrive at the adjoint system (5), which we reiterate:

$$\begin{cases} \partial_t \hat{I} + \nabla \cdot (v_t^{IJ} \hat{I}) + \nabla \cdot (P_t^{IJ} \hat{v}) = 0 \\ \partial_t \hat{P} + v_t^{IJ} \cdot \nabla \hat{P} - \nabla I \cdot \hat{v} = 0 \\ \hat{v} + K(\hat{I} \nabla I - P_t^{IJ} \nabla \hat{P}) = 0 \end{cases} \qquad (8)$$

Similarly, if we were to augment (7) with the EPdiff constraints for the $J \to I$ problem, and take the first variation with respect to $P_{s=0}^{JI}$, we would arrive at the analogous adjoint system for the $J \to I$ problem:

$$\begin{cases} \partial_t \hat{J} + \nabla \cdot (v_s^{JI} \hat{J}) + \nabla \cdot (P_s^{JI} \hat{v}) = 0 \\ \partial_t \hat{P} + v_s^{JI} \cdot \nabla \hat{P} - \nabla J \cdot \hat{v} = 0 \\ \hat{v} + K(\hat{J} \nabla J - P_s^{JI} \nabla \hat{P}) = 0 \end{cases} \qquad (9)$$

A brute force approach to optimizing (7) would be to optimize the $I \to J$ and $J \to I$ components of the problem separately and average the results. That is, optimize separate GSID models according to the GSID algorithm for both $I \to J$ and $J \to I$ problems, and after convergence, let $P_0^{sym} = \frac{1}{2}(P_{t=0}^{IJ} + (-P_{s=1}^{JI}))$ parameterize a geodesic that is informed by both of the reciprocal problems (see Eq. (10) to justify this averaging). Alternatively we leverage common information between the reciprocal problems to formulate an algorithm that requires roughly half as much work.

Although the orbits $\phi_t^{IJ} \cdot I$ and $\phi_s^{JI} \cdot J$ are different, there should be only one geodesic path of diffeomorphisms connecting the images; that is in fact the requirement of symmetry that we would like to enforce and exploit. If there is only one path connecting I and J, and the reciprocal problems simply construct that path from opposite end points, then the following trivial identifications can be made:

$$\begin{cases} s = 1 - t \\ P_s^{JI} = -P_{1-s}^{IJ} \\ v_s^{JI} = -v_{1-s}^{IJ} \end{cases} \qquad (10)$$

Further, because the paths ϕ_t^{IJ}, $\phi_t^{IJ,-1}$, ϕ_s^{JI}, and $\phi_s^{JI,-1}$ are constructed from velocities that satisfy identity (10), there should be some identification between them as well. ϕ_s^{JI} and $\phi_{1-s}^{IJ,-1}$ both map coordinates from image J to image I and correspond to the same point in time. Similarly, $\phi_s^{JI,-1}$ and ϕ_{1-s}^{IJ} both map coordinates from image I to image J, and correspond to the same point in time. Hence, these are the identifications we would like to make, however, before we can we must resolve a problem.

Numerically, ϕ_t^{IJ} is constructed as the solution to ODE (3) and is therefore specified with Lagrangian coordinates. $\phi_t^{IJ,-1}$ is constructed as the solution to the material derivative (4) and is therefore specified in Eulerian coordinates. Consequently, for the reciprocal problem, ϕ_s^{JI} is specified in Lagrangian coordinates and $\phi_s^{JI,-1}$ is specified in Eulerian coordinates. We cannot immediately make the appropriate identifications because the forward and inverse transformations we would like to identify have opposite coordinate specifications. This problem is resolved by the following simple compositions:

$$\begin{cases} \phi_s^{JI} = \phi_{1-s}^{IJ} \circ \phi_{1.0}^{IJ,-1} \\ \phi_s^{JI,-1} = \phi_{1.0}^{IJ} \circ \phi_{1-s}^{IJ,-1} \end{cases} \tag{11}$$

The transformations on the left and right sides of (11) map the same particles, in the same direction, at the same times.

Identities (10) and (11) indicate that the forward system variables for the $I \to J$ and $J \to I$ problems determine one another. This leads to the central idea of Symmetric Interleaved Geodesic Shooting in Diffeomorphisms (SIGSID): we solve the forward system (Eqs. (2), (3), and (4)) for the $I \to J$ problem, determine the forward system variables for the reciprocal problem through identities (10) and (11), then solve the backward system (Eq. (9)) for the $J \to I$ problem. We then update the momentum at *that* point, that is at $t = 1 = 1 - s$, according to:

$$P_{s=0}^{JI} = -P_{t=1}^{IJ} - \epsilon\big(\nabla J \cdot K(-P_{t=1}^{IJ}\nabla J) - \hat{P}_{s=0}^{JI}\big) \tag{12}$$

As we have updated the momentum at $s = 0$, on the subsequent iteration we solve the forward system for the $J \to I$ problem, use identities (10) and (11) to obtain the forward system variables for the reciprocal problem, solve the backward system for the $I \to J$ problem (Eq. (8)) and update the momentum at $s = 1 = 1 - t$. In this way, each iteration uses intensity and gradient information from *both* I and J and iterations which shoot the geodesic from either endpoint are interleaved. The algorithm is detailed in Algorithm 2.

The momentum may be output at either endpoint or both. The differences between GSID and SIGSID are detailed in Fig. 1. Regardless of whether the user inputs the images in the order I, J or J, I this algorithm will utilize the intensity and gradient information in both images in nearly an equal way. We hypothesize that the SIGSID algorithm will produce deformations ϕ_t and ϕ_t^{-1} that are significantly more robust to changing the order of the inputs than the GSID algorithm.

Algorithm 2. SIGSID
___
input: Images I and J to be registered
output: Initial momentum P_0
Initialization: Let $P_0 = 0$

1. Given P_0, solve the forward system: eqs. (2), (3), and (4)
2. Use eqs. (10) and (11) to obtain P_s^{JI}, v_s^{JI}, ϕ_s^{JI}, and $\phi_s^{JI,-1}$
3. Use $\phi_s^{JI,-1}$ to obtain J_s
4. Let $\hat{J}_{s=1} = I - J \circ \phi_{s=1}^{JI,-1}$ and $\hat{P}_{s=1} = 0$
5. Solve the backward system for the $J \to I$ problem, eqn. (9)
6. Update the momentum at $t = 1 \implies s = 0$ with eqn. (12)
7. Switch the labels of images I and J and repeat from step 1
___

3   Experiments and Results

If we let $s = 1.0$ in Eq. (11), then we get:

$$\begin{cases} \phi_{1.0}^{JI} = \phi_0^{IJ} \circ \phi_{1.0}^{IJ,-1} \\ \phi_{1.0}^{JI,-1} = \phi_{1.0}^{IJ} \circ \phi_0^{IJ,-1} \end{cases}$$

but $\phi_0^{IJ} = \phi_0^{IJ,-1} = Id$, which implies:

$$\begin{cases} \phi_{1.0}^{JI} = \phi_{1.0}^{IJ,-1} \\ \phi_{1.0}^{JI,-1} = \phi_{1.0}^{IJ} \end{cases}$$

which we can rearrange to:

$$\begin{cases} \phi_{1.0}^{JI} \circ \phi_{1.0}^{IJ} = Id \\ \phi_{1.0}^{JI,-1} \circ \phi_{1.0}^{IJ,-1} = Id \end{cases} \tag{13}$$

Of course, the symmetric compositions also hold:

$$\begin{cases} \phi_{1.0}^{IJ} \circ \phi_{1.0}^{JI} = Id \\ \phi_{1.0}^{IJ,-1} \circ \phi_{1.0}^{JI,-1} = Id \end{cases} \tag{14}$$

We choose Eqs. (13) and (14) to evaluate the level of symmetry achieved by both GSID and SIGSID. Hence, for a dataset of image pairs I_i and J_i for $i \in [0, 1, \ldots, n-1]$, we compute the $I_i \to J_i$ and $J_i \to I_i$ registration problems with GSID and with SIGSID. For an ideal symmetric algorithm, the Jacobian determinants of Eqs. (13) and (14) would be everywhere equal to 1.0:

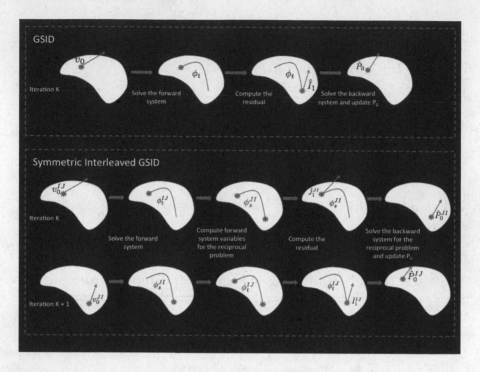

Fig. 1. Graphical comparison between GSID and Symmetric Interleaved GSID

$$\begin{cases} \left| D(\phi_{1.0}^{JI} \circ \phi_{1.0}^{IJ}) \right| = 1.0 \\ \left| D(\phi_{1.0}^{IJ} \circ \phi_{1.0}^{JI}) \right| = 1.0 \\ \left| D(\phi_{1.0}^{JI,-1} \circ \phi_{1.0}^{IJ,-1}) \right| = 1.0 \\ \left| D(\phi_{1.0}^{IJ,-1} \circ \phi_{1.0}^{JI,-1}) \right| = 1.0 \end{cases} \tag{15}$$

Due to discretization even SIGSID will not achieve this, but we take the extent to which the Jacobian determinants deviate from 1.0 as a measure of how symmetric the method is. We used 98 baseline and 24 month followup image pairs from the ADNI-2 data set. The image matching functional, model parameters, and number of iterations were identical for the GSID and SIGSID experiments. For GSID and SIGSID, and for each subject, we compute the following "symmetry scores" as scalar valued scores of how robust the method was to swapping the order of the inputs:

$$\begin{cases} \alpha^1 \text{ or } \beta^1 = \int_\Omega \text{abs}\left(\left| D(\phi_{1.0}^{JI} \circ \phi_{1.0}^{IJ}) \right| - 1.0 \right) dx \\ \alpha^2 \text{ or } \beta^2 = \int_\Omega \text{abs}\left(\left| D(\phi_{1.0}^{IJ} \circ \phi_{1.0}^{JI}) \right| - 1.0 \right) dx \\ \alpha^3 \text{ or } \beta^3 = \int_\Omega \text{abs}\left(\left| D(\phi_{1.0}^{JI,-1} \circ \phi_{1.0}^{IJ,-1}) \right| - 1.0 \right) dx \\ \alpha^4 \text{ or } \beta^4 = \int_\Omega \text{abs}\left(\left| D(\phi_{1.0}^{IJ,-1} \circ \phi_{1.0}^{JI,-1}) \right| - 1.0 \right) dx \end{cases} \tag{16}$$

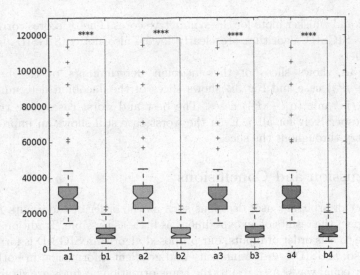

Fig. 2. Box and whisker plots comparing symmetry scores for GSID registrations (α^j) and SIGSID registrations (β^j). For all four cases $p \ll 10e^{-12}$ in a paired t-test

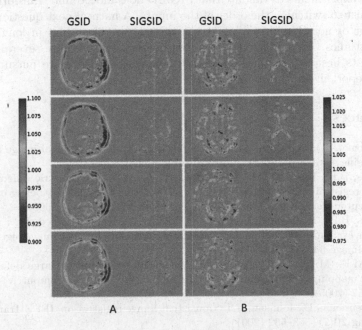

Fig. 3. Jacobian determinants corresponding to the components of Eq. (15) for the best (A) and worst (B) cases by difference in symmetry scores.

where Ω is the image domain, abs($\cdot$) is the absolute value, $|\cdot|$ is the determinant, D is the Jacobian operator, α_i^j corresponds to GSID registrations, β_i^j corresponds to the SIGSID registrations, and $i \in [0, 1, \ldots, 97]$ indexes the subject. Figure 2 shows box and whisker plots for the symmetry scores. The β_i^j scores corresponding to the SIGSID algorithm are clearly lower, also notice SIGSID produced fewer outliers.

Figure 3A shows slices of the Jacobian determinants of the best (i.e. $\max_i(\alpha_i^j - \beta_i^j)$) case and Fig. 3B shows slices of the Jacobian determinants of the worst (i.e. $\min_i(\alpha_i^j - \beta_i^j)$) cases. The best and worst cases were the same subjects respectively for all j. Even the worst case still shows an improvement in symmetry throughout the slice.

4   Discussion and Conclusions

The impact of arbitrary user decisions such as the order of the inputs I and J should impact the results of an experiment as little as possible. Traditional GSID is sensitive to this order of inputs; our proposed algorithm SIGSID is formulated to be less so. SIGSID uses the intensity and gradient information in both I and J in nearly equal ways. As a result, the transformations it finds are significantly less affected by changing the order of inputs. In this preliminary work, we have only done experiments to validate that SIGSID does indeed find transformations more robust to switching the order of the inputs. A natural next question to ask is whether or not this improvement in symmetry reduces bias in longitudinal atrophy studies. To properly address this question will require several careful experiments best left to their own study and write up; we are pursuing that work to report in a future publication.

References

1. Ashburner, J., Andersson, J.L.R., Friston, K.J.: High-dimensional image registration using symmetric priors. NeuroImage **9**, 619–628 (1999)
2. Avants, B.B., Epstein, C.L., Grossman, M., Gee, J.C.: Symmetric diffeomorphic image registration with cross-correlation: evaluating automated labeling of elderly and neurodegenerative brain. Med. Image Anal. **12**(1), 26–41 (2008)
3. Avants, B.B., Tustison, N.J., Song, G., Cook, P.A., Klein, A., Gee, J.C.: A reproducible evaluation of ants similarity metric performance in brain image registration. NeuroImage **54**(3), 2033–2044 (2011)
4. Beg, M.F., Miller, M.I., Trouvé, A., Younes, L.: Computing large deformation metric mappings via geodesic flows of diffeomorphisms. Int. J. Comput. Vis. **61**(2), 139–157 (2005)
5. Christensen, G.E., Johnson, H.J.: Consistent image registration. IEEE Trans. Med. Imaging **20**(7), 568–582 (2001)
6. Fleishman, G.M., Gutman, B.A., Fletcher, P.T., Thompson, P.M.: Simultaneous longitudinal registration with group-wise similarity prior. In: Ourselin, S., Alexander, D.C., Westin, C.-F., Cardoso, M.J. (eds.) IPMI 2015. LNCS, vol. 9123, pp. 746–757. Springer, Cham (2015). doi:10.1007/978-3-319-19992-4_59
7. Hua, X., Ching, C.R.K., Mezher, A., Gutman, B., Hibar, D.P., Bhatt, P., Leow, A.D., Jack Jr., C.R., Bernstein, M., Weiner, M.W., Thompson, P.M.: MRI-based brain atrophy rates in ADNI phase 2: acceleration and enrichment considerations for clinical trials. Neurobiology of Aging **37**, 26–37 (2016)

8. Hua, X., Hibar, D.P., Ching, C.R.K., Boyle, C.P., Rajagopalan, P., Gutman, B., Leow, A.D., Toga, A.W., Jack Jr., C.R., Harvey, D.J., Weiner, M.W., Thompson, P.M.: Unbiased tensor-based morphometry: improved robustness and sample size estimates for Alzheimer's disease clinical trials. NeuroImage **66**, 648–661 (2013)
9. Miller, M.I., Trouvé, A., Younes, L.: Geodesic shooting for computational anatomy. J. Math. Imaging Vis. **24**(2), 209–228 (2006)
10. Singh, N., Hinkle, J., Joshi, S., Fletcher, P.: A vector momenta formulation of diffeomorphisms for improved geodesic regression and atlas construction. In: Proceedings of the 2013 IEEE 10th International Symposium on Biomedical Imaging (ISBI), pp. 1219–1222 (2013)
11. Vemuri, P., Senjem, M.L., Gunter, J.L., Lundt, E.S., Tosakulwong, N., Weigand, S.D., Borowski, B.J., Bernstein, M.A., Zuk, S.M., Lowe, V.J., Knopman, D.S., Petersen, R.C., Fox, N.C., Thompson, P.M., Weiner, M.W., Jack Jr., C.R.: Accelerated vs. unaccelerated serial MRI based TBM-SyN measurements for clinical trials in Alzheimer's disease. NeuroImage **113**, 61–69 (2015)
12. Vialard, F.X., Risser, L., Rueckert, D., Cotter, C.J.: Diffeomorphic 3D image registration via geodesic shooting using an efficient adjoint calculation. Int. J. Comput. Vis. **97**(2), 229–241 (2012)
13. Yushkevich, P.A., Avants, B.B., Das, S.R., Pluta, J., Altinay, M., Craige, C.: Bias in estimation of hippocampal atrophy using deformation-based morphometry arises from asymmetric global normalization: an illustration in ADNI 3 t MRI data. NeuroImage **50**(2), 434–445 (2010)

Segmentation

Unsupervised Domain Adaptation in Brain Lesion Segmentation with Adversarial Networks

Konstantinos Kamnitsas[1,4](✉), Christian Baumgartner[1], Christian Ledig[1], Virginia Newcombe[2,3], Joanna Simpson[2], Andrew Kane[2], David Menon[2,3], Aditya Nori[4], Antonio Criminisi[4], Daniel Rueckert[1], and Ben Glocker[1]

[1] Biomedical Image Analysis Group, Imperial College London, London, UK
konstantinos.kamnitsas12@imperial.ac.uk
[2] Division of Anaesthesia, Department of Medicine, Cambridge University, Cambridge, UK
[3] Wolfson Brain Imaging Centre, Cambridge University, Cambridge, UK
[4] Microsoft Research Cambridge, Cambridge, UK

Abstract. Significant advances have been made towards building accurate automatic segmentation systems for a variety of biomedical applications using machine learning. However, the performance of these systems often degrades when they are applied on new data that differ from the training data, for example, due to variations in imaging protocols. Manually annotating new data for each test domain is not a feasible solution. In this work we investigate unsupervised domain adaptation using adversarial neural networks to train a segmentation method which is more robust to differences in the input data, and which does not require any annotations on the test domain. Specifically, we derive domain-invariant features by learning to counter an adversarial network, which attempts to classify the domain of the input data by observing the activations of the segmentation network. Furthermore, we propose a multi-connected domain discriminator for improved adversarial training. Our system is evaluated using two MR databases of subjects with traumatic brain injuries, acquired using different scanners and imaging protocols. Using our unsupervised approach, we obtain segmentation accuracies which are close to the upper bound of supervised domain adaptation.

1 Introduction

Great advancements have been achieved in machine learning, particularly with supervised learning algorithms, reaching human-level performance on applications that a few years ago would be considered extremely challenging. However, a common assumption in machine learning is that training and test data are drawn from the same probability distribution [19]. Methods are trained on data from a *source domain* $D_S = \{\mathcal{X}_S, P(X_S)\}$, where $\mathcal{X}_S$ is a feature space,

---

K. Kamnitsas—Part of this work was carried on when KK was an intern at Microsoft Research.

M. Niethammer et al. (Eds.): IPMI 2017, LNCS 10265, pp. 597–609, 2017.
DOI: 10.1007/978-3-319-59050-9_47

$X_S = \{x_{S1}, \ldots, x_{Sn}\}, x_{Si} \in \mathcal{X}_S$ the data and $P(X_S)$ the marginal distribution that their features follow. In an image segmentation problem, for example, X_S could be samples (voxels or patches) from multi-spectral MR scans, $\mathcal{X}_S$ is the feature space defined by the available MR sequences and $P(X_S)$ is the distribution of intensities in the sequences. In the developing stage of a supervised algorithm, given corresponding ground truth labels $Y_S = \{y_{S1}, \ldots, y_{Sn}\}, y_{Si} \in \mathcal{Y}_S$, such as segmentation masks, where $\mathcal{Y}_S$ the label space, a predictive function $f_S(x) = P_S(y|x)$ is learnt via training and configuration of hyper-parameters on the data (X_S, Y_S). $f_S(\cdot)$ tries to approximate the optimal function $f'_S(x), x \in \mathcal{X}_S$ that generated Y_S. At the time of deployment, however, these methods often under-perform or fail if the testing data come from a different *target domain* $D_T = \{\mathcal{X}_T, P(X_T)\}$, with $\mathcal{X}_T \neq \mathcal{X}_S$ and/or $P(X_T) \neq P(X_S)$. This is because the optimal predictive function $f'_T(x), x \in \mathcal{X}_T$ for D_T may differ from $f'_S(\cdot)$, and so the learnt $f_S(\cdot)$ will not perform well on D_T. The above scenario is common in biomedical applications due to variations in image acquisition, in particular, in multi-center studies. Training and testing data may differ in contrast, resolution, noise levels ($P(X_T) \neq P(X_S)$) or even type of sequences ($\mathcal{X}_T \neq \mathcal{X}_S$). Despite the rapid advancements in representation learning, this issue has been shown to affect even the latest models [18]. Generating labelled databases is time consuming and often expensive, and assuming annotations for training are available for each new domain is neither realistic nor scalable. Instead, it is desired to develop methods that can learn from existing databases and generalize well or adapt to the target domain without the need for additional training data.

Transfer learning (TL) [14] investigates development of predictive models by leveraging knowledge from potentially different but related domains and tasks. Even between tasks where label spaces $\mathcal{Y}_S$ and $\mathcal{Y}_T$ differ, TL can take advantage of similarities in the underlying structure of the mappings $f_S : \mathcal{X}_S \mapsto \mathcal{Y}_S$ and $f_T : \mathcal{X}_T \mapsto \mathcal{Y}_T$. A subclass of TL is *multi-task learning*, where a model is trained on multiple related tasks *simultaneously*. Most related to our work, *domain adaptation* (DA) is the subclass of TL that assumes $\mathcal{Y}_S = \mathcal{Y}_T$ and only the domains differ. It explores learning a function $f_a(\cdot)$ that performs well on both domains, under the basic assumption that such a function exists [1].

In this work we investigate *unsupervised domain adaptation* (UDA) [7]. In this setting we assume the availability of a labeled database $S = (X_S, Y_S)$ from source domain D_S, along with an *unlabeled* database $T = (X_T)$ from a different but related target domain D_T. We wish to model the unknown optimal function $f'_T(\cdot)$ for labelling X_T. However since no labels are available for D_T, $f'_T(\cdot)$ cannot be learnt. This is in contrast to supervised DA, which requires at least some labelled data for D_T. Instead, we try to learn a representation $h_a(x)$ that maps X_S and X_T to a feature space that is invariant to differences between the two domains, as well as a function $f_{ah}(\cdot)$ learnt using data $\{X_S, Y_S, X_T\}$, such that $f_a(x) = f_{ah}(h_a(x))$ approximates $f'_S(\cdot)$ and is closer to $f'_T(\cdot)$ than any function $f_S(\cdot)$ that can be learnt using only the source data (X_S, Y_S).

Contributions: In this work we develop a domain adaptation method based on adversarial neural networks [4,5]. We propose the adversarial training of a segmenter and a domain-classifier, which aims to make the representation learnt by the segmenter invariant to domain-specific factors. We describe and analyse the development of domain-adversarial networks for the purpose of segmentation, which to the best of our knowledge has not been previously performed. We investigate the adaptation of layers at various depths and propose multi-connected adversarial networks, which we show improve domain adaptation. We employ our system for the segmentation of traumatic brain injuries (TBI), investigating adaptation between databases acquired using two different scanners with difference in the available MR sequences. We show that without utilizing any labels in the target domain, our method closes the performance gap with respect to supervised learning with target labels to a large extent.

Related Work: TL and DA have attracted significant interest over the years. Comprehensive reviews of early works can be found in [1,7,14]. Popularity of TL increased with the wide adoption of neural networks when their features were found to be effective when transferred across tasks. For example, features learnt from natural images were used off-the-shelf for detecting peri-fissural nodules [3]. More commonly, TL is performed via pre-training on a source task, followed by fine-tuning for the target task via supervised training [16]. A representative example of TL via multi-task learning was presented in [12]. A network was trained simultaneously for segmentation of brain tissue, pectoral muscle and coronary arteries. These experiments show that much of a network's capacity can be shared between a variety of tasks. Note, all of the above require labels in D_T.

In contrast, DA explores the case where label spaces (Y_S, Y_T) are the same and little or no labelled data is available in D_T. In [13] the authors explored supervised DA with SVM-based adaptive classifiers in the scenario where source and target data are acquired with different protocols. This method, however, requires labelled target data. Unsupervised DA was tackled in [6] via instance weighting, but this relies on strong assumptions about the data distributions. [2] performed UDA with boosted decision stumps with a search for visual correspondences between source and target samples. This is not as flexible as our approach nor scales well to large databases. The authors in [2] question the feasibility of DA with neural networks on 3D data due to memory requirements. Here, we show that using adversarial 3D networks is indeed a viable approach.

2   Unsupervised Domain Adaptation with Adversarial Nets

The accuracy of a binary classifier that distinguishes between samples from two domains can serve as a proxy of the divergence of distributions $P(X_S)$ and $P(X_T)$, which otherwise is not straightforward to compute. This idea was first introduced in [1]. Inspired by this, the authors of [4] presented a method for simultaneously learning a domain-invariant representation and a task-related classifier by a single neural network. This is done by minimizing the accuracy of

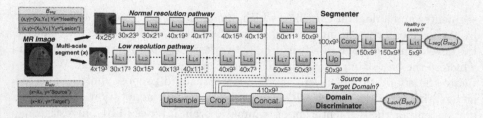

Fig. 1. Proposed multi-connected adversarial networks. Segmenter: we use the 3D CNN architecture presented in [8]. Dashed lines denote low resolution features. Input samples are multi-modal, although not depicted. Discriminator: We use a second 3D CNN for classifying the domain of input x, by processing activations at multiple layers of the segmenter. Red lines show the path of the adversarial gradients, from L_{adv} back to the segmenter. See text for details on architecture. (Color figure online)

an auxiliary network, a domain-discriminator, that processes a hidden representation of the main network and tries to classify the domain of the input sample. This approach formed the basis of our work. We below describe its extension for segmentation and our proposed multi-connected system.

2.1 Segmentation System with Domain Discriminator

Segmenter: At the core of our system is a fully convolutional neural network (CNN) for image segmentation [10]. Given an input x of arbitrary size, which can be a whole image or a sub-segment, this type of network predicts labels for multiple voxels in x, one for each stride of the network's receptive field over the input. The parameters of the network θ_{seg} are learnt by iteratively minimizing a segmentation loss $\mathcal{L}_{seg}$ using stochastic gradient descent (SGD). The loss is commonly the cross-entropy of the predictions on a training batch $B_{seg} = \{(x_1, y_1), \ldots, (x_{N_{seg}}, y_{N_{seg}})\}$ of N_{seg} samples. In our settings, (x_i, y_i) are sampled from the source database $S = (X_S, Y_S)$, for which labels Y_S are available. We borrowed the 3D multi-scale CNN architecture from [8], the segmenter depicted in Fig. 1, and adopt the same configuration for all meta-parameters.

Domain Discriminator: When processing an input x, the activations of any feature map (FM) in the segmenter encode a hidden representation $h(x)$. If samples come from different distributions $P(X_S) \neq P(X_T)$, e.g. due to different domains, and the filters of the segmenter are not invariant to the domain-specific variations, the distributions of the corresponding activations will differ as well, $P(h(X_S)) \neq P(h(X_T))$. This is expected when the segmenter is trained only on samples from S where learnt features will be specific to the source domain. Similar to [4], we choose a certain representation $h_a(x)$ from the segmenter and use a second network as a domain-classifier that takes $h_a(x)$ as input and tries to classify whether it comes from $P(h_a(X_S))$ or $P(h_a(X_T))$. This is equivalent to classifying the domain of x. Classification accuracy serves as an indication of how source-specific the representation $h_a(\cdot)$ is. The architecture we use for a domain classifier is a 3D CNN with five layers. The first four have 100 kernels of size 3^3. The last classification layer uses 1^3 kernels. This architecture has a receptive field of 9^3 with respect to its input $h_a(\cdot)$ and was chosen for compatibility with the size of feature maps in the 3 last layers of the segmenter.

We train this domain-discriminator simultaneously with the segmenter. For this, we form a second training batch $B_{adv} = \{(x_1, y_1^d), \ldots, (x_{N_{adv}}, y_{N_{adv}}^d)\}$. Equal number of samples x_i are extracted from X_S and X_T, so there is no bias towards either. y_i^d is a label that encodes the domain of x_i, used as the training target. B_{adv} is processed by the segmenter, at the same time with B_{seg} or interleaved to lower memory requirements, computing activations $h_a(x) \forall x \in B_{adv}$. These activations are then processed by the discriminator, which classifies the domain of each sample in B_{adv}. The discriminator's classification loss $\mathcal{L}_{adv}$ is minimized through optimization of the parameters θ_{adv}.

A complication arises for the joint training. The samples from S are shared in an SGD iteration for the two losses in the algorithm of [4]. However, many segmentation methods use weighted sampling in order to mitigate class-imbalance, for example by oversampling rare classes [8,12]. Such sampling requires segmentation masks that are not available for T whose samples are extracted randomly. In this case, the discriminator should not compare those against non-randomly extracted samples from S, as it could easily associate activations for the over-weighted classes with domain S and fail to learn useful domain-discriminative features. Hence, we resort to forming entirely separate batches. B_{adv} is formed of 20 image segments, randomly extracted from images in S and T. As done in [8], weighted sampling is used for extracting 10 segments from S to form B_{seg}. This ensures countering of class-imbalance for the segmenter, while being unbiased on the samples used for the discriminator.

Domain Adaptation via Adversarial Training: We aim at adapting the representation $h_a(\cdot)$ to become invariant to variations between S and T. To this end, we expose the accuracy of the domain-discriminator to the segmenter and let it alter its parameters such that its FMs that comprise $h_a(\cdot)$ do not contain cues about the input domain. This is done by incorporating the domain-discriminator's loss $\mathcal{L}_{adv}$ into the training objective of the segmenter, which now aims to simultaneously maximize the domain classification loss and minimize the segmentation loss $\mathcal{L}_{seg}$, or:

$$\mathcal{L}_{segAdv}(\theta_{seg}) = \mathcal{L}_{seg}(\theta_{seg}) - \alpha \mathcal{L}_{adv}(\theta_{seg}) \tag{1}$$

α is a positive weight that defines the relative importance of the domain adaptation task for the segmenter. This optimization is possible with regular SGD, as the adversarial networks are interconnected and gradients of $\mathcal{L}_{adv}$ can propagate back through the discriminator and into the segmenter. This process was implemented in [4] via a custom *gradient-reversal layer*, which is not needed if the optimization is formulated as in Eq. (1), as also noted by the authors.

2.2   Multi-connected Adversarial Networks

A natural question to arise concerns which layer(s) of the segmenter should be adapted. In [17], the authors investigated which of the last three fully connected layers of an AlexNet leads to better accuracy when adapted, concluding it is the last hidden layer that is optimal in their settings. Earlier layers are commonly not adapted as their features are considered rather generic and transferable across related tasks [4,11].

We argue that adapting only the last layers might not be ideal, especially for the case of segmentation. The accuracy of classification networks depends mostly on high-level patterns. For precise segmentation, however, fine patterns such as detailed texture and small contrast variations are likely to be important. These fine patterns are extracted in early layers and are more susceptible to image-quality variations between domains. Adapting top layers makes them invariant to such variations, but it is still a loss of capacity if such features have been already extracted by early layers, which may not be well adapted by the weakened adversarial gradients that reach them. On the other hand, if only early layers are adapted, assuming that the adaptation is not ideal and the features not entirely free of factors of variation between the two domains, the network could recover source-specific patterns at greater depth. For these reasons we propose an architecture where the domain discriminator is connected at multiple layers of the segmenter. First, this removes source-specific patterns early on but also disallows their recovery at deeper layers. Furthermore, the discriminator is enabled to process a large variety of features for discriminating between the domains, increasing its performance and thus the quality of the gradients for the domain adaptation. Finally, by seeing the whole adversarial network as an auxiliary cost function for the segmenter, this type of connections can be compared with deep-supervision [9], which allows better flow of the gradients incoming from $\mathcal{L}_{adv}$ throughout the segmenter and as such can improve learning of quality features. Our main results are based on feeding input $h_{in}(\cdot)$ to the discriminator from FMs of layers 4,6 and 8 of both high and low resolution pathways, as well as the 10-th hidden layer of the segmenter (cf. Fig. 1). After the FMs of the low resolution pathway are upsampled, all FMs are cropped to match the size of the deepest layer and concatenated. A detailed analysis of the effect of adapting different layers is presented in Sect. 3.4.

3   Experiments

3.1   Material

We make use of two databases with multi-spectral MR brain scans of patients with moderate to severe TBI, acquired within the first week of injury. The first database consists of 61 subjects, imaged on a 3-T Siemens Magnetom TIM Trio. The MR sequences are isotropic MPRAGE ($1\,mm^3$), axial FLAIR, T2 and Proton Density (PD) ($0.7 \times 0.7 \times 5\,mm$), and Gradient-Echo (GE) ($0.86 \times 0.86 \times 5\,mm$). The second database consists of 41 subjects, imaged on a 3-T Siemens Magnetom Verio. This database includes MPRAGE, FLAIR, T2 and PD sequences, acquired at the same resolution as in the first database. The important difference is that instead of GE, a Susceptibility Weighted Image (SWI) is available $(0.7 \times 0.7 \times 5\,\text{mm})$. On both databases, all visible lesions were manually annotated on the FLAIR and GE/SWI by clinical experts. We merge them into a single lesion mask, as we here focus on binary segmentation of abnormalities within the brain tissue. Extra-cerebral pathologies are treated as background. All images are skull-stripped, resampled to isotropic $1\,\text{mm}^3$ and affinely registered to MNI space. Image intensities under the brain masks are normalized to zero-mean and unit-variance, after windowing the lowest and top 2% of the intensity histograms.

Source (S) and Target (T) Databases: GE and SWI are commonly used in TBI studies due to their great sensitivity to haemorrhages. They enable detection of lesions invisible in other sequences, such as micro-bleeds. SWI is actually a type of GE that offers greater sensitivity and image quality [15]. See Fig. 2 for visual examples. For the purpose of this study, the first database, with GE available, is considered the *source* database S used to train the segmenter in a supervised manner. The second database, with SWI available, is considered the *target* database T on which we aim to successfully apply the trained segmenter. This corresponds to a typical scenario where a training database is generated on data coming from one clinical site, and new test data coming from another site with varying protocol. Motivated by their common property of being sensitive to blood and thus providing similar information for TBI segmentation, we consider GE and SWI as interchangeable for the same input channel to our system, unless stated otherwise. However the difference in appearance of GE and SWI images (cf. Fig. 2) contributes the largest variation between distributions $P(X_S)$ and $P(X_T)$. Further variations may be present due to the different scanners used for acquiring S and T. Using our method, we aim to learn features invariant to these domain differences without the need for any annotations on the target domain.

3.2 Configuration of the Training Schedule

A complication of adversarial training concerns the training schedule of the two connected networks, which influences the way they interact. The strength with which the segmenter is adapting its features in order to counter the domain-discriminator is controlled by the parameter α (cf. Eq. (1)). We set $\alpha = 0$ for the first $e_1 = 10$ epochs and let both networks learn independently. This allows the segmenter to initially learn features for the segmentation of S without being influenced by noisy adversarial gradients from an initially poorly performing domain-discriminator. After epochs e_1, when the discriminator's performance has increased, we start countering it to learn domain invariant features with the segmenter. For this, we increase α according to the linear schedule $\alpha = \alpha_{max} \frac{e_{curr} - e_1}{e_2 - e_1}$, where $e_2 = 35$ and α_{max} is the maximum weighting, so α equals α_{max} after epoch e_2. Finally, at epoch 43 we start refining the segmenter's features by gradually lowering its learning rate. The discriminator is optimized with constant learning rate 0.001. In the following, $\alpha_{max} = 0.05$ is used. In Sect. 3.4 we present a sensitivity analysis showing robust behaviour across a range of values for α_{max}. e_1, e_2 and the total duration of this piecewise linear schedule were determined empirically for satisfactory convergence without prolonging training time. Optimal settings are not fully explored yet and may vary between applications and the relative difficulty of each network's specific task.

3.3   Evaluation

We performed multiple experiments to obtain upper and lower bounds of baseline accuracy on the challenging task of TBI segmentation. We discuss experiments below, summarize results in Table 1 and give examples of segmentations in Fig. 2.

Table 1. Comparison of our method's performance on T with several baselines. Our system significantly closes the gap between the lower bound, when the segmenter is trained on S only, and the upper bound, when the segmenter is also trained with labelled data from T. Values are given in format *mean (std)*.

	DSC	Recall	Precision
Train on S	15.7(13.5)	80.4(12.3)	09.5(09.0)
Train on S (No GE/SWI)	59.7(22.1)	55.7(22.6)	69.7(21.5)
Train on S → UDA to T (ours)	62.7(19.8)	58.9(21.2)	71.6(18.4)
Train on T	63.5(20.2)	60.6(21.1)	71.5(19.8)
Train on S+T	66.5(17.7)	66.6(19.1)	69.4(19.0)
Train on S+T (GE/SWI diff chan.)	64.7(19.2)	65.7(20.2)	67.0(20.8)

Train on S, Test on T: We perform standard supervised training of the segmenter on S without adaptation. To segment T, motivated by the similarity between GE and SWI sequences, at test time we use SWI in the channel used for GE during training. Even though these sequences can serve similar purposes in the analysis of TBI by radiologists, this approach totally fails, proving them not directly interchangeable as input to a CNN.

Train on S (No GE/SWI), Test on T: We repeat the previous experiment but only use the common sequences of S and T in both training and testing, neglecting GE and SWI. The experiment was repeated twice to reduce random variations between training sessions. This corresponds to a practical scenario, where we need to segment T by only using annotated training data from S, and serves as the *lower bound* of accuracy for our system.

Train on T, Test on T: We perform a 2-fold validation using supervised training on half of T and testing on the other half. We use all sequences of T. The obtained performance is similar to what was reported in [8], although on a different database. This experiment provides another indication for the expected accuracy on this challenging segmentation task.

Train on S and T, Test on T: To obtain an *upper bound* of accuracy, we train the segmenter on all data of S and half the data of T, using their manual annotations. The same input channel is used for GE of S and SWI of T. We then test on the other half of data from T. The experiment is repeated for the other split of T. We balance the samples from the two domains in each batch B_{adv} to avoid biasing the segmenter towards S that has more subjects. With supervised training on T, the system learns to interchange GE and SWI successfully. This setting uses all available data from both domains, both images and manual annotations, and serves as an estimate of optimal, supervised transfer learning.

Train on S and T, Test on T (GE/SWI in Different Channels): We perform a sanity check that using GE and SWI in the same input channel is reasonable. We repeat the previous experiment but using a CNN with six channels, with separate ones for GE and SWI. The channel is filled with -4 when the sequence is not available, which corresponds to a very low value after our intensity normalization. From this the CNN learns when the sequence is missing and we found this to behave better than common zero-filling. The segmenter performs better than supervised training on T only. This indicates that information from both domains is used. However, knowledge transfer is not as strong as when GE and SWI, which share much information, are used in the same channel.

Proposed Unsupervised Domain Adaptation: We train the segmenter on all data of S and adapt the domains using half the subjects of T, but no labels. GE and SWI share the same input channel. We test accuracy on the other half of T. The experiment is repeated for the other fold. Our method learns filters invariant to the two imaging protocols and transfers knowledge from S to T, allowing the system to segment haemorrhages only visible on SWI without ever seeing a manual annotation from T (Fig. 2). This improves by 3% DSC over the non-adapted segmenter that uses only information from S and the common sequences, covering 44% of the difference between this practical lower bound and the upper bound achieved by supervised training with labels from both domains.

3.4   Analysis of the System

Effect of Adapting Layers at Different Depths: To investigate how depth of adapted layers affects our system, we repeat the experiment with domain adaptation from S to T, changing the layers at which the adversarial networks are connected. Results are shown on Fig. 3 and Table 2. Note that connections are added to both pathways of the segmenter at the same depth (for example, $L4$ means connections to the 4th layers of both pathways). Adapting shallow layers tends towards over-segmentation (increased recall but lower precision). It has been noticed that severe over-segmentation occurs without adaptation (Fig. 2). These observations indicate that source-specific features are possibly recovered between the adapted and the classification layer. Comparing $L2$ and

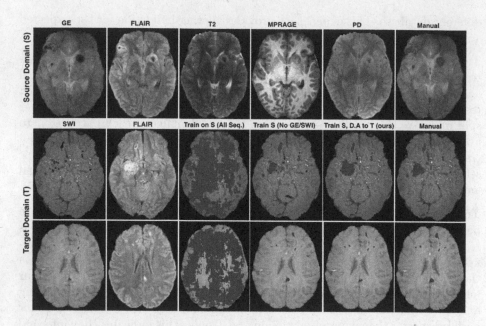

Fig. 2. (top) Example case from S. (middle/bottom) SWI and FLAIR of two subjects from T (T2, MPRAGE, PD also used but not shown). Notice that only GE and SWI show certain lesions, such as micro-bleeds. However, brain tissue appears differently in GE and SWI. Consequently, a model trained on S fails on T when SWI is naively used in place of GE (3rd col.). A model trained using only the four common sequences misses lesions visible only on SWI (4th col.). Our method mitigates these problems by learning features invariant to the imaging protocol (5th col.).

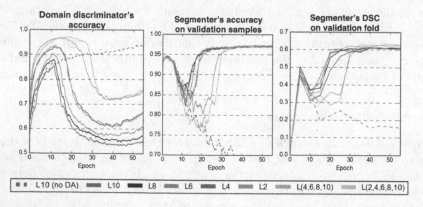

Fig. 3. Behaviour when the domain-discriminator is connected at different layers of the segmenter. Adaptation is performed after epoch 10 by linearly increasing α. Connections at earlier layers lead to higher performance of the discriminator but slower adaptation. Multiple connections increase performance. Note, features learnt at early layers during the refinement in the last stages of training seem more domain-discriminative.

Table 2. Final accuracy on T when the discriminator is connected at different depths of the segmenter. Shallow connections increase recall but significantly decrease precision. Multiple connections remove better the source-specific nuisances throughout the segmenter, closing the gap to the practical upper bound of 66.5% for UDA (Sect. 3.3) by approximately 1.5% DSC. Best configuration in bold.

	L10	L8	L6	L4	L2	**L(4,6,8,10)**	L(2,4,6,8,10)
DSC	61.3(21.0)	61.0(20.7)	61.2(19.2)	61.0(20.1)	60.4(20.2)	62.7(19.8)	62.7(19.5)
Recall	56.9(22.0)	57.3(21.6)	57.1(19.8)	59.1(20.0)	61.1(20.5)	58.9(21.2)	60.1(20.3)
Precision	71.9(20.8)	70.2(20.9)	69.9(20.8)	68.1(21.6)	64.3(21.9)	71.6(18.4)	69.8(20.0)

$L(2, 4, 6, 8, 10)$ shows that this is alleviated by multiple connections that enforce domain invariance throughout the segmenter. Since, however, behaviour of multi-connected adversarials is strongly defined by the shallowest connection, we avoid adapting the earliest layers, which offer less benefit but slow down convergence.

Effect of Adaptation's Strength via α_{max}: Here we investigate how sensitive is our method to α_{max}, which defines how strongly the segmenter counters the discriminator. Figure 4 shows that higher values lead to quicker adaptation but the accuracy is rather stable for a significant range of values $\alpha_{max} \in [0.05, 1.0]$. We note this range might differ for other applications and that smooth convergence is generally preferred for learning high quality features over steep schedules that alter the loss surface aggressively. Finally, we observe that strongly countering the discriminator does not guarantee better performance on T. A theoretical reason is that a more domain-invariant representation $h_a(x)$ likely encodes less information about x. This information loss increases the Bayes error rate and the entropy of the predictions by the learnt $f_a(x) = f_{ah}(h_a(x))$. After a certain level of invariance, this can outweigh the benefits of domain-adaptation [1,7].

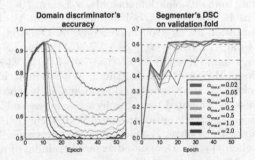

Fig. 4. The segmenter counters the domain-discriminator after epoch 10, when we linearly increase α from zero to α_{max} until epoch 35. Final accuracy on T was found rather stable for a wide range of values. Decrease greater than 1% DSC from the highest was found for values 0.02 and 2.0.

4   Conclusion

We present an unsupervised domain adaptation method for image segmentation based on adversarial training of two 3D neural networks. To the best of our knowledge this is the first work showing the plausibility and capabilities of such an approach on a biomedical imaging problem. Additionally, we propose multi-connected adversarial networks, which perform better by enabling flow of higher quality adversarial gradients throughout the adapted network. We investigate aspects of adversarial training such as the depth of the adapted layer and the strength of adaptation, providing valuable insights for development of future approaches. While unsupervised in the target domain, our method performs close to the accuracy of supervised baselines. We believe our work makes an important contribution in the context of multi-center studies where domain differences are a major limitation in current image analysis methods. Future work will investigate the capabilities of our approach to normalize different types of variations. An implementation of the proposed system will be made publicly available on https://biomedia.doc.ic.ac.uk/software/deepmedic/.

Acknowledgements. This work is supported by the EPSRC (grant No: EP/N023668/1) and partially funded by an European Union Framework Program 7 grant (CENTER-TBI; Agreement No: 60215). Part of this work was carried on when KK was an intern at Microsoft Research Cambridge. KK is also supported by the President's Ph.D. Scholarship of Imperial College London. VN is supported by an Academy of Medical Sciences/Health Foundation Clinician Scientist Fellowship. DM is supported by the Neuroscience Theme of the NIHR Cambridge Biomedical Research Centre and NIHR Senior Investigator awards. We gratefully acknowledge the support of NVIDIA Corporation with the donation of two Titan X GPUs.

References

1. Ben-David, S., Blitzer, J., Crammer, K., Kulesza, A., Pereira, F., Vaughan, J.W.: A theory of learning from different domains. Mach. Learn. **79**(1–2), 151–175 (2010)
2. Bermúdez-Chacón, R., Becker, C., Salzmann, M., Fua, P.: Scalable unsupervised domain adaptation for electron microscopy. In: Ourselin, S., Joskowicz, L., Sabuncu, M.R., Unal, G., Wells, W. (eds.) MICCAI 2016. LNCS, vol. 9901, pp. 326–334. Springer, Cham (2016). doi:10.1007/978-3-319-46723-8_38
3. Ciompi, F., de Hoop, B., van Riel, S.J., Chung, K., Scholten, E.T., Oudkerk, M., de Jong, P.A., Prokop, M., van Ginneken, B.: Automatic classification of pulmonary peri-fissural nodules in computed tomography using an ensemble of 2D views and a convolutional neural network out-of-the-box. MedIA **26**(1), 195–202 (2015)
4. Ganin, Y., Ustinova, E., Ajakan, H., Germain, P., Larochelle, H., Laviolette, F., Marchand, M., Lempitsky, V.: Domain-adversarial training of neural networks. J. Mach. Learn. Res. **17**(59), 1–35 (2016)
5. Goodfellow, I., Pouget-Abadie, J., Mirza, M., Xu, B., Warde-Farley, D., Ozair, S., Courville, A., Bengio, Y.: Generative adversarial nets. In: NIPS (2014)
6. Heimann, T., Mountney, P., John, M., Ionasec, R.: Learning without labeling: domain adaptation for ultrasound transducer localization. In: Mori, K., Sakuma, I., Sato, Y., Barillot, C., Navab, N. (eds.) MICCAI 2013. LNCS, vol. 8151, pp. 49–56. Springer, Heidelberg (2013). doi:10.1007/978-3-642-40760-4_7

7. Jiang, J.: A literature survey on domain adaptation of statistical classifiers (2008). http://sifaka.cs.uiuc.edu/jiang4/domain_adaptation/survey/da_survey.pdf
8. Kamnitsas, K., Ledig, C., Newcombe, V.F., Simpson, J.P., Kane, A.D., Menon, D.K., Rueckert, D., Glocker, B.: Efficient multi-scale 3D CNN with fully connected CRF for accurate brain lesion segmentation. MedIA **36**, 61–78 (2016)
9. Lee, C.Y., Xie, S., Gallagher, P., Zhang, Z., Tu, Z.: Deeply-supervised nets. In: AISTATS, vol. 2, p. 6 (2015)
10. Long, J., Shelhamer, E., Darrell, T.: Fully convolutional networks for semantic segmentation. In: CVPR (2015)
11. Long, M., Cao, Y., Wang, J., Jordan, M.: Learning transferable features with deep adaptation networks. In: ICML (2015)
12. Moeskops, P., Wolterink, J.M., Velden, B.H.M., Gilhuijs, K.G.A., Leiner, T., Viergever, M.A., Išgum, I.: Deep learning for multi-task medical image segmentation in multiple modalities. In: Ourselin, S., Joskowicz, L., Sabuncu, M.R., Unal, G., Wells, W. (eds.) MICCAI 2016. LNCS, vol. 9901, pp. 478–486. Springer, Cham (2016). doi:10.1007/978-3-319-46723-8_55
13. van Opbroek, A., Ikram, M.A., Vernooij, M.W., De Bruijne, M.: Transfer learning improves supervised image segmentation across imaging protocols. TMI **34**(5), 1018–1030 (2015)
14. Pan, S.J., Yang, Q.: A survey on transfer learning. IEEE Trans. Knowl. Data Eng. **22**(10), 1345–1359 (2010)
15. Shenton, M., Hamoda, H., Schneiderman, J., Bouix, S., Pasternak, O., Rathi, Y., Vu, M.A., Purohit, M., Helmer, K., Koerte, I., et al.: A review of magnetic resonance imaging and diffusion tensor imaging findings in mild traumatic brain injury. Brain Imaging Behav. **6**(2), 137–192 (2012)
16. Shin, H.C., Roth, H.R., Gao, M., Lu, L., Xu, Z., Nogues, I., Yao, J., Mollura, D., Summers, R.M.: Deep convolutional neural networks for computer-aided detection: Cnn architectures, dataset characteristics and transfer learning. TMI **35**(5), 1285–1298 (2016)
17. Tzeng, E., Hoffman, J., Zhang, N., Saenko, K., Darrell, T.: Deep domain confusion: maximizing for domain invariance. arXiv preprint (2014). arXiv:1412.3474
18. Ullman, S., Assif, L., Fetaya, E., Harari, D.: Atoms of recognition in human and computer vision. Proc. Nat. Acad Sci. **113**(10), 2744–2749 (2016)
19. Valiant, L.G.: A theory of the learnable. Commun. ACM **27**(11), 1134–1142 (1984). http://doi.acm.org/10.1145/1968.1972

Globally Optimal Coupled Surfaces for Semi-automatic Segmentation of Medical Images

Juan Eugenio Iglesias[✉]

Translational Imaging Group, University College London, London, UK
e.iglesias@ucl.ac.uk

Abstract. Manual delineations are of paramount importance in medical imaging, for instance to train supervised methods and evaluate automatic segmentation algorithms. In volumetric images, manually tracing regions of interest is an excruciating process in which much time is wasted labeling neighboring 2D slices that are similar to each other. Here we present a method to compute a set of discrete minimal surfaces whose boundaries are specified by user-provided segmentations on one or more planes. Using this method, the user can for example manually delineate one slice every n and let the algorithm complete the segmentation for the slices in between. Using a discrete framework, this method globally minimizes a cost function that combines a regularizer with a data term based on image intensities, while ensuring that the surfaces do not intersect each other or leave holes in between. While the resulting optimization problem is an integer program and thus NP-hard, we show that the equality constraint matrix is totally unimodular, which enables us to solve the linear program (LP) relaxation instead. We can then capitalize on the existence of efficient LP solvers to compute a globally optimal solution in practical times. Experiments on two different datasets illustrate the superiority of the proposed method over the use of independent, label-wise optimal surfaces ($\sim$5% mean increase in Dice when one every six slices is labeled, with some structures improving up to $\sim$10% in Dice).

1 Introduction

Image segmentation is the process of assigning meaningful labels to pixels (2D) or voxels (3D). In medical imaging, the set of labels corresponds to a number of biologically relevant regions of interest (ROIs), such as different organs, types of cells, etc., as well as a background, in most cases. Segmentation is a key preprocessing step for a wide array of subsequent analyses, such as volumetry or shape analysis, and is therefore one of the core problems in medical imaging.

As useful as traditional manual segmentation is, its usage is encumbered by the necessity that images have to be delineated by an expert, which leads to three main issues: (a) it is not reproducible; (b) it often requires expertise that might not be present at every research center; and (c) it is typically very time consuming – and thus expensive. This last limitation is particularly problematic in 3D data (in which multiple 2D slices are traced to create a 3D segmentation)

© Springer International Publishing AG 2017
M. Niethammer et al. (Eds.): IPMI 2017, LNCS 10265, pp. 610–621, 2017.
DOI: 10.1007/978-3-319-59050-9_48

for two reasons. First, the increasing resolution of medical images requires segmenting a larger number of 2D slices. And second, several iterations are often needed in order to ensure that segmentations made in a particular orientation are consistent and smooth when displayed in the orthogonal views. Moreover, 3D segmentation is typically a very inefficient process, since a lot of time is spent labeling 2D images that are very similar to their neighboring slices.

Some of the limitations of manual segmentation can be addressed with automated techniques. Most popular families of automatic segmentation methods are supervised and rely on training data, e.g., shape models [1], multi-atlas segmentation [2,3], probabilistic atlases [4], or voxel classifiers based on learning models such as support vector machines [5], random forests [6] or, more recently, deep neural networks (e.g., [7]). However, creating databases of labeled training data for supervised techniques still requires manually segmenting images. And even for unsupervised methods, manual delineations are needed to produce a gold standard with validation purposes.

A faster, more reproducible way of generating gold standards is through semi-automated segmentation, which represents a compromise between automated and manual methods: the user is required to provide a relatively small amount of input, which an automated algorithm subsequently uses to produce a dense segmentation of the whole image. In 2D, the popular live wire method [8,9] uses a shortest path algorithm to produce a continuous contour out of a set of points placed along the (possibly ill-defined) boundary of an object. The Grab-Cut algorithm [10] iteratively uses graph cuts [11] to create a segmentation of an object from a rectangular, user-provided bounding box. The Random Walker algorithm [12] uses a set of user-provided scribbles to compute a dense segmentation based on the probability that a random walker starting at each unlabeled pixel first reaches one of the prelabeled pixels. GeoS [13] also relies on scribbles to produce a geodesic distance map that, in the context of a conditional random field, yields the final segmentation. Many of these methods can be made interactive by allowing the user to modify his input while updating the output in real-time – if this is computationally feasible.

Extending the semi-automated methods described above to 3D is immediate in most cases. A notable exception is live wire, which requires finding a minimal surface joining user-specified contours. Such an extension has a direct, very useful application to semi-automated segmentation: a user can manually delineate one slice every n in a 3D volume (possibly with 2D semi-automated techniques) and then use this method to produce a smart "interpolation" of the segmentation for the unlabeled slices. This strategy effectively exploits the similarity between adjacent slices and can save large amounts of manual labeling effort.

After some attempts in the literature to reconstruct 2D surfaces from sets of 1D curves (e.g., [14]), Grady proposed an algorithm [15] to compute a globally minimal surface given its boundary. The solution is efficiently found by solving a minimum-cost flow problem [16]. Compared with other globally optimal surface algorithms, such as LOGISMOS [17] and its variants (all based on [18]), Grady's method has the advantages of being able to handle topological changes in the optimal surface; being agnostic to the type and modality of the input images; and not requiring a preliminary volumetric segmentation.

Generalizing Grady's method to multi-class segmentation is not straightforward. One can apply the algorithm one label at the time and combine the binary outputs into a multi-class segmentation, but this approach has three disadvantages. First, it requires handcrafting rules for handling conflicts (overlaps, holes) when merging segmentations. Second, it is suboptimal in terms of cost function. And third, the quality of the segmentation can in some cases be considerably worse than that of an algorithm that jointly computes the surfaces, e.g., high-contrast ROIs can help the segmentation of neighboring lower-contrast ROIs.

Here we present a generalization of Grady's algorithm to multiple ROIs. The method computes surfaces simultaneously for all labels while ensuring that no holes or overlaps are produced, and also inherits the ability to handle topological changes in the surfaces. We show that, despite the coupling between the surfaces, the globally optimal solution can still be obtained by solving a linear (rather than integer) program, which can be done in practical times with existing techniques.

2   Methods

2.1   Continuous Formulation of Joint Surface Fitting

In the continuous domain, the problem of joint surface fitting can be framed as a constrained optimization problem, illustrated in Fig. 1. Given a cuboid shaped 3D image domain Ω, let $\{\mathcal{U}_l : l = 1, \ldots, L\}$ represent user-provided segmentations for L different ROIs (including the background), defined on one or more planes. In our target application, there would be two parallel planes[1], but this does not need to be the case in our formulation. Let $\{\mathcal{R}_l = \delta\mathcal{U}_l : l = 1, \ldots, L\}$ represent the boundaries of the segmentations; note that each $\mathcal{R}_l$ can represent more than one contour, e.g., contours on different planes, as in Fig. 1. Finally, let $\{\mathcal{Z}_l : l = 1, \ldots, L\}$ represent the L surfaces to fit; note that $\mathcal{Z}_l$ is necessarily an open surface since it has a non-empty boundary $\mathcal{R}_l$. The problem is then:

$$\min_{\{\mathcal{Z}_l\}} \sum_{l=1}^{L} \left(\alpha \int_{\mathcal{Z}_l} dS + \int_{\mathcal{Z}_l} g_l(I, \hat{\boldsymbol{n}}; \beta) dS \right) \tag{1}$$

$$\text{s.t.} \quad \mathcal{B}(\mathcal{Z}_l) = \mathcal{R}_l, \quad \bigcup_{l=1}^{L} \text{Vol}(\mathcal{Z}_l \cup \mathcal{U}_l) = \Omega, \quad \bigcap_{l=\{l_1,l_2\}} \text{Vol}(\mathcal{Z}_l \cup \mathcal{U}_l) = \emptyset, \forall l_1 \neq l_2,$$

where dS is the area element; $\mathcal{B}$ is the boundary operator; $\text{Vol}(\mathcal{Z}_l \cup \mathcal{U}_l)$ is the 3D segmentation enclosed by $\mathcal{Z}_l \cup \mathcal{U}_l$; α, β are scalar constants; I represents the image intensities; and $\hat{\boldsymbol{n}}$ is the surface normal at each point (pointing towards the inside of the volume). The first term in Eq. 1 is a regularizer that penalizes the total surface area with relative weight α. The second term encourages the

---

[1] If there are more than two segmented slices, we can solve for one gap between labeled planes at the time because the boundary conditions decouple the problems.

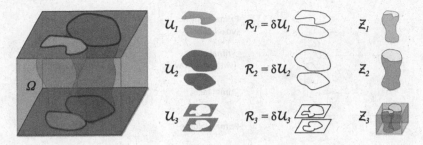

Fig. 1. We aim to find the open surfaces $\{\mathcal{Z}_l\}$ that: (a) globally minimize the cost function in Eq. 1; (b) are constrained to have boundaries $\{\mathcal{R}_l\}$ given by the contours of user-specified segmentations $\{\mathcal{U}_l\}$; and (c) do not intersect or leave holes in between.

surfaces to follow perpendicular image gradients, by means of a function g_l of the image intensities and the normal $\hat{n}$, parametrized by β. A frequent choice is:

$$g_l(I, \hat{n}; \beta) = \exp(-\beta \|\nabla_{\hat{n}} I\|^2), \tag{2}$$

which we use in this study. Note that the cost of a surface is independent of its label l in Eq. 2, but this does not need to be the case in general.

2.2 Discrete Formulation

We follow [15] to discretize the problem in Eq. 1, which enables us to compute a globally optimal solution. We assume that our image intensities are defined at the center of cuboid voxels. These centers correspond to the nodes of a 6-connected 3D lattice, which defines our primal graph (see Fig. 2). The (primal) nodes are connected by K primal[2] edges $\{e_k^p : k = 1, \ldots, K\}$, which have corresponding (label-dependent) weights $\boldsymbol{w}_l = [w_{l1}, \ldots, w_{lK}]^T$. In addition, we also consider the dual graph, in which nodes corresponds to volumes, edges to facets, and vice versa. The volumes of the dual graph correspond to the cuboids of the image voxels, such that the dual facets $\{f_k^d : k = 1, \ldots, K\}$ correspond to the faces of these cuboids (where our surfaces will be defined). The dual facets have a direct correspondence with the primal edges, and hence share the same weights w_{lk}. Note that it is crucial to include each primal edge/dual facet twice in $\{e_k^p\}$, $\{f_k^d\}$ and $\boldsymbol{w}_l$ with opposite orientations. This is because we need to discern whether the segmented ROI is on one side of the dual facet or the other, following the convention that the surface normal points toward the inside of the enclosed volume. In a similar fashion, we also consider the M dual edges $\{c_m^d : m = 1, \ldots, M\}$ with corresponding primal facets $\{f_m^p : m = 1, \ldots, M\}$.

To represent each surface, we use a discrete function $\boldsymbol{z}_l = [z_{l1}, \ldots, z_{lK}]^T$ that encodes whether dual facet f_k^d is part of the lth surface (or, equivalently, whether primal edge e_k^p intersects the surface), and with what multiplicity. Hence, we are replacing each continuous surface $\mathcal{Z}_l$ by a set of voxel faces represented by $\boldsymbol{z}_l$.

---

[2] We use superscript p for primal and superscript d for dual.

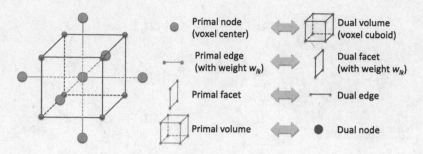

Fig. 2. Duality in 3D, 6-connected lattice. The image intensities are defined on the primal nodes. The surfaces we consider in this paper are given by sets of dual facets, which are equivalent to the faces of the cuboids representing image voxels.

Cost Function: We discretize the cost function by replacing integrals by sums in Eq. 1. If dual facet f_k^d is part of the lth surface, its contribution to the cost is:

$$w_{lk} = \text{Area}(f_k^d)\left(\alpha + \exp\left[-\beta(I_{j_1} - I_{j_2})^2\right]\right),$$

where I_{j_1} and I_{j2} are the image intensities at the primal nodes defining the corresponding primal edge e_k^p; and $\text{Area}(f_k^d)$ is the area of facet f_k^d, given by the voxel dimensions. In our case, due to the choice of g_l in Eq. 2, the weight is the same for both orientations of the edge, but this does not need to be the case in general. We have kept the weights $\{w_l\}$ separated in the notation (even if they are the same for all ROIs) for practical reasons in the implementation of the algorithm (Sect. 3.2 below). The total cost to minimize is then given by:

$$\min_{\{z_l\}} \quad \sum_l \boldsymbol{w}_l^T \boldsymbol{z}_l = \sum_l \sum_k w_{lk} z_{lk}. \tag{3}$$

Constraints: We need to consider two sets of constraints. First, we must ensure that the boundaries of the surfaces correspond to the contours of the specified 2D segmentations. This can be achieved through the edge-facet incidence matrix of the dual graph $\boldsymbol{B}$, which yields the discrete 3D boundary operator:

$$B_{mk} = \begin{cases} 1, & \text{if } e_m^d \text{ borders } f_k^d \text{ with coherent orientation,} \\ -1, & \text{if } e_m^d \text{ borders } f_k^d \text{ without coherent orientation,} \\ 0, & \text{otherwise,} \end{cases} \tag{4}$$

where orientation coherence is given by the right-hand rule. Next, we define the contour vectors $\{\boldsymbol{r}_l : l = 1, \ldots, L\}$, also on the dual graph, which represent the boundaries of the user-defined segmentations on one or more slices:

$$r_{lm} = \begin{cases} 1, & \text{if } e_m^d \text{ is on the } l^{\text{th}} \text{ contour with coherent orientation,} \\ -1, & \text{if } e_m^d \text{ is on the } l^{\text{th}} \text{ contour without coherent orientation,} \\ 0, & \text{otherwise.} \end{cases} \tag{5}$$

With these definitions of B and r_l, we can write the constraints simply as:

$$Bz_l = r_l, \quad \forall l. \tag{6}$$

The second set of constraint specifies that the union of the enclosed volumes needs to be equal to the image domain Ω, while the intersection must be the empty set. We define the matrix C and vector t as:

$$C_{kk'} = \begin{cases} 1, & \text{if } k' = k, \\ -1, & \text{if } k' = \tilde{k}(k), \\ 0, & \text{otherwise,} \end{cases}, \quad t_k = \begin{cases} 1, & \text{if } f_k^d \in \delta\Omega_{[\text{inwards}]}, \\ -1, & \text{if } f_k^d \in \delta\Omega_{[\text{outwards}]}, \\ 0, & \text{otherwise,} \end{cases} \tag{7}$$

where $\tilde{k}(k)$ is the index of facet $f_{\tilde{k}}^d$ with opposite orientation to f_k^d, whereas $\delta\Omega_{[\text{inwards}]}$ and $\delta\Omega_{[\text{outwards}]}$ are the sets of dual facets on the external boundary of Ω whose associated normals point towards the inside and outside of the image domain, respectively. We also define $C^* = [C \ C \cdots C]$, and $z^* = [z_1^T \cdots z_L^T]^T$. Then, the constraints can be encoded in the following system of linear equations:

$$C^* z^* = t. \tag{8}$$

Forcing $\sum_{l=1}^{L} \left(z_{lk} - z_{l\tilde{k}} \right)$ in Eq. 8 to be zero inside Ω ensures that, if a facet is part of a surface on one side, it must also be part of another on the other side, thus avoiding holes and overlaps in the segmentation. Forcing the sum to be ± 1 (depending on the orientation) on the walls ensures that the whole image domain will be covered by the surfaces. In practice, including one of the orientations in C and t is sufficient, since swapping k and $\tilde{k}$ yields the same constraints.

2.3   Integer Program and Linear Programming Relaxation

We can combine the cost function in Eq. 3 with the constraints defined in Eqs. 6 and 8 to define the following integer program (IP):

$$\begin{aligned} \min_{z^*} \quad & W^T z^* \\ \text{s.t.} \quad & Az^* = v \\ & z^* \succeq 0, \\ & z^* \in \mathbb{Z}^{L \times K}, \end{aligned} \tag{9}$$

where we have defined:

$$W = \begin{bmatrix} w_1 \\ w_2 \\ \vdots \\ w_L \end{bmatrix}, \quad A = \begin{bmatrix} B & 0 & \cdots & 0 \\ 0 & B & \cdots & 0 \\ \vdots & \vdots & \ddots & \vdots \\ 0 & 0 & \cdots & B \\ & & C^* & \end{bmatrix}, \quad v = \begin{bmatrix} r_1 \\ r_2 \\ \vdots \\ r_L \\ t \end{bmatrix}. \tag{10}$$

Integer programming is notoriously an NP-hard problem [19]. Therefore, solving (9) directly is impractical. However, it can be shown [20] that, if the equality constraint matrix A is totally unimodular[3] (TU) and the equality constraint vector v is integer valued, then the linear programming (LP) relaxation of the IP is guaranteed to produce an integer solution, which is equal to the solution of the original IP (note that this condition is sufficient, but not necessary).

Lemma. *The equality constraint matrix A in IP (9) is TU.*

Proof. It can be shown [21] that a sufficient condition for TU is that the columns of the matrix add up to zero while all its elements are in the set $\{-1, 0, 1\}$. Here, we first observe that the matrix B can be partitioned into $B = [B_1 | B_2]$, such that B_1 includes each dual facet only once – no matter with which of the two possible orientations. Then, if we sort the columns of B_2 such that they follow the same facet order as B_1, we have that $B_2 = -B_1$, since the columns correspond to the same facets but with opposite edge orientations. Hence, the columns of B add up to the zero vector. The columns of C^* also add up to the zero vector, since each row contains L elements equal to 1 and L equal to -1. Therefore, the columns of A also add up to zero (Eq. 10). Since all elements of A are in the set $\{-1, 0, 1\}$ (from the definitions of B and C^* in Eqs. 4 and 7), then A is TU.

Since A is TU and v is integer (see the definitions of r_l and t in Eqs. 5 and 7), the following LP relaxation yields the same solution as (9):

$$
\begin{aligned}
\min_{z^*} \quad & W^T z^* \\
\text{s.t.} \quad & A z^* = v \\
& z^* \succeq 0, \\
& z^* \in \mathbb{R}^{L \times K},
\end{aligned}
\tag{11}
$$

Linear programming has polynomial complexity, and efficient solvers exist to compute the globally optimal solution of (11) in practical times.

3 Experiments and Results

3.1 Data

We used two publicly available datasets in our experiments. The first dataset consists of 35 T1-weighted brain MRI scans from the 2013 MICCAI SATA challenge[4]. The images were acquired on a 3 T scanner with an MP-RAGE sequence at 1 mm isotropic resolution. Fourteen structures were labeled by experts in coronal plane: left and right amygdala, caudate, accumbens, hippocampus, putamen, thalamus and pallidum. We refer to these data as the "brain dataset".

The second dataset consists of five *ex vivo* MRI scans of single human hippocampi (3 right, 3 left) [22]. The scans were acquired on a 9.4 T scanner

---

[3] A matrix is TU if it is integer and every square submatrix has determinant 1 or -1.
[4] https://www.synapse.org/#!Synapse:syn3193805/wiki/217780.

with a multi-spin echo sequence at $0.2 \times 0.2 \times 0.3$ mm resolution (coronal). Five hippocampal subfields were manually delineated on the images by an expert: CA1; CA2 and CA3 (CA23); hilus of the dentate gyrus (DG:H); stratum radiatum, stratum lacunosum-moleculare and the vestigial hippocampal sulcus (SR+SLM+VHS); and stratum moleculare of the dentate gyrus (DG:SM). The manual segmentations were mostly made on the coronal plane, with verification in the sagittal plane. We refer to these images as the "hippocampal dataset".

3.2 Experimental Setup

We evaluated the performance of our algorithm as a function of n_{skip}, the number of unlabeled slices between each pair of labeled slices. As baseline approach, we applied Grady's algorithm to each label independently, and then merged the resulting L binary segmentations into a multi-label volume – if two segmentations overlapped in given region, we selected the label that gave the lowest cost (Eq. 3).

For each value of n_{skip}, we randomly sampled 10 and 50 stacks of $n_{\text{skip}} + 2$ coronal slices from each scan of the brain and hippocampal datasets, respectively. This yielded 600 test volumes (350 brain, 250 hippocampal), in which the segmentation was assumed to be known for the first and last slice. We then used the two competing methods to segment the rest of the slices in each volume, and measured the overlap with the ground truth using Dice scores. We merged the results of the left and right side of each ROI for simplicity of presentation.

Implementation Details: We min-max normalized the images to $[0, 255]$, and manually tuned the parameters (on a separate brain MRI dataset) to $\beta = 0.005$ and $\alpha = 10^{-5}/n_{\text{skip}}$. We solved the LP (11) with Gurobi 7.0 (www.gurobi.com). To handle the boundaries $\delta\Omega$ for which no segmentation was specified by the user (e.g., the "walls" completing the surface of the cuboid between two labeled slices), we assumed that the background ROI surrounded all others (which was the case in all our experiments) and set the costs w_{lk} of the corresponding surface facets (with the normal facing inwards) to a large negative constant:

$$
W = \begin{bmatrix} \tilde{w}_1 \\ \vdots \\ \tilde{w}_L \end{bmatrix}, \text{ where } \tilde{w}_{lk} = \begin{cases} -\infty, & \text{if } l = \text{background, } f_k^d \in \delta\Omega_{\text{[inwards]}} \text{ and } f_k^d \\ & \text{does not correspond to a segmented voxel} \\ w_{lk}, & \text{otherwise.} \end{cases}
$$

This setup also enabled us to drop the rows corresponding to the dual facets on $\delta\Omega$ from the C matrix (Eq. 7), speeding up convergence of the solver in practice.

3.3 Results

Figures 3 and 4 show the results for the brain and hippocampal datasets, respectively, whereas Figs. 5 and 6 display sample outputs for the two competing algorithms. In the brain dataset, the proposed method exploits the neighboring relationships between the structures in order to outperform the baseline algorithm for every ROI. The differences between the two methods become larger as

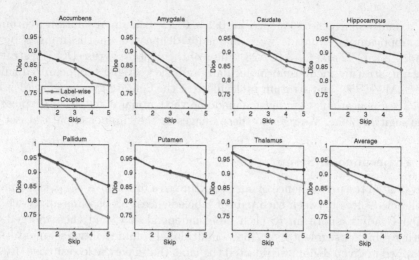

Fig. 3. Brain dataset: Dice score as a function of the number of unlabeled slices between manually segmented slices for each brain structure, as well as average across structures.

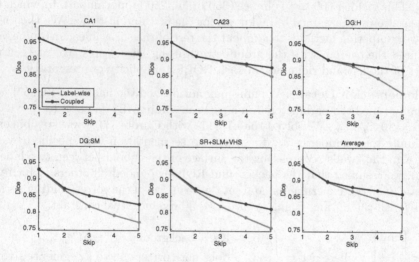

Fig. 4. Hippocampal dataset: Dice score as a function of the number of unlabeled slices between manually segmented slices for each subfield, as well as average across subfields.

the separation n_{skip} grows, averaging 5% Dice at $n_{skip} = 5$. The gap is particularly large (>11% at $n_{skip} = 5$) for the pallidum; this structure is often heavily undersegmented when processed on its own, but frequently emerges when segmented jointly with the neighboring, high-contrast putamen (as in Fig. 5).

The results are similar in the hippocampal dataset. For the larger, high-contrast CA1, both methods produce almost identical results. However, for the internal, lower-contrast subfields, the proposed method outperforms the baseline, averaging 4% higher Dice by $n_{skip} = 5$. The difference is largest for the stratum moleculare (DG:SM) and hilus (DG:H) of the dentate gyrus, which share a boundary that is practically invisible in the images (see example in Fig. 6).

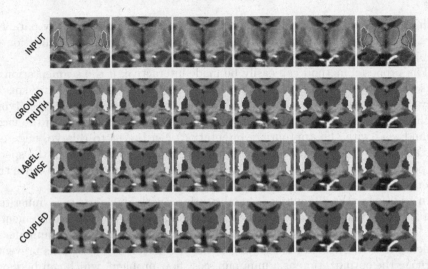

Fig. 5. Sample segmentations from brain dataset with $n_{skip} = 4$. Green is hippocampus, orange is putamen, blue is pallidum, dark red is thalamus, brown is caudate, and purple is amygdala. Note the missing pallidum in the baseline approach. (Color figure online)

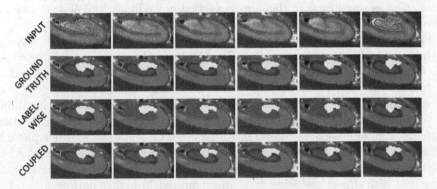

Fig. 6. Sample segmentations from the hippocampal dataset with $n_{skip} = 4$. Blue is CA1, white is CA23, red is DG:H, violet is DG:SM and pink is SR+SLM+VHS. Note the missing DG:SM in the baseline method. (Color figure online)

In absolute terms, the proposed algorithm yields satisfactory results (Dice above 85–90%) for many structures all the way to $n_{skip} = 5$ (hippocampus, putamen, thalamus, CA1, CA23, DG:H), and for most structures at $n_{skip} \leq 3$. Exceptions are ROIs with faint boundaries and poor reliability (e.g., amygdala, SR+SLM+VHS). However, even low values of n_{skip} can be very useful in practice, since they can save $100 \times n_{skip}/(1 + n_{skip})$ percent of manual labeling effort.

4   Conclusion

We have presented a semi-automated segmentation method that can compute a globally optimal set of discrete coupled surfaces, whose boundaries are specified by the contours of user-provided delineations on one or more (typically parallel) slices. The results have shown that the method outperforms the application of the binary version to each ROI independently.

The proposed method can easily be made interactive: if the segmentation is not satisfactory, feedback can be provided to correct the output. More specifically, the user can mark an oriented boundary between two voxels, specifying which label l should be found on a given side of it. Then, the weight of the facet at hand w_{lk} (with the appropriate orientation) can be set to a large, negative constant. This procedure effectively forces the surfaces to go through the specified points when the LP in (11) is solved to update the segmentation – since the solver is guaranteed to yield the global optimum.

In addition to the difficulties to handle surfaces with high curvature (inherited from [15]), the main limitation of the method is its computational requirements. The null-space of A in Eq. 10 does not yield a concatenation of volume-facet incidence matrices due to the coupling terms introduced by Eq. 8. This prevents rewriting the optimization as a minimum-cost flow problem, which can be more efficiently solved [15]. We were able to solve the LP relaxation relatively quickly in our experiments (minutes in the worst cases), but computation times grow quickly with image size. This is not a problem when "interpolating" segmentations across slices (a task the can be carried out offline), but it is a limiting factor for the interactive extension of the algorithm discussed above.

Future work will follow four directions. First, we will investigate ways of further simplifying the LP relaxation (Eq. 11). If we identify the graph for which A is the incidence matrix, we can device a faster optimization algorithm based on its dual graph. Second, we will implement and validate the interactive version of the algorithm. Third, we will evaluate the algorithm more extensively, including experiments with multiple orientations (e.g., 2.5D) and comparisons with other methods (e.g., alpha-expansion [11]). And fourth, we will explore other possible definitions of g_l (Eq. 2); while a simple exponential captures most visible edges (relying on the regularizer around ill-defined boundaries), ROI-specific weights computed with supervised edge detectors should yield higher performance.

As the amounts of available imaging data and their resolution grow, and as the requirements of labeled data to train state-of-the art supervised algorithms increase, we believe that semi-automated approaches like the method proposed in this paper will become increasingly important in medical image analysis.

Acknowledgement. This research was supported by the European Research Council (Starting Grant 677697, project BUNGEE-TOOLS), and would not have been possible without the suggestions from Dr. Leo Grady (HeartFlow, Inc.).

References

1. Cootes, T., Taylor, C., Cooper, D., Graham, J.: Active shape models-their training and application. Comput. Vis. Image Underst. **61**(1), 38–59 (1995)
2. Rohlfing, T., Brandt, R., Menzel, R., Maurer, C.R.: Evaluation of atlas selection strategies for atlas-based image segmentation with application to confocal microscopy images of bee brains. NeuroImage **21**(4), 1428–1442 (2004)

3. Iglesias, J.E., Sabuncu, M.R.: Multi-atlas segmentation of biomedical images: a survey. Med. Image Anal. **24**(1), 205–219 (2015)
4. Ashburner, J., Friston, K.J.: Unified segmentation. NeuroImage **26**, 839–851 (2005)
5. Boser, B.E., Guyon, I.M., Vapnik, V.N.: A training algorithm for optimal margin classifiers. In: Proceedings of the 5th Annual Workshop on Computational Learning Theory, pp. 144–152 (1992)
6. Breiman, L.: Random forests. Mach. Learn. **45**(1), 5–32 (2001)
7. Çiçek, Ö., Abdulkadir, A., Lienkamp, S.S., Brox, T., Ronneberger, O.: 3D U-Net: learning dense volumetric segmentation from sparse annotation. In: Ourselin, S., Joskowicz, L., Sabuncu, M.R., Unal, G., Wells, W. (eds.) MICCAI 2016. LNCS, vol. 9901, pp. 424–432. Springer, Cham (2016). doi:10.1007/978-3-319-46723-8_49
8. Falcão, A.X., Udupa, J.K., Samarasekera, S., Sharma, S., Hirsch, B.E., Lotufo, R.A.: User-steered image segmentation paradigms: live wire and live lane. Graph. Models Image Process. **60**(4), 233–260 (1998)
9. Mortensen, E.N., Barrett, W.A.: Interactive segmentation with intelligent scissors. Graph. Models Image Process. **60**(5), 349–384 (1998)
10. Rother, C., Kolmogorov, V., Blake, A.: GrabCut: interactive foreground extraction using iterated graph cuts. ACM Trans. Graph. **23**(3), 309–314 (2004)
11. Boykov, Y., Veksler, O., Zabih, R.: Fast approximate energy minimization via graph cuts. IEEE Trans. Pattern Anal. Mach. Intell. **23**(11), 1222–1239 (2001)
12. Grady, L.: Random walks for image segmentation. IEEE Trans. Pattern Anal. Mach. Intell. **28**(11), 1768–1783 (2006)
13. Criminisi, A., Sharp, T., Blake, A.: GeoS: geodesic image segmentation. In: Forsyth, D., Torr, P., Zisserman, A. (eds.) ECCV 2008. LNCS, vol. 5302, pp. 99–112. Springer, Heidelberg (2008). doi:10.1007/978-3-540-88682-2_9
14. Falcão, A.X., Udupa, J.K.: A 3D generalization of user-steered live-wire segmentation. Med. Image Anal. **4**(4), 389–402 (2000)
15. Grady, L.: Minimal surfaces extend shortest path segmentation methods to 3D. IEEE Trans. Pattern Anal. Mach. Intell. **32**(2), 321–334 (2010)
16. Sullivan, J.M.: A crystalline approximation theorem for hypersurfaces. Ph.D. thesis, Princeton (1990)
17. Yin, Y., Zhang, X., Williams, R., Wu, X., Anderson, D.D., Sonka, M.: LOGISMOS - layered optimal graph image segmentation of multiple objects and surfaces: cartilage segmentation in the knee joint. IEEE Trans. Med. Imaging **29**(12), 2023–2037 (2010)
18. Li, K., Wu, X., Chen, D.Z., Sonka, M.: Optimal surface segmentation in volumetric images-a graph-theoretic approach. IEEE Trans. Pattern Anal. Mach. Intell. **28**(1), 119–134 (2006)
19. Papadimitriou, C.H.: On the complexity of integer programming. J. ACM **28**(4), 765–768 (1981)
20. Grady, L.J., Polimeni, J.: Discrete Calculus: Applied Analysis on Graphs for Computational Science. Springer Science & Business Media, Berlin (2010)
21. Schrijver, A.: Theory of Linear and Integer Programming. Wiley, Hoboken (1998)
22. Yushkevich, P.A., Avants, B.B., Pluta, J., Das, S., Minkoff, D., Mechanic-Hamilton, D., Glynn, S., Pickup, S., Liu, W., Gee, J.C., Grossman, M., Detreb, J.: A high-resolution computational atlas of the human hippocampus from postmortem magnetic resonance imaging at 9.4 T. NeuroImage **44**(2), 385–398 (2009)

Joint Deep Learning of Foreground, Background and Shape for Robust Contextual Segmentation

Hariharan Ravishankar$^{(\boxtimes)}$, S. Thiruvenkadam, R. Venkataramani, and V. Vaidya

GE Global Research, Bangalore, India
hariharan.ravishankar@ge.com

Abstract. Encouraged by the success of CNNs in classification problems, CNNs are being actively applied to image-wide prediction problems such as segmentation, optic flow, reconstruction, restoration etc. These approaches fall under the category of fully convolutional networks [FCN] and have been very successful in bringing contexts into learning for image analysis. In this work, we address the problem of segmentation from medical images. Segmentation or object delineation from medical images/volumes is a fundamental step for subsequent quantification tasks key to diagnosis. Semantic segmentation has been popularly addressed using FCN (e.g. U-NET) with impressive results and has been the fore runner in recent segmentation challenges. However, there are a few drawbacks of FCN approaches which recent works have tried to address. Firstly, local geometry such as smoothness and shape are not reliably captured. Secondly, spatial context captured by FCNs while giving the advantage of a richer representation carries the intrinsic drawback of overfitting, and is quite sensitive to appearance and shape changes. To handle above issues, in this work, we propose a hybrid of generative modeling of image formation to jointly learn the triad of foreground (F), background (B) and shape (S). Such generative modeling of F, B, S would carry the advantages of FCN in capturing contexts. Further we expect the approach to be useful under limited training data, results easy to interpret, and enable easy transfer of learning across segmentation problems. We present ~8% improvement over state of art FCN approaches for US kidney segmentation and while achieving comparable results on CT lung nodule segmentation.

1 Introduction

Convolutional neural networks (CNNs) [7,10,14,18] have proven to be very successful in a wide range of visual tasks such as classification, recognition, characterization, tracking and segmentation. CNNs provide effective models for above vision learning tasks by incorporating spatial context and weight sharing between pixels across several hierarchical layers. Currently, CNNs are being actively applied to image-wide prediction problems such as segmentation [16],

---

The first two authors contributed equally.

© Springer International Publishing AG 2017
M. Niethammer et al. (Eds.): IPMI 2017, LNCS 10265, pp. 622–632, 2017.
DOI: 10.1007/978-3-319-59050-9_49

optic flow [8], reconstruction [12], restoration [5] etc. These approaches fall under the category of fully convolutional networks [FCN] and have been very successful in bringing contexts into learning for image analysis. Models based on FCN have now been applied successfully to various 2D/3D medical image segmentation problems (e.g. U-NET, [17]). FCNs have a few drawbacks which recent works have tried to address. Firstly, local geometry such as smoothness and topology are not reliably captured. Secondly, there is noticeable need for enough of representative training data to learn the multiple entities: foreground, background, shape, and the contextual interactions of above entities. With limited or not enough training data, failures are hard to interpret and it is not easy to handpick training data that can improve performance. Finally, it is hard to transfer weights learnt from FCN to new problems since the above entities are abstractly tied to each other for the current problem. The problem of local geometry was addressed recently in [2] imposing smoothness and topology priors for a multi-labeling problem of histology segmentation. Next, the problem of overfitting is tackled in [6], using parameter reduction due to very Deep networks with skip level connections, motivated by ResNets [9].

In this work, we propose an alternative refinement to the FCN framework compared to the above enhancements [2,9]. Segmentation and motion tracking using foreground/background modeling has a rich history e.g. [4,13] using DCNN, see survey [3] for traditional approaches. For example, in [13], a multistage FCN is proposed to integrate appearance and motion cues for crowd segmentation. Both appearance filters and motion filters are pre-trained stage-by-stage and then jointly optimized to give improved accuracy. Inspired by the above class of methods, we propose a novel approach to enhance FCN segmentation using a generative modeling of the triad of F, B and S. There are three distinct advantages from the proposed FCN framework: Firstly, by modeling the appearance F, B, challenging scenarios such as non-linear shading effects, artifacts, and loss of contrast are factored out leaving the learning and prediction of S more robust. Secondly, domain specific tuning of networks (e.g. data augmentation, complexity of the network) corresponding to F, B and S makes it easier to control the number of parameters and hence over fitting. Finally, weights corresponding to either of F, B and S models can be easily transferred across applications. We look at a few innovative FCN network architectures and loss functions to achieve the above. Broadly speaking, we consider three parallel FCN networks, each modeling one of F, B and S. Analogous to multi-task learning (e.g. [11,15]), the models are jointly learnt using weight sharing and through a novel loss function that ties the outputs together. Figure 1 shows the input image and also the predicted foreground, background texture and segmented shape from a longitudinal ultrasound B-mode scan of adult kidney.

For our experiments, we consider the applications of kidney segmentation from 2-D ultrasound images and 3-D CT lung nodule segmentation. Both the applications are clinically relevant and have varying challenges as explained in the Results section. We also present quantitative comparisons of our results with U-NET [17] on the above data. We show that we outperform U-NET by almost 8% on the kidney segmentation problem while achieving marginally higher and comparable results on lung nodule segmentation.

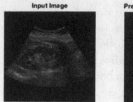
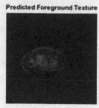
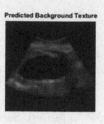
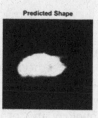

Fig. 1. (a) Input ultrasound B-mode kidney image (b) Synthesized foreground texture map (c) Synthesized background texture map (d) Predicted segmentation mask

2   Methods

CNNs provide effective models for several vision learning tasks by incorporating weight sharing between pixels across several hierarchical layers. The last layer is a fully connected layer whose outputs are used for regression/classification tasks. For image analysis tasks such as segmentation, one could use CNN in a sliding window fashion to predict the current pixel to be in the object or not. But such an approach has the disadvantage of being too slow and not being able to capture spatial context during pixel predictions.

Extending CNNs for pixel wise predictions are FCNs (e.g. [16,17] that essentially have hierarchical deconvolution layers that work on CNN feature maps to give an 'image' output. Each of these deconvolution layers have connections with the respective convolution layers to be able to preserve fine detail while upsampling. FCNs have the advantage of being really fast for pixel predictions being just feed forward operations along with the added utility of bringing spatial context into the predictions. In standard FCN formulations such as U-Net [17], given training examples of pairs of images and segmentations masks $I_k, S_k, k = 1, 2, \ldots, N$, the framework learns a predictor $\hat{S}_w[.]$ defined by parameters w that minimizes the training loss e.g. RMSE, $\frac{1}{N} \sum_{k=1}^{N} |S_k - \hat{S}_w[I_k]|^2$.

In our segmentation work, we extend FCNs to jointly model appearance (F and B) and shape (S). We learn the triad of predictors $\hat{F}_{w_1}[.], \hat{B}_{w_2}[.], \hat{S}_{w_3}[.], \hat{S}_{w_3} \in [0, 1]$ that minimize the following possibilities for the training loss, FBS_1 and FBS_2. Analogous to multi-task learning (e.g. [11,15]), FBS_1 can be seen to tie F, B, S together with shared weights while FBS_2 ties the models together using a loss function that mimics image formation.

In FBS_1, we seek *shared* parameters w_1, w_2, w_3 and $\hat{S}_{w_3} \in [0, 1]$ to minimize:

$$E_{FBS_1}[w_1, w_2, w_3] = \frac{1}{N} \sum_{k=1}^{N} |\hat{F}_{w_1}[I_k] - S_k.I_k|^2 + |\hat{B}_{w_2}[I_k] - (1 - S_k).I_k|^2$$

$$+ |\hat{S}_{w_3}[I_k] - S_k|^2 + E_{smth}[\hat{S}_{w_3}[I_k]] \tag{1}$$

The first two terms learn the foreground and background predictors respectively. Note that without sharing of weights between w_1, w_2, w_3, the first 3 terms are independent of each other and the shape predictor is no longer benefited by the appearance predictors and the appearance predictors in turn could just learn the identity mapping. Thus weight sharing is critical for the above formulation. E_{smth} is a smoothness prior (e.g. TV norm) on the shape predictor.

For ease of notation, we write e.g. $\hat{S}_{w_3}[I_k] = \hat{S}_k$. We look at a second formulation FBS_2 mimicking the image formation model. We seek parameters w_1, w_2, w_3 and $\hat{S}_{w_3} \in [0, 1]$ to minimize:

$$E_{FBS_2}[w_1, w_2, w_3] = \frac{1}{N} \sum_{k=1}^{N} |I - (\hat{S}_k \hat{F}_k + (1 - \hat{S}_k)\hat{B}_k)|^2$$
$$+ |I - (S_k \hat{F}_k + (1 - S_k)\hat{B}_k)|^2 + |\hat{S}_k - S_k|^2 + E_{smth}[\hat{S}_k] \tag{2}$$

The first term is the image formation model that ties the predictors $\hat{F}, \hat{B}, \hat{S}$. By itself, this term would not make sense since we have 3 unknowns. The 3rd term seeks a shape predictor $\hat{S}$ given the ground truth masks $S_k, k = 1, 2, \ldots, N$. With just the first and third terms, in the absence of a good initial guess for the weights w_1 and w_2, or w_3, it would be difficult to converge to good predictors $\hat{F}, \hat{B}, \hat{S}$. Thus, we add the second term; since we know the ground-truth mask S_k, we can use this to derive the foreground/background predictors as shown.

In both FBS_1 and FBS_2, the predictor $\hat{S}$ is influenced by the predictions of $\hat{F}, \hat{B}$ because of shared weights (FBS_1) and the choice of loss function (FBS_2). Consequently, the proposed approach is more robust to choice of training data due to complementarity of the foreground/background/shape predictors. In competing FCN methods such as U-Net, enough of training data is needed to abstract the foreground/background texture, the shape, and relations of texture with the shape. As seen in the above illustrative example on simulated data we created to study FCNs (Fig. 2), U-net has not been able to complete the shape (Green: Ground truth, Red: Result) in regions of poor contrast or complex background. FBS_1 has been able to complete the shape since the foreground and background texture models have been jointly learnt with shape.

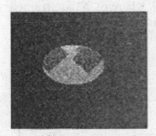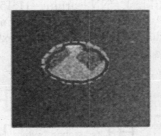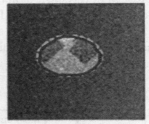

Fig. 2. Synthetic study example with contrast variation, weak edges and noise. (a) Input image (b) output of U-net (c) output of FBS_1. We see that results are better with joint appearance/shape modeling (FBS_1) (Color figure online)

3   Architectures

In this section, we explain how we realize the formulations described in previous sections using interesting FCN architectures. The vanilla U-NET architecture is shown in Fig. 3, which has become one of the most successful and popular approaches for medical image segmentation. U-NET is essentially a FCN with encoder-decoder blocks, with skip-level connections between responses from layers of the analysis arm to the synthesis arms as shown in Fig. 3.

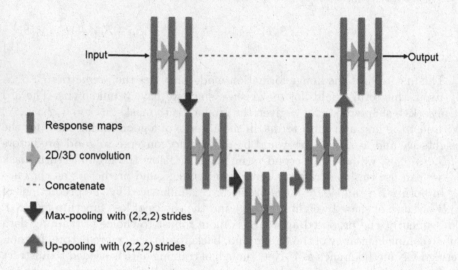

Fig. 3. U-NET architecture

3.1   Shared Weights Architecture

This architecture is an extension of U-NET with multiple outputs (Fig. 4). We proceed in the spirit of multi-task CNN learning [11,15], where FCNs are trained to simultaneously predict F, B and S based on our formulations from Eqs. (1) and (2). The intuition is that sharing weights for joint texture and shape prediction can lead to better generalization and robustness.

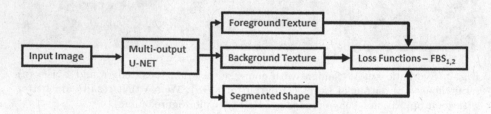

Fig. 4. Shared weights architecture

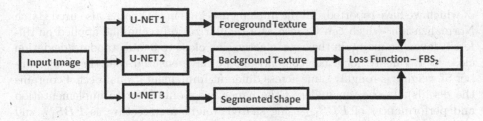

Fig. 5. Parallel architecture

3.2   Parallel Architecture

As discussed in Sect. 2, the weights corresponding to the three terms can be different and the parallel architecture in Fig. 5 attempts to model this scenario. The motivation for such an architecture can be attributed to the following reasons - (a) Even though U-NET attempts to get hierarchical, non-linear abstractions for texture and shape in an implicit fashion, the properties of these terms are very different and hence intuitively makes sense to model them using parallel networks. (b) This model also allows us to distribute the number of weights depending upon complexity of the term, for instance, background being a high entropy entity can be modeled using more weights than foreground. (c) Transferability across problems - depending upon tissue characteristics or background properties for similar, related problems, weights from the arms of relevance can be selectively transferred. We note that such an architecture may not be suitable for FBS_1 formulation as there is no single binding term that can jointly influence learning for F, B, S terms, with the independent parallel network implementation. However, this architecture is a natural fit for FBS_2 formulation, as it explicitly encodes the image synthesis model while allowing the flexibility to model the terms separately.

3.3   Implementation Details

We would like to point out that foreground and background texture modeling is a pixel-wise regression problem, while shape masks prediction is a binary classification problem. Hence, the output activation units of Figs. 4 and 5 have to be one of tanh, RelU or linear units for the two texture outputs and a sigmoid function for the shape term respectively. Note that terms on the FBS_1 formulation from Eq. (1) can have independent optimization metrics - the texture regression terms can be optimized for variants of L^2 norm and the binary shape term can be optimized using binary cross entropy as done in the baseline U-NET model. In our implementation, we used tanh units and mean-squared error for output activation and optimization metric for texture regression, respectively.

We experimented with different variants of dropout including (a) vanilla dropout - randomly drop inputs and (b) spatial dropout - the new variant of dropout tailored specifically for convolutional neural networks for zeroing entire feature maps. Our best results were obtained using spatial dropout, the results of which we have reported. All the implementations in this paper also used Batch Normalization -which can be seen as a regularization technique applied on different layers to maintain their mean activation close to 0 and standard deviation close to 1. Finally, for a fair comparison, we have ensured that the total number of weights is roughly same across different implementations (Sect. 4 contains the details). In the remainder of the paper, we would refer to implementation and performances of $FBS_{1,2}$ using shared weight architecture as $FBS_{1,2}^a$ and implementation of FBS_2 using parallel weight architecture as FBS_2^b.

4   Experiments and Results

In this section, we establish the efficacy of our approach on two challenging medical imaging segmentation problems. One is anatomy segmentation − kidney segmentation from 2-D ultrasound B-mode images and another problem is 3-D Lung Nodule segmentation from CT images.

4.1   Lung Nodule Segmentation from 3-D CT

Lung cancer contributes to a large proportion of cancer related fatalities. Like other cancer types, early detection of nodules through screening procedures is critical for treatment planning and recovery. Recently, low dose CT (LDCT) scan has emerged as the standard procedure for lung cancer screening. In addition to the clinical relevance, technical challenges like wide contrast variation and lack of clear shape or appearance features make this a challenging problem, which were amongst the reasons to choose lung nodule segmentation from 3-D LDCT images as one application for the proposed method.

Data. Lung Image Database Consortium (LIDC-IDRI) [1] contains a collection 1010 3-D LDCT volumes of patients with lung cancer. We work with a pre-selected subset of 93 volumes containing 267 lesions on which manual segmentations have been performed, of which 179 lesions were used for training, and remaining 88 was used for validation.

Table 1. Performance comparison for lung nodule in 3-D CT images

Architecture	Dice overlap on validation set in %
U-Net	65.54
$FBS1^a$	**66.68**

Performance. The main goal of this experiment was to demonstrate the applicability of our approach to 3-D problems and also to different modalities. We use Sect. 4.2 to illustrate nuances of our approach, exhaustive comparisons and intuitions towards generalization, transferability and other properties. For this problem, we implemented a baseline 6-layer deep U-Net architecture with

3-D convolution units. We also implemented Architectures FBS_1^a as explained in Sect. 3 for comparison. We use Dice overlap with ground truth as the performance comparison metric. Table 1 contains the performance comparison. It should be noted that performance is similar, while shared architecture implementation of formulation FBS_1 has slightly better performance achieving 1% more than U-NET. All the results are averaged over 5 runs. The comparative performance should not be surprising given that validation set also comes from the same population and the problems of overfitting are less critical. Even in such scenarios, explicit modeling of foreground and background texture adds value as shown by the marginal increase over vanilla U-NET.

4.2 Kidney Segmentation from U/S B-Mode Images

Automated methods for determining the morphology and size of kidney from 2-D or 3-D ultrasound images have many benefits - accelerated work flow, operator independence on measurements and improved clinical outcomes. However, automated kidney segmentation is extremely challenging due to large variability in kidney shape, weak boundaries and large variation in appearance of internal regions based on acquisition scan plane. Additionally, shape, size and texture of the kidney region could vary drastically depending on the age of the subject - adult or pediatric and healthy or diseased. Another important challenge for the segmentation algorithm is to work across different scan protocols – every site can have different probes, acquisition settings including depth, TGC, etc.

Data. The goal of this experiment is to demonstrate the robustness and generalization properties of the proposed approach over the state-of-the-art U-NETs. We consider two datasets of B-mode kidney images acquired from two different scanning sites, which we would refer to as Population 1 and Population 2, with 108 and 123 images respectively. Population 2 is significantly more difficult than Population 1 due to the presence of challenging subjects (healthy and non-healthy), larger age differences and varied probe and acquisition settings. We train on a subset of Population 1 (60 images) and validate it on the remainder of Population 1 (48 images) and the entire Population 2 (123 images). We compare performances for both the formulations $FBS_{1,2}$ and for all the different architecture implementations explained in previous sections.

Performance. We use Dice coefficient as the metric to compare our results with expert annotated ground truth. Figure 6 shows an illustrative example of a difficult ultrasound image for kidney segmentation. Multiple lines of shadow, deep fat layer, weak bottom edge and inconsistent kidney contrast are some factors that make this case challenging. Figure 6(c) shows the result our approach which achieves a dice overlap of 91% while U-NET result in Fig. 6(b) fails completely with dice overlap of 61%. Table 2 contains the aggregate results. All the results reported are averaged over five independent runs for every experiment. It should be noted that architecture FBS_1^a - shared weight architecture of FBS_1 outperforms U-NET by 8% difference. We would also like to highlight

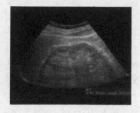 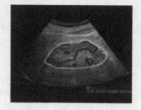 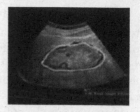

Fig. 6. Illustrative example on B-mode ultrasound kidney image. (a) Input image (b) U-NET segmentation result in red (ground truth - green) (c) FBS_1^a segmentation result in red (ground truth - green) (Color figure online)

Table 2. Performance comparison for kidney segmentation from U/S images

Architecture	Dice overlap with ground truth annotations in %		
	Validation set - population 1	Population 2	Mean over population 1 and 2
U-NET	75.90	62.18	66.03
FBS_1^a	**77.24**	**72.83**	**74.06**
FBS_2^a	75.02	66.28	68.74
FBS_2^b	68.98	59.89	62.44

that the difference in performance between U-NET and FBS_1^a on Population 1 is only 1.34%, however on more challenging, completely unseen Population 2, the improvement is 10%. This result clearly establishes the power of foreground, background modeling along with shape leading to better generalization and lesser over-fitting. Table 2 also shows that shared weight architecture for our second formulation - FBS_2^a also outperforms U-NET on Population 2 establishing the power of image synthesis formulations for segmentation. We mention that for FBS_2 in Eq. (2), we have not tuned the weights of relative contributions of different terms, which means that the cumulative cost could be dominated by the image synthesis terms than by shape error minimization term, explaining the lesser performance than FBS_1^a. Further, for the parallel architecture approach FBS_2^b, by enforcing the total number of parameters to be similar to U-Net and shared architectures (FBS_1^a, FBS_2^b), we have reduced the modeling capability of the S-arm by a factor of 3. This possibly explains the lesser performance of FBS_2^b. Improving the performance through better distribution of weights between the F, B, S arms along with better relative weighting of the terms, and demonstrating the value of transferability to related problems will be subject of our future work.

Finally, we show a palette of a few visual examples Fig. 7 for the kidney data. The second and third columns shown segmentation results from U-Net and FBS_1^a respectively for the input images (first column). The last two columns show the predicted foreground and background textures from FBS_1^a. The first two rows show examples where the proposed approach has done better than U-net while the third row shows over-segmentation in our approach.

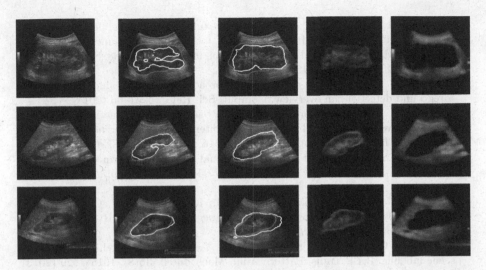

Fig. 7. A few examples on B-mode ultrasound kidney images. Columns: (a) Input image (b) U-NET segmentation result in green (ground truth - red) (c) FBS_1^a segmentation result in green (ground truth - red) (d) Synthesized foreground (e) Synthesized background (Color figure online)

5   Discussion

While U-NET has delivered impressive results on many challenging medical imaging segmentation tasks, it is still limited in its applicability in clinical applications because of lack of predictability in its output and correspondingly in its failure cases. We extend the FCN approaches by constructing a novel objective function which models texture and shape separately. The disentanglement of different properties allows us deeper insight into the model which in turn enables us to tune hyper-parameters and regularization approaches in a more meaningful manner. For instance, we could use shape regularizers only for the shape arm of the FBS_2^b architecture.

While a range of effective approaches for adding shape priors to traditional methods exist we find that integrating these methods into deep architectures poses new challenges. We are currently investigating adding shape priors to U-NET like architectures through dictionary learning approaches. Initial experiments have shown promise in enforcing smoothness of output and robustness of results. These characteristics are crucial in clinical applications where interpretability and failure modeling is crucial to technology acceptance.

References

1. The lung image database consortium (LIDC) and image database resource initiative (IDRI): a completed reference database of lung nodules on CT scans

2. BenTaieb, A., Hamarneh, G.: Topology aware fully convolutional networks for histology gland segmentation. In: Ourselin, S., Joskowicz, L., Sabuncu, M.R., Unal, G., Wells, W. (eds.) MICCAI 2016. LNCS, vol. 9901, pp. 460–468. Springer, Cham (2016). doi:10.1007/978-3-319-46723-8_53

3. Bouwmans, T.: Traditional and recent approaches in background modeling for foreground detection: an overview. Comput. Sci. Rev. **11**, 31–66 (2014)

4. Braham, M., Van Droogenbroeck, M.: Deep background subtraction with scene-specific convolutional neural networks. In: International Conference on Systems, Signals and Image Processing, 23–25 May 2016, Bratislava. IEEE (2016)

5. Chaudhury, S., Roy, H.: Can fully convolutional networks perform well for general image restoration problems? CoRR abs/1611.04481 (2016). http://arxiv.org/abs/1611.04481

6. Drozdzal, M., Vorontsov, E., Chartrand, G., Kadoury, S., Pal, C.: The importance of skip connections in biomedical image segmentation. CoRR abs/1608.04117 (2016). http://arxiv.org/abs/1608.04117

7. Farabet, C., Couprie, C., Najman, L., LeCun, Y.: Learning hierarchical features for scene labeling. IEEE Trans. Pattern Anal. Mach. Intell. **35**(8), 1915–1929 (2013)

8. Fischer, P., Dosovitskiy, A., Ilg, E., Häusser, P., Hazırbaş, C., Golkov, V., van der Smagt, P., Cremers, D., Brox, T.: FlowNet: Learning optical flow with convolutional networks. arXiv preprint arXiv:1504.06852 (2015)

9. He, K., Zhang, X., Ren, S., Sun, J.: Deep residual learning for image recognition. CoRR abs/1512.03385 (2015). http://arxiv.org/abs/1512.03385

10. Hong, S., You, T., Kwak, S., Han, B.: Online tracking by learning discriminative saliency map with convolutional neural network. arXiv preprint arXiv:1502.06796 (2015)

11. Huang, Y., Wang, W., Wang, L., Tan, T.: Multi-task deep neural network for multi-label learning. In: 2013 IEEE International Conference on Image Processing, pp. 2897–2900. IEEE (2013)

12. Jin, K.H., McCann, M.T., Froustey, E., Unser, M.: Deep convolutional neural network for inverse problems in imaging. CoRR abs/1611.03679 (2016). http://arxiv.org/abs/1611.03679

13. Kang, K., Wang, X.: Fully convolutional neural networks for crowd segmentation. arXiv preprint arXiv:1411.4464 (2014)

14. Krizhevsky, A., Sutskever, I., Hinton, G.E.: Imagenet classification with deep convolutional neural networks. In: Proceedings of the Advances in NIPS, pp. 1106–1114 (2012)

15. Li, X., Zhao, L., Wei, L., Yang, M., Wu, F., Zhuang, Y., Ling, H., Wang, J.: DeepSaliency: multi-task deep neural network model for salient object detection. CoRR abs/1510.05484 (2015). http://arxiv.org/abs/1510.05484

16. Long, J., Shelhamer, E., Darrell, T.: Fully convolutional networks for semantic segmentation. In: Proceedings of the IEEE Conference on Computer Vision and Pattern Recognition, pp. 3431–3440 (2015)

17. Ronneberger, O., Fischer, P., Brox, T.: U-Net: convolutional networks for biomedical image segmentation. In: Navab, N., Hornegger, J., Wells, W.M., Frangi, A.F. (eds.) MICCAI 2015. LNCS, vol. 9351, pp. 234–241. Springer, Cham (2015). doi:10.1007/978-3-319-24574-4_28

18. Simonyan, K., Zisserman, A.: Very deep convolutional networks for large-scale image recognition. arXiv preprint arXiv:1409.1556 (2014)

Automatic Vertebra Labeling in Large-Scale 3D CT Using Deep Image-to-Image Network with Message Passing and Sparsity Regularization

Dong Yang[1], Tao Xiong[2], Daguang Xu[3(✉)], Qiangui Huang[4], David Liu[3],
S. Kevin Zhou[3], Zhoubing Xu[3], JinHyeong Park[3], Mingqing Chen[3],
Trac D. Tran[2], Sang Peter Chin[2], Dimitris Metaxas[1], and Dorin Comaniciu[3]

[1] Department of Computer Science, Rutgers University, Piscataway, NJ 08854, USA
[2] Department of Electrical and Computer Engineering,
The Johns Hopkins University, Baltimore, MD 21218, USA
[3] Medical Imaging Technologies, Siemens Healthcare Technology Center,
Princeton, NJ 08540, USA
{daguang.xu,shaohua.zhou,dorin.comaniciu}@siemens-healthineers.com
[4] Department of Computer Science, University of Southern California,
Los Angeles, CA 90089, USA

Abstract. Automatic localization and labeling of vertebra in 3D medical images plays an important role in many clinical tasks, including pathological diagnosis, surgical planning and postoperative assessment. However, the unusual conditions of pathological cases, such as the abnormal spine curvature, bright visual imaging artifacts caused by metal implants, and the limited field of view, increase the difficulties of accurate localization. In this paper, we propose an automatic and fast algorithm to localize and label the vertebra centroids in 3D CT volumes. First, we deploy a deep image-to-image network (DI2IN) to initialize vertebra locations, employing the convolutional encoder-decoder architecture together with multi-level feature concatenation and deep supervision. Next, the centroid probability maps from DI2IN are iteratively evolved with the message passing schemes based on the mutual relation of vertebra centroids. Finally, the localization results are refined with sparsity regularization. The proposed method is evaluated on a public dataset of 302 spine CT volumes with various pathologies. Our method outperforms other state-of-the-art methods in terms of localization accuracy. The run time is around 3 seconds on average per case. To further boost the performance, we retrain the DI2IN on additional *1000+* 3D CT volumes from different patients. To the best of our knowledge, this is the first time more than *1000* 3D CT volumes with expert annotation are adopted in experiments for the anatomic landmark detection tasks. Our experimental results show that training with such a large dataset significantly improves the performance and the overall identification rate, for the first time by our knowledge, reaches *90%*.

D. Yang and T. Xiong contributed equally.

M. Niethammer et al. (Eds.): IPMI 2017, LNCS 10265, pp. 633–644, 2017.
DOI: 10.1007/978-3-319-59050-9_50

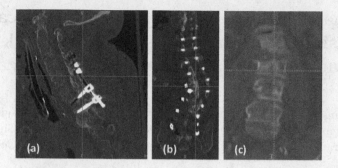

Fig. 1. Demonstration of pathological cases. (a) Surgical metal implants (b) Spine curvature (c) Limited FOV

1   Introduction

Automatic localization and labeling of vertebrae in 3D spinal imaging, e.g. computed tomography (CT) or magnetic resonance imaging (MRI), has become an essential tool for clinical tasks, including pathological diagnosis, surgical planning and post-operative assessment. Specific applications such as vertebrae segmentation, fracture detection, tumor detection, registration and statistical shape analysis can also benefit from the effective vertebrae detection and labeling algorithms. However, there are many challenges associated with designing an accurate and automatic algorithm, which arise from pathologies, image artifacts, and the limited field-of-view (FOV). For example, as shown in Fig. 1, the abnormal spine curvature and surgical metal implants significantly alter the appearance of vertebrae and reduce the image contrast. Spine-focused scans with small field-of-view (FOV) also add difficulty to the identification tasks due to lack of global spatial and contextual information.

To address these challenges, many approaches have been proposed for automatic localization and identification of vertebrae. Glocker *et al.* [1] presented a method based on regression forests and probabilistic graphic models. However, their method is likely to suffer from the narrow field-of-view because the broad contextual information is not always available. To overcome this limitation, Glocker *et al.* [2] proposed a randomized classification forest based approach which achieved reasonable localization and identification performances on pathological cases and those with limited FOV. Recently, deep learning has been employed in the applications of spine detection. Chen *et al.* [3] presented a joint convolutional neural network (J-CNN). This hybrid approach used a random forest classifier to coarsely localize the candidates before the J-CNN scanned the input CT volume for final results. By incorporating the pairwise information of neighboring vertebrae in J-CNN, it outperformed other methods [2]. Suzani *et al.* [4] proposed a deep feed-forward neural network to detect if an input image contained a specific vertebra. Although this work achieved high detection rates, it reported a large mean localization error compared with other works. Besides, instead of the direct 3D volumetric input, this work extracted

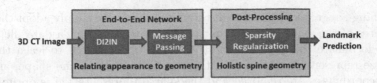

Fig. 2. Proposed method which consists of three major components: deep Image-to-Image Network (DI2IN), message passing and sparsity regularity.

1D features based on the local voxel intensities as the input of deep feed-forward neural network. In addition, no convolution or pooling operation was applied in the network. Payer *et al.* [5] proposed a composite neural network to build up the full connection between response maps of all landmarks with convolutional kernels. The spatial relationship of landmarks were implicitly embedded in the CNN model.

In order to overcome these limitations and to take advantage of deep neural networks, we present an approach, shown in Fig. 2, with the following contributions:

(a) *Deep Image-to-Image Network (DI2IN) for Voxel-Wise Regression*
    Without extracting features from input images, the proposed deep image-to-image architecture directly takes a 3D CT volume as input. The training of the proposed network is designed as multichannel voxel-wise regression (refer to Sect. 2.1). It generates the multichannel probability maps associated with different vertebra centers, which intuitively illustrate the location and label of vertebrae. Our neural network requires no coarse classifiers to remove the outliers for preprocessing. Instead, it automatically extracts contextual and spatial information by itself. By taking the advantage of fully convolutional implementation, the proposed network is significantly time-efficient, which sets it apart from the sliding window approaches.

(b) *Response Enhancement with Message Passing*
    Although the proposed deep image-to-image network generates confident probability maps, there is no guarantee that it will avoid false positives (outliers) due to the complexity of appearance (shown in Fig. 1). To resolve this problem, we adopt a message passing scheme within the probability maps of vertebra centers, which leverages the mutual relation of vertebrae. A chain-structure graphical model is introduced to depict the spatial relationship. Each node in the model represents a probability distribution of one vertebra center. During the passing scheme, the probability map of each vertebra center iteratively receives messages (encoded in the convolution operation) from all neighboring vertebrae (nodes) and absorbs them for further self-evolvement. The collected messages can not only enhance the response of correct location, but also suppress that of the false positives.

(c) *Refinement Using Sparse Representation*
    To further refine the coordinates of vertebrae, we incorporate a dictionary learning and sparse representation approach which utilizes the holistic structure of the spine and identifies the important set of coordinates. Instead of

learning a regression model to fit the spinal shape, we simply adopt the coordinates of the spine in the training samples to construct a data dictionary and formulate this problem as an ℓ_1 norm optimization to learn the best sparse representation. Based on the regularity of the spine shape, ambiguous coordinates are removed and the sparse representation is optimized in a subspace instead of all coordinates (refer to Sect. 2.2). Finally, the refined coordinates in each axis are reconstructed from the same subspace jointly, which further improves the localization and identification performance.

The rest of the paper is organized as follows: In Sect. 2, we introduce our deep image-to-image network architecture with message passing and refinement approach. In Sect. 3, the proposed framework is compared to previous state-of-the-art methods based on a public spine dataset. In Sect. 4, we present the conclusion and discussion.

2 Methodology

2.1 Deep Image-to-Image Network (DI2IN) for Multiple Landmark Localization

In this section, we present the proposed deep image-to-image network, which is multi-layer convolutional, to localize vertebra centroids. As shown in Fig. 3, the proposed network is deployed in a symmetric manner which can be treated equivalently as a convolutional encoder-decoder network. It is implemented in the fashion of voxel-wise end-to-end learning to enable efficient inference.

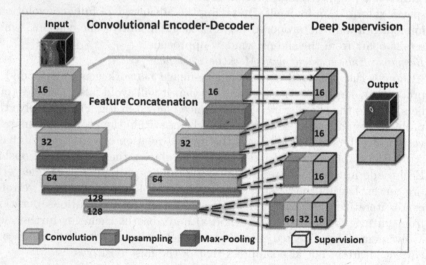

Fig. 3. Proposed deep image-to-image network (DI2IN). The front part is a convolutional encoder-decoder network with feature concatenation, and the backend is deep supervision network through multi-level. Numbers next to convolutional layers are the channel numbers.

The multichannel ground truth data is specially designed with the coordinates of vertebra centroid. A Gaussian distribution $I_{gt} = \frac{1}{\sigma\sqrt{2\pi}}e^{-\|x-\mu\|^2/2\sigma^2}$ is defined in each channel to represent the vertebra location. Vector $x \in \mathbb{R}^3$ represents the voxel coordinates in volume, vector μ is the ground truth location of vertebra centroid. Variance σ^2 is pre-defined which controls the scale of the Gaussian distribution. Each channel's prediction $I_{prediction}$ corresponds to a unique vertebra centroid. It has the same size as the input image. Therefore, the whole learning problem is formulated as multichannel voxel-wise regression. During the training, we apply the square loss $|I_{prediction} - I_{gt}|^2$ for each voxel at the output layer. We define the centroid detection as a regression task instead of classification. Because the highly imbalanced data in classification is inevitable and it causes the misleading classification accuracy.

Convolution, rectified linear unit (ReLU), and max-pooling layers are used in the encoder part of the proposed network. Pooling is critical as it helps increase the receptive field of neurons and lower the GPU memory consumption. With the larger receptive field, more contextual information is taken into consideration for each neuron in different layers. Therefore, the relative spatial position of vertebra centroids in prediction would be better interpreted. The decoder part is composed of the convolution, ReLU and upsampling layers. Upsampling layers are implemented with the bilinear interpolation to enlarge and densify the activation. It further enables the end-to-end voxel-wise training. The convolutional filter size is $1 \times 1 \times 1$ in the final output layer and $3 \times 3 \times 3$ for the other convolution layers. The max-pooling filter size is $2 \times 2 \times 2$. The stride in the convolution layers is set as 1 to maintain the same size in each channel. The pooling factor in pooling layers is set as 2 for downsampling by half in each dimension. The number of channels in each layers are marked next to the layers in Fig. 3. In upsampling layers, the input features are upsampled by a factor of 2 in x, y, z directions respectively. The network takes a 3D CT image (volume) as input and directly outputs multiple probability maps, with each map associated with one vertebra landmark (equivalent to vertebra centroid). The framework is more efficient at computing the probability maps as well as the centroid locations than the patch-wise classification or regression methods in [3,4].

Our DI2IN adopts several prevailing techniques [6–8,10,11] with necessary modification. We utilize the feature layer concatenation in DI2IN which is analogous with the one described in [7]. The shortcut bridges are built up directly from the encoder layers to decoder layers. It passes forward the feature maps from the encoder and is then concatenated with the decoder feature layers. The concatenated features are used as the input for next convolution layers. Following the concatenation, high and low level features are combined explicitly so that the network benefits from both the local and global contextual information. Deep supervision in neural network during the end-to-end training is shown in [8,10,11] to achieve excellent boundary detection and segmentation results. In the network, we introduce a more sophisticated deep supervision method to improve the performance. Several branches are bifurcated out from the main network from the intermediate layers of the decoder part. With proper upsampling factors and convolution operations, the output size of each channel of all branches matches the size of the input image. The supervision is introduced at the end of each branch i by computing a loss term l_i with the same ground truth data. To further leverage the results from different branches, the final output is determined by the convolution operation of output concatenation of all branches with ReLU. The total loss l_{total} is a combination of loss terms from all output layers which includes the output layers from all branches and the final output layer, as shown here:

$$l_{total} = \sum_i l_i + l_{final}$$

2.2   Probability Map Enhancement with Message Passing Scheme

Given the image I, the DI2IN generates one probability map $P(v_i|I)$ for the center of each individual vertebra i with high confidence. The vertebrae will be located at the peak positions v_i of probability maps. However, we find that these probability maps are not perfect yet: some probability maps don't have response or have very low response at the ground truth locations because of similar image appearances of several vertebrae (e.g. $T1$–$T12$). In order to handle the problem of missing response, we propose a message passing scheme to effectively enhance the probability maps by utilizing the prior knowledge of the spine structure.

The concept of message passing was first introduced in the context of probabilistic graphical models. It is used in the sum-product or max-product algorithms for exact inference of the marginal probabilities of nodes or the distribution mode in a tree-structured graph. Messages are passed iteratively between neighboring nodes to exchange information and optimize the overall probability distribution. Similarly, we introduce an MRF-like model, a chain-structure graph shown in Fig. 4, to express the spatial relationship among vertebrae, where each node in the graph represents one vertebra center v_i. Then we propose the following formulation to update the $P(v_i|I)$ during the iteration t of message passing.

$$P_{t+1}(v_i|I) = \frac{1}{Z}\left[\alpha \cdot \frac{\sum_{j\in\partial i} m_{j\to i}}{|\partial i|} + P_t(v_i|I)\right] \tag{1}$$

$$= \frac{1}{Z}\left[\alpha \cdot \frac{\sum_{j\in\partial i} P_t(v_j|I) * k(v_i|v_j)}{|\partial i|} + P_t(v_i|I)\right] \tag{2}$$

where ∂i is the neighbor of vertebra i in the graph, Z is a normalization constant, and $\alpha \in (0,1)$ is a discounted factor. The messages $m_{j\to i}$, defined as $P_t(v_j|I) * k(v_i|v_j)$, are passed along the chain shown in Fig. 4. $*$ is the convolution operation. $k(v_i|v_j)$ is a single convolution kernel which is learned from the ground truth distribution of vertebra i, j. Multi-dimensional convolution itself is capable to shift the mass of the probability map $P_t(v_i|I)$ to its neighborhood with a fixed orientation (kernel). If $P_t(v_i|I)$ is confident at its correct location, then the message $m_{j\to i}$ would be a strong prior for $P_{t+1}(v_j|I)$ at the correct

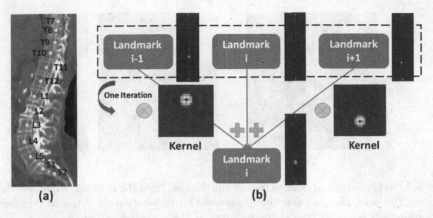

Fig. 4. (a) Chain-structure model for vertebra centers; (b) One iteration of message passing (landmarks represents vertebra centers): the neighbors' landmark probability maps help compensate the missing response of landmark i.

location of the vertebra j. After several iterations of message passing, the vertebra with missing response can be compensated with the aggregated messages from its neighboring vertebrae. The underlying assumption is that majority of the vertebra probability maps are confident and well distributed around the true locations, which is guaranteed by the powerful DI2IN in our method. The advantage of the proposed scheme is that it can be concatenated into the DI2IN for further end-to-end training (fine-tuning) when the iteration number is fixed. The location of each vertebra centroid can simply be determined by the location of the maximum value in the corresponding probability map.

Several recent works have deployed the message-passing concept for different landmark detection tasks. Chu et al. [12] proposed the passing scheme between the feature maps instead of landmark probability maps. Yang et al. [9] introduced a fully connected graphical model for message passing between probability maps. The hand-crafted features were adopted in the pair-wise terms of the messages. Payer et al. [5] also brought up the fully connected graphical model, applying one-time passing with pixel-wise dot-product for noise cancelling. In our proposed method, the passing is directly among the response maps along the chain-structure model. The response maps are gradually enhanced within several passing iterations, since one passing is not enough to make necessary adjustment for probability maps. Compared to the hand-craft features, the single convolutional kernel is eligible to generate messages between neighbors because the designed neighborhood is compact. In our framework, the missing response is the major issue instead of the noisy output, so the dot-product operation is not applicable and may hurt the output probabilities.

2.3 Sparse Representation for Landmark Refinement

As shown in Fig. 5, the DI2IN with message passing generates a clear probability map, where the high probability map indicates the potential location of the

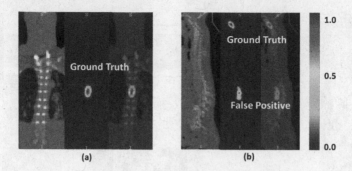

Fig. 5. Left: CT image. Middle: output of one channel from the network. Right: overlaid display. The prediction in (a) is close to ground truth location. In (b), a false positive response exists remotely besides the response at the correct location.

landmark (centroid of the vertebrae). However, sometimes due to image arti-facts and low image resolution, it is still difficult to guarantee there will be no false positive. In [3], a shape regression optimization model was used to refine the predicted vertebral centroids in the vertical axis. By minimizing an energy function, the optimized parameters are learned for each test sample to deter-mine the final coordinates of vertebrae. However, their model assumes that the coordinates distribution can be described in a quadratic form, and it was only applied for coordinates in the vertical axis.

Inspired by the previous works in sparse representation, we propose an ℓ_1 norm approach to help refine the coordinates in all x, y and z axes. Given a pre-generated shape-based dictionary $\mathbf{D}$ and the predicted coordinates vector of all centroids $\mathbf{v}$ in a testing sample, we adopt the ℓ_1 norm optimization to solve the sparse coefficient vector $\mathbf{a}$. The refined coordinates $\hat{\mathbf{v}}$ is defined as $\hat{\mathbf{v}} = \mathbf{D}\mathbf{a}$. In particular, the shape-based dictionary is learned from the training samples. For example, the dictionary $\mathbf{D}_z$ associated with the vertical axis is constructed by the z coordinates of all centroids of each sample in the training database. $\mathbf{v}_z$ denotes the predicted z coordinates of one sample in the testing database. The dictionaries $\mathbf{D}_x$ and $\mathbf{D}_y$ indicate the dictionaries associated with other axes and are learned in the same way.

The details are shown in Algorithm 1. First, we use dynamic programming to find the maximum descending subsequence in the predicted coordinates $\mathbf{v}_z$ since the vertical axis of the spine produces the most stable results. We define the subspace $\mathcal{S}$ of dictionary and the predicted coordinates vector based on the indices in the subsequence. For example, we only choose the atoms from dictionary $\mathbf{D}_z$ and $\mathbf{v}_z$ associated with the indices to generate a sub-dictionary $\mathbf{D}_{z,\mathcal{S}}$ and sub-vector $\mathbf{v}_{z,\mathcal{S}}$. Then we solve the optimization problem in Step 3 for x, y and z axes individually in the subspace $\mathcal{S}$ instead of the original space $\mathcal{S}_0$. Finally, all coordinates are reconstructed by the original dictionary (i.e., $\mathbf{D}_z$) and sparse vector (i.e., $\mathbf{a}_z$). Intuitively, we remove the ambiguous outliers in the preliminary predicted coordinates and then define a subspace without

Algorithm 1. The ℓ_1 Norm Refinement

Require: The dictionary $\mathbf{D}_x, \mathbf{D}_y$ and $\mathbf{D}_z \in \mathbb{R}^{M \times N}$, the predicted coordinates vector $\mathbf{v}_x, \mathbf{v}_y$ and $\mathbf{v}_z$ and the coefficient λ. M and N indicate the number of landmarks and size of items in dictionary, respectively.

1: Find the maximum descending subsequence in the predicted coordinates $\mathbf{v}_z$ by dynamic programming.
2: Add the indices associated with the maximum descending subsequence into the set $\mathcal{S}$ and define the subspace of the dictionary $\mathbf{D}_{x,\mathcal{S}}$, $\mathbf{D}_{y,\mathcal{S}}$, and $\mathbf{D}_{z,\mathcal{S}}$ and the predicted coordinates $\mathbf{v}_{x,\mathcal{S}}$, $\mathbf{v}_{y,\mathcal{S}}$ and $\mathbf{v}_{z,\mathcal{S}}$.
3: Solve the optimization problem below by ℓ_1 norm recovery for the vertical axis z:

$$\min_{\mathbf{a}_z} \frac{1}{2} ||\mathbf{v}_{z,\mathcal{S}} - \mathbf{D}_{z,\mathcal{S}} \mathbf{a}_z||_2^2 + \lambda ||\mathbf{a}_z||_1.$$

4: Solve the same optimization problem in Step 3 for $\mathbf{v}_{x,\mathcal{S}}$ and $\mathbf{v}_{y,\mathcal{S}}$, respectively.
5: Return the refined coordinates $\hat{\mathbf{v}}_x = \mathbf{D}_x \mathbf{a}_x$, $\hat{\mathbf{v}}_y = \mathbf{D}_y \mathbf{a}_y$ and $\hat{\mathbf{v}}_z = \mathbf{D}_z \mathbf{a}_z$.

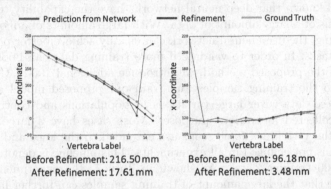

Before Refinement: 216.50 mm   Before Refinement: 96.18 mm
After Refinement: 17.61 mm   After Refinement: 3.48 mm

Fig. 6. Maximum errors of vertebra localization before and after the ℓ_1 norm refinement.

these outliers. Based on the subspace, we find the best sparse combination in the corresponding sub-dictionary. By taking advantage of the original dictionary, all coordinates are reconstructed and refined simultaneously as shown in Fig. 6.

3   Experiments

First, we evaluate the proposed method on the database introduced in [2] which consists of 302 CT scans of patients with varying types of pathologies. There are several unusual appearances in the database, such as the abnormal spine curvature and the bright visual artifacts caused by metal implants from the post-operative procedures. In addition, the field-of-view (FOV) of each CT image varies widely in terms of vertical cropping, image noise and physical resolution [1]. Most cases contain a portion of whole vertebrae while the global spine structure is visible only in a few cases. The large variations in pathologies and the limited FOV increase the complexity of vertebra appearance, and thus raise the difficulties of accurate spine localization and identification task. The ground truth is marked at the centroid of each vertebra, which is annotated by clinical experts. In previous works [1,3,4], there are two different settings on these 302 CT images: the first one uses 112 of the images as training and another 112 images as testing; the second one takes all images (242) in setting one with extra 18 images as training data and an additional 60 images as testing data. For a fair comparison, we follow the same database settings in our experiments. They are denoted as "Set 1" and "Set 2" respectively. We follow the evaluation metrics described in [2], in terms of the Euclidean distance error (in mm) and identification rates (Id.Rates) defined in [1]. Table 1 compares our evaluation performance with the number reported by previous approaches [2–4]. We obtain an overall average mean error of 9.1 mm and 8.6 mm and an identification rates of 80% and 85% on those two sets, respectively. Overall, our method outperforms the state-of-the-art methods on the same datasets in terms of mean error and identification rates.

It is well known that deep neural networks have the capability to represent the variations of a large amount of data. With large amounts of annotated data in the training, the deep neural network can usually achieve better performance on various tasks. In order to validate if more training data can boost the performance of the proposed method, we introduce additional 1000+ CT scans of patients into the training samples and train our proposed model again from scratch. These data cover large variations in populations and contrast phases which are collected for various purposes. Most cases have a large FOV and include all the vertebrae. Some scans are extended to the knee and head. The testing data is not changed in all experiments. This pipeline is denoted as "Our Method+1000 training data". As shown in Table 1, the experimental results demonstrate that the large amount of training samples can further improve the performance significantly. Our approach has achieved the best performance in almost all the metrics. On "Set 1", the Id. Rates of our method is 13% higher than the state-of-the-art method [2]. We also achieve more than 90% Id. Rates on "Set 2", which is 6% higher than the state-of-the-art method [3].

All experiments are conducted on a workstation equipped with an Intel 3.50 GHz CPU and a 12 GB Nvidia Titan X GPU. During the evaluation, the response maps of all output channels are compared with a heuristic threshold constant in an element-wise manner in order to distinguish valid response from random noise. Only the channels whose response maps contain elements with value greater than the threshold are considered. The vertebra centroids associated with these channels are then identified to be present in the image. The landmarks corresponding to the other response maps are considered as non-presented. The localization and identification of all vertebrae in one case is achieved simultaneously in an efficient way. The testing time of our method is around three seconds per case on average assisted with the GPU. The experimental results demonstrate that our proposed method for spine centroids localization and identification is not only effective in terms of accuracy, but also significantly time-efficient.

Table 1. Comparison of localization errors in mm and identification rates among different methods. "Set 1" has 112 CT images for training and 112 images for testing. "Set 2" uses all data in "Set 1" with extra 18 images for training and 60 images for testing. Our Method (DI2IN+MP+Sparsity) is trained and tested using default data setting in "Set 1" and "Set 2", while "+1000" indicates this model is trained with additional 1000 images and evaluated on the same testing data. Evaluation of results after each step are also listed for comparison, which shows that they improve the performance. "MP" and "Sparsity" denote message passing scheme and sparsity regularization respectively.

Region	Method	Set 1			Set 2		
		Mean	Std	Id.Rates	Mean	Std	Id.Rates
All	Glocker et al. [2]	12.4	11.2	70%	13.2	17.8	74%
	Suzani et al. [4]	18.2	11.4	-	-	-	-
	Chen et al. [3]	-	-	-	8.8	13.0	84%
	DI2IN	17.0	47.3	74%	13.6	37.5	76%
	DI2IN+MP	11.7	19.7	77%	10.2	13.9	78%
	DI2IN+MP+Sparsity	9.1	7.2	80%	8.6	7.8	85%
	DI2IN+1000	10.6	21.5	80%	7.1	11.8	87%
	DI2IN+MP+1000	9.4	16.2	82%	6.9	8.3	89%
	DI2IN+MP+Sparsity+1000	**8.5**	**7.7**	**83%**	**6.4**	**5.9**	**90%**
Cervical	Glocker et al. [2]	7.0	4.7	80%	6.8	10.0	89%
	Suzani et al. [4]	17.1	8.7	-	-	-	-
	Chen et al. [3]	-	-	-	**5.1**	8.2	92%
	DI2IN+MP+Sparsity	6.6	3.9	83%	5.6	**4.0**	92%
	DI2IN+MP+Sparsity+1000	**5.8**	**3.9**	**88%**	5.2	4.4	**93%**
Thoracic	Glocker et al. [2]	13.8	11.8	62%	17.4	22.3	62%
	Suzani et al. [4]	17.2	11.8	-	-	-	-
	Chen et al. [3]	-	-	-	11.4	16.5	76%
	DI2IN+MP+Sparsity	9.9	7.5	74%	9.2	7.9	81%
	DI2IN+MP+Sparsity+1000	**9.5**	**8.5**	**78%**	**6.7**	**6.2**	**88%**
Lumbar	Glocker et al. [2]	14.3	12.3	75%	13.0	12.5	80%
	Suzani et al. [4]	20.3	12.2	-	-	-	-
	Chen et al. [3]	-	-	-	8.4	8.6	88%
	DI2IN+MP+Sparsity	10.9	9.1	80% ·	11.0	10.8	83%
	DI2IN+MP+Sparsity+1000	**9.9**	**9.1**	**84%**	**7.1**	**7.3**	**90%**

4   Conclusion

In this paper, we proposed an effective and fast automatic method to localize and label vertebra centroids in 3D CT volumes. Our method outperforms other state-of-the-art methods of spine labeling in terms of various evaluation metrics. For the future study, we plan to investigate various DI2IN architectures (e.g. ResNet) and other sophisticated refinement approaches to further improve the localization and identification performance.

Disclaimer: This feature is based on research, and is not commercially available. Due to regulatory reasons its future availability cannot be guaranteed.

References

1. Glocker, B., Feulner, J., Criminisi, A., Haynor, D.R., Konukoglu, E.: Automatic localization and identification of vertebrae in arbitrary field-of-view CT scans. In: Ayache, N., Delingette, H., Golland, P., Mori, K. (eds.) MICCAI 2012. LNCS, vol. 7512, pp. 590–598. Springer, Heidelberg (2012). doi:10.1007/978-3-642-33454-2_73

2. Glocker, B., Zikic, D., Konukoglu, E., Haynor, D.R., Criminisi, A.: Vertebrae localization in pathological spine CT via dense classification from sparse annotations. In: Mori, K., Sakuma, I., Sato, Y., Barillot, C., Navab, N. (eds.) MICCAI 2013. LNCS, vol. 8150, pp. 262–270. Springer, Heidelberg (2013). doi:10.1007/978-3-642-40763-5_33

3. Chen, H., Shen, C., Qin, J., Ni, D., Shi, L., Cheng, J.C.Y., Heng, P.-A.: Automatic localization and identification of vertebrae in spine CT via a joint learning model with deep neural networks. In: Navab, N., Hornegger, J., Wells, W.M., Frangi, A.F. (eds.) MICCAI 2015. LNCS, vol. 9349, pp. 515–522. Springer, Cham (2015). doi:10.1007/978-3-319-24553-9_63

4. Suzani, A., Seitel, A., Liu, Y., Fels, S., Rohling, R.N., Abolmaesumi, P.: Fast automatic vertebrae detection and localization in pathological CT scans - a deep learning approach. In: Navab, N., Hornegger, J., Wells, W.M., Frangi, A.F. (eds.) MICCAI 2015. LNCS, vol. 9351, pp. 678–686. Springer, Cham (2015). doi:10.1007/978-3-319-24574-4_81

5. Payer, C., Štern, D., Bischof, H., Urschler, M.: Regressing heatmaps for multiple landmark localization using CNNs. In: Ourselin, S., Joskowicz, L., Sabuncu, M.R., Unal, G., Wells, W. (eds.) MICCAI 2016. LNCS, vol. 9901, pp. 230–238. Springer, Cham (2016). doi:10.1007/978-3-319-46723-8_27

6. Badrinarayanan, V., Kendall, A., Cipolla, R.: Segnet: a deep convolutional encoder-decoder architecture for image segmentation. arXiv preprint. arXiv:1511.00561 (2015)

7. Ronneberger, O., Fischer, P., Brox, T.: U-Net: convolutional networks for biomedical image segmentation. In: Navab, N., Hornegger, J., Wells, W.M., Frangi, A.F. (eds.) MICCAI 2015. LNCS, vol. 9351, pp. 234–241. Springer, Cham (2015). doi:10.1007/978-3-319-24574-4_28

8. Xie, S., Tu, Z.: Holistically-nested edge detection. In: Proceedings of the IEEE International Conference on Computer Vision, pp. 1395–1403 (2015)

9. Yang, W., Ouyang, W., Li, H., Wang, X.: End-to-end learning of deformable mixture of parts and deep convolutional neural networks for human pose estimation. In: CVPR (2016)

10. Merkow, J., Kriegman, D., Marsden, A., Tu, Z.: Dense volume-to-volume vascular boundary detection. arXiv preprint arXiv:1605.08401 (2016)

11. Dou, Q., Chen, H., Jin, Y., Yu, L., Qin, J., Heng, P.-A.: 3D deeply supervised network for automatic liver segmentation from CT volumes. In: Ourselin, S., Joskowicz, L., Sabuncu, M.R., Unal, G., Wells, W. (eds.) MICCAI 2016. LNCS, vol. 9901, pp. 149–157. Springer, Cham (2016). doi:10.1007/978-3-319-46723-8_18

12. Chu, X., Ouyang, W., Li, H., Wang, X.: Structured feature learning for pose estimation. arXiv preprint arXiv:1603.09065 (2016)

General Image Analysis

A Deep Cascade of Convolutional Neural Networks for MR Image Reconstruction

Jo Schlemper[1](✉), Jose Caballero[1], Joseph V. Hajnal[2], Anthony Price[2], and Daniel Rueckert[1]

[1] Imperial College London, London, UK
jo.schlemper11@imperial.ac.uk
[2] King's College London, London, UK

Abstract. The acquisition of Magnetic Resonance Imaging (MRI) is inherently slow. Inspired by recent advances in deep learning, we propose a framework for reconstructing MR images from undersampled data using a deep cascade of convolutional neural networks to accelerate the data acquisition process. We show that for Cartesian undersampling of 2D cardiac MR images, the proposed method outperforms the state-of-the-art compressed sensing approaches, such as dictionary learning-based MRI (DLMRI) reconstruction, in terms of reconstruction error, perceptual quality and reconstruction speed for both 3-fold and 6-fold undersampling. Compared to DLMRI, the error produced by the method proposed is approximately twice as small, allowing to preserve anatomical structures more faithfully. Using our method, each image can be reconstructed in 23 ms, which is fast enough to enable real-time applications.

Keywords: Deep learning · Convolutional neural network · Magnetic Resonance Imaging · Image reconstruction

1 Introduction

In many clinical scenarios, medical imaging is an indispensable diagnostic and research tool. One such important modality is Magnetic Resonance Imaging (MRI), which is non-invasive and offers excellent resolution with various contrast mechanisms to reveal different properties of the underlying anatomy. However, MRI is associated with a slow acquisition process. This is because data samples of an MR image are acquired sequentially in *k-space* and the speed at which *k*-space can be traversed is limited by underlying MR physics. A long data acquisition procedures impose significant demands on patients, making the tool expensive and less accessible. One possible approach to accelerate the acquisition process is to undersample *k*-space, which in theory provides an acceleration rate proportional to a reduction factor of a number of k-space traversals required. However, undersampling in *k*-space violates the Nyquist-Shannon theorem and generates aliasing artefacts when the image is reconstructed. The main challenge

© Springer International Publishing AG 2017
M. Niethammer et al. (Eds.): IPMI 2017, LNCS 10265, pp. 647–658, 2017.
DOI: 10.1007/978-3-319-59050-9_51

in this case is to find an algorithm that takes into account the undersampling undergone and can compensate missing data with a-priori knowledge on the image to be reconstructed.

Using Compressed Sensing (CS), images can be reconstructed from sub-Nyquist sampling, assuming the following: firstly, the acquired images must be *compressible*, i.e. they have a sparse representation in some transform domain. Secondly, one must ensure *incoherence* between the sampling and sparsity domains to guarantee that the reconstruction problem has a unique solution and that this solution is attainable. In practice, this can be achieved with random sub-sampling of k-space, which translates aliasing patterns in the image domain into patterns that can be regarded as correlated noise. Under such assumptions, images can then be reconstructed through nonlinear optimization or iterative algorithms. The class of methods which applies CS to the MR reconstruction problem is termed CS-MRI [13]. A natural extension of these has been to enable more flexible representations with *adaptive* sparse modelling, where one attempts to obtain the optimal representation from data directly. This can be done by exploiting, for example, dictionary learning (DL) [17].

To achieve more aggressive undersampling, several strategies can be considered. One way is to further exploit the inherent redundancy of the MR data. For example, in dynamic imaging, one can make use of spatio-temporal redundancies [2,9,16]. Similarly, when imaging a full 3D volume, one exploit redundancy from adjacent slices [6]. An alternative approach is to exploit sources of explicit redundancy of the data and solve an overdetermined system. This is the fundamental assumption underlying parallel imaging [24]. Similarly, one can make use of multi-contrast information [7] or the redundancy generated by multiple filter responses of the image [14]. These explicit redundancies can also be used to complement the sparse modelling of inherent redundancies [8,12].

Recently, deep learning has been successful at tackling many computer vision problems. Deep neural network architectures, in particular convolutional neural network (CNN), are becoming the state-of-the-art technique for various imaging problems including image classification [4], object localisation [18] and image segmentation [19]. Deep architectures are capable of extracting features from data to build increasingly abstract representations that are useful for the end-goal being considered, replacing the traditional approach of carefully hand-crafting features and algorithms. For example, it has already been demonstrated that CNNs outperform sparsity-based methods in super-resolution [3], not only for its quality but also in terms of the reconstruction speed [21]. One of the contributions of our work is to explore the application of CNNs in undersampled MR reconstruction and investigate whether they can exploit data redundancy through learned representations. In fact, CNNs have already been applied to compressed sensing from random Gaussian measurements [11]. Despite the popularity of CNNs, there has only been preliminary research on CNN-based MR image reconstruction [22,25], hence the applicability of CNNs to this problem is yet to be qualitatively and quantitatively assessed in detail.

In this work we consider reconstructing 2D static images with Cartesian sampling using CNNs. Similar to the formulations in CS-MRI, we view the reconstruction problem as a de-aliasing problem in the image domain. However, reconstructing an undersampled MR image is challenging because the images typically have low signal-to-noise ratio, yet often high-quality reconstructions are needed for clinical applications. To resolve this issue, we propose a very deep network architecture which forms a cascade of CNNs. Our cascade network closely simulates the iterative reconstruction of DL-based methods, however, our approach allows end-to-end optimisation of the reconstruction algorithm. We show that under the Cartesian undersampling scheme, our CNN approach is capable of producing high-quality reconstructions of 2D cardiac MR images, outperforming DL-based MRI reconstruction (*DLMRI*) [17]. Moreover, using the proposed method, each images can be reconstructed in about 23 ms, which enables the real-time applications.

2   Problem Formulation

Let $\mathbf{x} \in \mathbb{C}^N$ represent a complex-valued MR image composed of $\sqrt{N} \times \sqrt{N}$ pixels stacked as a column vector. Our problem is to reconstruct $\mathbf{x}$ from $\mathbf{y} \in \mathbb{C}^M$, the measurements in k-space, such that:

$$\mathbf{y} = \mathbf{F}_u \mathbf{x} \tag{1}$$

Here $\mathbf{F}_u \in \mathbb{C}^{M \times N}$ is an undersampled Fourier encoding matrix. For undersampled k-space measurements $(M \ll N)$, the system of Eq. (1) is underdetermined and hence the inversion process is ill-defined. In order to reconstruct $\mathbf{x}$, one must exploit a-priori knowledge of its properties, which can be done by formulating an unconstrained optimisation problem:

$$\min_{\mathbf{x}} \quad \mathcal{R}(\mathbf{x}) + \lambda \|\mathbf{y} - \mathbf{F}_u \mathbf{x}\|_2^2 \tag{2}$$

$\mathcal{R}$ expresses regularisation terms on $\mathbf{x}$ and λ allows the adjustment of data fidelity based on the noise level of the acquired measurements $\mathbf{y}$. For CS-based methods, the regularisation terms $\mathcal{R}$ typically involve ℓ_0 or ℓ_1 norms in the sparsifying domain of $\mathbf{x}$. Our formulation is inspired by DL-based reconstruction approaches, in which the problem is formulated as:

$$\min_{\mathbf{x}, \mathbf{D}, \{\boldsymbol{\gamma}_i\}} \quad \sum_i \left(\|\mathbf{R}_i \mathbf{x} - \mathbf{D}\boldsymbol{\gamma}_i\|_2^2 + \nu \|\boldsymbol{\gamma}_i\|_0 \right) + \lambda \|\mathbf{y} - \mathbf{F}_u \mathbf{x}\|_2^2 \tag{3}$$

Here $\mathbf{R}_i$ is an operator which extracts an image patch at i, $\boldsymbol{\gamma}_i$ is the corresponding sparse code with respect to a dictionary $\mathbf{D}$. In this approach, the regularisation terms enforce $\mathbf{x}$ to be approximated by the reconstructions from the sparse code of patches. By taking the same approach, for our CNN formulation, we enforce $\mathbf{x}$ to be well-approximated by the CNN reconstruction:

$$\min_{\mathbf{x}, \boldsymbol{\theta}} \quad \|\mathbf{x} - f_{\text{cnn}}(\mathbf{x}_u | \boldsymbol{\theta})\|_2^2 + \lambda \|\mathbf{F}_u \mathbf{x} - \mathbf{y}\|_2^2 \tag{4}$$

Here f_{cnn} is the forward mapping of the CNN parameterised by $\boldsymbol{\theta}$, which takes in the zero-filled reconstruction $\mathbf{x}_u = \mathbf{F}_u^H \mathbf{y}$ and directly produces a reconstruction as an output. Since $\mathbf{x}_u$ is heavily affected by aliasing from sub-Nyquist sampling, the CNN reconstruction can therefore be seen as solving de-aliasing problem in the image domain.

The approach of Eq. (4), however, is limited in the sense that the CNN reconstruction and the data fidelity are two independent terms. In particular, since the CNN operates in the image domain, it is trained to reconstruct the image without a-priori information of the acquired data in k-space. However, if we already know some of the k-space values, then the CNN should be discouraged from modifying them. Therefore, by incorporating the data fidelity in the learning stage, the CNN should be able to achieve better reconstruction. This means that the output of the CNN is now conditioned on Ω, an index set indicating which k-space measurements have been sampled in $\mathbf{y}$. Then, our final reconstruction is given simply by the output, $\mathbf{x}_{\text{cnn}} = f_{\text{cnn}}(\mathbf{x}_u | \boldsymbol{\theta}, \lambda, \Omega)$. Given training data $\mathcal{D}$ of input-target pairs $(\mathbf{x}_u, \mathbf{x}_t)$, we can train the CNN to produce an output that attempts to accurately reconstruct the fully-sampled data by minimising an objective function:

$$\mathcal{L}(\boldsymbol{\theta}) = \sum_{(\mathbf{x}_u, \mathbf{x}_t) \in \mathcal{D}} \ell(\mathbf{x}_t, \mathbf{x}_{\text{cnn}}) \qquad (5)$$

where ℓ is a loss function. In this work, we consider an element-wise squared loss, which is given by $\ell(\mathbf{x}_t, \mathbf{x}_{\text{cnn}}) = \|\mathbf{x}_t - \mathbf{x}_{\text{cnn}}\|_2^2$.

3   Data Consistency Layer

In order to incorporate the data fidelity in the network architecture, we first note the following: for a fixed $\boldsymbol{\theta}$, Eq. (4) has a closed-form solution in k-space, given as in [17]:

$$\hat{\mathbf{x}}_{\text{rec}}(k) = \begin{cases} \hat{\mathbf{x}}_{\text{cnn}}(k) & \text{if } k \notin \Omega \\ \frac{\hat{\mathbf{x}}_{\text{cnn}}(k) + \lambda \hat{\mathbf{x}}_u(k)}{1+\lambda} & \text{if } k \in \Omega \end{cases} \qquad (6)$$

where $\hat{\mathbf{x}}_{\text{cnn}} = \mathbf{F} f_{\text{cnn}}(\mathbf{x}_u | \boldsymbol{\theta})$, $\hat{\mathbf{x}}_u = \mathbf{F} \mathbf{x}_u$ and $\mathbf{F}$ is the Fourier encoding matrix. The final image is reconstructed by applying the inverse of the encoding matrix $\mathbf{x}_{\text{rec}} = \mathbf{F}^{-1} \hat{\mathbf{x}}_{\text{rec}}$. In the noiseless setting (i.e. $\lambda \to \infty$), we simply replace the ith predicted coefficient by the original coefficient if it has been sampled. For this reason, this operation is called *data consistency step* in k-space (DC).

Since the DC step has a simple expression, we can in fact treat it as a layer operation of the network, which we denote as *DC layer*. When defining a layer of a network, the rules for forward and backward passes must be specified. This is because CNN training can effectively be performed through stochastic gradient descent, where one updates the network parameters $\boldsymbol{\theta}$ to minimise the objective function $\mathcal{L}$ by descending along the direction given by the derivative $\partial \mathcal{L} / \partial \boldsymbol{\theta}^T$. For this, it is necessary to define the gradients of each network layer relative to the network's output. In practice, one uses an efficient algorithm called *backpropagation* [20], where the final gradient is given by the product of all the Jacobians of the layers contributing to the output. Hence, in general, it suffices to specify a layer operation f_L for the forward pass and derive the Jacobian of the layer with respect to the layer input $\partial f_L / \partial \mathbf{x}^T$ for the backward pass.

Forward Pass. The data consistency in k-space can be simply decomposed into three operations: Fourier transform, data consistency and inverse Fourier transform. In our case, we take our Fourier transform to be a two-dimensional (2D) discrete Fourier transform (DFT) of the 2D image representation of $\mathbf{x}$, which is written as $\hat{\mathbf{x}} = \mathbf{F}\mathbf{x}$ in matrix form. The inverse transformation is defined analogously, where $\mathbf{x} = \mathbf{F}^{-1}\hat{\mathbf{x}}$. The data consistency f_{dc} performs the element-wise operation defined in Eq. (6). We can write it in matrix form as:

$$f_{dc}(\hat{\mathbf{x}}, \hat{\mathbf{x}}_u, \lambda) = \Lambda\hat{\mathbf{x}} + \frac{\lambda}{1+\lambda}\hat{\mathbf{x}}_u \tag{7}$$

Here Λ is a diagonal matrix of the form:

$$\Lambda_{kk} = \begin{cases} 1 & \text{if } k \notin \Omega \\ \frac{1}{1+\lambda} & \text{if } k \in \Omega \end{cases} \tag{8}$$

Combining the three operations defined above, we can obtain the forward pass of the layer performing data consistency in k-space:

$$f_L(\mathbf{x}, \hat{\mathbf{x}}_u, \lambda) = \mathbf{F}^{-1}\Lambda\mathbf{F}\mathbf{x} + \frac{\lambda}{1+\lambda}\mathbf{F}^{-1}\hat{\mathbf{x}}_u \tag{9}$$

Backward Pass. In general, one requires *Wirtinger calculus* to derive a gradient in complex domain [1], however, in our case, the derivation greatly simplifies due to the linearity of the DFT matrix and the data consistency operation. The Jacobian of the DC layer with respect to the layer input $\mathbf{x}$ is therefore given by:

$$\frac{\partial f_L}{\partial \mathbf{x}^T} = \mathbf{F}^{-1}\Lambda\mathbf{F} \tag{10}$$

There are several points that deserve further explanation: firstly, unlike many other applications where CNNs process real-valued data, MR images are complex-valued and the network needs to account for this. One possibility would be to design the network to perform complex-valued operations. A simpler approach, however, is to accommodate the complex nature of the data with real-valued operation in a dimensional space twice as large (i.e. we replace $\mathbb{C}^N$ by $\mathbb{R}^{2N}$). In the latter case, the derivations above still hold due to the fundamental assumption in Wirtinger calculus. Secondly, even though the DC layer does not have any additional parameters to be optimised, it allows end-to-end training of CNN, hence benefiting our final reconstruction.

4 Cascading Network

For CS-based methods, in particular for DLMRI, the optimisation problem is solved using a coordinate-descent type algorithm, alternating between the de-aliasing step and the data consistency step until convergence. In contrast, with CNNs, we are performing one step de-aliasing and the same network cannot be used to de-alias iteratively. While CNNs may be powerful enough to learn one step reconstruction, such network could indicate signs of overfitting, unless we have vast amounts of training data. In addition, training such networks may require a long time as well as careful fine-tuning steps. It is therefore best to be able to use CNNs for iterative reconstruction approaches.

A simple solution is to train a second CNN which learns to reconstruct from the output of the first CNN. In fact, we can concatenate a new CNN on the output of the previous CNN to build extremely deep networks which iterate between intermediate de-aliasing and the data consistency reconstruction. We term this a *cascading network*. In fact, one can essentially view this as unfolding the optimisation process of DLMRI. If each CNN expresses the dictionary learning reconstruction step, then the cascading CNN can be seen as a direct extension of DLMRI, where the whole reconstruction pipeline can be optimised from training.

5 Architecture and Implementation

Incorporating all the new elements mentioned above, we can devise our cascading network architecture. Our CNN takes in a two-channeled image $\mathbb{R}^{\sqrt{n} \times \sqrt{n} \times 2}$, where each channel stores real and imaginary parts of the undersampled image. Based on literature, we used the following network architecture for CNN, illustrated in Fig. 1: it has $n_d - 1$ convolution layers C_i, which are all followed by Rectifier Linear Units (ReLU) as a choice of nonlinearity. For each of them, we used a kernel size $k = 3$ [23] and the number of filters were set to $n_f = 64$. The network is followed by another convolution layer C_{rec} with kernel size $k = 3$ and $n_f = 2$, which projects the extracted representation back to image domain. We also used *residual connection* [5], which sums the output of the CNN module with its input. Finally, we form a cascading network by using the DC layers interleaved with the CNN reconstruction modules. For our experiment, we chose $n_d = 5$ and $n_c = 5$. We found that our choice of hyperparameters work sufficiently well, however, by no means were they optimised. Hence the result is likely to be improved by changing the architecture and varying the parameters such as kernel size and stride [19, 26].

As mentioned, pixel-wise squared error was used as our objective function. The minibatch size was set to 10, however, for the deeper models with large number of cascades, the minibatch size was reduced to fit the model on a single GPU memory. We initialised our network weights using He initialisation [5]. Adam optimiser [10] was used to train all models, with the parameters $\alpha = 10^{-4}, \beta_1 = 0.9$ and $\beta_2 = 0.999$. We also added ℓ_2 weight decay of 10^{-7}. The network was implemented in Python using Theano and Lasagne libraries.

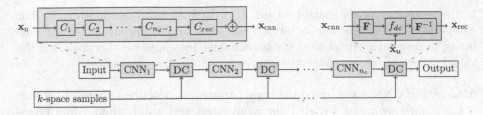

Fig. 1. A cascade of CNNs. The depth of architecture and the depth of cascade is denoted by n_d and n_c respectively.

6 Experimental Results

6.1 Setup

Dataset. Our method was evaluated using the cardiac MR dataset used in [2], consisting of 10 fully sampled short-axis cardiac cine MR scans. Each scan contains a single slice SSFP acquisition with 30 temporal frames with a 320×320 mm field of view and 10 mm slice thickness. The raw data consists of 32-channel data with sampling matrix size 192×190, which was zero-filled to the matrix size 256×256. The data was combined into a single complex-valued image using SENSE [15] with no undersampling, retrospective gating and the coil sensitivity maps normalised to a body coil image. The images were then retrospectively undersampled using Cartesian undersampling masks, where we fully sampled along the frequency-encoding direction but undersample in the phase-encoding direction. The strategy was adopted from [9]: for each frame we acquired eight lowest spatial frequencies. The sampling probability of other frequencies along the phase-encoding direction was determined by a zero-mean Gaussian distribution. The acceleration rates are stated with respect to the matrix size of the raw data. Note that similarly to previous studies, [2,17], since the raw data was combined prior to the simulation, the coil sensitivities were not directly addressed in our reconstruction. This is set for future investigation, where we plan to incorporate the explicit redundancy created by parallel imaging into our model.

Although the dataset is a dynamic sequence, we restrict our experiments to the 2D case only. Therefore, each time frame was treated as an independent image, yielding a total of 300 images. We found that applying rigid transformations as a data augmentation was crucial, as without it, the network quickly overfitted the training data. Moreover, for a fixed undersampling rate, we generated an undersampling mask on-the-fly to allow the network to learn diverse patterns of aliasing artefact.

Metric. We evaluated our method by reconstructing undersampled images from 3-fold and 6-fold acceleration rates. We used mean squared error (MSE) as our quantitative measure. During our experiment, we noticed that even for the same undersampling rate, different undersampling masks yield considerable differences in the reconstruction's signal-to-noise. To take this into consideration for fair comparison, we assigned an arbitrary but fixed undersampling mask for each image in test data. Apart from the quantitative measure, we also inspected the visual aspect of the reconstructed images for qualitative assessment.

Models. For CNN, we selected the hyperparameters described above. To ensure a fair comparison, we reported the aggregated test result from 2-fold cross-validation (i.e. train on five subjects and test on the other five). For each iteration of the cross validation, the network was initialised using He initialisation, trained end-to-end. For 6-fold undersampling, we initialised the network using the parameters obtained from the trained models from 3-fold acceleration and fine-tuned using Adam optimiser. Each network converged within 3 days on GeForce TITAN X.

We compared our method to DLMRI, a representative of the state-of-the-art CS-based methods. For DLMRI, we simplified the implementation of DLTG from [2], with patch size 6 × 6. We switched off any de-aliasing along the temporal axis. Since DLMRI is quite time consuming, in order to obtain the results within a reasonable amount of time, we trained a joint dictionary for all time frames within the subject and reconstructed them in parallel. Note that we did not observe any decrease in performance from this approach. For each subject, we ran 400 iterations and obtained the final reconstruction.

6.2   Results

The means of the reconstruction errors across 10 subjects are summarised in Table 1. For both 3-fold and 6-fold acceleration, one can see that CNN consistently outperformed DLMRI, and that the standard deviation of the error made by CNN was smaller. The reconstruction from 3-fold acceleration can be found in Fig. 2. It can be seen that the CNN approach produced a smaller overall error. The CNN reconstruction produced a more homogeneous reconstruction. On the other hand, DLMRI gave a blocky reconstruction. In some cases, both CNN and DLMRI suffered from small losses of important anatomical structures in their reconstructions (orange), but CNN was able to recover more details (red). The reconstructions from 6-fold acceleration is in Fig. 3. Although both methods suffered from significant loss of structures (orange), CNN was still capable of better preserving the texture than DLMRI (red). On the other hand, DLMRI created extremely block-like artefacts due to over-smoothing. 6× undersampling for these

Table 1. DLMRI vs. CNN across 10 scans

	3-fold	6-fold
Models	MSE (SD) × 10^{-3}	MSE (SD) × 10^{-3}
DLMRI	2.12 (1.27)	6.31 (2.95)
CNN	**0.89 (0.46)**	**3.42 (1.65)**

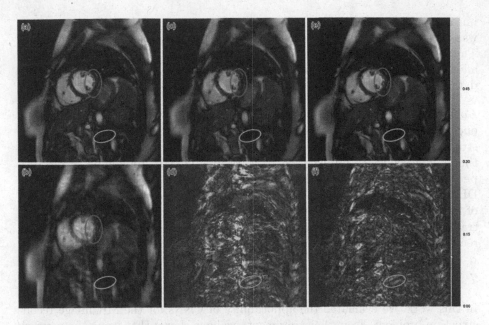

Fig. 2. The comparison of reconstruction from DLMRI and CNN. (a) The original, (b) 3× undersampled, (c)–(d) DLMRI reconstruction and its error map ×5 and (e)–(f) CNN reconstruction and its error map ×5. (Color figure online)

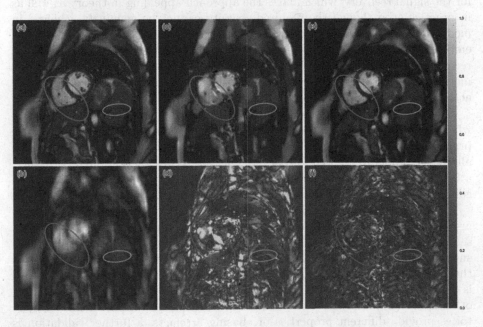

Fig. 3. The comparison of reconstructions from DLMRI and CNN. (a) The original, (b) 6× undersampled, (c)–(d) DLMRI reconstruction and its error map ×5 and (e)–(f) CNN reconstruction and its error map ×5. (Color figure online)

images typically approaches the limit of sparsity-based methods, however, CNN was able to predict some anatomical details which was not possible by DLMRI. This could be due to the fact that CNN has more free parameters to tune with, allowing the network to learn complex but more accurate transformations of data.

Comparison of Reconstruction Speed. While training CNN is time consuming, once it is trained, the inference can be done extremely quickly on a GPU. Reconstructing each slice took 23 ± 0.1 ms on GeForce GTX 1080, which enables real-time applications. To produce the above results, DLMRI took about 6.1 ± 1.3 h per subject on CPU. Even though we do not have a GPU implementation of DLMRI, it is expected to take longer than 23 ms because DLMRI requires dozens of iterations of dictionary learning and sparse coding steps. Using a fixed, pre-trained dictionary could remove this bottleneck, in exchange of lowering the reconstruction capacity.

7   Discussion and Conclusion

In this work, we evaluated the applicability of CNNs for the MR image reconstruction problem. From the experiment, we have shown that using the network with interleaved data consistency stages, we can obtain a model which can reconstruct images sufficiently well. The CS framework offers mathematical guarantee for the signal recovery, which makes the approach appealing in theory as well as in practice even though the required sparsity cannot be genuinely achieved in medical imaging. However, even though this is not the case for CNNs, we have empirically shown that a CNN-based approach can outperform DL-based MR reconstruction. In addition, at very aggressive undersampling rates, the CNN method was capable of reconstructing most of the anatomical structures more accurately, while CS-based methods do not guarantee such behaviour.

The limitation of this work is that the data was first reconstructed by SENSE, which was then used to simulated the acquisition process. It is, however, more practical to consider images with sensitivity map of the surface coils, which allows the model to be used for parallel imaging reconstruction directly. In fact, a better approach is to exploit the redundancy of the coil sensitivity maps and combine directly into our model, which will be addressed in our future work.

In this work, we were able to show that the network can be trained using arbitrary Cartesian undersampling masks of the fixed sampling rate rather than selecting a fixed number of undersampling masks for training and testing. This suggests that the network was capable of learning a generic strategy to de-alias the images. A further investigation should consider how tolerant the network is for different undersampling rates. Furthermore, it is interesting to consider other sampling patterns such as radial and spiral trajectories. As these trajectories provide different properties of aliasing artefacts, a further validation is appropriate to determine the flexibility of our approach.

Finally, Although CNNs can only learn local representations which should not affect global structure, it remains to be determined how the CNN approach operates when there is a pathology present in images, or other more variable content. We have performed a two-fold cross-validation to ensure that the network can handle unseen data acquired through the same acquisition protocol. Generalisation properties must be evaluated carefully on a larger dataset, however, CNNs are flexible in a way such that one can incorporate application specific priors to its objective to allocate more importance on preserving any features of interest in the reconstruction, provided that such expert knowledge is available at training time. For example, analysis of cardiac images in clinical settings often employs segmentation and/or registration. Multi-task learning is a promising approach to further improve the utility of CNN-based MR reconstructions.

Acknowledgment. The work was partially funded by EPSRC Programme Grant (EP/P001009/1).

References

1. Amin, M., Murase, K.: Learning Algorithms in Complex-Valued Neural Networks Using Wirtinger Calculus. Wiley Online Library, Hoboken (2013)
2. Caballero, J., Price, A.N., Rueckert, D., Hajnal, J.V.: Dictionary learning and time sparsity for dynamic MR data reconstruction. IEEE Trans. Med. Imaging **33**(4), 979–994 (2014)
3. Dong, C., Loy, C.C., He, K., Tang, X.: Image super-resolution using deep convolutional networks. IEEE Trans. Pattern Anal. Mach. Intell. **38**(2), 295–307 (2016)
4. He, K., Zhang, X., Ren, S., Sun, J.: Deep residual learning for image recognition. arXiv preprint arXiv:1512.03385 (2015)
5. He, K., Zhang, X., Ren, S., Sun, J.: Delving deep into rectifiers: surpassing human-level performance on imagenet classification. In: Proceedings of the IEEE International Conference on Computer Vision, pp. 1026–1034 (2015)
6. Hirabayashi, A., Inamuro, N., Mimura, K., Kurihara, T., Homma, T.: Compressed sensing MRI using sparsity induced from adjacent slice similarity. In: 2015 International Conference on Sampling Theory and Applications (SampTA), pp. 287–291. IEEE (2015)
7. Huang, J., Chen, C., Axel, L.: Fast multi-contrast MRI reconstruction. Magn. Reson. Imaging **32**(10), 1344–1352 (2014)
8. Jin, K.H., Lee, D., Ye, J.C.: A novel k-space annihilating filter method for unification between compressed sensing and parallel MRI, pp. 327–330 (2015)
9. Jung, H., Ye, J.C., Kim, E.Y.: Improved k-t BLAST and k-t SENSE using FOCUSS. Magn. Reson. Med. **52**, 3201–3226 (2007)
10. Kingma, D., Ba, J.: Adam: a method for stochastic optimization. arXiv preprint arXiv:1412.6980 (2014)
11. Kulkarni, K., Lohit, S., Turaga, P., Kerviche, R., Ashok, A.: ReconNet: non-iterative reconstruction of images from compressively sensed measurements. In: Proceedings of the IEEE Conference on Computer Vision and Pattern Recognition, pp. 449–458 (2016)
12. Liang, D., Liu, B., Wang, J., Ying, L.: Accelerating SENSE using compressed sensing. Magn. Reson. Med. **62**(6), 1574–1584 (2009)
13. Lustig, M., Donoho, D.L., Santos, J.M., Pauly, J.M.: Compressed sensing MRI. IEEE Signal Process. Mag. **25**(2), 72–82 (2008)

14. Peng, X., Liang, D.: MR image reconstruction with convolutional characteristic constraint (CoCCo). IEEE Signal Process. Lett. **22**(8), 1184–1188 (2015)
15. Pruessmann, K.P., Weiger, M., Scheidegger, M.B., Boesiger, P., et al.: SENSE: sensitivity encoding for fast MRI. Magn. Reson. Med. **42**(5), 952–962 (1999)
16. Quan, T.M., Jeong, W.K.: Compressed sensing reconstruction of dynamic contrast enhanced MRI using GPU-accelerated convolutional sparse coding. In: 2016 IEEE 13th International Symposium on Biomedical Imaging (ISBI), pp. 518–521. IEEE (2016)
17. Ravishankar, S., Bresler, Y.: MR image reconstruction from highly undersampled k-space data by dictionary learning. IEEE Trans. Med. Imaging **30**(5), 1028–1041 (2011)
18. Ren, S., He, K., Girshick, R., Sun, J.: Faster R-CNN: towards real-time object detection with region proposal networks. In: Advances in Neural Information Processing Systems, pp. 91–99 (2015)
19. Ronneberger, O., Fischer, P., Brox, T.: U-Net: convolutional networks for biomedical image segmentation. In: Navab, N., Hornegger, J., Wells, W.M., Frangi, A.F. (eds.) MICCAI 2015. LNCS, vol. 9351, pp. 234–241. Springer, Cham (2015). doi:10.1007/978-3-319-24574-4_28
20. Rumelhart, D.E., Hinton, G.E., Williams, R.J.: Learning representations by back-propagating errors. Cogn. Model. **5**(3), 1 (1988)
21. Shi, W., Caballero, J., Huszár, F., Totz, J., Aitken, A.P., Bishop, R., Rueckert, D., Wang, Z.: Real-time single image and video super-resolution using an efficient sub-pixel convolutional neural network. In: Proceedings of the IEEE Conference on Computer Vision and Pattern Recognition, pp. 1874–1883 (2016)
22. Sun, J., Li, H., Xu, Z., et al.: Deep ADMM-net for compressive sensing MRI. In: Advances In Neural Information Processing Systems, pp. 10–18 (2016)
23. Szegedy, C., Liu, W., Jia, Y., Sermanet, P., Reed, S., Anguelov, D., Erhan, D., Vanhoucke, V., Rabinovich, A.: Going deeper with convolutions. In: Proceedings of the IEEE Conference on Computer Vision and Pattern Recognition, pp. 1–9 (2015)
24. Uecker, M., Lai, P., Murphy, M.J., Virtue, P., Elad, M., Pauly, J.M., Vasanawala, S.S., Lustig, M.: ESPIRiT - an eigenvalue approach to autocalibrating parallel MRI: where SENSE meets GRAPPA. Magn. Reson. Med. **71**(3), 990–1001 (2014)
25. Wang, S., Su, Z., Ying, L., Peng, X., Zhu, S., Liang, F., Feng, D., Liang, D.: Accelerating magnetic resonance imaging via deep learning. In: 2016 IEEE 13th International Symposium on Biomedical Imaging (ISBI), pp. 514–517. IEEE (2016)
26. Yu, F., Koltun, V.: Multi-scale context aggregation by dilated convolutions. arXiv preprint arXiv:1511.07122 (2015)

Population Based Image Imputation

Adrian V. Dalca[1,2(✉)], Katherine L. Bouman[1], William T. Freeman[1,3],
Natalia S. Rost[4], Mert R. Sabuncu[2,5], and Polina Golland[1]

[1] Computer Science and Artificial Intelligence Lab, MIT, Cambridge, USA
adalca@csail.mit.edu
[2] Martinos Center for Biomedical Imaging, Massachusetts General Hospital, HMS,
Charlestown, MA, USA
[3] Google Research, Cambridge, MA, USA
[4] Department of Neurology, Massachusetts General Hospital, HMS, Boston, USA
[5] School of Electrical and Computer Engineering, Cornell, Ithaca, USA

Abstract. We present an algorithm for creating high resolution anatomically plausible images consistent with acquired clinical brain MRI scans with large inter-slice spacing. Although large databases of clinical images contain a wealth of information, medical acquisition constraints result in sparse scans that miss much of the anatomy. These characteristics often render computational analysis impractical as standard processing algorithms tend to fail when applied to such images. Highly specialized or application-specific algorithms that explicitly handle sparse slice spacing do not generalize well across problem domains. In contrast, our goal is to enable application of existing algorithms that were originally developed for high resolution research scans to significantly undersampled scans. We introduce a model that captures fine-scale anatomical similarity across subjects in clinical image collections and use it to fill in the missing data in scans with large slice spacing. Our experimental results demonstrate that the proposed method outperforms current upsampling methods and promises to facilitate subsequent analysis not previously possible with scans of this quality.

1 Introduction

Increasingly open acquisition efforts in clinical practice are driving dramatic increases in the number and size of patient cohorts in clinical archives. Unfortunately, clinical volumes are typically of dramatically lower resolution than the research scans that motivate most methodological development. Specifically, while individual slices in the scan can be of high resolution, slice spacing is often significantly larger, resulting in missing voxels, as illustrated in Fig. 1. This presents significant challenges for even basic tasks, such as skull stripping and registration, which are often necessary for downstream analysis [4,9]. We present a novel method for constructing high resolution anatomically plausible volumetric images consistent with the available slices in sparsely sampled clinical scans. The restored images promise to enable computational analysis of clinical scans with existing techniques originally developed for isotropic research scans.

© Springer International Publishing AG 2017
M. Niethammer et al. (Eds.): IPMI 2017, LNCS 10265, pp. 659–671, 2017.
DOI: 10.1007/978-3-319-59050-9_52

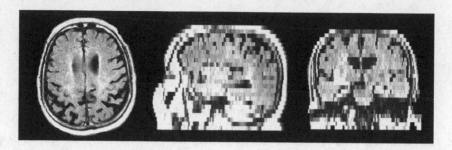

Fig. 1. Axial, saggital and coronal slices from an example scan in our clinical dataset.

Importantly, our method does not require any high resolution scans or expert annotations, but instead imputes the missing structure by learning from the available collection of clinical scans.

Our work is motivated by a study that includes brain MRI scans of thousands of stroke patients acquired within 48 h of stroke onset. The study aims to quantify white matter disease burden, necessitating skull stripping and deformable registration into a common coordinate frame [16]. The volumes are severely under-sampled (0.85 mm × 0.85 mm × 6 mm) due to clinical constraints of acute stroke care, as illustrated in Fig. 1. Such undersampling is typical of modalities that aim to characterize tissue properties such as T2-FLAIR, even in research studies like ADNI2 [9].

Since clinically acquired scans violate many algorithms' underlying assumptions, even basic tasks present significant challenges [6,20,21]. In undersampled scans, the image is no longer smooth, and the anatomical structure may change substantially between consecutive slices (Fig. 1). Application-specific algorithms promise to address these problems for certain clinical scans but do not generalize well across applications and imaging modalities. In contrast, we harness the data available in a given clinical image collection to reconstruct the high resolution images that represent plausible anatomy from the low resolution scans (Fig. 2). The resulting images can then be analyzed by widely used algorithms that require nearly isotropic high resolution input. The imputed data acts as a medium for improving analysis tasks. For example, although imputed data should not be used in the clinical evaluation, the brain mask obtained through skull stripping of the restored scans can be applied to the original clinical scan for further analysis.

Prior Work. Traditional image restoration, or superresolution, techniques depend on having enough information in a single scan to synthesize data. Unfortunately, clinical slices are often sampled too sparsely for functional interpolation, such as linear, cubic or spline [19], to succeed. Similarly, patch-based methods that rely on redundancy within a single scan to "hallucinate" missing fine scale structure [13–15] fail to produce anatomically plausible reconstructions at this level of sparsity. Superresolution algorithms that use multiple images of

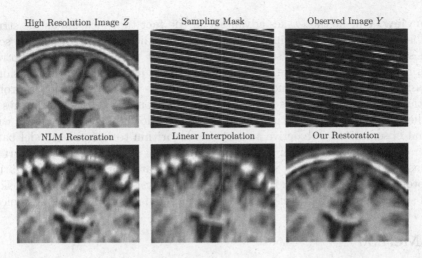

High Resolution Image Z · Sampling Mask · Observed Image Y

NLM Restoration · Linear Interpolation · Our Restoration

Fig. 2. Problem setup and preview of the results. Top row: (unobserved) isotropic image Z that we seek to recover is sampled according to the sampling mask which produces observed image Y. Bottom row: restoration results for non-local means (NLM) upsampling, linear interpolation, and our method, respectively. The most dramatic improvement can be seen in restorations of the skull, dura matter, and ventricles.

the same subject to improve a single scan [2,10,15] are unsuitable for clinical data where multiple similar acquisitions are not commonly available.

Nonparametric upsampling methods proposed to tackle the problem of super-resolution often rely on an external dataset of high resolution data or cannot handle extreme undersampling present in clinical scans. For example, some methods fill in missing data by matching a low resolution patch from the scan with a high resolution patch from the training dataset [3,7,10,11,18]. A recent approach to improve resolution from a collection of scans with sparse slices jointly upsamples all images using non-local means [17]. However this method has only been demonstrated on slice spacing of roughly three times the in-plane resolution, and in our experience similar non-parametric methods fail to upsample clinical scans with more significant undersampling.

Parametric methods and low dimensional embeddings have been used to model the common structure of image patches from full resolution images, but are typically not designed to handle missing data. Specifically, priors [22] and Gaussian Mixture Models [23] have been used in both medical and natural images for classification [1] and denoising [5,23]. The procedures used for training these models rely on having full resolution patches with no missing data. Unfortunately, high (full) resolution training datasets are not readily available for many image contrasts and scanners, and may not adequately represent pathology or other properties of clinical populations. Acquiring the appropriate high resolution data is often infeasible, and here we explicitly focus on the realistic medical scenario where only low resolution image sets are available.

Overview. Our method takes advantage of the fact that local fine scale structure is intrinsically shared in a population of medical images, and each scan with sparse slices captures some partial aspect of this structure. We borrow ideas from Gaussian Mixture Model (GMM) patch priors [23], low dimensional Gaussian embeddings [8], and missing data models [8,12] to develop a probabilistic model that describes sparse 3D patches from all volumetric images in a collection around a particular location using a low-dimensional GMM with partial observations. We derive an iterative algorithm to learn the model parameters. We demonstrate our algorithm using scans from the ADNI cohort as well as the motivating stroke study, and also illustrate a preliminary illustration of potential improvements in the down-stream analysis using an example task of skull stripping. Finally, we discuss initialization tradeoffs and modelling choices.

2   Method

We employ a Gaussian Mixture Model (GMM) to capture local structure in sparse 3D patches in the vicinity of a particular location across the entire collection. We treat a patch as a high dimensional manifestation of a low dimensional representation, with the intuition that the covariation within image patches has small intrinsic dimensionality relative to the number of voxels in the patch. In this section, we describe the model, the resulting learning algorithm, and our image restoration procedure.

2.1   Generative Model

Let $\{Y_1, \ldots, Y_N\}$ be an image collection of scans with large slice separation, roughly aligned into a common atlas space (we use affine transformations in our experiments). For each image Y_i in the collection, only a few slices are known, and we seek to restore the anatomically plausible high resolution volume by imputing the missing voxel values.

We capture local structure using image patches. We assume a constant patch shape, and use y_i to denote a D-length vector that contains voxels of the image patch centered at a certain location of image Y_i. We perform inference at each location independently. We model the set of patches $\mathcal{Y} = \{y_i\}$ at a common location as drawn from a K-component multivariate GMM. If generated by cluster k, patch y_i is a high dimensional observation of a low dimensional patch representation x_i of length d:

$$y_i = \mu_k + W_k x_i + \epsilon_i, \quad \text{where} \tag{1}$$
$$x_i \sim \mathcal{N}(0, I_{D \times D}),$$
$$\epsilon_i \sim \mathcal{N}(0, \sigma_k^2 I_{D \times D}), \quad \text{and} \quad \epsilon_i \perp\!\!\!\perp x_i.$$

Here patch μ_k is the mean of cluster k, matrix W_k shapes the covariance structure of the cluster, and σ_k^2 is the variance of image noise. The likelihood of all patches at this location under the mixture model is

$$p(\mathcal{Y}; \{\mu_k\}, \{W_k\}, \{\sigma_k^2\}, \pi) = \prod_i \sum_k \pi_k \mathcal{N}(y_i; \mu_k, C_k), \tag{2}$$

where $C_k = W_k W_k^T + \sigma_k^2 I_{D \times D}$ and π is a vector of cluster proportions.

Let $\mathcal{O}_i$ be the set of observed voxels, i.e., from the known slices, in patch y_i, and $y_i^{\mathcal{O}_i}$ be the corresponding vector of their intensity values:

$$y_i^{\mathcal{O}_i} = \mu_k^{\mathcal{O}_i} + W_k^{\mathcal{O}_i} x_i + \epsilon_i, \tag{3}$$

where $W_k^{\mathcal{O}_i}$ comprises rows of W_k that correspond to the observed voxel set $\mathcal{O}_i$. The likelihood of the *observed* data is therefore

$$p(\mathcal{Y}^{\mathcal{O}}; \{W_k\}, \{\mu_k\}, \{\sigma_k^2\}, \pi) = \prod_i \sum_k \pi_k \mathcal{N}(y_i^{\mathcal{O}_i}; \mu_k^{\mathcal{O}_i}, C_k^{\mathcal{O}_i \mathcal{O}_i}), \tag{4}$$

where $\mathcal{Y}^{\mathcal{O}} = \{y_i^{\mathcal{O}_i}\}$, and matrix $C_k^{\mathcal{O}_i \mathcal{O}_i}$ extracts the rows and columns of C_k that correspond to the observed voxel subset $\mathcal{O}_i$.

2.2   Learning

We learn the maximum likelihood estimates of the parameters $\{\mu_k\}, \{W_k\}, \{\sigma_k^2\}$ and π under the likelihood (4). As traditional Expectation Maximization for our model does not lead to closed form update equations, we employ the Expectation Conditional Maximization (ECM) [8,12] variant of the Generalized Expectation Maximization, where parameter updates depend on the previous parameter estimates. Due to space limitations, we omit the derivations and provide the resulting updates along with their interpretations.

The **expectation step** updates the class memberships based on the observed voxels of the patches at this location:

$$\gamma_{ik} \triangleq p(k|y_i^{\mathcal{O}_i}; \{W_k\}, \{\mu_k\}, \{\sigma_k^2\}, \pi) \leftarrow \frac{\pi_k \mathcal{N}(y_i^{\mathcal{O}_i}; \mu_k^{\mathcal{O}_i}, C_k^{\mathcal{O}_i \mathcal{O}_i})}{\sum_k \pi_k \mathcal{N}(y_i^{\mathcal{O}_i}; \mu_k^{\mathcal{O}_i}, C_k^{\mathcal{O}_i \mathcal{O}_i})}. \tag{5}$$

Next, we compute the statistics of the low dimensional representation x for each patch as "explained" by each cluster:

$$\widehat{x}_{ik} \triangleq E[x_i|k] = ((W_k^{\mathcal{O}_i})^T W_k^{\mathcal{O}_i} + \sigma_k^2 I_{D \times D})^{-1} (W_k^{\mathcal{O}_i})^T (y_i^{\mathcal{O}_i} - \mu_k^{\mathcal{O}_i}), \tag{6}$$

$$S_{ik} \triangleq E[x_i x_i^T|k] - \widehat{x}_{ik}\widehat{x}_{ik}^T = \sigma_k^2 ((W_k^{\mathcal{O}_i})(W_k^{\mathcal{O}_i})^T + \sigma_k^2 I_{D \times D})^{-1}. \tag{7}$$

The **maximization step** uses the observed voxels to update the model parameters. We let $\mathcal{P}_j$ be the set of patches in which voxel j is observed, y_i^j be the jth element of vector y_i, and W_k^j be the jth row of matrix W_k. We update the mean as the average residual of the predicted patch voxels $W_k^j \widehat{x}_{ik}$ and the observed values y_i:

$$\mu_k^j \leftarrow \frac{\sum_{i \in \mathcal{P}_j} \gamma_{ik}(y_i^j - W_k^j \widehat{x}_{ik})}{\sum_{i' \in \mathcal{P}_j} \gamma_{i'k}}. \tag{8}$$

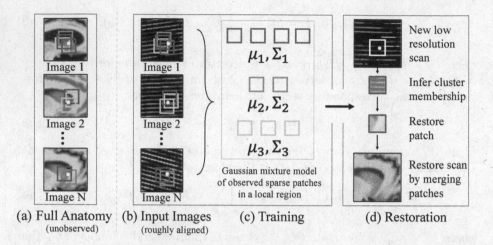

(a) Full Anatomy **(b) Input Images**   **(c) Training**   **(d) Restoration**
(unobserved)   (roughly aligned)

Fig. 3. Image imputation. (a) Full resolution images, for illustration only. These are unobserved by the algorithm. (b) Sparse planes acquired in clinical scans. (c) During learning, we train a GMM that captures the low dimensional nature of patch variability at a particular location (white dot). (d) Given an image from the collection, or a new image, we infer the most likely cluster for each 3D patch, and restore the missing data using the learned model and the observed voxels. We quilt the final volume from overlapping restored patches. 2D images are shown for illustration only, the algorithms operate fully in 3D.

The covariance factors and residual variance are updated based on the statistics of low dimensional representation from (6) and (7):

$$W_k^j \leftarrow \left[\sum_{i \in \mathcal{P}_j} \gamma_{ik}(\widehat{x}_{ik}\widehat{x}_{ik}^T + S_{ik})\right]^{-1} \sum_{i \in \mathcal{P}_j} \gamma_{ik}(y_i^j - \mu_k^j)\widehat{x}_{ik}^T \qquad (9)$$

$$\sigma_k^2 \leftarrow \frac{1}{\sum_j \sum_{i \in \mathcal{P}_j} \gamma_{ik}} \sum_j \sum_{i \in \mathcal{P}_j} \gamma_{ik}\left[(y_i^j - W_k^j\widehat{x}_{ik} - \mu_k^j)^2 + W_k^j S_{ik}(W_k^j)^T\right]. \quad (10)$$

Finally, we update the cluster proportions:

$$\pi_k = \frac{1}{N}\sum_i \gamma_{ik}. \qquad (11)$$

Throughout learning, we work in the atlas space, and approximate voxels as either observed or missing in this space by thresholding interpolation weights and ignoring interpolation effects due to affine alignment. Intuitively, learning such a model with sparse data is possible because each image patch provides a slightly different subset of voxel observations that contribute to the parameter estimation (Fig. 3). The estimation can be extended to carry out the learning by appropriately transforming model parameters into the subject-specific space in order to optimally use the observed voxels, but this leads to computationally prohibitive updates.

In our experiments, all subject scans have the same acquisition direction. Despite different affine transformations to the atlas space for each subject, some voxel *pairs* are still never observed in the same patch, resulting in missing entries of the covariance. Representing covariance using a low-rank approximation helps to alleviate this lack of observations:

2.3 Restoration

To restore an individual patch y_i, we first estimate the most likely cluster $\widehat{k}$ for patch y_i by selecting the cluster with the highest membership γ_{ik}. We then estimate the low dimensional representation $\widehat{x}_{i\widehat{k}}$ given the observed voxels $y_i^{\mathcal{O}_i}$ using (6). Finally, we reconstruct the high resolution patch:

$$z_i = \mu_{\widehat{k}} + W_{\widehat{k}}\widehat{x}_{i\widehat{k}} \qquad (12)$$

using the estimates of the model parameters $\mu_{\widehat{k}}$ and $W_{\widehat{k}}$. We average overlapping restored patches using standard techniques and form the restored volume Z_i [13].

2.4 Implementation

We stack together the affinely registered sparse images from the entire collection and split the stack into overlapping subvolumes of $18 \times 18 \times 18$ voxels in the isotropically sampled common atlas space. Subvolumes are centered 9 voxels apart in each direction. Within each subvolume, we learn the mixture model parameters. Instead of selecting just one patch from each volume at a given location, we collect all overlapping patches within the subvolume centered at that location. This aggregation provides more data for each model, which is crucial when working with severely undersampled volumes. Moreover, it offers robustness in the face of image misalignment. Given the learned parameters at each location, we restore all overlapping patches within a subvolume. We use a cubic patch of size $9 \times 9 \times 9$ voxels, and found $K = 5$ clusters and $d = 21$ to be sufficient. We use a hierarchical implementation, where the subvolume parameters are trained at three iterative scales.

While learning is performed in the common atlas space, we restore each volume in its original subject space to limit effects of interpolation. We apply the inverse of the estimated subject-specific affine transformation to the cluster statistics, and use them to restore patches via (12) in the original subject space.

Our implementation is freely available at https://github.com/adalca/papago.

3   Experiments

We demonstrate the proposed imputation algorithm on two datasets and evaluate the results both visually and quantitatively. We also include a preliminary example of how imputation can aid in a skull stripping task.

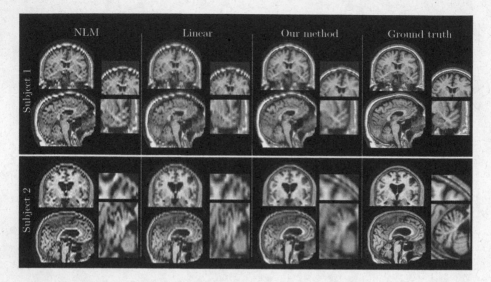

Fig. 4. Representative ADNI restorations. Representative reconstruction by NLM, linear interpolation, and our method, and the original high resolution images for two representative subjects in the study. Our method reconstructs more anatomically plausible substructures as can be especially seen in the close-up panels, for example in the skull or temporal lobe.

3.1   Data

ADNI Dataset. We evaluate our algorithm using 326 T1-weighted brain MR images from ADNI [9]. We downsample the isotropic $1\,\text{mm}^3$ images to slice separation of $5\,\text{mm}$ ($1\,\text{mm} \times 1\,\text{mm}$ in-plane), and use these low resolution images as input. All subjects are affinely registered to a T1 atlas. The original images serve as the ground truth for quantitative comparisons.

Clinical Dataset. We also demonstrate our algorithm on a clinical set of 127 T2-FLAIR brain MR scans in a stroke patient cohort. These scans are severely anisotropic ($0.85 \times 0.85\,\text{mm}$ in-plane, slice separation of $6\,\text{mm}$). All subjects are affinely registered to a T2-FLAIR atlas and intensity normalized. The slices are resampled to $1.2\,\text{mm} \times 1.2\,\text{mm}$ resolution.

3.2   Evaluation

We compare our algorithm to three upsampling methods: nearest neighbour (NN) interpolation, linear interpolation, and non-local means (NLM) upsampling [13]. For ADNI images, we found the hierarchical implementation was unnecessary and only ran the final scale of our algorithm. We compare the reconstructions to the original isotropic volumes both visually and quantitatively (ADNI images only). We use mean squared error MSE $(Z, Z_o) = \frac{1}{N} \sum (Z - Z_o)^2$

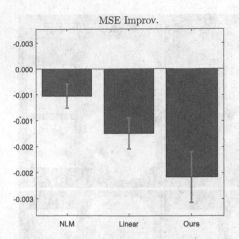
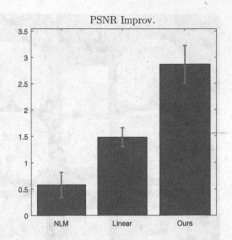

Fig. 5. Reconstruction accuracy statistics. Accuracy improvement over nearest neighbor interpolation for different image restoration methods. Left: MSE (lower is better), Right: PSNR (higher is better). Our method performs significantly better. For Nearest neighbor interpolation, MSE $= 0.004\pm0.001$ and PSNR $= 23.7\pm1.1$. All statistics were computed over 40 scans randomly chosen from the ADNI dataset. Image intensities are scaled to a $[0, 1]$ range.

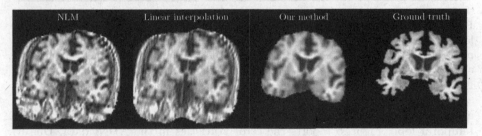

Fig. 6. Skull stripping example. Example of a skull stripping failure for linear and NLM interpolation. Skull stripping dramatically improves when applied to the imputed image for this example.

of the reconstructed image Z relative to the original high resolution scan Z_o, and peak signal to noise ratio PSNR $= \log_{10} \frac{max(Z_o)}{MSE(Z, Z_o)}$. Both metrics are commonly used in measuring the quality of reconstruction of compressed or noisy signals. Additionally, we illustrate a preliminary example application where skull stripping fails using the original scan and improves dramatically if an imputed image is used.

3.3   Results

Figure 4 illustrates representative restored images for typical subjects in the ADNI dataset. Our method produces more plausible structure both in coronal and saggital slices. The method restores anatomical structures that are almost

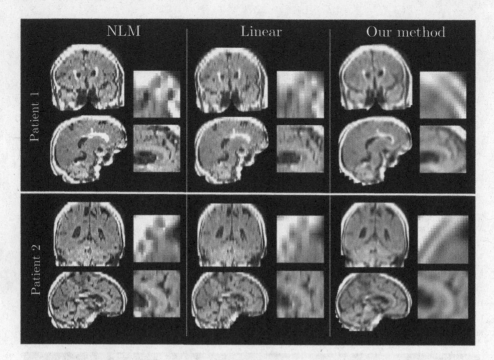

Fig. 7. Representative clinical restorations. Reconstruction using NLM, linear interpolation and our method for two representative subjects. Our method reconstructs more plausible substructures, as can be especially seen in the close-up panels of the skull and periventricular regions.

entirely missing in the other reconstructions, such as the dura or the sulci of the temporal lobe. Figure 5 reports the error statistics in the ADNI data. Due to high variability among subject scans, we report improvements of each method over the nearest neighbor interpolation baseline in the same scan. Our algorithm offers significant improvement compared to the linear interpolation and NLM.

We also show a preliminary result where imputed data facilitates downstream image analysis. Specifically, the first step in many analysis pipelines is brain extraction – isolating the brain from the rest of the anatomy. Typical algorithms assume that the brain consists of a single connected component separated from the skull and dura by cerebral spinal fluid [20], and often fail on sparsely sampled scans that no longer have clear contrast between these regions. Figure 6 illustrates an example result where the brain extraction fails on the original subject scan but succeeds on our reconstructed image.

Figure 7 illustrates representative restoration improvements in the clinical population. Our method produces more plausible structure, as can be especially seen in the close-up panels focusing on anatomical details.

4   Discussion and Conclusions

We propose an image imputation method that employs a large collection of low-resolution images to infer fine-scale anatomy of a particular subject. We introduce a model that captures structural similarity across subjects in large clinical image collections, and fills in the missing data in low resolution scans. The method produces anatomically plausible volumetric images consistent with sparsely sampled input scans.

Latent Structure. In this paper, we explicitly model and estimate the latent low-dimensional embedding for each patch. Additionally, we also explored an alternative choice that instead models each missing voxel as a latent variable. The resulting ECM algorithm estimates the expected missing voxel statistics directly, and then updates the cluster parameters. The most notable difference between this formulation and simpler algorithms that iteratively fill in missing voxels and then estimate GMM model parameters is in the estimation of the expected data covariance, which captures the covariance of the missing and observed data (c.f. [12], Chap. 8). We found that this variant often got stuck in local minima and had difficulty moving away from the initial missing voxel estimates, and was an order of magnitude slower than the presented method. We provide both implementations in our code.

Initialization. In contrast to the classical EM algorithm, the M-step of the ECM algorithm employs previous parameter estimates to perform parameter updates. This makes the initialization more challenging compared to the classical GMM learning, where initializing cluster memberships is sufficient, and also leads to slower convergence than simpler GMMs. We experimented with several initialization schemes, and provide them in our implementation. The experimental results are initialized by first learning a simple GMM from the linearly interpolated volumes, and using the resulting parameter as initializations for our method. This leads to results that improve on the linear interpolation but still maintain slightly blocky effects caused by interpolation. More agnostic initializations, such as random parameter values, lead to more realistic anatomy but noisier final estimates. Different methods perform well in different regions of the brain. Future research will further investigate the effects of initialization on the resulting reconstruction.

Restoration Method. Our restoration method, assumes that the observed voxels are noisy manifestations of low dimensional patch representations, and reconstructs the entire patch, including the observed voxels, leading to smoother images. We also explored an alternative reconstruction method of filling in just the missing voxels given the observed voxels (not shown). This formulation imputes the most likely missing voxels assuming the observed voxels are true observations, leading to sharper but noisier patches. The two restoration methods therefore yield images with different characteristics. This tradeoff is a function of the noise in the original acquisition: higher noise in the clinical acquisition leads to noisier reconstructions using the alternative method, whereas in the ADNI dataset the two methods perform similarly.

Varying Resolution. The proposed method can be used for general image imputation using datasets of various resolutions. For example, while acquiring a large high resolution dataset for a clinical study is often infeasible, our algorithm will naturally make use of any additional image data available. Even a small number of acquisitions in different directions or higher resolution than the study scans promise to improve accuracy of the resulting reconstruction.

Slice Thickness. In many clinical datasets the slice spacing is unknown or varies by site, scanner or acquisition. Therefore, throughout our model we simply treat the original data as high resolution planes. Explicitly modeling varying slice thickness is an interesting direction of future research.

Our method does not require high volumetric resolution scans or expert annotations, but can instead build the missing structure by learning from collections of clinical scans of similar quality to that of the input image. This enables the use of untapped clinical data for large scale scientific studies, promising to facilitate novel clinical analyses.

Acknowledgements. We acknowledge the following funding sources: NIH NINDS R01NS086905, NIH NICHD U01HD087211, NIH NIBIB NAC P41EB015902, NIH R41AG052246-01, 1K25EB013649-01, 1R21AG050122-01, and Wistron Corporation.

References

1. Bhatia, K.K., Rao, A., Price, A.N., Wolz, R., Hajnal, J.V., Rueckert, D.: Hierarchical manifold learning for regional image analysis. TMI **33**(2), 444–461 (2014)
2. Carmi, E., Liu, S., Alon, N., Fiat, A., Fiat, D.: Resolution enhancement in MRI. Magn. Reson. Imaging **24**(2), 133–154 (2006)
3. Coupé, P., Manjón, J.V., Fonov, V., Pruessner, J., Robles, M., Collins, L.D.: Patch-based segmentation using expert priors: application to hippocampus and ventricle segmentation. NeuroImage **54**(2), 940–954 (2011)
4. Di Martino, A., Yan, C.G., Li, Q., Denio, E., Castellanos, F.X., Alaerts, K., et al.: The autism brain imaging data exchange: towards a large-scale evaluation of the intrinsic brain architecture in autism. Mol. Psychiatry **19**(6), 659–667 (2014)
5. Elad, M., Aharon, M.: Image denoising via sparse and redundant representations over learned dictionaries. IEEE TMI **15**(12), 3736–3745 (2006)
6. Hill, D.L., Batchelor, P.G., Holden, M., Hawkes, D.J.: Medical image registration. Phys. Med. Biol. **46**(3), R1 (2001)
7. Iglesias, J.E., Konukoglu, E., Zikic, D., Glocker, B., Leemput, K., Fischl, B.: Is synthesizing MRI contrast useful for inter-modality analysis? In: Mori, K., Sakuma, I., Sato, Y., Barillot, C., Navab, N. (eds.) MICCAI 2013. LNCS, vol. 8149, pp. 631–638. Springer, Heidelberg (2013). doi:10.1007/978-3-642-40811-3_79
8. Ilin, A., Raiko, T.: Practical approaches to principal component analysis in the presence of missing values. J. Mach. Learn. Res. **11**, 1957–2000 (2010)
9. Jack, C.R., Bernstein, M.A., Fox, N.C., Thompson, P., Alexander, G., Harvey, D., et al.: The Alzheimer's disease neuroimaging initiative (ADNI): MRI methods. J. Magn. Reson. Imaging **27**(4), 685–691 (2008)
10. Jog, A., Carass, A., Prince, J.L.: Improving magnetic resonance resolution with supervised learning. In: ISBI, pp. 987–990. IEEE (2014)

11. Konukoglu, E., van der Kouwe, A., Sabuncu, M.R., Fischl, B.: Example-based restoration of high-resolution magnetic resonance image acquisitions. In: Mori, K., Sakuma, I., Sato, Y., Barillot, C., Navab, N. (eds.) MICCAI 2013. LNCS, vol. 8149, pp. 131–138. Springer, Heidelberg (2013). doi:10.1007/978-3-642-40811-3_17
12. Little, R.J., Rubin, D.B.: Statistical Analysis with Missing Data. Wiley, Hoboken (2014)
13. Manjón, J.V., Coupé, P., Buades, A., Fonov, V., Louis Collins, D., Robles, M.: Non-local MRI upsampling. Med. Image Anal. **14**(6), 784–792 (2010)
14. Manjón, J.V., Coupé, P., Buades, A., Louis Collins, D., Robles, M.: New methods for MRI denoising based on sparseness and self-similarity. Med. Image Anal. **16**(1), 18–27 (2012)
15. Plenge, E., Poot, D.H.J., Niessen, W.J., Meijering, E.: Super-resolution reconstruction using cross-scale self-similarity in multi-slice MRI. In: Mori, K., Sakuma, I., Sato, Y., Barillot, C., Navab, N. (eds.) MICCAI 2013. LNCS, vol. 8151, pp. 123–130. Springer, Heidelberg (2013). doi:10.1007/978-3-642-40760-4_16
16. Rost, N.S., Fitzpatrick, K., Biffi, A., Kanakis, A., Devan, W., Anderson, C.D., Cortellini, L., Furie, K.L., Rosand, J.: White matter hyperintensity burden and susceptibility to cerebral ischemia. Stroke **41**(12), 2807–2811 (2010)
17. Rousseau, F., Kim, K., Studholme, C.: A groupwise super-resolution approach: application to brain MRI. In: ISBI, pp. 860–863. IEEE (2010)
18. Rousseau, F., Habas, P.A., Studholme, C.: A supervised patch-based approach for human brain labeling. IEEE Tran. Med. Imag. **30**(10), 1852–1862 (2011)
19. Schoenberg, I.J., Schoenberg, I.J.: Cardinal Spline Interpolation, vol. 12. SIAM, Philadelphia (1973)
20. Ségonne, F., Dale, A.M., Busa, E., Glessner, M., Salat, D., Hahn, H.K., Fischl, B.: A hybrid approach to the skull stripping problem in MRI. Neuroimage **22**(3), 1060–1075 (2004)
21. Sridharan, R., et al.: Quantification and analysis of large multimodal clinical image studies: application to stroke. In: Shen, L., Liu, T., Yap, P.-T., Huang, H., Shen, D., Westin, C.-F. (eds.) MBIA 2013. LNCS, vol. 8159, pp. 18–30. Springer, Cham (2013). doi:10.1007/978-3-319-02126-3_3
22. Yang, J., Wright, J., Huang, T.S., Ma, Y.: Image super-resolution via sparse representation. IEEE Trans. Image Process. **19**(11), 2861–2873 (2010)
23. Zoran, D., Weiss, Y.: Natural images, Gaussian mixtures and dead leaves. In: Advances in Neural Information Processing Systems, pp. 1736–1744 (2012)

VTrails: Inferring Vessels with Geodesic Connectivity Trees

Stefano Moriconi[1(✉)], Maria A. Zuluaga[1], H. Rolf Jäger[2],
Parashkev Nachev[2], Sébastien Ourselin[1,3], and M. Jorge Cardoso[1,3]

[1] Translational Imaging Group, CMIC, University College London, London, UK
`stefano.moriconi.15@ucl.ac.uk`
[2] Institute of Neurology, University College London, London, UK
[3] Dementia Research Centre, University College London, London, UK

Abstract. The analysis of vessel morphology and connectivity has an
impact on a number of cardiovascular and neurovascular applications by
providing patient-specific high-level quantitative features such as spatial
location, direction and scale. In this paper we present an end-to-end approach to extract an acyclic vascular tree from angiographic data by solving a connectivity-enforcing anisotropic fast marching over a voxel-wise
tensor field representing the orientation of the underlying vascular tree.
The method is validated using synthetic and real vascular images. We
compare VTrails against classical and state-of-the-art ridge detectors for
tubular structures by assessing the connectedness of the vesselness map
and inspecting the synthesized tensor field as proof of concept. VTrails
performance is evaluated on images with different levels of degradation:
we verify that the extracted vascular network is an acyclic graph (i.e. a
tree), and we report the extraction accuracy, precision and recall.

1 Introduction

Vessel morphology and connectivity is of clinical relevance in cardiovascular and
neurovascular applications. In clinical practice, the vascular network and its
abnormalities are assessed by inspecting intensity projections, or image slices
one at a time, or using multiple views of 3D rendering techniques. In a number
of conditions, the connected vessel segmentation is required for intervention or
treatment planning [18]. A schematic representation of the vascular network has
an impact in interventional neuroradiology and in vascular surgery by providing
patient-specific high-level quantitative features (spatial localization, direction
and scale). In vascular image analysis these features are used for segmentation and labelling [13], with the final aim of reconstructing a physical vascular
model for hemodynamic simulations, or catheter motion planning, or identifying (un)safe occlusion points [6]. With this view, previous studies addressed the
problem of extracting a connected vascular network in a disjoint manner. First,
[8,12] proposed tubular enhancing methods in 3D with the aim of better con-
trasting vessels over a background: by using the eigendecomposition of either

© Springer International Publishing AG 2017
M. Niethammer et al. (Eds.): IPMI 2017, LNCS 10265, pp. 672–684, 2017.
DOI: 10.1007/978-3-319-59050-9_53

the Hessian matrix, or the image gradient projected on a unit sphere boundary, a scalar *vesselness* measure is obtained, which represents a vascular saliency map. Secondly, given the vascular saliency map, local disconnected branches or fragmented centerlines, [6,11,16] proposed a set of methods to recover a connected network: 'cores' identify and track furcating branches, whereas vascular graphs are recovered using minimum spanning tree algorithms on image-intensity features, or using graph kernels (subtree patterns) matched on a similarity metric. Alternatively, geometrical models embedding shape priors, or probabilistic models based on image-related features were employed to recover the connected vessel centerlines and prune artifacts from an initial set of segments. A different approach is proposed in [2], where the connected centerlines are recovered *a-posteriori* as medial axes of the 3D surface model which segments the lumen.

Given the varying complexity of the vascular network in healthy and diseased subjects and the lack of an extensive connected ground-truth for complex vascular networks of several anatomical compartments, the accurate and exhaustive extraction of the vessel connectivity remains however a challenging task.

Here we propose *VTrails*, a novel method that addresses vascular connectivity under a unified mathematical framework. VTrails enhances the connectedness of furcating, fragmented and tortuous vessels through scalar and high-order vascular features, which are employed in a greedy connectivity paradigm to determine the final vascular network. In particular, the vascular image is filtered first with a Steerable Laplacian of Gaussian Swirls filterbank, synthesizing simultaneously a connected vesselness map and an associated tensor field. Under the assumption that vessels join by minimal paths, VTrails then infers the unknown fully-connected vascular network as the minimal cost acyclic graph connecting automatically extracted seed nodes.

2 Methods

We introduce in Sect. 2.1 a Steerable Laplacian of Gaussian Swirls (SLoGS) filterbank used to reconstruct simultaneously the vesselness map and the associated tensor field. The SLoGS filterbank is first defined, then a multiscale image filtering approach is described using a locally selective overlap-add method [15]. The connected vesselness map and the tensor field are integrated over scales.

In Sect. 2.2, an anisotropic level-set combined with a connectivity paradigm extracts the fully-connected vascular tree using the synthesized connected vesselness map and tensor field.

2.1 SLoGS Curvilinear Filterbank

With the aim of enhancing the connectivity of fragmented, furcating and tortuous vessels, we propose a multi-resolution analysis/synthesis filterbank of Steerable Laplacian of Gaussian Swirls, whose elongated and curvilinear Gaussian kernels recover a smooth, connected and orientation aware vesselness map with local maxima at vessels' mid-line.

Steerable Laplacian of Gaussian Swirls (SLoGS). Similarly to [1] and without losing generality, given an image $V : \mathbb{R}^3 \to \mathbb{R}$, the respective SLoGS vesselness response is obtained as $V_{SLoGS,s} := V_s * K$, for any given scale s and any predefined SLoGS filtering kernel $K \colon \mathbb{R}^3 \to \mathbb{R}$. Here we formulate and derive the SLoGS filtering kernel K by computing the second-order directional derivative in the gradient direction of a curvilinear Gaussian trivariate function $\Gamma \colon \mathbb{R}^3 \times \mathbb{R}_+^3 \times \mathbb{R}^3 \to \mathbb{R}$. The gradient direction and its perpendicular constitute the first-order gauge coordinates system (ω, v). These are defined as $\omega = \frac{\nabla \Gamma}{\|\nabla \Gamma\|}$, and $v = \omega_\perp$, with the spatial gradient ∇. The function Γ has the form

$$\Gamma(\mathbf{x}, \boldsymbol{\sigma}, \mathbf{c}) = \frac{1}{\sqrt{2\pi\sigma_1^2}} e^{-\frac{x_1^2}{2\sigma_1^2}} \frac{1}{\sqrt{2\pi\sigma_2^2}} e^{-\frac{\left(x_2 + c_0 x_1 + c_1 x_1^2\right)^2}{2\sigma_2^2}} \frac{1}{\sqrt{2\pi\sigma_3^2}} e^{-\frac{\left(x_3 + c_2 x_1^3\right)^2}{2\sigma_3^2}}, \quad (1)$$

where $\mathbf{x} = x_1 \underline{i} + x_2 \underline{j} + x_3 \underline{k}$, with $\{\underline{i}, \underline{j}, \underline{k}\}$ the Euclidean image reference system, $\boldsymbol{\sigma}$ modulates the elongation and the cross-sectional profiles of the Gaussian distribution, and the curvilinear factor $\mathbf{c}$ accounts for planar asymmetry and two levels of curvilinear properties (i.e. bending and tilting orthogonally to the elongation of the distribution) by means of quadratic- and cubic-wise bending of the support, respectively. For any $\boldsymbol{\sigma}$ and $\mathbf{c}$, $\Gamma(\mathbf{x}, \boldsymbol{\sigma}, \mathbf{c})$ represents therefore the smooth impulse response of the Gaussian kernel. By operating a directional derivative on Γ along ω, i.e. $\mathcal{D}_\omega$, we obtain the SLoGS filtering kernel K as

$$K = \mathcal{D}_\omega \left[\mathcal{D}_\omega \Gamma\right] = \mathcal{D}_\omega \left[\omega^t \nabla \Gamma\right] \triangleq \omega^t H(\Gamma) \omega, \text{ where } H(\Gamma) = \begin{pmatrix} \Gamma_{\underline{i}\underline{i}} & \Gamma_{\underline{i}\underline{j}} & \Gamma_{\underline{i}\underline{k}} \\ \Gamma_{\underline{j}\underline{i}} & \Gamma_{\underline{j}\underline{j}} & \Gamma_{\underline{j}\underline{k}} \\ \Gamma_{\underline{k}\underline{i}} & \Gamma_{\underline{k}\underline{j}} & \Gamma_{\underline{k}\underline{k}} \end{pmatrix} \quad (2)$$

is the Hessian matrix of the Gaussian kernel. Given that Γ is twice continuously differentiable, $H(\Gamma)$ is well defined. Since $H(\Gamma)$ is symmetric, an orthogonal matrix Q exists, so that $H(\Gamma)$ can be diagonalized as $H(\Gamma) = Q \Lambda Q^{-1}$. The eigenvectors $\underline{q}_l$ form the columns of Q, whereas the eigenvalues λ_l, with $l = 1, 2, 3$, constitute the diagonal elements of Λ, so that $\Lambda_{ll} = \lambda_l$ and $\|\lambda_1\| \leq \|\lambda_2\| \leq \|\lambda_3\|$. Given a point $\mathbf{x}$, $K(\mathbf{x})$ can be reformulated as $K(\mathbf{x}) = \omega^t \left(Q \Lambda Q^{-1}\right) \omega$. Geometrically, the columns of Q represent a rotated orthonormal basis in $\mathbb{R}^3$ relative to the image reference system so that $\underline{q}_l$ are aligned to the principal directions of Γ at any given point $\mathbf{x}$. The diagonal matrix Λ characterizes the topology of the hypersurface in the neighbourhood of $\mathbf{x}$ (e.g. flat area, ridge, valley or saddle point in 2D) and modulates accordingly the variation of slopes, being the eigenvalues λ_l the second-order derivatives along the principal directions of Γ. Factorizing $K(\mathbf{x})$, we obtain: $K(\mathbf{x}) = (\omega^t Q) \Lambda (Q^{-1} \omega)$, so that the gradient direction ω is mapped onto the principal directions of Γ for any point $\mathbf{x}$. Solving (2)

$$K(\mathbf{x}) = \frac{1}{\Gamma_{\underline{i}}^2 + \Gamma_{\underline{j}}^2 + \Gamma_{\underline{k}}^2} \begin{pmatrix} \Gamma_{\underline{i}} \\ \Gamma_{\underline{j}} \\ \Gamma_{\underline{k}} \end{pmatrix}^t \overbrace{\begin{pmatrix} q_{11} & q_{21} & q_{31} \\ q_{12} & q_{22} & q_{32} \\ q_{13} & q_{23} & q_{33} \end{pmatrix}}^{Q} \underbrace{\begin{pmatrix} \lambda_1 & 0 & 0 \\ 0 & \lambda_2 & 0 \\ 0 & 0 & \lambda_3 \end{pmatrix}}_{\Lambda} \underbrace{\begin{pmatrix} q_{11} & q_{12} & q_{13} \\ q_{21} & q_{22} & q_{23} \\ q_{31} & q_{32} & q_{33} \end{pmatrix}}_{Q^{-1} = Q^t} \begin{pmatrix} \Gamma_{\underline{i}} \\ \Gamma_{\underline{j}} \\ \Gamma_{\underline{k}} \end{pmatrix} =$$

$$= \sum_{l=1}^{3} \gamma_l \lambda_l = \gamma_1 \frac{\partial^2}{\partial \underline{q_1}^2} \Gamma + \gamma_2 \frac{\partial^2}{\partial \underline{q_2}^2} \Gamma + \gamma_3 \frac{\partial^2}{\partial \underline{q_3}^2} \Gamma \triangleq \gamma LoG(\Gamma), \text{ where} \quad (3)$$

$$\gamma_1 = \frac{(\Gamma_i q_{11} + \Gamma_j q_{12} + \Gamma_k q_{13})^2}{\Gamma_i^2 + \Gamma_j^2 + \Gamma_k^2}, \quad \gamma_2 = \frac{(\Gamma_i q_{21} + \Gamma_j q_{22} + \Gamma_k q_{23})^2}{\Gamma_i^2 + \Gamma_j^2 + \Gamma_k^2}, \quad \text{and} \quad \gamma_3 = \frac{(\Gamma_i q_{31} + \Gamma_j q_{32} + \Gamma_k q_{33})^2}{\Gamma_i^2 + \Gamma_j^2 + \Gamma_k^2}$$

modulate the respective components of the canonical Laplacian of Gaussian (*LoG*) filter oriented along the principal directions of Γ. It is clear that given any arbitrary orientation Ω as an orthonormal basis similar to Q, the proposed dictionary of filtering kernels can steer by computing the rotation transform, which maps the integral orientation basis of each Gaussian kernel $\Phi_\Gamma = \frac{\int (\Gamma(\mathbf{x}) \cdot Q(\mathbf{x})) d\mathbf{x}}{\| \int (\Gamma(\mathbf{x}) \cdot Q(\mathbf{x})) d\mathbf{x} \|}$ on Ω. Together with the SLoGS filtering kernel K, we determine the second-moment matrix T associated to the filter impulse response Γ by adopting the ellipsoid model in the continuous neighborhood of $\mathbf{x}$. A symmetric tensor $T(\mathbf{x})$ is derived from the eigendecomposition of $H(\Gamma)$ as $T(\mathbf{x}) = Q \, \Psi \, Q^{-1}$, where Ψ is the diagonal matrix representing the canonical unitary volume ellipsoid

$$\Psi = \left(\prod_{l=1}^3 \psi_l \right)^{-\frac{1}{3}} \begin{pmatrix} \psi_1 & 0 & 0 \\ 0 & \psi_2 & 0 \\ 0 & 0 & \psi_3 \end{pmatrix}, \quad \text{being} \quad \psi_1 = \frac{|\lambda_1|}{\sqrt{|\lambda_2 \lambda_3|}}, \quad \psi_2 = \frac{|\lambda_2|}{|\lambda_3|}, \quad \text{and} \quad \psi_3 = 1 \quad (4)$$

the respective semiaxes' lengths. Conversely from $H(\Gamma)$, which is indeterminate, the tensor field T is a symmetric positive definite (SPD) matrix for any $\mathbf{x} \in \mathbb{R}^3$. Here, the definition of the tensor kernel T in (4) can be further reformulated exploiting the intrinsic log-concavity of Γ. By mapping $\Gamma \mapsto \tilde{\Gamma} = -\log(\Gamma)$, a convex quadratic form is obtained, so that $H(\tilde{\Gamma})$ is an SPD, as the modelled tensor T. In either case, the manifold of tensors can be mapped into a set of 6 independent components in the Log-Euclidean space, which greatly simplifies the computation of Riemannian metrics and statistics. We refer to [3] for a detailed methodological description. The continuous and smooth tensor field T inherits the steerable property. Similarly to diffusion tensor MRI, the kernel shows a preferred diffusion direction for a given energy potential, e.g. the scalar function Γ itself (Fig. 1). This allows to define an arbitrary dictionary of filtering kernels (DFK) that embeds anisotropy and high-order directional features to scalar curvilinear templates, which enhances and locally resembles typical,

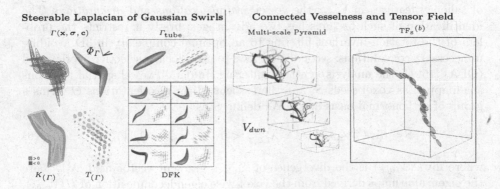

Fig. 1. SLoGS filterbank: definition of a Dictionary of Filtering Kernels and synthesis of the Tensor Field within the overlap-add block b at the given scale s.

smooth vessel patterns. Together with the arbitrary SLoGS DFK, we also intro-
duce an extra pair of non-curvilinear kernels for completeness. These are the
pseudo-impulsive δLoG, an isotropic derivative filter given by the Laplacian of
Gaussian of $\Gamma_\delta(\mathbf{x}, \boldsymbol{\sigma}, \mathbf{c} = \mathbf{0})$, representing a Dirac delta function for $\boldsymbol{\sigma} \to 0$.
Also, the uniformly flat νLoG is another isotropic degenerate case, where the
Laplacian of Gaussian derives from $\Gamma_\nu(\mathbf{x}, \boldsymbol{\sigma}, \mathbf{c} = \mathbf{0})$, which is assumed to be a
uniform, constant-value kernel for $\boldsymbol{\sigma} \to \infty$. The purpose of introducing the extra
kernels is to better contrast regions that most likely relate to vessel boundaries
and to image background, respectively. Although δLoG and νLoG have singular-
ities, ideally they represent isotropic degenerate kernels. Therefore we associate
pure isotropic tensors for any given $\mathbf{x} \in \mathbb{R}^3$, so that $T_{\delta LoG}(\mathbf{x}) = T_{\nu LoG}(\mathbf{x}) = I_3$
(Identity). The respective directional kernel bases $\Phi(\delta LoG) = \Phi(\nu LoG)$ are
undetermined.

Connected Vesselness Map and the Tensor Field. The idea is to convolve
finite impulse response SLoGS with the discrete vascular image in a scale- and
rotation-invariant framework, to obtain simultaneously the connected vesselness
maps and the associated tensor field. For simplicity, the filtering steps will be
presented for a generic scale s. Scale-invariance is achieved by keeping the size
of the small compact-support SLoGS fixed, while the size of the vascular image
V varies accordingly with the multi-resolution pyramid. Also, different σ will
produce SLoGS kernels with different spatial band-pass frequencies. V is down-
sampled at the arbitrary scale s as proposed in [7] to obtain V_{dwn}. An early
saliency map of tubular structures V_{tube} is then determined as

$$V_{tube} = \sum_\Omega V_{tube}^{(\Omega)}, \quad \text{where} \quad V_{tube}^{(\Omega)} = \max\left(0, V_{dwn} * K_{tube}^{(\Omega)}\right). \tag{5}$$

K_{tube} is derived from the discretized tubular kernel $\Gamma_{tube}(\mathbf{x}, \sigma_1 > \sigma_2 = \sigma_3, \mathbf{c} = \mathbf{0})$
(Fig. 1), whereas Ω is defined as a group of orthonormal basis in $\mathbb{R}^3$, using an
icosphere at arbitrary subdivision level n to determine the orientation sampling
in 3D. V_{tube} is meant to provide an initial, coarse, although highly-sensitive set
of saliency features in V_{dwn}: the vessel *spatial locations* and *orientations*. The
identification of such features has two advantages; firstly it restricts the problem of the rotation-invariant filtering to an optimal complexity in 3D avoiding
unnecessary convolutions; secondly it allows to use a locally selective overlap-add
(OLA) [15] for the analysis/synthesis filtering. In detail, vessel spatial locations
are mapped as voxel seeds $\tilde{S}$, and the associated set of orientations Θ forms a
group of orthonormal basis in $\mathbb{R}^3$. We define $\tilde{S}$ as

$$\tilde{S} = \text{div}\left(\nabla V_{tube}\right)_{<0} \wedge \lambda_{1,2,3}^{V_{tube}} < 0 \wedge V_{tube} \geq Q_p(V_{tube}^+), \tag{6}$$

where $\text{div}\left(\nabla V_{tube}\right)$ is the divergence of V_{tube}'s gradient vector field, $\lambda_{1:3}^{V_{tube}}$ are
the eigenvalue maps derived from the voxel-wise eigendecomposition of $H(V_{tube})$,
and $Q_p(V_{tube}^+)$ is the pth quantile of the positive V_{tube} samples' pool. With $\tilde{S}$, the
orientations Θ are automatically determined as the set of eigenvectors associated

to $\lambda_{1:3}^{V_{tube}}$. The greater the intensity threshold $Q_p(V_{tube}^+)$, the greater the image noise-floor rejection, the lower the number of seeds and the fewer the details extracted from V_{tube}. Also, the cardinality of $\tilde{S}$ and Θ is a trade-off for the convolutional complexity in each OLA filtering step. The analysis/synthesis filtering can be embedded in a fully parallel OLA, by considering an overlapping grid of 3D cubic blocks spanning the domain of V_{dwn}, and by processing each block b so that at least one seed exists within it. The integral connected vesselness map $CVM_s^{(b)}$, for each block b at any given scale s, has the form

$$CVM_s^{(b)} = \sum_{K \in DFK} \sum_{\theta \in \Theta^{(b)}} V_S^{(b,K,\theta)}, \quad \text{where} \quad V_S^{(b,K,\theta)} = \max\left(0, \left(V_{dwn}^{(b)} \cdot \mathcal{H}\right) * K^{(\theta)}\right). \quad (7)$$

Here, $V_S^{(b,K,\theta)}$ is the convolutional filter response given the considered SLoGS kernel. In detail, $V_{dwn}^{(b)}$ is the down-sampled image in b, $\mathcal{H}$ is the 3D OLA Hann weighting window, and $K^{(\theta)}$ is the steered filtering kernel along $\theta \in \Theta^{(b)}$, those being the seeds' orientations in b. Note that in the discrete domain each voxel has a spatial indexed location $\mathbf{b} \in b$. The anisotropic tensor field $TF_s^{(b)}$ is synthesized and normalized in the Log-Euclidean space as the integral *weighted-sweep* of each steered tensor patch within the block b, and has the form

$$TF_{s,(LE)}^{(b)} = \frac{1}{W} : \sum_{K \in \left\{\begin{array}{c} DFK, \\ \delta LoG, \\ \nu LoG \end{array}\right\}} \sum_{\theta \in \Theta^{(b)}} \underbrace{\left(\sum_{\lfloor \mathbf{b} \rceil \subset b} \overbrace{V_S^{(\mathbf{b},K,\theta)} \cdot \Gamma_{(K)}^{(\theta)} \cdot \Xi}^{\text{weights}} \cdot \overbrace{T_{K,(LE)}^{(\theta)}}^{\text{patch}} \right)}_{\text{within-block patch sweep}}, \quad \text{so that}$$

$$\det\left(TF_s^{(b)}(\mathbf{b})\right) = \mathcal{H}(\mathbf{b}), \quad \text{and} \quad W = \left(\sum_{K \in \left\{\begin{array}{c} DFK, \\ \delta LoG, \\ \nu LoG \end{array}\right\}} \sum_{\theta \in \Theta^{(b)}} \sum_{\lfloor \mathbf{b} \rceil \subset b} V_S^{(\mathbf{b},K,\theta)} \cdot \Gamma_{(K)}^{(\theta)} \cdot \Xi \right), \quad (8)$$

where W is the integral normalizing weight-map accounting for all vessel, boundary and background components; $V_S^{(\mathbf{b},K,\theta)}$ is the modulating SLoGS filter response at $\mathbf{b}$ as in (7); $\Gamma_{(K)}^{(\theta)}$ is the steered Gaussian impulse response associated to the kernel $K \in \{DFK, \delta Log, \nu LoG\}$; Ξ is the Hann smoothing window in the neighbourhood $\lfloor \mathbf{b} \rceil$ centred at $\mathbf{b}$, and $T_{K,(LE)}^{(\theta)}$ is one of the 6 components of the discrete steered tensors patch T in the Log-Euclidean space. Note that all 6 tensorial components are equally processed, and that the neighbourhood $\lfloor \mathbf{b} \rceil$ and the SLoGS tensors patch $T_{K,(LE)}^{(\theta)}$ have the same size. In (8), $TF_{s,(LE)}^{(b)}$ integrates also the isotropic contributions from vessel boundaries and background to better contrast the tubular structures' anisotropy and to reduce synthetic artifacts surrounding the vessels (Fig. 1). In particular, $TF_{s,(LE)}^{(b)}$ is averaged with an identically null tensor patch in the Log-Euclidean space in correspondence of boundaries and background, and $V_S^{(\mathbf{b},K,\theta)}|_{\{\delta LoG, \nu LoG\}}$ is computed as in (7), where the image negative of $V_{dwn}^{(b)}$ is considered. Lastly, the connected vesselness maps and the associated synthetic tensor field are reconstructed by adding adjacent overlapping blocks in the OLA 3D grid for the given scale s.

Integration Over Multiple Scales. Each scale-dependent contribution is up-sampled and cumulatively integrated with a weighted sum

$$CVM = \sum_s \tfrac{1}{s} CVM_s, \text{ and, } TF_{(LE)} = \tfrac{1}{CVM} \sum_s \left(\tfrac{1}{s} CVM_s\right) \cdot T_{s,(LE)}. \qquad (9)$$

Vesselness contributions are weighted here by the inverse of s, emphasizing responses at spatial low-frequencies. We further impose that the Euclidean TF has unitary determinant at each image voxel; for stability, the magnitude of the tensors is decoupled from the directional and anisotropic features throughout the whole multi-scale process, since tensors' magnitude is expressed by CVM. Note that with the proposed method we do not aim at segmenting vessels by thresholding the resulting CVM, we rather provide a measure of vessels' connectedness with maximal response at the centre of the vascular structures.

2.2   Vascular Tree of Geodesic Minimal Paths

Following the concepts first introduced in [4], we formulate an anisotropic front propagation algorithm that combined with an acyclic connectivity paradigm joins multiple sources $\tilde{S} \mapsto S$ propagating concurrently on a Riemannian speed potential $\mathcal{P}$. Since we want to extract geodesic minimal paths between points, we minimize an energy functional $\mathcal{U}(\mathbf{x}) = \min_\pi \int_\pi \mathcal{P}\left(\pi(\mathbf{x}), \pi'(\mathbf{x})\right) d\mathbf{x}$ for any possible path π between two generic points along its geodesic length, so that $\|\nabla\mathcal{U}(\mathbf{x})\| = 1$, and $\mathcal{U}(S) = 0$. The solution to the Eikonal partial differential equation is given here by the anisotropic Fast Marching (aFM) algorithm [4], where front waves propagate from S on $\mathcal{P}$, with $\mathcal{P}\left(\pi, \pi'\right) = \sqrt{\pi'^t \cdot \mathcal{M} \cdot \pi'}$ describing the infinitesimal distance along π, relative to the anisotropic tensor $\mathcal{M}$. In our case, $\mathcal{M} = TF$, and $\pi' \propto \frac{1}{CVM}$. Note that the anisotropic propagation is a generalised version of the isotropic propagation medium, $\mathcal{M} \equiv I_3$. The acyclic connectivity paradigm is run until convergence together with the aFM to extract the vascular tree of multiple connected geodesics Π.

Anisotropic FM and Acyclic Connectivity Paradigm. Geodesic paths are determined by back-tracing $\mathcal{U}$ when different regions collide. The connecting geodesic π is extracted minimizing $\mathcal{U}$ at the collision grid-points. The aFM maps, i.e. $\mathcal{U}$; the *Voronoi index map* $\mathcal{V}$, representing the label associated to each propagating seed; and the *Tag* $\mathcal{T}$, representing the state of each grid-point (Front, Visited, Far), are then updated within the collided regions, so that these merge as one and the front is consistent with the unified resulting region. This is continued until all regions merge.

Initialization. The seeds $\tilde{S}$ are aligned towards the vessels' mid-line with a constrained gradient descent, resulting in an initial set of sources S. All 26-connected components $\pi_p^{(S)} \in S$ initialize the aFM maps, i.e., $\mathcal{U}(\pi_p^{(S)}) = 0$, $\mathcal{V}(\pi_p^{(S)}) = p$, $\mathcal{T}(\pi_p^{(S)}) = $ *Front*, and constitute also the initial geodesics $\pi_p^{(S)} \to \Pi$.

Fast Marching Step. The aFM maps are updated by following an informative propagation scheme. We refer to [4] for the 3D aFM step considering the 48 simplexes in the 26-neighbourhood of the *Front* grid-point with minimal $\mathcal{U}$.

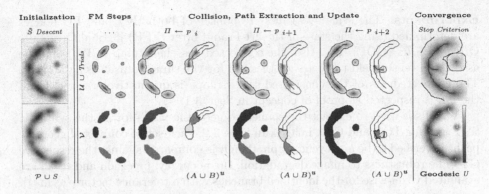

Fig. 2. Sequential acyclic connectivity paradigm on a synthetic 2D image.

Path Extraction. Collision is detected when *Visited* grid-points of different regions are adjacent. A connecting π is determined by linking the back-traced minimal paths from the collision grid-points to their respective sources $\pi_A, \pi_B \in \Pi$ with a gradient descent on $\mathcal{U}$ (Fig. 2). The associated integral geodesic length $U_\pi = \int_{\pi_A}^{\pi_B} \mathcal{U} d\pi$ is computed and the connectivity in Π is updated in the form of an adjacency list. Lastly, the grid-points of the extracted π are further considered as path seeds in the updating scheme, since furcations can occur at any level of the connecting minimal paths.

Fast Updating Scheme. A nested *aFM* is run only in the union of the collided regions $(A \cup B)$ using a temporary independent layer of *aFM* maps, where $\tilde{\mathcal{U}}(\pi) = 0$, $\tilde{\mathcal{T}}(\pi) = Front$, and $\tilde{\mathcal{T}}_{\overline{(A \cup B)}} = Visited$. Ideally, the nested *aFM* is run until complete domain exploration, however, to speed up the process, the propagation domain is divided into the solved and ***unsolved*** sub-regions, and the update is focused on the latter $(A \cup B)^u$ (Fig. 2). The boundary geodesic values of $(A \cup B)^u$ equal the geodesic distances $\mathcal{U}$ at the collision grid-points. Lastly, the *aFM* maps are updated as: $\mathcal{U}_{(A \cup B)^u} = \min\{\mathcal{U}_{(A \cup B)^u}, \tilde{\mathcal{U}}_{(A \cup B)^u}\}$, $\mathcal{V}_{(A \cup B)} = \min\{\mathcal{V}_A, \mathcal{V}_B\}$, and $\mathcal{T}_{(A \cup B)^u} = \tilde{\mathcal{T}}_{(A \cup B)^u}$.

3   Experiments and Results

Dataset. A 3D hand-crafted tortuous and convoluted phantom (HCP) is designed to account for complex vessel patterns, i.e. branching, kissing vessels, scale and shape variations induced by pathologies. Also a set of 20 synthetic vascular trees (SVT) ($64 \times 64 \times 64$ voxels) were generated using VascuSynth [10] considering two levels of additional noise (N_1: $\mathcal{N}(0,5)$ + Shadows: 1 + Salt&Pepper: 1‰; N_2: $\mathcal{N}(0,10)$ + Shadows: 1 + Salt&Pepper: 2‰). Together with the synthetic data, a cerebral Phase Contrast MRI (PC) ($0.86 \times 0.86 \times 1.0$ mm), a cerebral Time of Flight MRI (TOF) ($0.36 \times 0.36 \times 0.5$ mm) and a carotid CTA ($0.46 \times 0.46 \times 0.45$ mm) were used. Vascular network ground-truths (GT) are given in the form of connected raster centerlines for all the synthetic images and for both TOF and CTA.

Experiments. The scalar vesselness responses of both HCP and PC images are determined using the state-of-the-art Frangi filter (FFR) [8], and Optimally Oriented Flux (OOF) [12]. Also, the connected vesselness map (*CVM*) and the associated tensor field (*TF*) are synthesized for the same dataset using VTrails. The connectedness of the considered scalar maps is qualitatively assessed and the *TF* is inspected as proof of concept in Sect. 3.1.

VTrails is used to extract the connected geodesic paths for all the synthetic SVT and for TOF and CTA images. In Sect. 3.2, each set of connected geodesic paths is verified to be an acyclic graph, then it is compared against the respective GT. The robustness to image degradation, the accuracy, precision and recall are evaluated voxel-wise for the identified branches with a tolerance factor ϱ as in [1].

3.1 Connectedness of the Vesselness Map

Figure 3 shows the connectedness of vessels recovered from state-of-the-art vascular enhancers and curvilinear ridge detectors FFR and OOF together with the proposed *CVM* for the synthetic HCP and the real PC images. On the synthetic phantom, FFR shows a fragmented and rough vesselness response in correspondence of irregularly shaped sections of the structure. Also, the response at the bifurcation is not smoothly connected with the branches (triangular loop). Conversely, OOF recovers the phantom connectedness at the branch-point, and the vesselness response is consistent along the tortuous curvilinear section, however ghosting artifacts are observed as the shape of the phantom becomes irregular (C-like) or differs from a cylindrical tube. Also, close convoluted structures, which change scale rapidly in the HCP, produce inconsistent responses of OOF (Fig. 3). *CVM* shows here a strongly connected vesselness response in correspondence of both regular and irregular tubular sections, with local maxima at structures' mid-line. The connectedness of the structures is emphasized regardless the

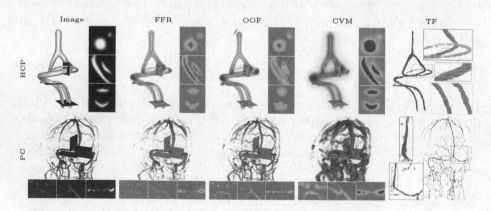

Fig. 3. Vesselness response maps for Frangi, OOF, and proposed scalar CVM with associated tensor field on a digital phantom example and on data of a phase contrast cerebral venogram.

complexity of the shape, and it resolves spatially the tortuous curvilinear 'kissing vessels' without additional ghosting artifacts, despite the smooth profile.

Similar results are observed on the PC dataset: FFR has a poor connected response in the noisy and low-resolution image. Vessels are overall enhanced, however thin and fragmented structures remain disconnected. Overall, the vesselness response is not uniform within the noisy structures, where maximal values are often off-centred. A more consistent response is obtained from OOF, where the connectedness of vessels is improved. Maximal response is observed at the mid-line of vessels, however, noise rejection is poor. *CVM* strongly enhances here the vessel connectivity. The fragmented vessels of PC have a continuous and smooth response in *CVM* with higher values and a more defined profile. Large vessels shows solid connected regions with local maxima at mid-line as in OOF. Conversely from OOF, *CVM* shows improved noise rejection in the background.

The respective tensor fields (*TF*) synthesized on both HCP and PC show consistent features. The *TF*'s characteristics are in line with the connectedness of *CVM*: enhanced and connected vessels are associated with high anisotropy, whereas background areas show a predominant isotropic component.

3.2   Connected Geodesic Paths as Vascular Tree

Representative examples of degraded synthetic images from SVT and the respective GT are shown in Fig. 4 together with the connected graphs extracted by VTrails. Analogously, the same set of images are reported for the real images TOF and CTA in Fig. 4. Qualitatively, the extracted set of connected geodesic paths shows remarkable matching with the provided GT in all cases. First, we verify the acyclic nature of the graph. We found no cycles, degenerate graphs and unconnected nodes, meaning that the extracted connected geodesic paths represent a connected geodesic tree. Precision and recall are then evaluated for the identified branches. Also, error distances are determined as the connected tree's binary distance map evaluated at GT. Average errors ($\bar{\varepsilon}$) precision and recall are reported (mean $\pm$ SD) in Table 1. Note that no pruning of any spurious branches is performed in the analysis.

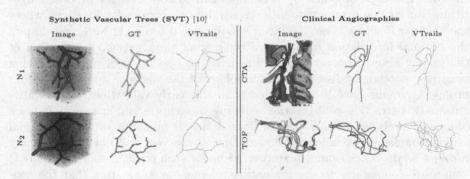

Fig. 4. Comparison of the vascular connected trees against the relative ground-truth for a representative set of synthetic data, and for a carotid CTA and for a middle cerebral artery TOF MRI. Note that main branches are correctly identified and connected.

Table 1. Connectivity tree error distances, precision and recall (mean±SD): (left) synthetic vascular tree at degradation levels N_1 and N_2; (right) TOF and CTA. Note the invariance of all metrics regardless the degradation level.

		Synthetic Vascular Trees [10]		Clinical Angiographies	
		N_1	N_2	TOF	CTA
$\bar{\varepsilon}$	[voxels]	2.15 ± 0.65	2.09 ± 0.37	[mm] 1.07 ± 2.65	1.1 ± 1.63
ϱ			2	1.42	1.57
Precision		$88.21 \pm 2.58\%$	$87.93 \pm 2.56\%$	77.12%	89.67%
Recall		$68.31 \pm 7.44\%$	$69.18 \pm 3.69\%$	89.49%	83.97%

4   Discussion and Conclusions

We presented VTrails, a novel connectivity-oriented method for vascular image analysis. The proposed method has the advantage of introducing the SLoGS filterbank, which simultaneously synthesizes a connected vesselness map and the associated tensor field in the same mathematically coherent framework. Interestingly, recent works [9,17] are exploring Riemannian manifolds of tensors for high-order vascular metrics, however the coherent definition of a tensor field is not trivial for an arbitrary scalar image, as its topology cannot be generally approximated simply by an ellipsoid model [14]. The steerability property of SLoGS stands out as key feature for *i.* reducing the dimensionality of the kernels parameters in 3D, *ii.* determining the filterbank's rotation-invariance and *iii.* optimizing the 3D filtering complexity in the OLA. Also, the combined rotation- and curvature-invariance of the filtering process results in branch-points that coincide with the locally integrated center of mass of the multiple SLoGS filter responses. This explains the strong response in the *CVM* at the branch-point in Fig. 3. Regarding the acyclic connectivity paradigm employed in VTrails, we experimentally verified that the resulting set of connected geodesic paths Π forms a tree. The assumption of a vascular tree provides a natural and anatomically valid constraint for 3D vascular images, with few rare exceptions, such as the complete circle of Willis [5]. It is important to note that the proposed algorithm can include extra anatomical constraints to correct for locations where the vascular topology is not acyclic or where noise it too high. Note that despite the optimal formulation of the anisotropic front propagation, a limitation of the greedy acyclic connectivity paradigm is the possibility of miss-connecting branches, potentially disrupting the topology of the vascular network. Overall, promising results have been reported from this early validation, with a fully-automatic extraction configuration. Missing branches occur in correspondence of small vessels, where the effect of degradation is predominant: tiny terminal vessels completely occluded by the corrupting shadows will not automatically produce seeds, hence cannot be recovered under such configuration. Globally, $\bar{\varepsilon}$ values are comparable to the evaluation tolerance ϱ, suggesting that the connected geodesic paths extracted by VTrails lie in the close neighbourhood of the vessels' centerlines. Moreover, the reported values are comparable regardless the level of degradation. Future developments will address the optimization of the *CVM* integration strategy in Sect. 2.1 to account for an equalized response over the vascular spatial frequency-bands. Also, the topological analysis of vascular networks on a population of subjects will be investigated in future works to better embed priors in the acyclic connectivity paradigm.

Acknowledgements. The study is co-funded from the EPSRC grant (EP/H046410/1), the Wellcome Trust and the National Institute for Health Research (NIHR) University College London Hospitals (UCLH) Biomedical Research Centre.

References

1. Annunziata, R., Kheirkhah, A., Hamrah, P., Trucco, E.: Scale and curvature invariant ridge detector for tortuous and fragmented structures. In: Navab, N., Hornegger, J., Wells, W.M., Frangi, A.F. (eds.) MICCAI 2015. LNCS, vol. 9351, pp. 588–595. Springer, Cham (2015). doi:10.1007/978-3-319-24574-4_70
2. Antiga, L., Piccinelli, M., Botti, L., Ene-Iordache, B., Remuzzi, A., Steinman, D.A.: An image-based modeling framework for patient-specific computational hemodynamics. Med. Biol. Eng. Comput. **46**, 1097 (2008)
3. Arsigny, V., Fillard, P., Pennec, X., Ayache, N.: Log-euclidean metrics for fast and simple calculus on diffusion tensors. Magn. Reson. Med. **56**, 411–421 (2006)
4. Benmansour, F., Cohen, L.D.: Tubular structure segmentation based on minimal path method and anisotropic enhancement. Int. J. Comput. Vis. **92**, 192–210 (2011)
5. Bergman, R.A., Afifi, A.K., Miyauchi, R.: Illustrated encyclopedia of human anatomic variation: Circle of Willis. www.anatomyatlases.org/AnatomicVariants/
6. Bullitt, E., Aylward, S., Liu, A., Stone, J., Mukherji, S.K., Coffey, C., Gerig, G., Pizer, S.M.: 3D graph description of the intracerebral vasculature from segmented MRA and tests of accuracy by comparison with x-ray angiograms. In: Kuba, A., Šáamal, M., Todd-Pokropek, A. (eds.) IPMI 1999. LNCS, vol. 1613, pp. 308–321. Springer, Heidelberg (1999). doi:10.1007/3-540-48714-X_23
7. Cardoso, M.J., Modat, M., Vercauteren, T., Ourselin, S.: Scale factor point spread function matching: beyond aliasing in image resampling. In: Navab, N., Hornegger, J., Wells, W.M., Frangi, A.F. (eds.) MICCAI 2015. LNCS, vol. 9350, pp. 675–683. Springer, Cham (2015). doi:10.1007/978-3-319-24571-3_81
8. Frangi, A.F., Niessen, W.J., Vincken, K.L., Viergever, M.A.: Multiscale vessel enhancement filtering. In: Wells, W.M., Colchester, A., Delp, S. (eds.) MICCAI 1998. LNCS, vol. 1496, pp. 130–137. Springer, Heidelberg (1998). doi:10.1007/BFb0056195
9. Gülsün, M.A., Funka-Lea, G., Sharma, P., Rapaka, S., Zheng, Y.: Coronary centerline extraction via optimal flow paths and CNN Path pruning. In: Ourselin, S., Joskowicz, L., Sabuncu, M.R., Unal, G., Wells, W. (eds.) MICCAI 2016. LNCS, vol. 9902, pp. 317–325. Springer, Cham (2016). doi:10.1007/978-3-319-46726-9_37
10. Hamarneh, G., Jassi, P.: VascuSynth: simulating vascular trees for generating volumetric image data with ground-truth segmentation and tree analysis. Comput. Med. Imag. Graph. **34**, 605–616 (2010)
11. Kwitt, R., Pace, D., Niethammer, M., Aylward, S.: Studying cerebral vasculature using structure proximity and graph kernels. In: Mori, K., Sakuma, I., Sato, Y., Barillot, C., Navab, N. (eds.) MICCAI 2013. LNCS, vol. 8150, pp. 534–541. Springer, Heidelberg (2013). doi:10.1007/978-3-642-40763-5_66

12. Law, M.W.K., Chung, A.C.S.: Three dimensional curvilinear structure detection using optimally oriented flux. In: Forsyth, D., Torr, P., Zisserman, A. (eds.) ECCV 2008. LNCS, vol. 5305, pp. 368–382. Springer, Heidelberg (2008). doi:10.1007/978-3-540-88693-8_27

13. Lesage, D., Angelini, E.D., Bloch, I., Funka-Lea, G.: A review of 3D vessel lumen segmentation techniques: models, features and extraction schemes. Med. Image Anal. **13**, 819–845 (2009)

14. Lin, Q.: Enhancement, extraction, and visualization of 3D volume data (2003)

15. Oppenheim, A.V., Schafer, R.W.: Discrete-Time Signal Processing. Pearson Higher Education, New York (2010)

16. Schaap, M., Manniesing, R., Smal, I., Walsum, T., Lugt, A., Niessen, W.: Bayesian tracking of tubular structures and its application to carotid arteries in CTA. In: Ayache, N., Ourselin, S., Maeder, A. (eds.) MICCAI 2007. LNCS, vol. 4792, pp. 562–570. Springer, Heidelberg (2007). doi:10.1007/978-3-540-75759-7_68

17. Wang, C., Oda, M., Hayashi, Y., Yoshino, Y., Yamamoto, T., Frangi, A.F., Mori, K.: Tensor-based graph-cut in riemannian metric space and its application to renal artery segmentation. In: Ourselin, S., Joskowicz, L., Sabuncu, M.R., Unal, G., Wells, W. (eds.) MICCAI 2016. LNCS, vol. 9902, pp. 353–361. Springer, Cham (2016). doi:10.1007/978-3-319-46726-9_41

18. Zuluaga, M.A., Rodionov, R., Nowell, M., Achhala, S., Zombori, G., Mendelson, A.F., Cardoso, M.J., Miserocchi, A., McEvoy, A.W., Duncan, J.S., Ourselin, S.: Stability, structure and scale: improvements in multi-modal vessel extraction for SEEG trajectory planning. Int. J. Comput. Assist. Radiol. Surg. **10**, 1227–1237 (2015)

Author Index

686   Author Index

Printed in the United States
By Bookmasters